Medicinal Chemistry: Computational Methods to Support Drug Design

Medicinal Chemistry: Computational Methods to Support Drug Design

Editor: Holly Lambert

AMERICAN
MEDICAL PUBLISHERS
www.americanmedicalpublishers.com

AMERICAN
MEDICAL PUBLISHERS
www.americanmedicalpublishers.com

Cataloging-in-Publication Data

Medicinal chemistry : computational methods to support drug design / edited by Holly Lambert.
p. cm.
Includes bibliographical references and index.
ISBN 979-8-88740-255-0
1. Drugs--Design. 2. Drugs--Design--Data processing. 3. Drug development.
4. Pharmaceutical chemistry--Data processing. 5. Cheminformatics. I. Lambert, Holly.
RS420 .M43 2023
615.6--dc23

American Medical Publishers,
41 Flatbush Avenue,
1st Floor, New York,
NY 11217, USA

ISBN 979-8-88740-255-0 (Hardback)

Contents

Preface

Medicinal chemistry is the study of molecular aspects of drug actions. It encompasses molecules, their structures, designs, and their pharmacological activities. A molecule's potency is determined by its structure. The structural activity relationship is a sub-branch of medicinal chemistry that estimates a molecule's potential to display any pharmacological activity. Computational methods play a significant role in the development of molecules that are therapeutically significant. These methods can be categorized into ligand-based and structure-based methods. Ligand-based methods make use of ligand information for the prediction of activity based on the similarities and dissimilarities compared to previously known active ligands. Generally utilized ligand-based methods include quantitative structure-activity relationships, molecular descriptors, and ligand-based pharmacophores. These methods are analogous towards high-throughput screening, where information regarding ligand and target structure both is important. Structure-based methods include ligand design methods, pharmacophore, and ligand docking. This book contains some path-breaking studies in the field of medicinal chemistry. It will provide interesting topics for research on the computational methods for drug design, which interested readers can take up. This book will serve as a reference source for a broad spectrum of readers.

Significant researches are present in this book. Intensive efforts have been employed by authors to make this book an outstanding discourse. This book contains the enlightening chapters which have been written on the basis of significant researches done by the experts.

Finally, I would also like to thank all the members involved in this book for being a team and meeting all the deadlines for the submission of their respective works. I would also like to thank my friends and family for being supportive in my efforts.

Editor

1

Predicting Synergism of Cancer Drug Combinations Using NCI-ALMANAC Data

Pavel Sidorov[1], *Stefan Naulaerts*[1,2], *Jérémy Ariey-Bonnet*[1], *Eddy Pasquier*[1] *and Pedro J. Ballester*[1*]

[1] CRCM, INSERM, Cancer Research Center of Marseille, Institut Paoli-Calmettes, Aix-Marseille Univ, CNRS, Marseille, France, [2] Department of Tumor Immunology, Institut de Duve, Bruxelles, Belgium

***Correspondence:**
Pedro J. Ballester
pedro.ballester@inserm.fr

Drug combinations are of great interest for cancer treatment. Unfortunately, the discovery of synergistic combinations by purely experimental means is only feasible on small sets of drugs. *In silico* modeling methods can substantially widen this search by providing tools able to predict which of all possible combinations in a large compound library are synergistic. Here we investigate to which extent drug combination synergy can be predicted by exploiting the largest available dataset to date (NCI-ALMANAC, with over 290,000 synergy determinations). Each cell line is modeled using primarily two machine learning techniques, Random Forest (RF) and Extreme Gradient Boosting (XGBoost), on the datasets provided by NCI-ALMANAC. This large-scale predictive modeling study comprises more than 5,000 pair-wise drug combinations, 60 cell lines, 4 types of models, and 5 types of chemical features. The application of a powerful, yet uncommonly used, RF-specific technique for reliability prediction is also investigated. The evaluation of these models shows that it is possible to predict the synergy of unseen drug combinations with high accuracy (Pearson correlations between 0.43 and 0.86 depending on the considered cell line, with XGBoost providing slightly better predictions than RF). We have also found that restricting to the most reliable synergy predictions results in at least 2-fold error decrease with respect to employing the best learning algorithm without any reliability estimation. Alkylating agents, tyrosine kinase inhibitors and topoisomerase inhibitors are the drugs whose synergy with other partner drugs are better predicted by the models. Despite its leading size, NCI-ALMANAC comprises an extremely small part of all conceivable combinations. Given their accuracy and reliability estimation, the developed models should drastically reduce the number of required *in vitro* tests by predicting *in silico* which of the considered combinations are likely to be synergistic.

Keywords: chemoinformatics, drug synergy, machine learning, QSAR (qualitative structure-activity relationships), predictive (QSPR) models

INTRODUCTION

Drug combinations are a well-established form of cancer treatment (Bayat Mokhtari et al., 2017). Administering more than one drug can provide many benefits: higher efficacy, lower toxicity, and at least delayed onset of acquired drug resistance (Sugahara et al., 2010; Holohan et al., 2013; Crystal et al., 2014). Serendipitous discovery in the clinic has been a traditional source of effective drug combinations (Zoli et al., 2001; Kurtz et al., 2015). Yet systematic large-scale efforts to identify them have only recently been pursued, with a growing number of preclinical experimental efforts to identify synergistic combinations (Zoli et al., 2001; Budman et al., 2012; Lieu et al., 2013; Kashif et al., 2015; Yu et al., 2015; Kischkel et al., 2017) being reported in literature. The sheer number of available and possible drug-like molecules (Polishchuk et al., 2013) and an exponential number of their combinations, however, make the process of finding new therapeutic combinations by purely experimental means highly inefficient.

An efficient way of discovering molecules with previously unknown activity on a given target is using *in silico* prediction methods. Quantitative Structure-Activity Relationship (QSAR) models establish a mathematical relationship between the chemical structure of a molecule, encoded as a set of structural and/or physico-chemical features (descriptors), and its biological activity on a target. Such methods have been successfully used in a wide variety of pharmacology and drug design projects (Cherkasov et al., 2014), including cancer research (Chen et al., 2007; Mullen et al., 2011; Ali and Aittokallio, 2018). QSAR models are traditionally built using simple linear models (Sabet et al., 2010; Pick et al., 2011; Speck-Planche et al., 2011, 2012) to predict the activity of individual molecules against a molecular target. In the last 15 years, non-linear machine learning methods, such as Neural Network (NN) (González-Díaz et al., 2007), Support Vector Machine (SVM) (Doucet et al., 2007) or Random Forest (RF) (Singh et al., 2015), have also been employed to build QSAR models. More recently, QSAR modeling has also achieved accurate prediction of compound activity on non-molecular targets such as cancer cell lines (Kumar et al., 2014).

To extend QSAR modeling beyond individual molecules, the set of features from each molecule in the combination must be integrated. Various ways exist to encode two or more molecules as a feature vector, e.g., SIRMS descriptors (Kuz'min et al., 2008) for properties of combinations or the CGR approach for chemical reactions (de Luca et al., 2012). Rigorous validation strategies for the resulting models have been developed too (Muratov et al., 2012). The most common representation of a drug pair is, however, the concatenation of features from both molecules (Bulusu et al., 2016). On the other hand, modeling drug combinations requires the quantification of their synergy. Several metrics exist to quantify synergy (Foucquier and Guedj, 2015) (e.g., Bliss independence Bliss, 1939, Loewe additivity Chou and Talalay, 1984, Highest single agent approach Greco et al., 1995 or Chou-Talalay Method Chou, 2010). These are implemented in various commercial and publicly available software kits for the analysis of combination data, e.g., Combenefit (Di Veroli et al., 2016), CompuSyn (http://www.combosyn.com) or CalcuSyn (http://www.biosoft.com/w/calcusyn.htm).

One major roadblock in drug synergy modeling has been the lack of homogeneous data (i.e., datasets generated with the same assay, experimental conditions and synergy quantification). This has been, however, alleviated by the recent availability of large datasets from High-Throughput Screening (HTS) of drug combinations on cancer cell lines. For instance, Merck has released an HTS synergy dataset (O'Neil et al., 2016), covering combinations of 38 drugs and their activity against 39 cancer cell lines (more than 20,000 measured synergies). This dataset has been used to build predictive regression and classification models using multiple machine learning methods (Preuer et al., 2018). AstraZeneca carried out a screening study, spanning 910 drug combinations over 85 cancer cell lines (over 11,000 measured synergy scores), which was subsequently used for a DREAM challenge (Li et al., 2018; Menden et al., 2019). Very recently, the largest publicly available cancer drug combination dataset has been provided by the US National Cancer Institute (NCI). This NCI-ALMANAC (Holbeck et al., 2017) tested over 5,000 combinations of 104 investigational and approved drugs, with synergies measured against 60 cancer cell lines, leading to more than 290,000 synergy scores (ComboScores).

NCI-ALMANAC datasets have recently been modeled to predict the best growth inhibition of a given drug combination—cell line tuple (Xia et al., 2018). However, the question remains of how well ComboScores can be predicted on each NCI-60 cell line, which is important given that ComboScore-based screening has led to the identification of novel synergistic drug combinations *in vivo* (Holbeck et al., 2017). Here we present a large-scale study addressing this question. We build an individual model for each cell line using the popular RF algorithm (Breiman, 2001). We also build a second model per cell line using XGBoost (XGB for short) (Chen and Guestrin, 2016), a recent machine learning method that has helped to win numerous Kaggle competitions (Chen and Guestrin, 2016) as well as to generate highly predictive QSAR models (Sheridan et al., 2016). We validate these models for commonly-encountered prediction scenarios: e.g., unseen drug combination or unseen drug partner. We also introduce and validate reliability estimation techniques to further improve prediction of drug combination synergy. Lastly, we assess the suitability of NCI-ALMANAC datasets for predictive modeling depending on the screening center where they were generated.

METHODS

Data

NCI-ALMANAC is the largest-to-date phenotypic drug combination HTS. It contains the synergy measurements of pairwise combinations of 104 FDA approved drugs on the 60 cancer cell lines forming the NCI-60 panel (Shoemaker, 2006). The drugs include a wide array of small organic compound families, as well as several inorganic molecules (cisplatin and related platinum-organic compounds, arsenic trioxide). A similarity clustering dendrogram (**Figure 1**) shows the high diversity of the drugs in NCI-ALMANAC. Indeed, only 3 clusters comprising 8 drugs are formed with a Tanimoto score threshold of 0.8 (Vinblastine with Vincristine, Sirolimus and Everolimus, and Daunorubicin-Doxorubicin-Idarubicin-Epirubicin clusters), while the remaining 96 drugs have smaller similarity among them.

NCI-ALMANAC aggregates synergy data from three screening centers: NCI's Frederick National laboratory for Cancer Research (screening center code 1A, 11,259 synergy determinations), SRI International (FF, 146,147 determinations),

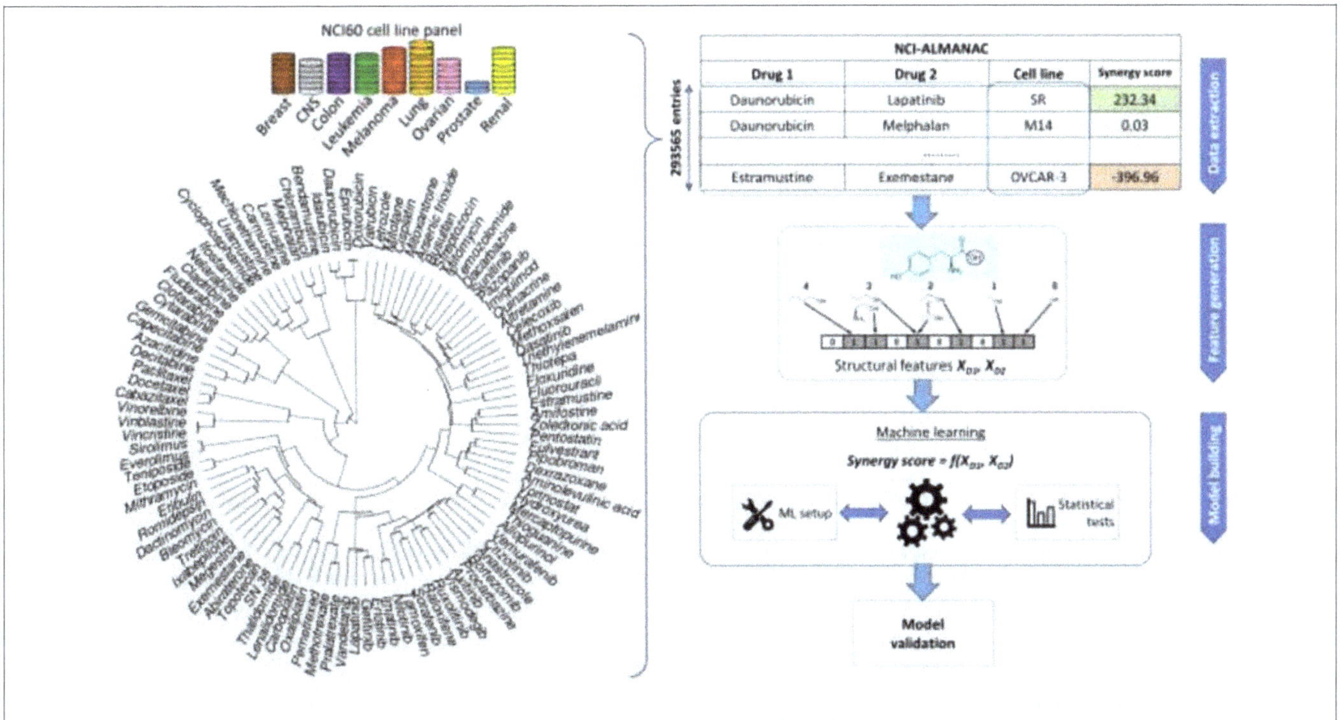

FIGURE 1 | Sketch of the workflow for drug combination modeling. Training data comes from NCI-ALMANAC, which comprises over 290,000 synergy measurements from pairs of 104 drugs tested on the 60 cell lines. Structural and physico-chemical features are calculated for each drug from its chemical structure. Similarity clustering diagram for 104 NCI-ALMANAC drugs is on the left. Each drug is characterized by MFPC features complemented with physico-chemical features, using the Tanimoto score on these features as the similarity metric. Hierarchical agglomerative clustering was carried out (ward.D2 algorithm in the R hclust function). Closely related compounds form tight clusters (e.g., doxorubicin and its analogs, analogs of paclitaxel, etc). By contrast, naturally inorganic compounds such as cisplatin and arsenic trioxide appear as outliers (the highest similarity coefficient to other drugs being 0.156 and 0.125, respectively). The concatenated vectors of the two drugs are the features utilized to build and test predictive models with machine learning techniques. The predictive accuracies of the models are determined by multiple cross-validation experiments.

and University of Pittsburgh (FG, 136,129 determinations). The synergy of drug pairs is measured in these screening centers against the NCI-60 panel, which includes cell lines from nine cancer types: leukemia, melanoma, non-small-cell lung, colon, central nervous system, ovarian, renal, prostate, and breast. In total, synergy is measured for 293,565 drug combination—cell line tuples, which represents a matrix completeness of 91.35%. Each center follows its own protocol, and some drugs are absent from the combination pool depending on the screening center. Since there is no overlap between drug combination—cell line tuples between the three centers, it is not possible to estimate inter-center batch effects, and therefore we must use data from different screening centers separately.

The combination benefit is quantified in NCI-ALMANAC by the so-called ComboScore (a modified version of the Bliss independence model). From the entire dose-response matrix of the considered drug combination and cell line tuple, the gain (or loss) of the effect achieved by the combination over the theoretically expected value if the effect was additive is calculated. Positive values of ComboScore indicate a synergistic effect of the combination, whereas the negative correspond to an antagonistic effect (those purely additive obtain a zero ComboScore).

Further description of NCI-ALMANAC data is available at **Supplementary Information**.

Features

For the use in machine learning, the structures of compounds must be encoded as vectors of numerical features known in chemoinformatics as molecular descriptors (Todeschini and Consonni, 2000). Several types of chemical structure features have been considered in this work: (1) Morgan FingerPrints (MFP) are topological descriptors describing the connectivity of the molecular structure, which take values 0 or 1, depending on whether the pattern is present in the molecule or not (Rogers and Hahn, 2010). They have been calculated with RDKit library (Lamdrum, 2015) using the following parameters—length is 256 bits, radius is 2. (2) Morgan FingerPrint Counts (MFPC) are a non-binary version of MFP that takes integer values equal to the number of times the pattern is detected in the molecule (256 features per drug, also calculated with RDKit). (3) MACCS keys encode presence or absence of 166 predetermined substructural fragments as binary vectors (calculated with RDKit). (4) ISIDA fragments encode structure as a vector of numbers of occurrences of substructural fragments of given nature and topology in the molecule (Varnek et al., 2005), which are calculated with ISIDA/Fragmentor (Ruggiu et al., 2015). Only one type of fragments is considered here: sequences of atoms and bonds of length 2 to 6 (1,325 features per drug in total). (5) SIRMS fragments are the number of occurrences of 4-atom fragments

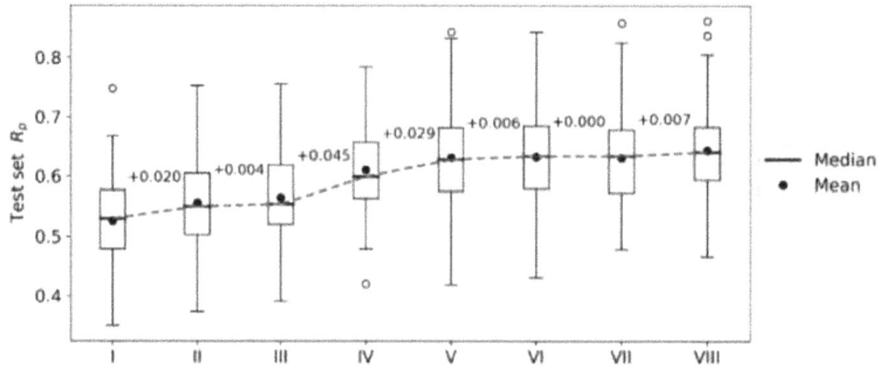

FIGURE 2 | Performance gain across cell lines for each introduced modeling choice during the exploratory analysis of FG data. Each boxplot represents the distribution of the cell line models' test set performances (R_p) at any given step. Analysis steps are carried out sequentially: I—RF, 1,000 trees with all n features tried to split a node, 80% training set, 20% test set, MACCS (Molecular ACCess System) keys as features; II—MFPC (Morgan fingerprint counts) are used as features instead; III—physico-chemical features are added for each drug; IV—training set rows are duplicated with the reverse order of drugs (data augmentation); V-–90% training set, 10% test set are used instead of the initial 80/20 partition; VI—RF with 250 trees with n/3 features tried to split a node; VII—XGB models with recommended settings; VIII—tuned XGB models. Note that I-V employ RF with same values for its hyperparameters (RF tuned in VI) and V-VIII use the same training and test sets. Modeling choices introducing the largest improvements are the choice of molecular features and the data augmentation strategies.

of varying topology in a molecule, including bonded and non-bonded atoms (Kuz'min et al., 2008). Calculated with SiRMS python library (github.com/DrrDom/sirms), it led to 1,454 features per drug. In addition to these sets, 7 physico-chemical features are calculated by RDkit: total polar surface area (TPSA), molecular weight, logP, number of aliphatic and aromatic rings, H-bond donors and acceptors.

Machine Learning (ML) Workflow

Models are built using two ML algorithms: Random Forest (RF) (Svetnik et al., 2003) and Extreme Gradient Boosting (XGBoost; XGB for short) (Sheridan et al., 2016). The entire modeling workflow is sketched in **Figure 1**. Further details about how ML models were built are available at the **Supplementary Information.**

Predictive Performance Metrics

To evaluate the performance of a model, the following metrics are calculated from observed y_{obs} and predicted y_{pred} ComboScore values:

Root Mean Squared Error (*RMSE*)

$$RMSE = \sqrt{\frac{\sum_N \left(y_{i,\,obs} - y_{i,\,pred}\right)^2}{N}}$$

Coefficient of determination (R^2) (Leach and Gillet, 2007)

$$R^2 = 1 - \frac{\sum_N \left(y_{i,\,obs} - y_{i,\,pred}\right)^2}{\sum_N \left(y_{i,\,obs} - \overline{y_{obs}}\right)^2} = 1 - \frac{RMSE^2}{Var\left(y_{obs}\right)};$$

$$\overline{y_{obs}} = \frac{1}{N}\sum_{i=1}^{N} y_{i,obs}$$

Pearson's correlation coefficient (R_p)

$$R_p = \frac{\sum_N (y_{i,\,obs} - \overline{y_{obs}})(y_{i,\,pred} - \overline{y_{pred}})}{\sqrt{\sum_N (y_{i,\,obs} - \overline{y_{obs}})^2}\sqrt{\sum_N (y_{i,\,pred} - \overline{y_{pred}})^2}}$$

Spearman's rank-order correlation coefficient (R_s)

$$R_s = R_p(\text{rank}\, y_{obs},\, \text{rank}\, y_{pred})$$

We use R_p between observed and predicted values of ComboScore of a dataset not used to train the model as a primary metric of its accuracy. For proper estimation of the generalization error, these metrics are always calculated here on a test set not used to train or select the model.

RESULTS

Exploratory Modeling of NCI-ALMANAC Data

First, we perform an exploratory modeling on the FG datasets in order to determine optimal settings for synergy prediction by assessing various types of features, data augmentation schemes and machine learning methods. The summary of performance improvements is shown on **Figure 2**. The best median R_p across cell lines for RF was obtained with 250 trees, a third of the features evaluated at each tree node, training data augmentation and MFPC fingerprints complemented by physico-chemical properties (256 and 7 features per drug, respectively). The gain of performance with RF is substantial: the median R_p increases from 0.530 (I) to 0.634 (VI).

XGB models are generated with the same features and data set partitions. Changing the machine learning algorithm from RF to XGB does not improve the median test set R_p, although both minimum and maximum R_p are higher with XGB (boxplots

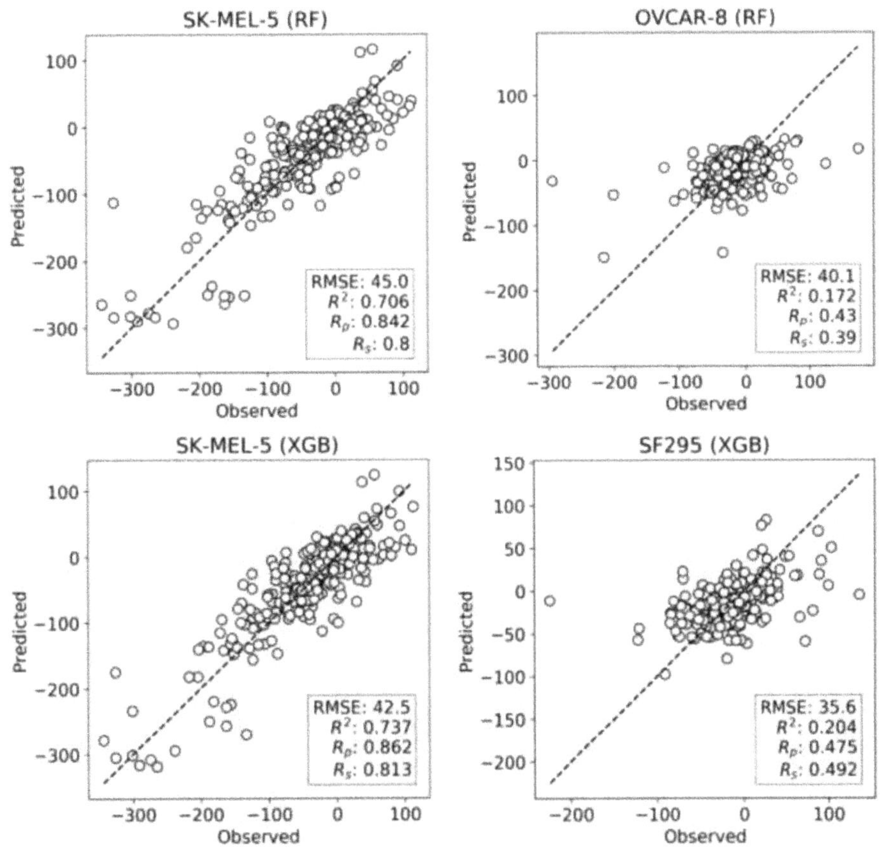

FIGURE 3 | Observed vs. predicted ComboScore for all the drug combinations in the test set. This is presented for the best- and worst-performing models with both ML methods, RF, and XGB (these models correspond hence to the extremes of **Figure 2**'s boxplots VI and VIII, respectively). On the left column, the best-performing cell line models from each method. On the right side, the worst-performing cell line models. All performance metrics are shown. Each point represents a drug combination in that test set.

VI and VII in **Figure 2**, respectively). After tuning of XGB hyperparameters per cell line, a small gain in overall performance is obtained: the median R_p of tuned XGB rises to 0.641 (boxplot VIII). In comparison, Y-randomization (Tropsha et al., 2003) tests using the same learning algorithm did only obtain a median R_p of −0.016 (−0.024 when using RF). **Figure 3** shows the degree of accuracy achieved by each algorithm for the best and the worst predicted cell line. The cell lines with the worst predictions (OVCAR-8 for RF and SF295 for XGB) have substantially smaller variance in observed ComboScore than those with the best predictions (SK-MEL-5 for both algorithms).

Estimating the Reliability of Drug Synergy Predictions

For prospective use of models, it is paramount to calculate not only predicted drug combination synergies, but also how reliable these predictions are (Mathea et al., 2016). With this purpose, we have applied a RF-specific reliability prediction approach, where the degree of agreement between the diverse trees in the forest serves as a reliability score. This is quantified here as the standard deviation (SD) of the RF tree predictions (250 per drug combination and cell line) and referred to as tree_SD. tree_SD has been pointed out as one of the most powerful metrics to assess the reliability of predictions in regression problems (Mathea et al., 2016). We thus assemble test subsets with the 25% most reliable ComboScore predictions per cell line (i.e., combinations with the 25% lowest tree_SD scores). Likewise, we assemble test subsets with 25% least reliable predictions per cell line.

Figure 4 presents the test set performances of each cell line model on the three scenarios: 25% most reliable predictions, all predictions regardless of estimated reliability and 25% least reliable predictions. The top and bottom 25% predictions in terms of reliability obtain the lowest and highest RMSE in every cell line, which demonstrates the accuracy and generality of tree_SD as a reliability score for drug synergy predictions. Test set RMSE varies greatly across cell lines, e.g., models built on leukemia cell lines obtain in general higher error. This, however, comes from the higher range of ComboScores observed in these cell lines. Indeed, the larger this range, the higher the range of predicted ComboScores is, which combined tend to make RMSE larger. Similar RMSE is only obtained on the K-562 leukemia cell line, which is consistent with the fact that it has the lowest range among leukemia cell lines and similar to that of other cancer types.

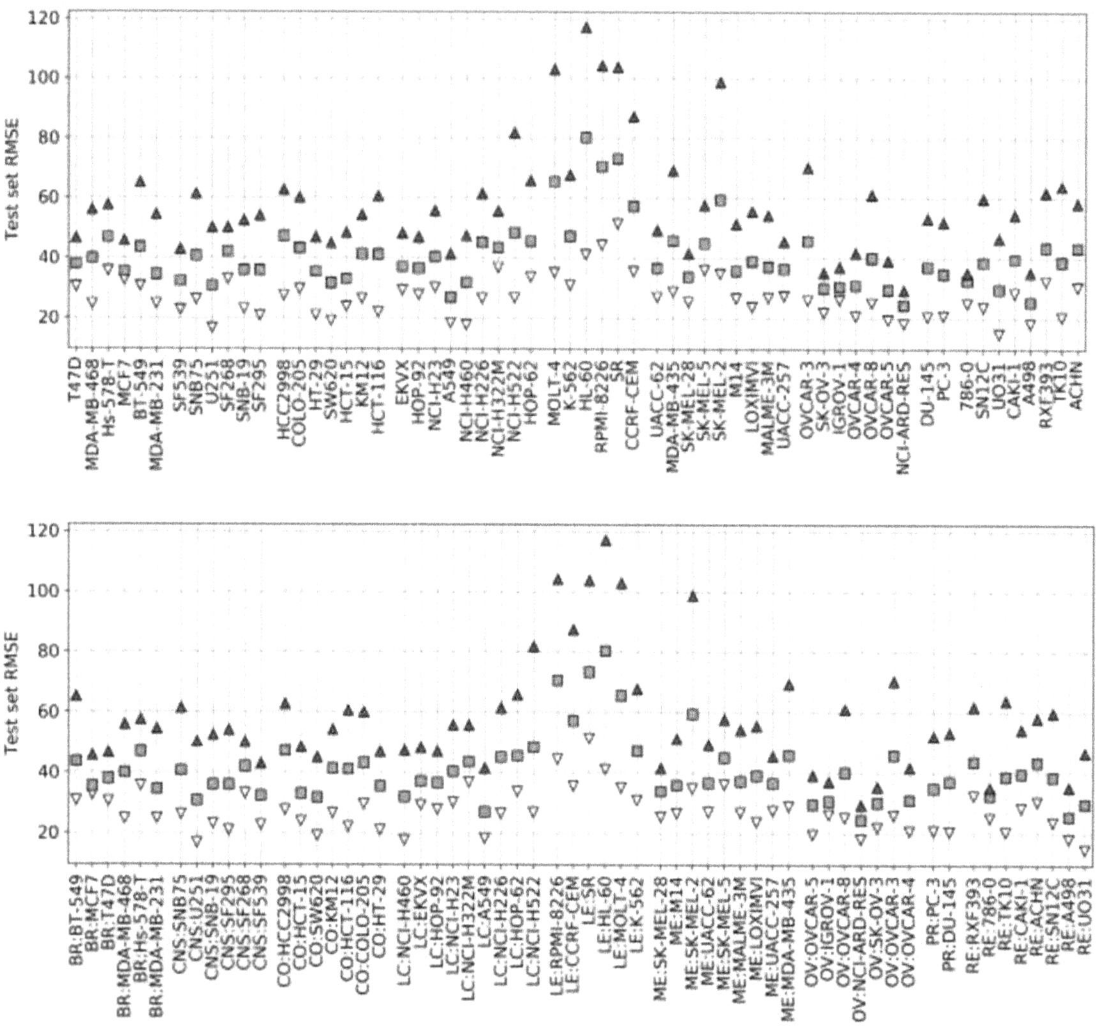

FIGURE 4 | Ten percent test set RMSE of RF cell line models trained on 90% of the FG data. Gray squares represent the model's RMSE on all the test combinations (RF predictions as usual). Black triangles mark the RMSE of the 25% least reliable (highest tree_SD) combos, whereas white inverted triangles correspond to the RMSE of the 25% most reliable (lowest tree_SD). In each cell line, the reliability score tracks test RMSE and hence it can be used to identify *a priori* the most accurate predictions. Each cell line name in the horizontal axis is preceded by its cancer type ID: breast (BR), central nervous system (CNS), colon (CO), non-small-cell lung (LC), leukemia (LE), melanoma (ME), ovarian (OV), prostate (PR), and renal (RE).

Reliability estimation is evaluated in terms of RMSE rather than R_p. While RMSE is not as intuitive as correlation, correlations may be misleading when comparing performances of models across test sets with distinct variances. **Figure 5** illustrates this issue with the test performances of HL-60 models, which benefit the most from reliability estimation. The test set with the most reliable combinations is predicted with half the RMSE of the entire test set (RMSE of 41 vs. 80) and a third of the least reliable combinations (RMSE of 41 vs. 117). This more accurate prediction can be visually observed too, but the other metrics (R^2, R_p, and R_s) do not capture this increase in accuracy due to substantially different ComboScore variance between the compared test sets. Importantly, RF with reliability prediction provides a much larger reduction in RMSE than that introduced by XGB (bottom right), both with respect to RF without reliability prediction (bottom left). These results strongly suggest that, in cases where it is not necessary to test all positive predictions (here synergistic drug combinations), selecting the most reliable predictions is more effective than using the most suitable ML algorithm.

Performance in Predicting Synergies With Drugs Not Included in NCI-ALMANAC

The random data splits that we have used so far may overestimate the model's performance in the case of drug combinations. This would be due to the presence of the two drugs in the combination in both training and test sets, albeit with other partners (Muratov et al., 2012). In order to assess to which extent this is the case, we also carry out Leave-One-Drug-Out (LODO)

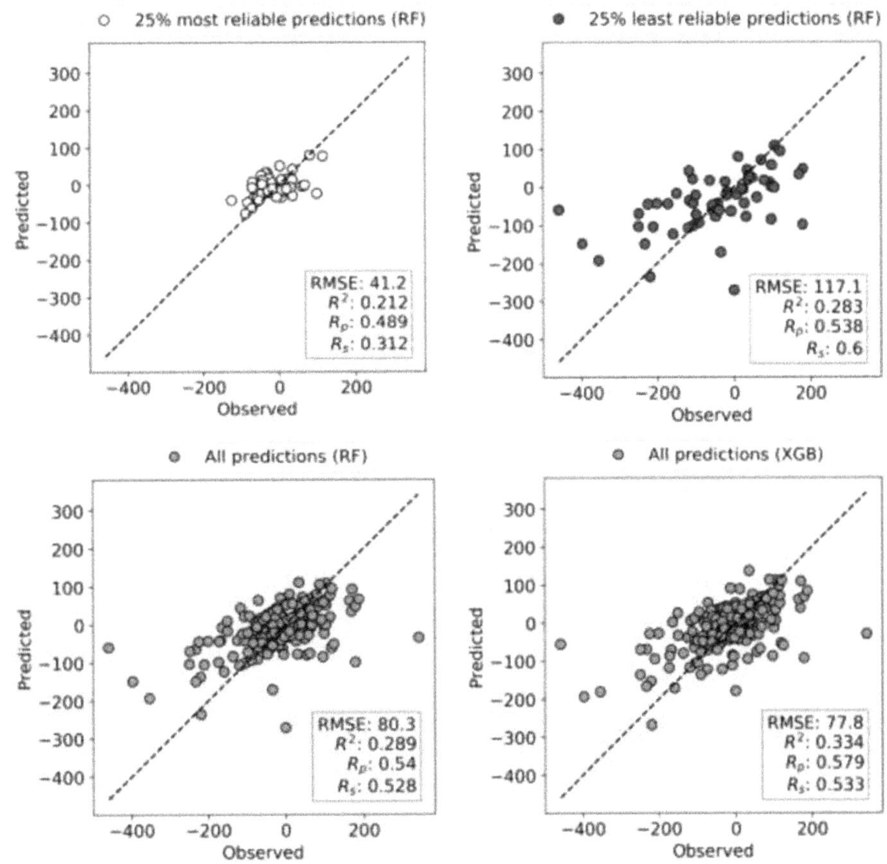

FIGURE 5 | Observed vs. Predicted ComboScore plots for HL-60 leukemia cell line test set (10% of data). Models are built on 90% of FG dataset corresponding to this cell line using RF and XGB methods, both tuned. Each circle is now a drug combination from the entire test set, with its shade of gray indicating one of the three scenarios (as in **Figure 4**). All performance metrics are displayed in each plot. The subset with the most reliable ComboScore RF predictions (top left plot) achieves half the RMSE of the entire test set (bottom right). Importantly, this is a much larger reduction in RMSE than that introduced by XGB (bottom right) with respect to RF (bottom left). Furthermore, the most reliable predicted ComboScores (top right) obtain a third of the RMSE of the least reliable predictions (top left).

cross-validation experiments for each cell line. In LODO cross-validation, every combination containing the considered left-out drug is placed in its test set, and the model is built on the remaining combinations tested on that cell line. Thus, there are as many folds as drugs in the dataset. In this way, the LODO cross-validation simulates the model's behavior when presented with a new chemical entity outside of the model's scope, as if it was not included in the dataset.

Figure 6 shows the outcome of LODO cross-validation for XGB per cell line. We henceforth use XGB with the recommended values for hyperparameters, as tuning them for each LODO cross-validation fold and cell line is prohibitive and would only provide marginal gains (see **Figure 2**). LODO results show that combinations associated with 75% of the left-out drugs can be predicted with an accuracy of at least $R_p = 0.3$ against any cell line. This accuracy raises to at least $R_p = 0.5$ for 50% of the left-out drugs. The latter is not much worse than the median R_p across cell lines when using 90/10 data partitions ($R_p = 0.641$ as shown in **Figure 2**'s boxplot VIII). k-fold cross-validation results are available for comparison in **Supplementary Figure 3**.

Figure 7 shows the analysis for LODO cross-validations in terms of RMSE. About 75% of models demonstrate at least moderate accuracy (RMSE < 50). The exceptions are mostly leukemia cell line models, which obtain higher RMSE due to having the highest variances in ComboScores among cancer types. An important result is that using RF models restricted to the most reliable predictions allows us to reduce the error of prediction further in every cell line (RMSE < 40), in full agreement with the findings from random 90/10 partitions (see **Figure 4**) and also outperforming the best models without reliability prediction.

Analyzing LODO results per left-out drug instead of per cell line reveals that synergy prediction is much worse for certain left-out drugs in each cancer type. LODO performance of each drug across cell lines is shown in **Supplementary Figure 4**. This figure shows that models for arsenic trioxide, highly dissimilar to other drugs, have the lowest performance across cell lines and partner drugs (median R_p of models concerning this drug is -0.28). Conversely, partners of tyrosine kinase inhibitors, well-represented in these datasets (e.g., Imatinib, Nilotinib or

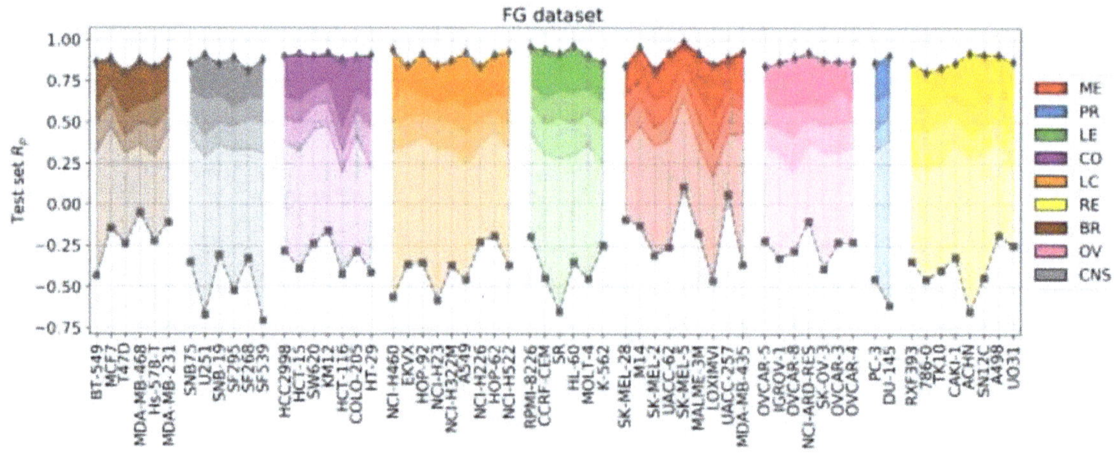

FIGURE 6 | LODO cross-validation results using XGB with the recommended values for their hyperparameters on the FG dataset. Distribution of models' performances is shown by cancer type (color code). Each colored zone represents 25% of models per cell line: from dense zone—top performing 25%; to light zone—bottom quartile. The method performs with at least moderate accuracy ($R_p > 0.30$) in 75% of left-out drugs (the top 3 quartiles) across cell lines. Left-out drugs within the top quartile, darkest shade among the four employed per cell line, are predicted with a R_p ranging from 0.471 (HCT-116) to 0.986 (SK-MEL-5). Although there are no large differences in how well different cancer types are predicted, left-out drugs on melanoma (ME, in red) and leukemia (LE, in green) cell lines obtain slightly higher average performance (median R_p of drug-out models for corresponding cell lines are 0.554 and 0.524, respectively).

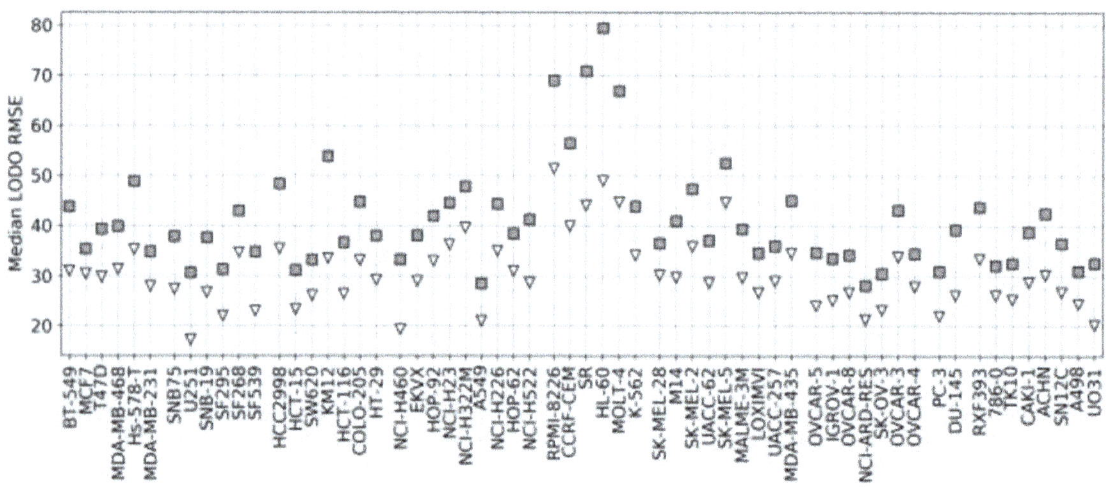

FIGURE 7 | Median RMSE in LODO cross-validation for XGB with the recommended values for their hyperparameters (gray squares) and RF top 25% most reliable predictions (white inverted triangles) for each cell line (grouped by cancer type). As the plot shows, combinations with one left-out drug can be predicted with at least moderate accuracy across cell lines (RMSE < 50 for XGB, RMSE < 40 for RF with reliability estimation; both being approximate thresholds).

Lapatinib), are predicted with high accuracy (e.g., models for imatinib have median $R_p = 0.82$). Topoisomerase inhibitors (Teniposide and Etoposide) are also among the best-predicted left-out drugs. These *in silico* models could be used to anticipate how the synergies of a drug in combination with its partner drugs would vary across NCI-60 cell lines. However, since high accuracy is only obtained on those left-out drugs well-represented in NCI-ALMANAC, such selectivity predictions should only be accurate for drugs with similar chemical structure to those in NCI-ALMANAC. As models predicting drug-induced cell line response have been shown to improve by integrating drug features with multi-omics cell features (Menden et al., 2013; Xia et al., 2018), we expect that predicting drug synergy across cell lines will also improve by following such multi-task learning approach on this closely related problem.

Comparing Predictive Models Built With Data From Different Screening Centers

So far we have exclusively employed data from the FG screening center, which represents about half of NCI-ALMANAC data. Practically all the remaining ComboScores come from the FF screening center and are also determined with a 3 × 3 grid of

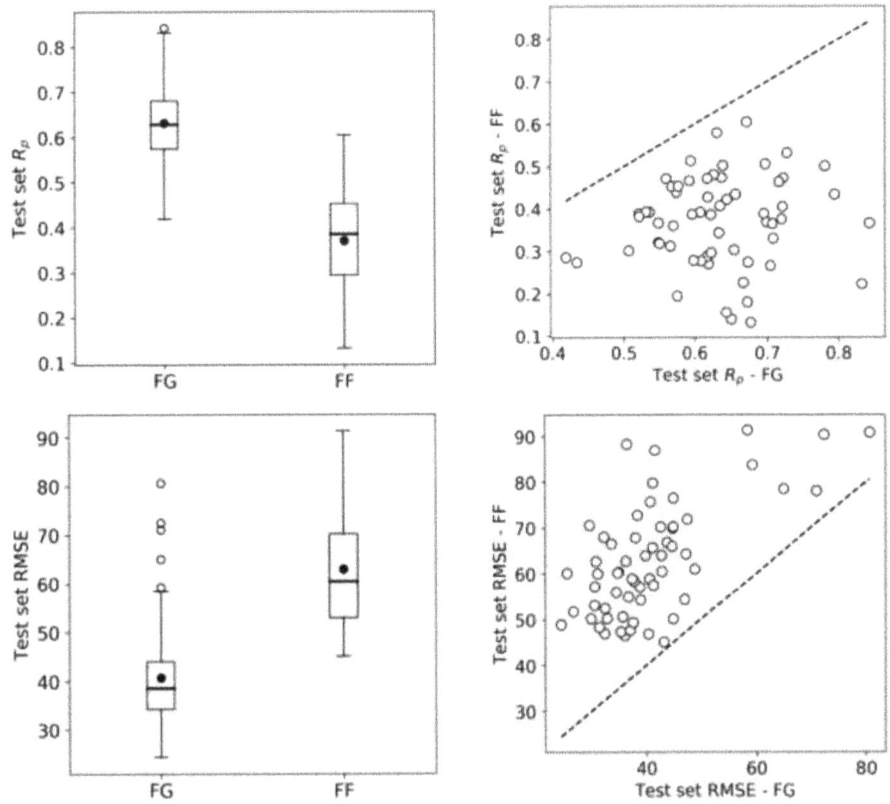

FIGURE 8 | RF model performance comparison for FG and FF datasets. Models are built following the final setup in the exploratory analysis (a 90/10 data partition is employed for each cell line); MFPC with physico-chemical features as well as data augmentation are also used). On the left, boxplots for cell line models test set R_P's (top row) and RMSE (bottom row) for both centers data. On the right, R_P (top row) and RMSE (bottom row) of models trained on FG dataset against models trained on FF dataset, each point shows the two model performances for the cell line. FF models obtain consistently lower performance than FG models. As the same modeling workflow was used, this strongly suggests that FF data is less predictive than FG data.

non-zero concentrations. Thus, we evaluate here the predictive potential of FF datasets. We start by building RF models from FF data using the same 90/10 partitions as with FG. Surprisingly, FF-based models obtained worse performance in every cell line (**Figure 8**) and thus were objectively worse at predicting ComboScores.

In trying to understand this unexpected result, we started by investigating whether this was due to modeling differences, but this was not the case. First, FF training sets are slightly larger than FG datasets (see **Supplementary Table 1**), which theoretically favors better performance on FF. Furthermore, using tuned XGB models led to essentially the same result (median R_p of 0.641 for FG vs. 0.368 for FF) as shown in **Figure 8** with RF. In addition to these non-linear methods, we also used Elastic Net (EN), but FF models were still substantially less predictive than FG models (median R_p of 0.37 for FG vs. 0.23 for FF). When we carried out LODO cross-validations instead of 90/10 partitions, the same trend was observed (**Supplementary Figures 5, 6** also show worse performance of FF-based LODO than that of FG-based LODO in **Figure 6**).

To shed light into this issue, we looked at the only factor that we can compare between these screening centers: the relative growth inhibition (PERCENTGROWTH) induced by a given concentration of a drug tested individually. Interestingly, by counting the different test dates, we observed that FG had on average tested a non-combined drug 3.77 times per cell line, whereas FF almost doubled this number (7.13 times per cell line). A higher number of tests is not in itself worrisome if the growth inhibition of the drug-concentration-cell line tuple is similar between dates. However, if the measurements from these tests are substantially different, this is a problem because the set of ComboScores determined with variable measurements from the same tuple will be inconsistent as well. Consequently, synergy differences between such combinations will not only come from their intrinsic properties, but also from unrelated experimental variability.

To show that higher growth inhibition variability in FF data results in less predictive models, we analyzed five drugs (Thioguanine, Chlorambucil, Altretamine, Fluorouracil, and Melphalan) with a high number of different test dates in both centers. We first consider the drugs on a cell line were only FG models obtain high average accuracy in predicting synergy (NCI/ADR-RES) and subsequently on another where both FF and FG models are on average predictive (NCI-H322M). On each

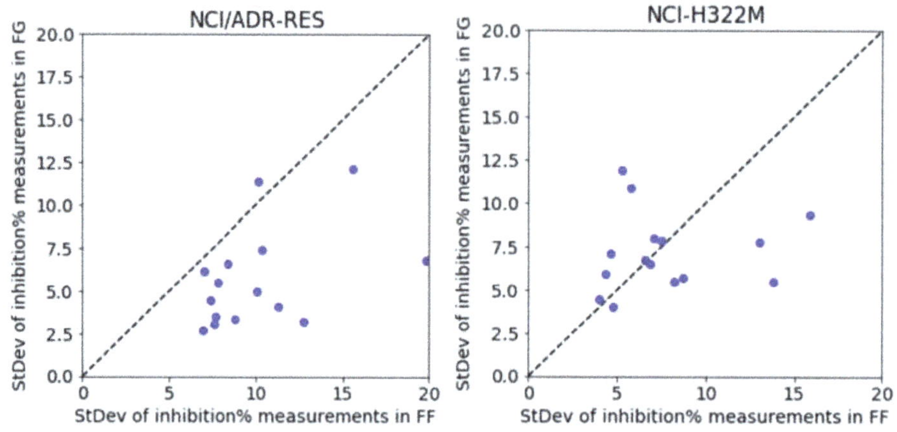

FIGURE 9 | RF model performance comparison for FG and FF datasets. Models are built following the final setup in the exploratory analysis (i.e., a 90/10 data partition is employed for each cell line; MFPC with physico-chemical features as well as data augmentation are also used). We analyzed five drugs (Thioguanine, Chlorambucil, Altretamine, Fluorouracil, and Melphalan) with a high number of different test dates in both centers. On the left, the results with the cell line that is worst predicted by RF with FF data (NCI/ADR-RES with $R_p = 0.14$ in 90/10 partition), which is much better predicted with FG ($R_p = 0.65$, using the same partition). This plot shows the standard deviation of the values of each set from FG against those from FF.

cell line, each drug has a set of growth inhibition replicates per concentration and screening center (i.e., 15 sets per screening center). The performance on NCI/ADR-RES using FF data is indeed poor ($R_p = 0.14$ in 90/10 partition by RF), but it is much better predicted using FG data ($R_p = 0.65$, using the same partition and method). Fourteen of the fifteen sets have higher standard deviation of growth inhibition with FF data (**Figure 9**), which is consistent with the lower accuracy in predicting synergy obtained with this dataset. Conversely, we repeated this operation with NCI-H322M where synergy is well-predicted by RF with both FF ($R_p = 0.61$ in 90/10 partition) and FG data ($R_p = 0.66$, on the same partition). The standard deviations from both screening centers are now similar (**Figure 9**). Taken together, these experiments suggest that the reason why FF data results in less predictive models is the noise introduced in ComboScore determination by larger variability of growth inhibition measurements.

DISCUSSION

NCI-ALMANAC is an extremely valuable resource for the discovery of novel synergistic drug combinations on NCI-60 cell lines. First, it is by far the largest-to-date HTS of drug combinations, therefore allowing *in silico* models with much higher accuracy and broader domain of applicability in predicting the synergy of other combinations. Second, some of the synergistic drug combinations discovered *in vitro* by NCI-ALMANAC were subsequently tested on human tumor mouse xenografts of the same cell line. 48% of them were also synergistic in at least one of these *in vivo* models (Holbeck et al., 2017), which led to the launch of two clinical trials so far (NCT02211755 and NCT02379416).

In this study, we have found that it is possible to predict the synergy of unseen drug combinations against NCI-60 panel cell lines with high accuracy by exploiting NCI-ALMANAC data. We have established a general ML workflow (types of structural features, data preprocessing strategy, ML method) to generate such models. When trained on FG data, predicted synergies from these models match observable synergies with R_p correlations comprised between 0.43 and 0.86 depending on the considered cell line. Incidentally, these regression problems must be highly non-linear, as EN leads to substantially less predictive models than XGB or RF.

Some cell lines and drug combinations can be predicted with higher accuracy than others. For example, models for the SK-MEL-5 cell line perform best with any method (**Figure 6**). However, if we use RMSE instead of R_p to reduce the influence of the ComboScore range, models for the NCI-ARD-RES are now best (gray squares in **Figure 7**). Another explanatory factor for this variability is the adequacy of the employed ML technique to the problem instance to solve (each cell line constitutes here a different problem instance). Even if training set size, features and classifier are the same, the modeled relationship between drug synergy and features depend on training set composition and cell line properties (implicitly). It is well-established that the performance of supervised learning algorithms varies depending on the problem instance in ways that cannot be anticipated without doing the actual numerical experiments (Fernández-Delgado et al., 2014). LODO cross-validation also revealed both best and worst partner drugs. These differences are mainly due to the number of similar partner drugs. For example, it is difficult to predict synergy of combinations containing arsenic trioxide because its 103 partner drugs are highly dissimilar in terms of chemical structure and physico-chemical properties. Indeed, machine learning from dissimilar data instances tend to be less accurate, although here the dissimilarity can be partial as arsenic trioxide's partner can be similar to other NCI-ALMANAC drugs. On the other hand, combinations containing some other drugs are better represented in NCI-ALMANAC and hence tend to be predicted with higher accuracy. This is the case of various alkylating agents, tyrosine kinase inhibitors and topoisomerase inhibitors (**Supplementary Figure 4**).

Recent QSAR and drug combination modeling studies have evaluated the application of the latest machine learning algorithms (e.g., XGBoost, Deep Neural Network). These studies have found that these algorithms provide better performance on average across targets than RF. However, these gains are small and hence do not always justify the much greater resources required for hyperparameter tuning (Sheridan et al., 2016; Preuer et al., 2018). Performance gains have also been found small here with NCI-ALMANAC data, as the average test set R_P of XGBoost across the 60 cell lines is just +0.007 larger than with RF. An important result is that restricting to the most reliable RF predictions provides much greater predictive accuracy than that introduced by a more suitable learning algorithm (e.g., XGBoost). It is surprising that this powerful technique is so uncommonly used, as has already been pointed out (Sheridan, 2013; Mathea et al., 2016). In fact, we are not aware of any other previous study applying reliability estimation to the prediction of drug synergy on cancer cell lines. Here reliability prediction permitted to reduce the RMSE by up to 50% depending on the cell line. This is particularly exciting for virtual screening problems, where only a small subset of the predictions can be tested *in vitro*. In this scenario, it is useful to identify those combinations that are not only predicted to be synergistic, but also reliable because this should provide higher hit rates. Lastly, highly synergistic combinations predicted with low reliability should also be tested, as the corresponding measurements would be those broadening the applicability domain of future models the most.

We have also found that using FG datasets leads to substantially more predictive models than FF datasets. This result is robust in that it is observed with various types of models (XGB, RF, EN). Moreover, it occurs in spite of the availability of slightly more training data. Further investigation revealed that there are many more measurements of growth inhibition and with greater variability in FF than in FG. This in turn introduces more noise into ComboScore determinations in FF, thus impairing its modeling. Inconsistencies between centers measuring the response of cancer cell lines to drugs have been observed before (Haibe-Kains et al., 2013). There has been intense controversy about the extent, sources and impact of these inconsistencies (Stransky et al., 2015; Geeleher et al., 2016; Safikhani et al., 2016, 2017). In any case, it is clear that data permits the development of predictive models regardless of the screening center (Ammad-ud-din et al., 2014; Covell, 2015; Fang et al., 2015; Naulaerts et al., 2017), as it has also been the case here with NCI-ALMANAC. Owing to this controversy on datasets from multiple screening centers, a better understanding of their limitations and the identification of protocols to generate them with improved consistency has emerged (Haverty et al., 2016). These protocols will ultimately permit that merging datasets from different screening centers result in further predictive accuracy.

CONCLUSION

While NCI-ALMANAC measured the synergies of over 5,000 combinations per cell line, this still represents a minuscule part of all conceivable combinations. Even if we restricted ourselves to the set of 12,000 drug molecules estimated to have reached clinical development or undergone significant preclinical profiling (Janes et al., 2018), almost 72 million combinations per cell line would have to be tested *in vitro* to identify the most synergistic among them. Therefore, the developed *in silico* models are of great importance because these can drastically reduce the number of required *in vitro* tests by predicting which of the considered combinations are likely to be synergistic.

AUTHOR CONTRIBUTIONS

PB conceived the study and wrote the manuscript. PS implemented the software and carried out the numerical experiments with the assistance of SN. All authors commented and proposed improvements to the manuscript.

FUNDING

ANR Tremplin-ERC grant n° N° ANR-17-ERC2-0003-01 (PB).

ACKNOWLEDGMENTS

The initially submitted version of this manuscript was previously released as a Pre-Print at https://www.biorxiv.org/content/10.1101/504076v1 (Sidorov et al., 2018).

REFERENCES

Ali, M., and Aittokallio, T. (2018). Machine learning and feature selection for drug response prediction in precision oncology applications. *Biophys. Rev.* 11, 31–39. doi: 10.1007/s12551-018-0446-z

Ammad-ud-din, M., Georgii, E., Gönen, M., Laitinen, T., Kallioniemi, O., Wennerberg, K., et al. (2014). Integrative and personalized QSAR analysis in cancer by kernelized Bayesian matrix factorization. *J. Chem. Inf. Model.* 54, 2347–2359. doi: 10.1021/ci500152b

Bayat Mokhtari, R., Homayouni, T. S., Baluch, N., Morgatskaya, E., Kumar, S., Das, B., et al. (2017). Combination therapy in combating cancer. *Oncotarget* 8, 38022–38043. doi: 10.18632/oncotarget.16723

Bliss, C. I. (1939). The toxicity of poisons applied jointly I. *Ann. Appl. Biol.* 26, 585–615. doi: 10.1111/j.1744-7348.1939.tb06990.x

Breiman, L. (2001). Random forests. *Mach. Learn.* 45, 5–32. doi: 10.1023/A:1010933404324

Budman, D. R., Calabro, A., Rosen, L., and Lesser, M. (2012). Identification of unique synergistic drug combinations associated with downexpression of survivin in a preclinical breast cancer model system. *Anticancer Drugs* 23, 272–279. doi: 10.1097/cad.0b013e32834ebda4

Bulusu, K. C., Guha, R., Mason, D. J., Lewis, R. P., Muratov, E., Kalantar Motamedi, Y., et al. (2016). Modelling of compound combination effects and applications to efficacy and toxicity: state-of-the-art, challenges and perspectives. *Drug Discov. Today* 21, 225–238. doi: 10.1016/j.drudis.2015.09.003

Chen, J., Shen, Y., Liao, S., Chen, L., and Zheng, K. (2007). DFT-based QSAR study and molecular design of AHMA derivatives as potent anticancer agents. *Int. J. Quantum Chem.* 107, 1468–1478. doi: 10.1002/qua.21285

Chen, T., and Guestrin, C. (2016). "XGBoost: a scalable tree boosting system," in *Proceedings of the 22nd ACM SIGKDD International Conference on Knowledge Discovery and Data Mining—KDD '16* (New York, NY: ACM Press), 785–794. Available online at: https://dl.acm.org/citation.cfm?id=2939672&picked=prox

Cherkasov, A., Muratov, E. N., Fourches, D., Varnek, A., Baskin, I. I., Cronin, M., et al. (2014). QSAR modeling: where have you been? where are you going to? *J. Med. Chem.* 57, 4977–5010. doi: 10.1021/jm4004285

Chou, T.-C. (2010). Drug combination studies and their synergy quantification using the chou-talalay method. *Cancer Res.* 70, 440–446. doi: 10.1158/0008-5472.CAN-09-1947

Chou, T.-C., and Talalay, P. (1984). Quantitative analysis of dose-effect relationships: the combined effects of multiple drugs or enzyme inhibitors. *Adv. Enzyme Regul.* 22, 27–55. doi: 10.1016/0065-2571(84)90007-4

Covell, D. G. (2015). Data mining approaches for genomic biomarker development: applications using drug screening data from the cancer genome project and the cancer cell line encyclopedia. *PLoS ONE* 10:e0127433. doi: 10.1371/journal.pone.0127433

Crystal, A. S., Shaw, A. T., Sequist, L. V., Friboulet, L., Niederst, M. J., Lockerman, E. L., et al. (2014). Patient-derived models of acquired resistance can identify effective drug combinations for cancer. *Science* 346, 1480–1486. doi: 10.1126/science.1254721

de Luca, A., Horvath, D., Marcou, G., Solov'ev, V., and Varnek, A. (2012). Mining chemical reactions using neighborhood behavior and condensed graphs of reactions approaches. *J. Chem.Inf. Model.* 52, 2325–2338. doi: 10.1021/ci300149n

Di Veroli, G. Y., Fornari, C., Wang, D., Mollard, S., Bramhall, J. L., Richards, F. M., et al. (2016). Combenefit: an interactive platform for the analysis and visualization of drug combinations. *Bioinformatics* 32, 2866–2868. doi: 10.1093/bioinformatics/btw230

Doucet, J.-P., Barbault, F., Xia, H., Panaye, A., and Fan, B. (2007). Nonlinear SVM approaches to QSPR/QSAR studies and drug design. *Curr. Comput. Aided-Drug Des.* 3, 263–289. doi: 10.2174/157340907782799372

Fang, Y., Qin, Y., Zhang, N., Wang, J., Wang, H., and Zheng, X. (2015). DISIS: prediction of drug response through an iterative sure independence screening. *PLoS ONE* 10:e0120408. doi: 10.1371/journal.pone.0120408

Fernández-Delgado, M., Cernadas, E., Barro, S., and Amorim, D. (2014). Do we need hundreds of classifiers to solve real world classification problems? *J. Mach. Learn. Res.* 15, 3133–3181. Available online at: http://jmlr.org/papers/v15/delgado14a.html

Foucquier, J., and Guedj, M. (2015). Analysis of drug combinations: current methodological landscape. *Pharmacol. Res. Perspect.* 3:e00149. doi: 10.1002/prp2.149

Geeleher, P., Gamazon, E. R., Seoighe, C., Cox, N. J., and Huang, R. S. (2016). Consistency in large pharmacogenomic studies. *Nature* 540, E1–E2. doi: 10.1038/nature19838

González-Díaz, H., Bonet, I., Terán, C., De Clercq, E., Bello, R., García, M. M., et al. (2007). ANN-QSAR model for selection of anticancer leads from structurally heterogeneous series of compounds. *Eur. J. Med. Chem.* 42, 580–585. doi: 10.1016/J.EJMECH.2006.11.016

Greco, W. R., Bravo, G., and Parsons, J. C. (1995). The search for synergy: a critical review from a response surface perspective. *Pharmacol. Rev.* 47, 331–385.

Haibe-Kains, B., El-Hachem, N., Birkbak, N. J., Jin, A. C., Beck, A. H., Aerts, H. J., et al. (2013). Inconsistency in large pharmacogenomic studies. *Nature* 504, 389–393. doi: 10.1038/nature12831

Haverty, P. M., Lin, E., Tan, J., Yu, Y., Lam, B., Lianoglou, S., et al. (2016). Reproducible pharmacogenomic profiling of cancer cell line panels. *Nature* 533, 333–337. doi: 10.1038/nature

Holbeck, S. L., Camalier, R., Crowell, J. A., Govindharajulu, J. P., Hollingshead, M., Anderson, L. W., et al. (2017). The National Cancer Institute ALMANAC: a comprehensive screening resource for the detection of anticancer drug pairs with enhanced therapeutic activity. *Cancer Res.* 77, 3564–3576. doi: 10.1158/0008-5472.can-17-0489

Holohan, C., Van Schaeybroeck, S., Longley, D. B., and Johnston, P. G. (2013). Cancer drug resistance: an evolving paradigm. *Nat. Rev. Cancer* 13, 714–726. doi: 10.1038/nrc3599

Janes, J., Young, M. E., Chen, E., Rogers, N. H., Burgstaller-Muehlbacher, S., Hughes, L. D., et al. (2018). The ReFRAME library as a comprehensive drug repurposing library and its application to the treatment of cryptosporidiosis. *Proc. Natl. Acad. Sci. U.S.A.* 155, 10750–10755. doi: 10.1073/pnas.1810137115

Kashif, M., Andersson, C., Hassan, S., Karlsson, H., Senkowski, W., Fryknäs, M., et al. (2015). *In vitro* discovery of promising anti-cancer drug combinations using iterative maximisation of a therapeutic index. *Sci. Rep.* 5:14118. doi: 10.1038/srep14118

Kischkel, F. C., Eich, J., Meyer, C. I., Weidemüller, P., Krapfl, J., Yassin-Kelepir, R., et al. (2017). New *in vitro* system to predict chemotherapeutic efficacy of drug combinations in fresh tumor samples. *PeerJ* 5:e3030. doi: 10.7717/peerj.3030

Kumar, R., Chaudhary, K., Singla, D., Gautam, A., and Raghava, G. P. (2014). Designing of promiscuous inhibitors against pancreatic cancer cell lines. *Sci. Rep.* 4:4668. doi: 10.1038/srep04668

Kurtz, S. E., Traer, E., Martinez, J., Park, A., Wagner, J., Pandya, R., et al. (2015). Identification of effective targeted drug combinations using functional *ex vivo* screening of primary patient specimens. *Blood* 126:865. Available online at: http://www.bloodjournal.org/content/126/23/865

Kuz'min, V. E., Artemenko, A. G., and Muratov, E. N. (2008). Hierarchical QSAR technology based on the Simplex representation of molecular structure. *J. Comput. Aided. Mol. Des.* 22, 403–421. doi: 10.1007/s10822-008-9179-6

Lamdrum, G. (2015). *RDKit: Open-source Cheminformatics.* Available online at: http://www.rdkit.org/ (accessed April 3, 2015).

Leach, A. R., and Gillet, V. J. (2007). *An Introduction To Chemoinformatics.* Dordrecht: Springer Netherlands.

Li, H., Li, T., Quang, D., and Guan, Y. (2018). Network Propagation Predicts Drug Synergy in Cancers. *Cancer Res.* 78, 5446–5457. doi: 10.1158/0008-5472.CAN-18-0740

Lieu, C. H., Tan, A.-C., Leong, S., Diamond, J. R., and Eckhardt, S. G. (2013). From bench to bedside: lessons learned in translating preclinical studies in cancer drug development. *JNCI J. Natl. Cancer Inst.* 105, 1441–1456. doi: 10.1093/jnci/djt209

Mathea, M., Klingspohn, W., and Baumann, K. (2016). Chemoinformatic classification methods and their applicability domain. *Mol. Inform.* 35, 160–180. doi: 10.1002/minf.201501019

Menden, M. P., Iorio, F., Garnett, M., McDermott, U., Benes, C. H., Ballester, P. J., et al. (2013). Machine learning prediction of cancer cell sensitivity to drugs based on genomic and chemical properties. *PLoS ONE* 8:e61318. doi: 10.1371/journal.pone.0061318

Menden, M. P., Wang, D., Mason, M. J., Szalai, B., Bulusu, K. C., Guan, Y., et al. (2019). Community assessment to advance computational prediction of cancer drug combinations in a pharmacogenomic screen. *Nat. Commun.* 10:2674. doi: 10.1038/s41467-019-09799-2

Mullen, L. M. A., Duchowicz, P. R., and Castro, E. A. (2011). QSAR treatment on a new class of triphenylmethyl-containing compounds as potent anticancer agents. *Chemom. Intell. Lab. Syst.* 107, 269–275. doi: 10.1016/J.CHEMOLAB.2011.04.011

Muratov, E. N., Varlamova, E. V., Artemenko, A. G., Polishchuk, P. G., and Kuz'min, V. E. (2012). Existing and developing approaches for QSAR analysis of mixtures. *Mol. Inform.* 31, 202–221. doi: 10.1002/minf.201100129

Naulaerts, S., Dang, C. C., and Ballester, P. J. (2017). Precision and recall oncology: combining multiple gene mutations for improved identification of drug-sensitive tumours. *Oncotarget* 8:20923. doi: 10.18632/oncotarget.20923

O'Neil, J., Benita, Y., Feldman, I., Chenard, M., Roberts, B., Liu, Y., et al. (2016). An unbiased oncology compound screen to identify novel combination strategies. *Mol. Cancer Ther.* 15, 1155–1162. doi: 10.1158/1535-7163.MCT-15-0843

Pick, A., Müller, H., Mayer, R., Haenisch, B., Pajeva, I. K., Weigt, M., et al. (2011). Structure-activity relationships of flavonoids as inhibitors of breast cancer resistance protein (BCRP). *Bioorg. Med. Chem.* 19, 2090–2102. doi: 10.1016/J.BMC.2010.12.043

Polishchuk, P. G., Madzhidov, T. I., and Varnek, A. (2013). Estimation of the size of drug-like chemical space based on GDB-17 data. *J. Comput. Aided. Mol. Des.* 27, 675–679. doi: 10.1007/s10822-013-9672-4

Preuer, K., Lewis, R. P. I., Hochreiter, S., Bender, A., Bulusu, K. C., and Klambauer, G. (2018). DeepSynergy: predicting anti-cancer drug synergy with deep learning. *Bioinformatics* 34, 1538–1546. doi: 10.1093/bioinformatics/btx806

Rogers, D., and Hahn, M. (2010). Extended-connectivity fingerprints. *J. Chem. Inf. Model.* 50, 742–754. doi: 10.1021/ci100050t

Ruggiu, F., Marcou, G., Solov 'ev, V., Horvath, D., and Varnek, A. (2015). *ISIDA Fragmentor2015—User Manual.*

Sabet, R., Mohammadpour, M., Sadeghi, A., and Fassihi, A. (2010). QSAR study of isatin analogues as *in vitro* anti-cancer agents. *Eur. J. Med. Chem.* 45, 1113–1118. doi: 10.1016/J.EJMECH.2009.12.010

Safikhani, Z., El-Hachem, N., Smirnov, P., Freeman, M., Goldenberg, A., Birkbak, N. J., et al. (2016). Safikhani et al. reply. *Nature* 540, E2–E4. doi: 10.1038/nature19839

Safikhani, Z., Smirnov, P., Freeman, M., El-Hachem, N., She, A., Rene, Q., et al. (2017). Revisiting inconsistency in large pharmacogenomic studies. *F1000Res.* 5:2333. doi: 10.12688/f1000research.9611.3

Sheridan, R. P. (2013). Using random forest to model the domain applicability of another random forest model. *J. Chem. Inf. Model.* 53, 2837–2850. doi: 10.1021/ci400482e

Sheridan, R. P., Wang, W. M., Liaw, A., Ma, J., and Gifford, E. M. (2016). Extreme gradient boosting as a method for quantitative structure–activity relationships. *J. Chem. Inf. Model.* 56, 2353–2360. doi: 10.1021/acs.jcim.6b00591

Shoemaker, R. H. (2006). The NCI60 human tumour cell line anticancer drug screen. *Nat. Rev. Cancer* 6, 813–823. doi: 10.1038/nrc1951

Sidorov, P., Naulaerts, S., Ariey-Bonnet, J., Pasquier, E., and Ballester, P. (2018). Predicting synergism of cancer drug combinations using NCI-ALMANAC data. *bioRxiv* 10:504076. doi: 10.1101/504076

Singh, H., Singh, S., Singla, D., Agarwal, S. M., and Raghava, G. P. (2015). QSAR based model for discriminating EGFR inhibitors and non-inhibitors using Random forest. *Biol. Direct* 10:10. doi: 10.1186/s13062-015-0046-9

Speck-Planche, A., Kleandrova, V. V., Luan, F., and Cordeiro, M. N. (2011). Multi-target drug discovery in anti-cancer therapy: fragment-based approach toward the design of potent and versatile anti-prostate cancer agents. *Bioorg. Med. Chem.* 19, 6239–6244. doi: 10.1016/J.BMC.2011.09.015

Speck-Planche, A., Kleandrova, V. V., Luan, F., and Cordeiro, M. N. (2012). Chemoinformatics in anti-cancer chemotherapy: multi-target QSAR model for the *in silico* discovery of anti-breast cancer agents. *Eur. J. Pharm. Sci.* 47, 273–279. doi: 10.1016/J.EJPS.2012.04.012

Stransky, N., Ghandi, M., Kryukov, G. V., Garraway, L. A., Lehár, J., Liu, M., et al. (2015). Pharmacogenomic agreement between two cancer cell line data sets. *Nature* 528, 84–87. doi: 10.1038/nature15736

Sugahara, K. N., Teesalu, T., Karmali, P. P., Kotamraju, V. R., Agemy, L., Greenwald, D. R., et al. (2010). Coadministration of a tumor-penetrating peptide enhances the efficacy of cancer drugs. *Science* 328, 1031–1035. doi: 10.1126/science.1183057

Svetnik, V., Liaw, A., Tong, C., Culberson, J. C., Sheridan, R. P., and Feuston, B. P. (2003). Random forest: a classification and regression tool for compound classification and QSAR modeling. *J. Chem. Inf. Comput. Sci.* 43, 1947–1958. doi: 10.1021/ci034160g

Todeschini, R., and Consonni, V. (2000). *Handbook of Molecular Descriptors.* Weinheim: Wiley-VCH Verlag GmbH.

Tropsha, A., Gramatica, P., and Gombar, V. (2003). The importance of being earnest: validation is the absolute essential for successful application and interpretation of QSPR models. *QSAR Comb. Sci.* 22, 69–77. doi: 10.1002/qsar.200390007

Varnek, A., Fourches, D., Hoonakker, F., and Solov'ev, V. P. (2005). Substructural fragments: an universal language to encode reactions, molecular and supramolecular structures. *J. Comput. Aided. Mol. Des.* 19, 693–703. doi: 10.1007/s10822-005-9008-0

Xia, F., Shukla, M., Brettin, T., Garcia-Cardona, C., Cohn, J., Allen, J. E., et al. (2018). Predicting tumor cell line response to drug pairs with deep learning. *BMC Bioinformatics* 19:3. doi: 10.1186/s12859-018-2509-3

Yu, D., Kahen, E., Cubitt, C. L., McGuire, J., Kreahling, J., Lee, J., et al. (2015). Identification of synergistic, clinically achievable, combination therapies for osteosarcoma. *Sci. Rep.* 5:16991. doi: 10.1038/srep16991

Zoli, W., Ricotti, L., Tesei, A., Barzanti, F., and Amadori, D. (2001). *In vitro* preclinical models for a rational design of chemotherapy combinations in human tumors. *Crit. Rev. Oncol. Hematol.* 37, 69–82. doi: 10.1016/S1040-8428(00)00110-4

2

ChEMBL-Likeness Score and Database GDBChEMBL

*Sven Bühlmann and Jean-Louis Reymond**

Department of Chemistry and Biochemistry, University of Bern, Bern, Switzerland

Correspondence:
Jean-Louis Reymond
jean-louis.reymond@dcb.unibe.ch

The generated database GDB17 enumerates 166.4 billion molecules up to 17 atoms of C, N, O, S and halogens following simple rules of chemical stability and synthetic feasibility. However, most molecules in GDB17 are too complex to be considered for chemical synthesis. To address this limitation, we report GDBChEMBL as a subset of GDB17 featuring 10 million molecules selected according to a ChEMBL-likeness score (CLscore) calculated from the frequency of occurrence of circular substructures in ChEMBL, followed by uniform sampling across molecular size, stereocenters and heteroatoms. Compared to the previously reported subsets FDB17 and GDBMedChem selected from GDB17 by fragment-likeness, respectively, medicinal chemistry criteria, our new subset features molecules with higher synthetic accessibility and possibly bioactivity yet retains a broad and continuous coverage of chemical space typical of the entire GDB17. GDBChEMBL is accessible at http://gdb.unibe.ch for download and for browsing using an interactive chemical space map at http://faerun.gdb.tools.

Keywords: chemical space exploration, molecular database, enumeration algorithm, chemical space mapping, virtual screening

INTRODUCTION

Innovation at the level of chemical structures is an essential part of drug discovery. Novelty often results from chemical intuition however this approach is increasingly difficult as the number of known molecules increases. Novelty is similarly limited in virtual combinatorial libraries (Leach and Hann, 2000; Hu et al., 2011; van Hilten et al., 2019) and generative models trained with known molecules (Chen et al., 2018; Elton et al., 2019) because these systems mostly shuffle known patterns, which produces many technically new but often not fundamentally innovative molecules. To circumvent this limitation, we have initiated the exhaustive enumeration of all possible organic molecules following simple rules of chemical stability and synthetic feasibility, and reported large databases enumerating molecules up to 11 (Fink et al., 2005; Fink and Reymond, 2007), 13 (Blum and Reymond, 2009), and 17 atoms (Ruddigkeit et al., 2012, 2013), as well as of possible ring systems up to 30 atoms (Visini et al., 2017a). Analyzing the resulting generated databases (GDBs) shows that there are many orders of magnitude more possible molecules spanning a much broader structural diversity than already known ones (Reymond, 2015; Awale et al., 2017b).

One of the defining features of the GDB databases is the exponential increase in the number of possible molecules as function of increasing molecular size and complexity elements, such as stereocenters and heteroatoms, implying that most possible molecules are in fact far too complex to be considered as realistic synthetic targets. To address this problem we have designed subsets of our largest database GDB17 by limiting complexity elements using simplification criteria, such as fragment-likeness (Congreve et al., 2003), producing the fragment database FDB17, and medicinal chemistry rules for functional groups and complexity (Mignani et al., 2018), producing the medicinal chemistry aware database GDBMedChem (Visini et al., 2017b; Awale et al., 2019). These approaches however also constrain the diversity of GDB molecules, which partly defeats the purpose of exploring chemical space broadly.

Herein we report an alternative approach to create subsets of GDB17 based on the frequency of occurrence of substructures from known molecules independent of the overall molecular structure (**Figure 1A**). We define a "ChEMBL-likeness" score (CLscore) by considering which substructures in a molecule also occur in molecules from the public database ChEMBL (Gaulton et al., 2017), using a subset of molecules with reported high confidence datapoint of activity on single protein targets, a type of ChEMBL subset which we have used previously for target prediction (Awale and Reymond, 2019; Poirier et al., 2019). We then filter the entire GDB17 with a cut-off value for CLscore, followed by uniform sampling of the resulting subset across molecular size, stereocenters and heteroatoms as done previously with FDB17 and GDBMedChem, to obtain a ChEMBL-like subset of 10 million molecules forming the database GDBChEMBL. This database covers chemical space as broadly as but more continuously than FDB17 and GDBMedChem yet features a much higher synthetic accessibility as judged by a calculated synthetic accessibility score (Ertl and Schuffenhauer, 2009), might contain molecules with a higher probability of bioactivity, and in any case provides a very different starting point to serve as a source of inspiration for molecular design.

RESULTS AND DISCUSSION

ChEMBL-Likeness Score

Our definition of CLscore is related to the synthetic accessibility score (SAscore) (Ertl and Schuffenhauer, 2009) and natural product likeness score (NPscore) (Jayaseelan et al., 2012) of a molecule, which are calculated from the occurrence frequencies of its substructures in PubChem and fragments from natural products, respectively, combined with additional functional group rules. Here we focus on 457,139 compounds recorded in ChEMBL24 as being active on single protein targets (IC_{50} or $EC_{50} \leq 10\,\mu M$) with high confidence datapoints (Awale and Reymond, 2019; Poirier et al., 2019). To design our CLscore we consider circular substructures, called molecular shingles, because they form the basis for molecular fingerprints ECFP4 and MHFP6 which perform best in benchmarking studies (Riniker and Landrum, 2013; Probst and Reymond, 2018).

The frequency of occurrence of the 636,979 molecular shingles up to a diameter of six bonds found in our ChEMBL subset follows a power law distribution (**Figure 1C**). To compute the CLscore of a molecule, we assign to each of its shingles (S) a shingle value calculated from the logarithm of its frequency of occurrence f_S in our ChEMBL subset, considering only shingles occurring at least 100 times in this subset (141,261 shingles, 22.2% of the total). We then sum all shingle values and divide the sum by the total number of shingles in the molecule (Equation 1).

$$\mathrm{CLscore} = \frac{\sum_{i=1}^{m} \log_{10}(f_S)_i}{N} \quad \left|\; \begin{array}{l} \mathrm{CLscore} := \mathrm{ChEMBL-likeness\ score} \\ S := \mathrm{shingle in molecular\ structure} \\ f_S := \mathrm{abundance of molecular shingle in\ ChEMBL} \\ N := \mathrm{total number of shingles in molecular\ structure} \\ m := \mathrm{number of shingles shared with\ ChEMBL} \end{array} \right.$$

The histogram of CLscore for the 457,139 ChEMBL reference molecules is approximately Gaussian with a peak at CLscore = 3.9 (**Figure 1B**). DrugBank (Law et al., 2014) and particularly ZINC (Sterling and Irwin, 2015) peak at a similar CLscore, showing that these three databases consist of molecules built from the same type of substructures. By contrast GDB17 and its subsets FDB17 and GDBMedChem have a much lower CLscore distribution peaking at CLscore = 2.7, reflecting the fact that GDB molecules are very different from ChEMBL molecules. CLscore values correlate with SAscore values, reflecting the similar principles underlying both scores, and suggesting that molecules with high CLscore should also be synthetically accessible (**Figure 1D**).

GDBChEMBL Database

Calculating CLscores on the entire GDB17 (166.4 billion SMILES) and keeping molecules with CLscore $\geq$ 3.3, a cut-off value which retains 78.3% of our ChEMBL subset, eliminates 84.3% of GDB17. The remaining 26.2 billion molecules are then binned in triplet value bins considering heavy atom count (HAC 1-17), stereocenter count (0–4, $\geq$ 5) and heteroatom count (0–8, $\geq$ 8). There are 538 different triplet value bins, which are occupied by 1 to 1.6×10^9 molecules. Uniform sampling finally yields a final set of 10 million molecules evenly distributed across molecular size, stereochemical complexity and polarity, forming the database GDBChEMBL (**Figure 1E**).

As a consequence of uniform sampling, the heavy atom count (HAC) profile of GDBChEMBL resembles that of FDB17 and GDBMedChem and is relatively flat compared to the very steep peak at HAC = 17 in the parent database GDB17 (**Figure 2A**). Uniform sampling also explains the rotatable bond count (RBC) profile in GDB subsets compared to GDB17 (**Figure 2B**), as well as the fact that the profiles of the three GDB subsets across these parameters are generally more similar to the profile of molecules up to 17 atoms in ChEMBL (ChEMBL17) and to natural products (UNPD17) (Banerjee et al., 2015) than to the profile of GDB17.

GDBChEMBL displays a very broad distribution in terms of hydrogen bond donor atoms (HBD, **Figure 2C**), hydrogen bond acceptor atoms (HBA, **Figure 2D**) and nitrogen plus oxygen atom count (N+O, **Figure 2E**) due to the absence of heteroatom capping criteria in selecting GDBChEMBL compared to FDB17 and GDBMedChem, for which fragment-likeness criteria, respectively, caps on the number of functional groups were applied. Similar differences are visible in topological polar surface area (TPSA, **Figure 2F**) and calculated octanol/water partition coefficient (alogP, **Figure 2G**). The broader distribution of polarity parameters in GDGChEMBL compared to GDB17 results from uniform sampling since the procedure gives relatively more importance to molecules with extreme size and polarity values.

Synthetic accessibility is better (lower SAscore) in GDBChEMBL than for GDB17, FDB17, or GDBMedChem,

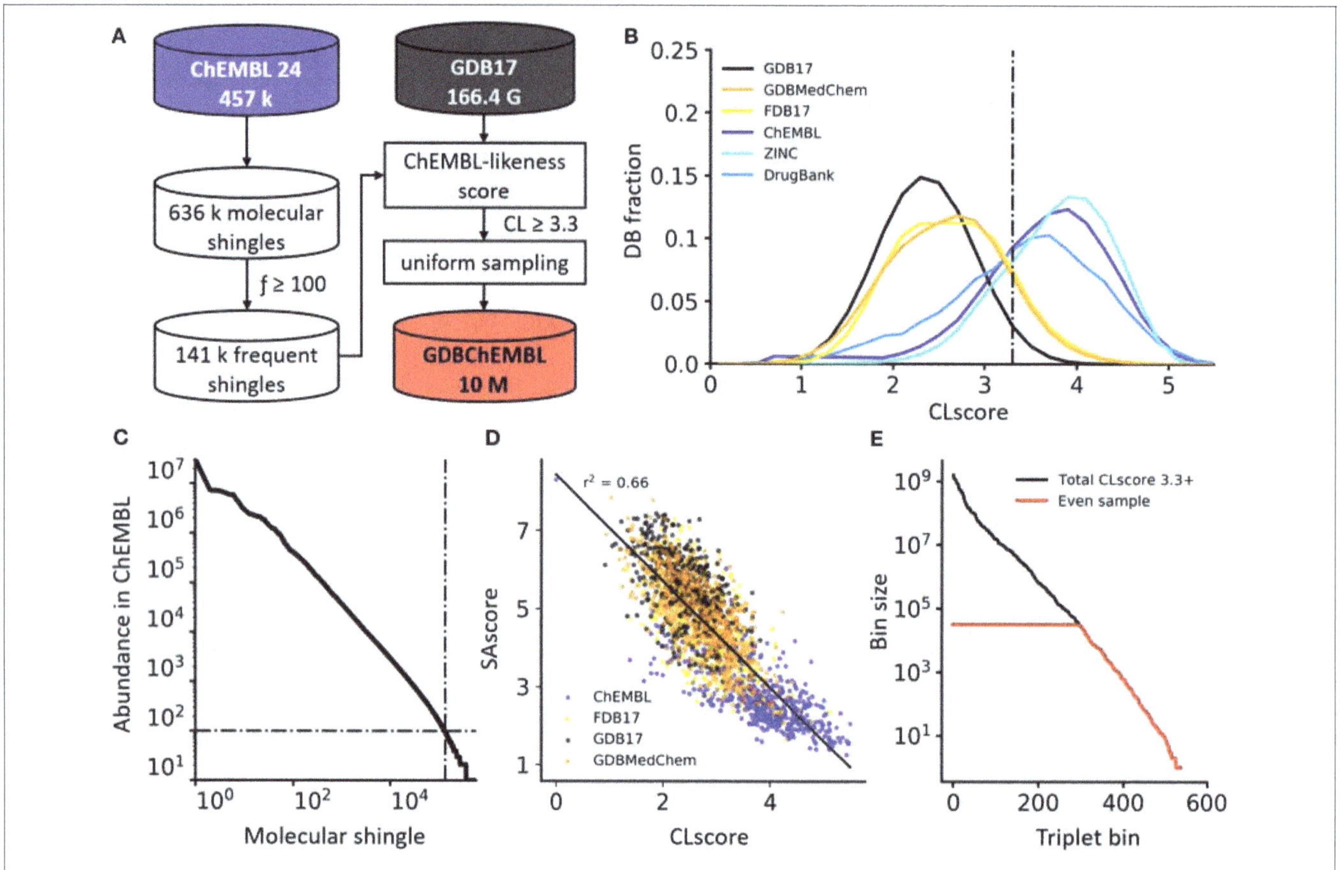

FIGURE 1 | (A) Generation process of GDBChEMBL. **(B)** CLscore distributions for GDB17, its subsets FDB17 and GDBMedChem, and public databases ChEMBL, ZINC, and DrugBank. **(C)** Frequency distribution of molecular shingles up to a diameter of 6 bonds in ChEMBL. **(D)** SAscore vs. CLscore in various databases. A lower SAscore indicates higher synthetic accessibility, and a higher CLscore indicates higher similarity to ChEMBL molecules. **(E)** Occupancy of triplet value bins (HAC, stereocenters, heteroatoms) in all GDB17 cpds with CLscore ≥3.3 (black line) and after uniform sampling forming GDBChEMBL (red line).

reflecting the correlation between CLscore and SAscore noted above (**Figure 2H**). Similar to GDB17 and its other subsets, GDBChEMBL displays a much higher fraction of sp^3 atoms than ChEMBL (fsp^3, **Figure 2I**). As a consequence GDB molecules are closer to natural products, which is reflected in the NPscore profile (**Figure 2J**). Despite of these differences and similarities in SAscore and NPscore, it must be noted that GDB17 and its subsets stand out by the fact that they contain fewer aromatic and more heterocyclic molecules than ChEMBL and natural products (**Figure 2K**).

Visualization and Similarity Searching

To gain an overview of GDBChEMBL we computed Molecular Quantum Number (MQN) fingerprint values (Nguyen et al., 2009), performed a principal component analysis (Rosén et al., 2009), and visualized the resulting 3D-map in the interactive web-based application faerun (Probst et al., 2018). In this 3D-map accessible at http://faerun.gdb.tools, each point represents one or more molecules present at the corresponding position and can be color-coded according to a molecular property selected from the faerun menu.

Comparing MQN maps of GDBChEMBL, FDB17 and GDBMedChem shows that each of the three GDB17 subset cover a similar range of properties, however coverage by GDBChEMBL is more continuous, as is well visible in the vertical stripe at right containing all acyclic molecules (**Figures 3A–C**). Note that CLscore values are not correlated with MQN properties, which is not surprising considering that ChEMBL substructure span a broad range of properties (**Figure 3D**). Color-coding by the calculated logP value (alogP, **Figure 3E**) and by rotatable bond count (RBC, **Figure 3F**) illustrate the distribution of molecules in the MQN map.

The fact that molecules in GDBChEMBL are substantially different from those in the other subsets FDB17 and GDBMedChem can be shown by retrieving 1,000 MQN-nearest neighbors of nicotine from each database, and representing each dataset in a similarity map (Medina-Franco et al., 2007; Raghavendra and Maggiora, 2007; Awale and Reymond, 2015) using the molecular shape and pharmacophore fingerprint Xfp (Awale and Reymond, 2014), computed with the web-based application WebMolCS (Awale et al., 2017a). This visualization shows that each database provides different types of nicotine analogs (**Figure 3G**) with a good number of high

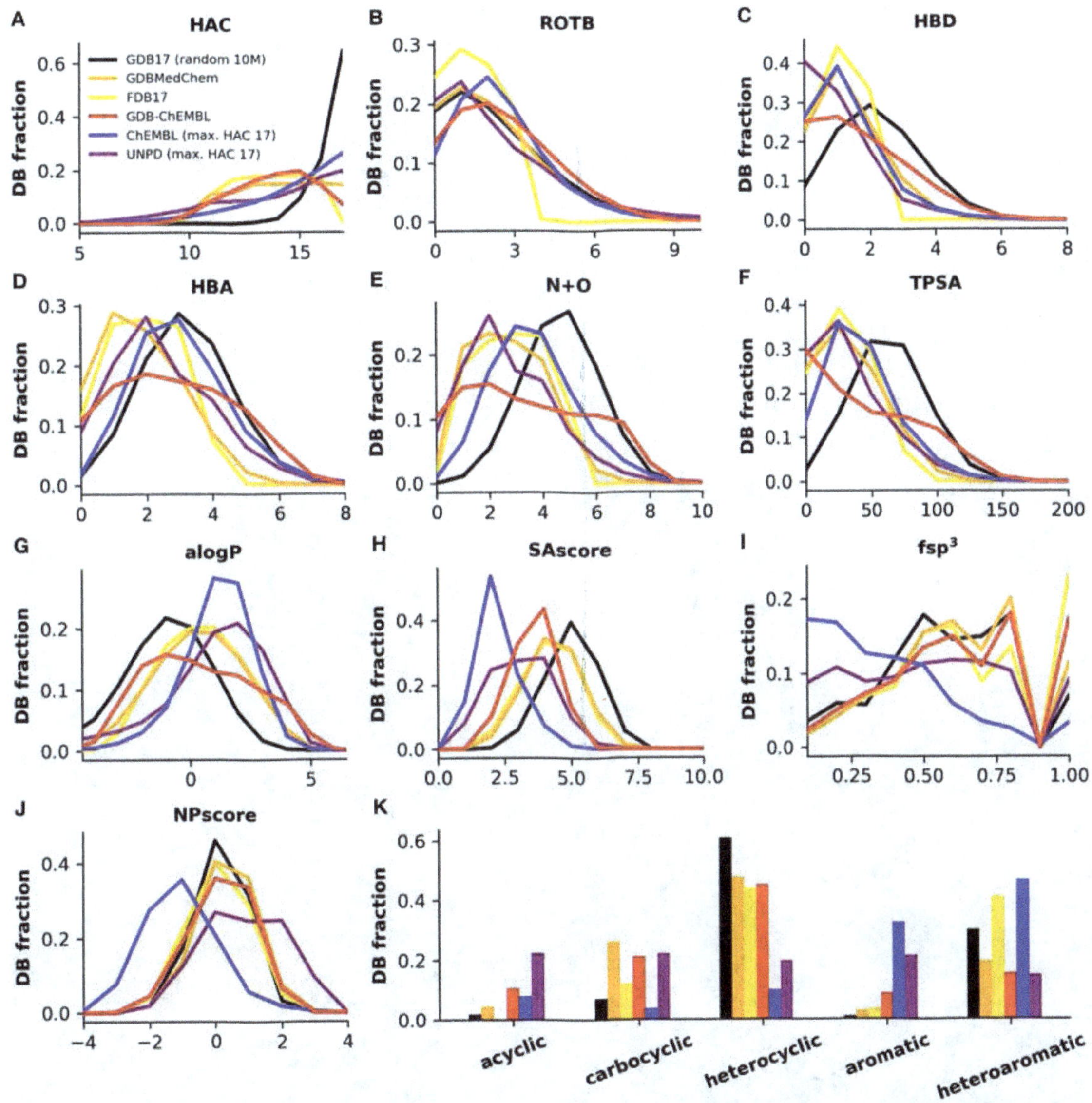

FIGURE 2 | (A) Heavy atom count (HAC), **(B)** rotatable bonds (ROTB), **(C)** hydrogen bond donors (HBD), **(D)** hydrogen bond acceptors (HBA), **(E)** nitrogen plus oxygen count (N+O), **(F)** topological polar surface area (TPSA), **(G)** computed partition coefficient (aLogP), **(H)** synthetic accessibility score (SAscore), **(I)** Fraction of sp^3 hybridized atoms (fsp^3), **(J)** natural product likeness score (NPscore), and **(K)** fraction of structures by ring class. Property histograms for GDB17 (black), GDBMedChem (orange), FDB17 (yellow), GDBChEMBL (red), ChEMBL (cpds with HAC $\leq$ 17, blue) and natural products (cpds with HAC $\leq$ 17, purple).

similarity analogs (**Figure 3H**). To facilitate similarity searches in GDBChEMBL, we have implemented a similarity search portal by which nearest neighbor searches of any molecule can be performed in GDBChEMBL using MQN, ECFP4, or a combined MQN-MHFP6 similarity, as described previously for GDBMedChem (Awale et al., 2019).

CONCLUSION

The data above demonstrate a substructure-based approach to select molecules from the generated database GDB17. As selection criterion we defined a ChEMBL-likeness score (CLscore) from the frequency occurrence of circular substructures, called molecular shingles, in a subset of the database ChEMBL consisting of compounds active on single protein targets with high confidence datapoints. This selection reduced GDB17 by 84.3%, leaving 26.2 billion molecules, which we sampled uniformly across molecular size, stereochemistry and heteroatoms to form GDBChEMBL comprising 10 million molecules.

Property profiles, chemical space maps and similarity searches show that GDBChEMBL is very different from our earlier GDB subsets FDB17 and GDBMedChem and spans chemical space more continuously. At the same time, the correlation between CLscore and the synthetic accessibility score (SAscore) implies that GDBChEMBL molecules will be on average easier

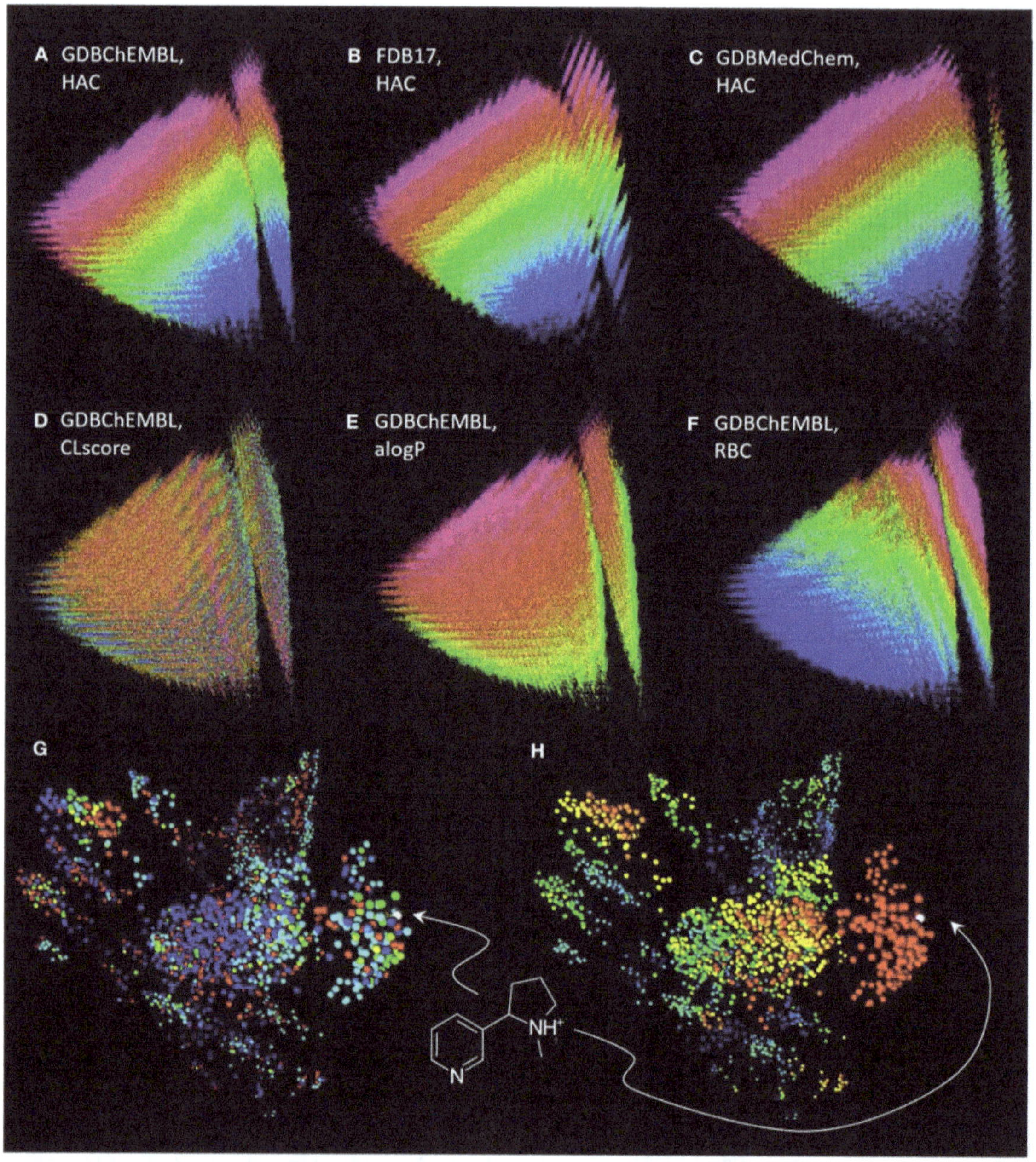

FIGURE 3 | Chemical space maps of GDBChEMBL, FDB17, and GDBMedChem. **(A)** PCA 3D-map of GDBChEMBL in MQN-space, color coded by heavy atom count; **(B)** same as a for FDB17; **(C)** same as a for GDBMedChem; **(D)** GDBChEMBL color-coded by CLscore value; **(E)** GDBChEMBL color-coded by calculated octanol/water partition coefficient alogP; **(F)** GDBChEMBL color-coded by rotatable bond count; **(G)** similarity map of MQN-nearest neighbors of nicotine from GDBChEMBL (red), FDB17 (cyan), and GDBMedChem (blue). Points in green and yellow indicate molecules shared by two databases. **(H)** Same as g color-coded by Xfp-similarity to nicotine. MQN maps a to f are accessible at http://faerun.gdb.tools. The similarity map of nicotine analogs g and h is accessible at: http://gdbtools.unibe.ch:8080/webMolCS/.

to synthesize than molecules from FDB17 and GDBMedChem, which have significantly lower CLscore and higher SAscores. We anticipate that the requirements for GDBChEMBL molecules to share a minimum number of substructures with molecules of known bioactivities from ChEMBL will also facilitate target prediction and the selection of interesting GDB molecules for synthesis and testing.

METHODS

Preparative Steps

ChEMBL Shingle Extraction

The ChEMBL (v 24.1) database was downloaded from https://www.ebi.ac.uk/chembl/. Data points for extraction of molecular shingles were selected by applying the same restrictions that were used for extraction of training data for our Polypharmacology Browser PPB2 (Visini et al., 2017b). Structures were normalized to their major protonation state at pH 7.4 using ChemAxon cxcalc (v. 18.23.0). Molecular shingles for radii 1–3 were created using RDkit (2019.03.4) and converted to rooted, canonical, aromatic SMILES strings without retaining stereochemistry information. In association with abundancy in the ChEMBL, the SMILES substructures were stored as pickled python dictionary. Molecular substructures that were found <100 times were not stored.

CLscore Calculation

Scoring of GDB17 molecular structures was achieved by decomposition to molecular shingles in the exact same way as described for ChEMBL reference shingle extraction. For a specific query structure, all shingles are uniquely counted, then looked up in the ChEMBL reference database and upon match, logarithmic abundancy is summed up. The final CLscore is given by the ratio of total logarithmic abundancies of matched unique shingles to total unique shingles in the query structure. All respective scripts are accessible at: https://github.com/reymond-group/GDBChEMBL.

GDBChEMBL Generation

All 166.4 billion molecular structures of GDB17 were decomposed to unique substructures in the same way as described for ChEMBL reference molecules. Only structures with CLscore ≥3.3 were stored. The final GDBChEMBL was obtained by distribution of all filtered 26.2 billion structures to 538 property triplet bins (heavy atom, heteroatom and stereocenter count). Property information was gathered using RDKit. Bins with 5+ hetero atoms and/or 8+ chiral atoms were merged. The actual even sampling was performed by sorting all property bins by size and defining target structure count as 10 million. Iteratively, remaining target count was divided by count of remaining bins, keeping all bins of size smaller than the current number to sample randomly. For each step, number of previously selected structures was subtracted from target count until random sample per remaining bins was lower than bin size. At this point, sample size was kept constant for all further bins.

Visualizing GDBChEMBL in Faerun

Property color coded 3D maps for GDBChEMBL, FDB17, and GDBMedChem were generated using FUn (doc.gdb.tools/fun), an in-house developed framework for interactive visualization of chemical spaces on the web. Datasets were given as plain text, consisting of the four columns (space-separated): SMILES-string, numeric ID, 42 MQN descriptors (semicolon-separated) and further molecular properties used for map coloring (semicolon-separated). Next, the preprocessing toolchain was used to project the 42-dimensional MQN-space to 3D by applying Principal Component Analysis (PCA) and to generate all further files needed for visualization. Finally, the Underdark server was run using docker with Faerun visualization containers mapped.

Similarity Searching in GDBChEMBL

For better accessibility, GDBChEMBL is provided as a web-based interactive similarity search tool. The implementation uses HTML, Bootstrap, JavaScript, and the python Flask framework. Search times were reduced using Annoy trees (Approximate Nearest Neighbors Oh Yeah, https://github.com/spotify/annoy) which were created for the 42-dimensional MQN property space, as well as for 256-bit ECfp4. A third search option, MQN-MHFP6, initially searches using the MQN Annoy tree followed by resorting after Jaccard distance to query molecule in the MHFP6 fingerprint space (https://github.com/reymond-group/mhfp). The search tool is available at: gdb.unibe.ch/tools.

AUTHOR CONTRIBUTIONS

SB designed and realized the study and wrote the paper. J-LR designed and supervised the study and wrote the paper.

FUNDING

This work was supported financially by the Swiss National Science Foundation.

REFERENCES

Awale, M., Probst, D., and Reymond, J. L. (2017a). WebMolCS: a web-based interface for visualizing molecules in three-dimensional chemical spaces. *J. Chem. Inf. Model.* 57, 643–649. doi: 10.1021/acs.jcim.6b00690

Awale, M., and Reymond, J.-L. (2019). Polypharmacology browser PPB2: target prediction combining nearest neighbors with machine learning. *J. Chem. Inf. Model.* 59, 10–17. doi: 10.1021/acs.jcim.8b00524

Awale, M., and Reymond, J. L. (2014). Atom pair 2D-fingerprints perceive 3D-molecular shape and pharmacophores for very fast virtual screening of ZINC and GDB-17. *J. Chem. Inf. Model.* 54, 1892–1897. doi: 10.1021/ci500232g

Awale, M., and Reymond, J. L. (2015). Similarity mapplet: interactive visualization of the directory of useful decoys and ChEMBL in high dimensional chemical spaces. *J. Chem. Inf. Model.* 55, 1509–1516. doi: 10.1021/acs.jcim.5b00182

Awale, M., Sirockin, F., Stiefl, N., and Reymond, J.-L. (2019). Medicinal chemistry aware database GDBMedChem. *Mol. Informatics* 38:1900031. doi: 10.1002/minf.201900031

Awale, M., Visini, R., Probst, D., Arus-Pous, J., and Reymond, J. L. (2017b). Chemical space: big data challenge for molecular diversity. *Chimia* 71, 661–666. doi: 10.2533/chimia.2017.661

Banerjee, P., Erehman, J., Gohlke, B.-O., Wilhelm, T., Preissner, R., and Dunkel, M. (2015). Super natural II—a database of natural products. *Nucleic Acids Res.* 43, D935–D939. doi: 10.1093/nar/gku886

Blum, L. C., and Reymond, J. L. (2009). 970 Million druglike small molecules for virtual screening in the chemical universe database GDB-13. *J. Am. Chem. Soc.* 131, 8732–8733. doi: 10.1021/ja902302h

Chen, H., Engkvist, O., Wang, Y., Olivecrona, M., and Blaschke, T. (2018). The rise of deep learning in drug discovery. *Drug Discovery Today* 23, 1241–1250. doi: 10.1016/j.drudis.2018.01.039

Congreve, M., Carr, R., Murray, C., and Jhoti, H. (2003). A rule of three for fragment-based lead discovery? *Drug Discovery Today* 8, 876–877. doi: 10.1016/S1359-6446(03)02831-9

Elton, D. C., Boukouvalas, Z., Fuge, M. D., and Chung, P. W. (2019). Deep learning for molecular design—a review of the state of the art. *Mol. Syst. Des. Eng.* 4, 828–849. doi: 10.1039/C9ME00039A

Ertl, P., and Schuffenhauer, A. (2009). Estimation of synthetic accessibility score of drug-like molecules based on molecular complexity and fragment contributions. *J. Cheminf.* 1:8. doi: 10.1186/1758-2946-1-8

Fink, T., Bruggesser, H., and Reymond, J. L. (2005). Virtual exploration of the small-molecule chemical universe below 160 daltons. *Angew. Chem. Int. Ed. Engl.* 44, 1504–1508. doi: 10.1002/anie.200462457

Fink, T., and Reymond, J. L. (2007). Virtual exploration of the chemical universe up to 11 atoms of C, N, O, F: assembly of 26.4 million structures (110.9 million stereoisomers) and analysis for new ring systems, stereochemistry, physicochemical properties, compound classes, and drug discovery. *J. Chem. Inf. Model.* 47, 342–353. doi: 10.1021/ci600423u

Gaulton, A., Hersey, A., Nowotka, M., Bento, A. P., Chambers, J., Mendez, D., et al. (2017). The ChEMBL database in 2017. *Nucleic Acids Res.* 45, D945–D954. doi: 10.1093/nar/gkw1074

Hu, Q., Peng, Z., Kostrowicki, J., and Kuki, A. (2011). LEAP into the Pfizer Global Virtual Library (PGVL) space: creation of readily synthesizable design ideas automatically. *Methods Mol. Biol.* 685, 253–276. doi: 10.1007/978-1-60761-931-4_13

Jayaseelan, K. V., Moreno, P., Truszkowski, A., Ertl, P., and Steinbeck, C. (2012). Natural product-likeness score revisited: an open-source, open-data implementation. *BMC Bioinformatics* 13:106. doi: 10.1186/1471-2105-13-106

Law, V., Knox, C., Djoumbou, Y., Jewison, T., Guo, A. C., Liu, Y., et al. (2014). DrugBank 4.0: shedding new light on drug metabolism. *Nucleic Acids Res.* 42, D1091–D1097. doi: 10.1093/nar/gkt1068

Leach, A. R., and Hann, M. M. (2000). The *in silico* world of virtual libraries. *Drug Discov. Today* 5, 326–336. doi: 10.1016/S1359-6446(00)01516-6

Medina-Franco, J. L., Maggiora, G. M., Giulianotti, M. A., Pinilla, C., and Houghten, R. A. (2007). A similarity-based data-fusion approach to the visual characterization and comparison of compound databases. *Chem. Biol. Drug Des.* 70, 393–412. doi: 10.1111/j.1747-0285.2007.00579.x

Mignani, S., Rodrigues, J., Tomas, H., Jalal, R., Singh, P. P., Majoral, J.-P., et al. (2018). Present drug-likeness filters in medicinal chemistry during the hit and lead optimization process: how far can they be simplified? *Drug Discovery Today* 23, 605–615. doi: 10.1016/j.drudis.2018.01.010

Nguyen, K. T., Blum, L. C., van Deursen, R., and Reymond, J.-L. (2009). Classification of organic molecules by molecular quantum numbers. *ChemMedChem* 4, 1803–1805. doi: 10.1002/cmdc.2009 00317

Poirier, M., Awale, M., Roelli, M. A., Giuffredi, G. T., Ruddigkeit, L., Evensen, L., et al. (2019). Identifying lysophosphatidic acid acyltransferase β (LPAAT-β) as the target of a nanomolar angiogenesis inhibitor from a phenotypic screen using the polypharmacology browser PPB2. *ChemMedChem* 14, 224–236. doi: 10.1002/cmdc.201800554

Probst, D., and Reymond, J.-L. (2018). A probabilistic molecular fingerprint for big data settings. *J. Cheminf.* 10:66. doi: 10.1186/s13321-018-0321-8

Probst, D., Reymond, J.-L., and Wren, J. (2018). FUn: a framework for interactive visualizations of large, high-dimensional datasets on the web. *Bioinformatics* 34, 1433–1435. doi: 10.1093/bioinformatics/btx760

Raghavendra, A. S., and Maggiora, G. M. (2007). Molecular basis sets - a general similarity-based approach for representing chemical spaces. *J. Chem. Inf. Model.* 47, 1328–1240. doi: 10.1021/ci600552n

Reymond, J.-L. (2015). The chemical space project. *Acc. Chem. Res.* 48, 722–730. doi: 10.1021/ar500432k

Riniker, S., and Landrum, G. A. (2013). Open-source platform to benchmark fingerprints for ligand-based virtual screening. *J. Cheminf.* 5:26. doi: 10.1186/1758-2946-5-26

Rosén, J., Gottfries, J., Muresan, S., Backlund, A., and Oprea, T. I. (2009). Novel chemical space exploration via natural products. *J. Med. Chem.* 52, 1953–1962. doi: 10.1021/jm801514w

Ruddigkeit, L., Blum, L. C., and Reymond, J. L. (2013). Visualization and virtual screening of the chemical universe database GDB-17. *J. Chem. Inf. Model.* 53, 56–65. doi: 10.1021/ci300535x

Ruddigkeit, L.;, van Deursen, R., Blum, L. C., and Reymond, J. L. (2012). Enumeration of 166 billion organic small molecules in the chemical universe database GDB-17. *J. Chem. Inf. Model.* 52, 2864–2875. doi: 10.1021/ci300415d

Sterling, T., and Irwin, J. J. (2015). ZINC 15 – ligand discovery for everyone. *J. Chem. Inform. Model.* 55, 2324–2337. doi: 10.1021/acs.jcim.5b00559

van Hilten, N., Chevillard, F., and Kolb, P. (2019). Virtual compound libraries in computer-assisted drug discovery. *J. Chem. Inf. Model.* 59, 644–651. doi: 10.1021/acs.jcim.8b00737

Visini, R., Arus-Pous, J., Awale, M., and Reymond, J. L. (2017a). Virtual exploration of the ring systems chemical universe. *J. Chem. Inf. Model.* 57, 2707–2718. doi: 10.1021/acs.jcim.7b00457

Visini, R., Awale, M., and Reymond, J. L. (2017b). Fragment database FDB-17. *J. Chem. Inf. Model.* 57, 700–709. doi: 10.1021/acs.jcim.7b00020

3

In silico Guided Drug Repurposing: Discovery of New Competitive and Non-competitive Inhibitors of Falcipain-2

Lucas N. Alberca[1], *Sara R. Chuguransky*[1], *Cora L. Álvarez*[2], *Alan Talevi*[1*] and *Emir Salas-Sarduy*[3]

[1] *Laboratory of Bioactive Compounds Research and Development (LIDeB), Department of Biological Sciences, Exact Sciences College, Universidad Nacional de La Plata, La Plata, Argentina,* [2] *Departamento de Biodiversidad y Biología Experimental, Facultad de Farmacia y Bioquímica, Facultad de Ciencias Exactas y Naturales, Consejo Nacional de Investigaciones Científicas y Técnicas, Instituto de Química y Fisico-Química Biológicas (IQUIFIB) "Prof. Alejandro C. Paladini", Universidad de Buenos Aires, Buenos Aires, Argentina,* [3] *Instituto de Investigaciones Biotecnológicas "Dr. Rodolfo Ugalde", Universidad Nacional de San Martín, CONICET, Buenos Aires, Argentina*

Correspondence:
Alan Talevi
alantalevi@gmail.com

Malaria is among the leading causes of death worldwide. The emergence of *Plasmodium falciparum* resistant strains with reduced sensitivity to the first line combination therapy and suboptimal responses to insecticides used for Anopheles vector management have led to renewed interest in novel therapeutic options. Here, we report the development and validation of an ensemble of ligand-based computational models capable of identifying falcipain-2 inhibitors, and their subsequent application in the virtual screening of DrugBank and Sweetlead libraries. Among four hits submitted to enzymatic assays, two (odanacatib, an abandoned investigational treatment for osteoporosis and bone metastasis, and the antibiotic methacycline) confirmed inhibitory effects on falcipain-2, with Ki of 98.2 nM and 84.4 μM. Interestingly, Methacycline proved to be a non-competitive inhibitor ($\alpha = 1.42$) of falcipain-2. The effects of both hits on falcipain-2 hemoglobinase activity and on the development of *P. falciparum* were also studied.

Keywords: malaria, *Plasmodium falciparum*, falcipain-2, drug repositioning, virtual screening, drug rescue, odanacatib, methacycline

INTRODUCTION

Despite decades of successful interventions aimed at reducing its incidence and mortality, malaria continues being one of global leading causes of death, being the main global cause globally in the 5- to 14-year-old population and the third cause among children below five (World Health Organization (WHO), 2017; Ritchie and Roser, 2018). The most recent estimates from the World Health Organization (WHO) report around 216 million cases and 445,000 related deaths worldwide in 2016 (Ritchie and Roser, 2018). The emergence of *Plasmodium falciparum* drug-resistant strains with reduced sensitivity to the first line artemisinin combination therapy and suboptimal response to insecticides used for vector management pose a threat to control interventions (Satimai et al., 2012; Ajayi and Ukwaja, 2013; Kisinza et al., 2017). Accordingly, novel therapeutic options are urgently required.

Falcipains are *P. falciparum* cysteine proteases involved in different processes of the erythrocytic cycle of the parasite, including hydrolysis of host hemoglobin and erythrocyte invasion and rupture. Four falcipains have so far been identified, with falcipain-2 and falcipain-3 constituting promising targets in the search for novel therapies due to their significant hemoglobinase capacity (Marco and Coterón, 2012; Bekono et al., 2018).

Drug repurposing involves finding novel medical uses for existing drugs, including approved, investigational, discontinued, and shelved therapeutics. Repurposing a drug has several advantages in comparison to *de novo* drug discovery, since the new therapeutic indication is built on already available pharmacokinetic, toxicological, and manufacturing data, thus leading to therapeutic solutions in a expedite manner (Ferreira and Andricopulo, 2016; Corsello et al., 2017). While the best-known examples of successful repurposing have been serendipitous or arose from intelligent exploitation of side effects (Corsello et al., 2017; Talevi, 2018), the drug discovery community has recently focused on systematic, large-scale repurposing efforts, including the use of genomic tools, and *in silico* and *high-throughput* screening (Jin and Wong, 2015; Talevi, 2018; Yella et al., 2018). The Virtual lock-and-key approach (Lauria et al., 2011, 2014; Tutone et al., 2017) and the BIOlogical Target Assignation method (Lauria et al., 2014) can be mentioned among many other interesting examples of the use of computational resources to deepen the rational basis of drug repurposing programs.

Here, we have implemented a computer-aided drug repurposing campaign to discover new inhibitors of falcipain-2. Four hits were acquired and tested against the enzyme, with two of them confirming inhibitory activity. The abandoned drug odanacatib displayed competitive inhibition, while the antibiotic methacycline also showed inhibitory effects through non-competitive inhibition.

MATERIALS AND METHODS

Dataset Collection

P. falciparum falcipain-2 inhibitors were compiled from literature. A total of 515 compounds previously assayed against falcipain-2 were collected from over 20 original articles, conforming the dataset used for model calibration and validation (Domínguez et al., 1997; Chiyanzu et al., 2003; Shenai et al., 2003; Desai et al., 2004, 2006; Greenbaum et al., 2004; Fujii et al., 2005; Goud et al., 2005; Micale et al., 2006; Valente et al., 2006; Biot et al., 2007; Chipeleme et al., 2007; Li et al., 2009; Hans et al., 2010; Praveen Kumar et al., 2011; Shah et al., 2011; Huang et al., 2012; Luo et al., 2012; Conroy et al., 2014; Ettari et al., 2014; Jin et al., 2014; Wang et al., 2014; Weldon et al., 2014; Bertoldo et al., 2015; Mundra and Radhakrishnan, 2015a,b; Sharma et al., 2015; Singh et al., 2015; Schmidt et al., 2016). Such compounds were labeled as ACTIVE or INACTIVE according to their reported inhibitory data. The ACTIVE category included compounds with $IC_{50} \leq 5\,\mu M$, plus compounds with a percentage of inhibition $\geq$ 50% against the enzyme at $10\,\mu M$ or $\geq$ 80% at $20\,\mu M$ (when a single-point inhibition assay was reported). When none of the previous conditions were met, the compound was labeled as INACTIVE. Considering such criteria, the dataset includes 122 active compounds and 393 inactive compounds. Such dataset was curated using the standardization tool available in Instant JCHEM v. 17.2.6.0 (Chemaxon). The molecular diversity of the whole dataset and within each category can be appreciated in the heatmap displayed in **Figure 1**, which shows, for every compound pair, the Tanimoto distance computed using ECFP_4 molecular fingerprints. The heatmap was built using Gitools v. 2.3.1 (Perez-Llamas and Lopez-Bigas, 2011) and Tanimoto distances were calculated using ScreenMD—Molecular Descriptor Screening v. 5.5.0.1 (ChemAxon). The dataset is included as **Supplementary Data Sheet 1**.

Dataset Partition

It has been observed that rational/representative splitting of datasets into training and test sets tends to produce models with better predictivity (Golbraikh et al., 2003; Leonard and Roy, 2006; Martin et al., 2012). In the present study, a representative sampling procedure was thus used to divide the datasets into: (a) a training set, that was used to calibrate the models and; (b) a test set, that was used to independently assess model predictivity. Such representative partition of the dataset resulted from a serial combination of two clustering procedures. First, we have used the hierarchical clustering method included in LibraryMCS software (version 17.2.13.0–ChemAxon), which relies on the Maximum Common Substructure (MCS). A compound from each of the resulting cluster was randomly chosen and used as a seed to perform a non-hierarchical clustering using the k-means algorithm, as implemented in Statistica 10 Cluster Analysis module (Statsoft). Hierarchical clustering allowed deciding on an initial partition of n molecules into k groups, and this

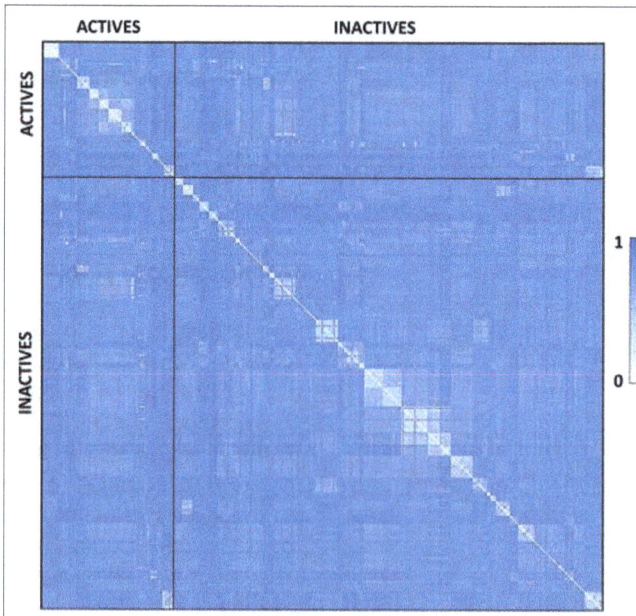

FIGURE 1 | Dissimilarity heatmap of the whole dataset. Light areas indicate high similarity between the compared compounds while dark blue areas indicate low similarity between the compared compounds.

preliminary clustering was then optimized through the non-hierarchical procedure, as suggested by Everitt et al. (2011). We have previously used this combined approach for representative dataset partitioning, with good results (Alberca et al., 2016, 2018; Gantner et al., 2017). The clustering procedure was performed separately for the ACTIVE and INACTIVE categories.

75% of the compounds in each cluster of the ACTIVE category were kept for the training set (making a total of 91 compounds); an equal number of compounds were taken from the INACTIVE category clusters (23% of each INACTIVE cluster). We have under-sampled the INACTIVE category, so that a balanced training sample (comprising an identical proportion of active and inactive examples) was obtained and model bias toward predicting the larger category was avoided. The remaining 31 active and 302 inactive compounds were assigned to test set (333 compounds in total), which was later used for external validation of the models.

Molecular Descriptor Calculation and Modeling Procedure

3,668 conformation-independent descriptors were computed with Dragon 6.0 software. A random subspace-based method was applied to obtain 1,000 descriptor subsets of 200 potential independent variables each. In the random subspace approach, the molecular descriptors are randomly sampled, and each model is trained on one subset of the feature space (Yu et al., 2012; El Habib Daho and Chikh, 2015); as a result, individual models do not over-focus on features that display high explanatory power in the training set.

A dummy variable (class label) was used as dependent variable. It was assigned observed values of 1 for compounds within the ACTIVE category and observed values of 0 for compounds in the INACTIVE one. Using a Forward Stepwise procedure and a semi-correlation approach (Toropova and Toropov, 2017), 1,000 linear classifiers were obtained, one from each of the random subsets of features. In order to avoid overfitting, only one molecular descriptor every 12 training instances was allowed into each model, with no more than 12 independent variables per model. Also, a maximal Variance Inflation Factor of 2 was tolerated. No descriptor with regression coefficient with p-value above 0.05 was allowed into the model. R language and environment was used for all data analysis. The R package data table (https://cran.r-project.org/package=data.table) was used to handle datasets.

The robustness and predictive ability of the models were initially estimated through randomization and Leave-Group-Out cross-validation tests. In the case of randomization, the class label was randomized across the compounds in the training set. The training set with the randomized dependent variable was then used to train new models from the descriptor selection step. Such procedure was repeated 10 times within each descriptor subset and the 95% confidence interval was built around the mean accuracy of the randomized models. It is expected that the randomized models will perform poorly compared to the real ones. Regarding the Leave-Group-Out cross-validation, random stratified subsets comprising 10 active compounds and 10 inactive compounds were removed from the training set in each cross-validation round, and the model was regenerated using the remaining compounds as training examples. The resulting model was used to predict the class label for the 20 removed compounds. The procedure was repeated 10 times, with each of the training set compounds removed at least once. The results were informed as the average percentage of good classifications (accuracy) across the folds, and this was compared to the accuracy of the model for the original training set and also, as advised by Gramatica (2013), to the No-Model error rate or risk (NOMER%), i.e., the error provided in absence of model:

$$NOMER\% = \frac{(n - nm)}{n} \times 100$$

where n is the total number of objects and nm is the number of objects of the most represented class.

Finally, the predictivity of each individual model was assessed through external validation, using the 333-compound test set that was already described in section Dataset Collection. A diversity of statistical parameters commonly used to assess the performance of classificatory models (Roy and Mitra, 2011; Gramatica, 2013) were estimated for both the training and test sets: sensitivity (Se, i.e., true positive rate), specificity (Sp, i.e., true negative rate), accuracy (Acc, i.e., overall percentage of good classifications), positive and negative predictivity and the F-measure, which is defined as follows (Roy and Mitra, 2011):

$$F - measure = \frac{2 \times Se \times (1 - Sp)}{Se + (1 - Sp)}$$

Ensemble Learning

Classifier ensembles are known to provide better generalization and accuracy than single model classifiers (El Habib Daho and Chikh, 2015; Carbonneau et al., 2016; Min, 2016). Here, we have used two retrospective virtual screening campaigns to assess the performance of individual classifiers and classifier ensembles. As described in the next subsection, the first retrospective virtual screen allowed assessing the performance of individual classifiers and provided the basis to decide which individual models would be selectively combined in the model ensemble and how they would be combined. The second retrospective virtual screen served to the sole purpose of assessing the performance of the chosen model ensemble.

The best individual classifiers were selected and combined using the area under the ROC curve metric (AUC ROC) in the first retrospective screen as criterion of performance. To choose the ideal number of models to be included in the ensemble, systematic combinations of the 2 to 100 best performing classifiers were analyzed (the two best-performing models were combined, then the three best-performing models, the four best-performing models, and so on up to a total of 100 models included in the ensemble). Four combination schemes were applied to obtain a combined score: MIN operator (which returns the minimum score among the individual scores of the combined models); Average Score; Average Ranking and; Average Voting. Voting was computed according to the equation previously used by Zhang and Muegge (2006). AUC ROCs were obtained with the pROC package (Robin et al., 2011); the Delong method was used to statistically compare the AUC ROCs. BEDROC and RIE (1%) were also computed (Truchon and Bayly, 2007). For that purpose, we resorted to the R package enrichvs (enrichment assessment of virtual screening approaches; Yabuuchi et al., 2011) and the online tool ROCKER (Lätti et al., 2016).

Retrospective Screening Campaigns

Through simulated ranking experiments, Truchon and Bayly (2007) demonstrated that the AUC ROC metric is dependent on the ratio of active compounds/inactive compounds, and the standard deviation of the metric converges to a constant value when small yields of actives (Ya) of the screened library are used (Ya below 0.05 seem to provide more robust results). Reasonably small Ya also ensures that the saturation effect is constant or absent. A high number of decoys (around 1,000 or higher) and a small Ya contribute to a controlled statistical behavior (Truchon and Bayly, 2007). Accordingly, to estimate the enrichment performance of our models and model ensembles in a real virtual screening scenario, we have performed retrospective virtual screening experiments. For that purpose, we have seeded known active compounds among a large number of decoys obtained with the help of the Directory of Useful Decoys Enhanced (DUD-E; Mysinger et al., 2012), a widely used benchmarking tool which allows the obtention of putative inactive compounds paired to known active compounds by physicochemical properties (e.g., molecular weight, logP, number of rotatable bonds, among others), but topologically dissimilar to such active compounds. In this way, two chemical libraries for such pilot screens were obtained. The first one, that we will call DUDE-A, was compiled by using the active compounds from the test set as queries in the DUD-E website. Such active compounds were later dispersed among the so-obtained paired decoys (putative inactive compounds). As a result, DUDE-A contained 31 known active compounds dispersed among 1500 DUD-E decoys and displayed a Ya of 0.020. DUDE-A was used to estimate the performance of the individual models in a virtual screening experiment and to choose the best individual models that would be included in the ensemble (i.e., to train the ensembles). It was also applied to choose which score threshold would be applied in prospective virtual screening campaigns. A second library, called DUDE-B, was obtained to validate the ensemble that showed the best performance in the DUDE-A screen. For that purpose, we compiled from literature 33 recently reported active compounds against FP-2 (IC50 $\leq 5\,\mu$M; Nizi et al., 2018; Stoye et al., 2019). The DUDE-B library was generated by merging these 33 active compounds with 4,337 decoys from the DUD-E website. The calculated Ya for DUDE-B is about 0.007.

Building Positivity Predictive Value Surfaces and Choosing an Adequate Score Threshold Value

A practical concern when implementing *in silico* screens involves estimating the actual probability that a predicted hit will confirm its activity when submitted to experimental testing (Positive Predictive Value, PPV). Estimation of such probability is however precluded due to its dependency on the Ya of the screened library, which is not known *a priori*:

$$PPV = \frac{Se\ Ya}{Se\ Ya + (1 - Sp)\,(1 - \ Ya)}$$

where *Se* represents the sensitivity associated to a given score cutoff value and *Sp* represents the specificity. The former equation was applied to build PPV surfaces. In order to choose an optimal cutoff value to select predicted hits in prospective virtual screening experiments, 3D plots showing the interplay between PPV, the Se/Sp ratio and Ya were built for each individual model and for each model ensemble. This approach has recently been reported by our group (Alberca et al., 2018). Using DUDE-A (described in previous subsection), Se and Sp were computed in all the range of possible cutoff score values. Though there is no guarantee that the Se and Sp associated to each score value for DUDE-A will be the same when applying the classifiers to other libraries, e.g., in the prospective virtual screening campaign, since controlled statistical behavior is observed for database sizes of 1,000 compounds or more and Ya below 0.05, we can reasonably assume that the ROC curve and derived metrics will be similar when applying the models to classify other large chemical databases with low Ya. Taking into consideration that in real virtual screening applications Ya is ignored a priori but invariably low, Ya was varied between 0.001 and 0.010. The R package plotly (https://cran.r-project.org/package=plotly) was used to obtain all the PPV graphs. Visual analysis of the resulting PPV surfaces allowed us to select a score threshold value with a desired range of PPV.

Prospective Virtual Screening

Based on visual inspection of the resulting of PPV graphs, we have applied in a prospective virtual screen an 11-model ensemble using the MIN operator to combine individual classifiers. Based on PPV surface analysis, we chose a score threshold that provides a PPV $\geq$ 20% at Ya = 0.01.

We have used the 11-model ensemble to screen two databases: (a) DrugBank 4.0, an online database containing extensive information about the US Food and Drug Administration (FDA) approved, experimental, illicit and investigational drugs (Law et al., 2014); (b) SWEETLEAD, a curated database of drugs approved by other international regulatory agencies, plus compounds isolated from traditional medicinal herbs and regulated chemicals (Novick et al., 2013). Both databases were curated using Standardizer 16.10.10.0 (ChemAxon). The following actions were applied to obtain homogeneous representations of the molecular structure for the subsequent virtual screen: (1) Strip salts; (2) Remove Solvents; (3) Clear Stereo; (4) Remove Absolute Stereo; (5) Aromatize; (6) Neutralize; (7) Add Explicit Hydrogens; and (8) Clean 2D. Duplicated structures were removed using Instant JCHEM v. 17.2.6.0. Four hits were selected for experimental evaluation, using the following criteria: (a) no previous report of falcipain-2 inhibition; (b) availability through local suppliers; (c) cost. Methacycline, benzthiazide, and bendroflumethiazide were acquired from Sigma-Aldrich. Odanacatib (99% HPLC) was acquired from AK Scientific (Y0388).

Molecular Docking

To gain insight into the possible mode of action of the active hits, we studied their possible interactions with falcipain-2 by docking simulations. The structure of the enzyme was obtained from the Protein data bank. We retrieved the available experimental structure of the target in complex with an inhibitor, the epoxysuccinate E64, that shows 2.9 Å of resolution (PDB code: 3BPF; Kerr et al., 2009). Among the four chains crystalized, we selected the B chain for the simulations. We used AutoDockTools4 software to remove the inhibitor and the crystallographic water molecules off the pdb file, and to add the hydrogen atoms of the protein.

Autodock4 was used for docking simulations. The docking software and conditions were selected based on the previous investigation by Mugumbate et al. (2013). The authors showed the capacity of this software to replicate the experimental pose of E64 in the re-docking experiment and to identify known inhibitors from non-inhibitors through the docking scores. Our own results of the re-docking E64 into the binding site of FP-2 were similar to such previous investigations, since Autodock4 was able to reproduce the experimental pose with a RMSD value of 1.84 Å.

Odanacatib was docked into the active site of the enzyme. Calculations were conducted with a grid of 40X40X40 grid points, centered on the experimental ligand E64 (coordinates: −36.75, 31.05, −47.07 in x, y, and z, respectively) and with a spacing between grid point of 0.39 Å. We used the default Autodock4 parameters for a population of 150, 50 genetic algorithm runs, 2.5×10^6 evaluations and 27,000 maximum generations.

Regarding non-competitive inhibitor methacycline, we first used DoGSiteScore server (Volkamer et al., 2012) to detect possible binding pockets in the protein. The server proposed two regions of binding, besides the known catalytic binding site of the enzyme. Methacycline was docked in both regions and the best results were achieved in the area delimited by CYS39, SER41, TRP43, GLU67, GLN68, LEU70, VAL71, ASP72, CYS73, SER74, PHE75, ASN77, TYR78, GLY79, CYS80, TYR106, VAL107, SER108, ASP109, ALA110, PRO111, ASN112. The simulation was conducted in the conditions described before for odanacatib and E64, except for the position of the grid, which was centered on the side chain on VAL71, specifically in the carbon atom defined as CG1.

Falcipain-2 Expression and Refolding

Falcipain-2 (MEROPS ID: C01.046) was expressed as inclusion bodies in BL21(DE3) *Escherichia coli* strain, purified by IMAC under denaturing conditions (final purity: 91%) and refolded to active enzyme as previously described (Pradines et al., 2001).

Falcipain-2 Kinetic Assay

Falcipain-2 activity was assayed fluorometrically with Z-LR↓AMC (Bachem) as substrate in 100 mM acetate buffer pH 5.5 containing 5 mM DTT and 0.01% Triton X-100, as this is expected to increase enzyme stability and reduce the number of false positives (Jadhav et al., 2010). Assays (final reaction volume ~80 μL) were performed at 30°C in solid black 384-well plates (Corning) at fixed enzyme concentration (3.3 nM). Except stated otherwise, fluorogenic substrate was added at final concentration of 5 μM (~1 x K_M) to match balanced assay conditions (Copeland, 2005). The release of 7-amino-4-methylcoumarin was monitored continuously for 60 min with a FilterMax F5 Multimode Microplate Reader (Molecular Devices) using standard 360 nm excitation and 465 nm emission filter set. Enzyme activity was estimated as the slope of the linear region of the resultant progress curves. Under the described conditions, falcipain-2 activity showed no significant changes in the presence of DMSO (0–8%) and the Selwyn test (Selwyn, 1965) indicated that enzyme remained stable during the assay.

Falcipain-2 Inhibition Assay

1 μL of each compound (2.5 mM in DMSO), N-(trans-epoxysuccinyl)-l-leucine 4-guanidinobutylamide (E-64, Sigma-Aldrich) (10 μM in DMSO) or DMSO were dispensed into each well. Then, 40 μL of activity buffer containing falcipain-2 (6.6 nM) were added to each well, plates were homogenized (30 seg, orbital, medium intensity) and each well subjected to a single autofluorescence read (exc/ems = 360/465 nm). Plates were incubated in darkness for 15 min at 30°C and then 40 μL of Z-LR-AMC (10 μM in assay buffer) were added to each well to start the reaction. After homogenization (30 seg, orbital, medium intensity), the fluorescence of AMC (exc/ems = 360/465 nm) was acquired kinetically for each well (12 read cycles, one cycle every 300 s). Fluorescence measurements were used to determine the slope (dF/dt) of progress curves by linear regression and inhibition percentage (%Inh) was calculated for each compound according to:

$$\%Inh = 100 \cdot [1 - (dF/dt^{WELL} - \mu^{C-})/(\mu^{C+} - \mu^{C-})]$$

where dF/dt^{WELL} represents the slope of each compound well and μ^{C+} and μ^{C-} the average of falcipain-2 + DMSO (no-inhibition) and substrate (no-enzyme) controls, respectively.

Compounds were re-tested in a dose-response manner (final concentration ranging from 375 μM to 44.7 pM) using identical assay conditions. 6 μL of compounds stock (10 mM in DMSO), E-64 (10 μM in DMSO), and DMSO were added to the first wells (column 1), followed by addition of 34 μL of activity buffer. After addition of 20 μL of buffer to subsequent wells, 24 serial 2-fold dilutions were made horizontally. Then, 40 μL of activity buffer containing falcipain-2 (6.6 nM) were added to each well, except for those corresponding to C-; completed with 40 μL of activity buffer. After homogenization, incubation, and autofluorescence measurement, 20 μL of Z-LR-AMC substrate (20 μM in activity buffer) were added. Data collection and processing were performed exactly as described above. At the concentration tested, no significant autofluorescence (360/465 nm) was apparent for the investigated compounds.

Percentage of falcipain-2 residual activity was calculated for each condition according to:

$$\%Res.Act = 100 \cdot \left[\frac{(dF/dt^{WELL} - \mu^{C-})}{(\mu^{C+} - \mu^{C-})} \right]$$

Half-maximal inhibitory concentration (IC_{50}) and Hill slope parameters were estimated by fitting experimental data from dose-response curves to the four-parameter Hill equation by using GraphPad Prism program (version 5.03).

Determining Reversibility, Mode of Inhibition, and Ki

Reversibility and time dependence of falcipain-2 inhibition by investigational compounds was assayed as previously described (Morrison, 1969). In brief, odanacatib (15 μM) and falcipain-2 (330 nM) were incubated at 30 °C for 60 min in activity buffer. Two microliters of the mix were rapidly added to 200 μL of Z-LR-AMC (5 μM in activity buffer) pre-incubated at the same temperature. Immediately after mixing, AMC fluorescence (λexc/ems = 355/460 nm, sensitivity = 550 V) was continuously monitored every second using a thermostated (30°C) Aminco Bowman Series 2 spectrofluorometer (Thermo Spectronic). In the case of the methacycline, the final inhibitor concentration in the mixture with falcipain-2 was 330 μM. For falcipain-2 control, the equivalent volume of DMSO vehicle was pre-incubated with the enzyme. To determine the kinetics of inhibition onset, falcipain-2 (3.3 nM final concentration) was added to 200 μL of reaction mix (previously tempered at 30°C) containing activity buffer, odanacatib (0.15 μM) and Z-LR-AMC (5 μM). Immediately after mixing, AMC release was monitored as indicated above. For methacycline (33 μM final concentration in the reaction mix), the experiment was exactly the same.

The identification of the mode of inhibition was performed as indicated previously. For odanacatib, falcipain-2 activity was determined for at least six different substrate concentrations (ranging from 62.5 to 1.95 μM) in the absence and presence of three fixed doses of inhibitor: 0.15, 0.5, and 2.5 μM. Data were re-arranged to estimate percentage of falcipain-2 residual activity for each condition and the values for IC_{50} and Hill slope were estimated by fitting experimental data to the four-parameter Hill equation by using GraphPad Prism. To estimate Ki, kinetic data were arranged in the form of Michaelis curves (dF/dt vs. $[Z\text{-}LR\text{-}AMC]_0$) and globally fitted to the competitive inhibition equation present in GraphPad Prism (version 5.03). Finally, to estimate Ki by using the tight-binding inhibition approach (Morrison, 1969), data were transformed to fractional velocity vs. inhibitor concentration and re-analyzed by global fitting to the Morrison equation by using GraphPad Prism (version 5.03).

To identify the mode of inhibition of methacycline, dose-response curves (0–625 μM) were performed as described above at six different substrate concentrations (ranging from 1 to 50 μM) and fitted as indicated above to estimate the values of IC_{50} and Hill slope. Finally, kinetic data were arranged in the form of Michaelis curves (dF/dt vs. $[Z\text{-}LR\text{-}AMC]_0$) and globally fitted to the mixed inhibition equation present in GraphPad Prism (version 5.03) for the simultaneous estimation of α and Ki.

Determining the Sensitivity of Methacycline Inhibition to RedOx Potential

The inhibitory activity of decreasing concentrations (375 μM−91.6 pM) of methacycline were determined in activity buffer containing DTT (0.1–10 mM) or L-cysteine (0.1–10 mM) as indicated above. Resultant dose-response curves were fitted as previously indicated to estimate the values of IC_{50} and Hill slope.

Densitometric Estimation of the Inhibition of Falcipain-2 Hemoglobinase Activity

Increasing concentrations of methacycline (200 μM, 500 μM, and 1 mM) and odanacatib (0.5, 5, and 50 μM) were preincubated with falcipain-2 (132 nM) for 30 min at 37°C in buffer 100 mM NaAc, 10 mM DTT pH 5.5. Then, human hemoglobin (H7379, Sigma-Aldrich) was added to a final concentration of 100 μg/mL to initiate reaction (final assay volume = 50 μL). E64 (10 μM) and DMSO were used as negative and positive controls, respectively. Also, a blank (no falcipain-2) control was included. In all cases, the final concentration of DMSO was 10%. Mixes were incubated without agitation for 3 h at 37°C to allow the enzymatic reaction to proceed. Then, reactions were stopped by addition of 15 μL of 5xSDS–PAGE sample buffer + 7.5 μL of DTT (1 M) and boiled for 5 min. Samples (22.5 μL, equivalent to 1.5 μg of hHb) were electrophoretically resolved by SDS-PAGE on a 15% acrylamide gel and Coomassie stained. The amount of undegraded hHb, observed as a doublet of around 15 kDa, was estimated densitometrically by using ImageJ 1.38d software (Nation al Institutes of Health, USA).

Evaluation of Antiparasitic Activity

Human erythrocytes were obtained from volunteer donors with a procedure approved by CEIC (Committee for Ethics on Clinical Investigation, Facultad de Farmacia y Bioquímica, Universidad de Buenos Aires EXP-UBA: 0048676/2017). Human erythrocytes infected with the NF54 strain of *P. falciparum* were cultivated in RPMI 1640 medium supplemented with 0.5% albumax II (Invitrogen), 22 mM glucose, 25 mM HEPES, 0.65 mM hypoxanthine, and 50 mg/mL gentamicin. Cultures were maintained at 37°C by routine passage at 5% hematocrit with a maximum parasitemia of 5% in a 90% N_2/5% O_2/5% CO_2 atmosphere as previously described (Alvarez et al., 2014).

When needed, ring-stage parasites were synchronized by using sorbitol treatment (Aley et al., 1986). After 24 h synchronization, cultures of infected erythrocytes at trofozoite-stage were treated with various concentrations of odanacatib, methacycline and E-64 for 48 h. Briefly, 100 μL of synchronous trophozoite-stage infected erythrocytes cultures were plated in 96-well at 4% hematocrit and 1% parasitemia. 100 μL of odanacatib (200, 20, or 2 μM), methacycline (1,000, 100, or 20 μM), E-64 (50, 10, or 2 μM), DMSO (vehicle control), or RPMI 1640 medium (control) were dispensed into each well to achieve final hematocrit of 2%, 0.5% parasitemia and the final concentration of each compound tested in a final volume of 200 μL. Parasitemia was evaluated by light microscopy counting infected forms of the parasite (ring, trophozoite, and schizont-stages) in a thick blood smear stained with Giemsa. A total of ~1,500 erythrocytes distributed in at least 15 random microscopic fields were evaluated of each smear and the parasitemia was calculated as (infected erythrocytes / total erythrocytes)*100. Then, each treatment was normalized to control parasitemia and expressed as percentage.

Significance was determined using one-way Analysis of Variance followed by a Tukey Multiple Comparison Test. Computations were carried out using PRISM statistical software (GraphPad Software, Inc., version 6). A p-value < 0.05 was considered significant. The number of determinations (n) for independent preparations (N) are indicated.

RESULTS

A ligand-based virtual screening approach was used to discover falcipain-2 inhibitors. 1,000 individual linear classifiers were obtained by applying a random subspace approximation on a pool of more than 3,000 Dragon molecular descriptors. The individual models were internally and externally validated.

Results of the internal validation are shown in **Table 1**. Regarding the Leave-Group-Out, results for each individual classifier are informed as the average accuracy across the folds, which is in all cases above 80% and close to the correspondent accuracy on the training set, suggesting the models are robust. Since the proportions of the active and inactive compounds in the training set are identical (as are in each of the Leave-Group-Out folds) the correspondent NOMER% (associated to random classification) is 50%, well below the behavior of the models in the cross-validation.

Regarding the randomization results, **Table 1** shows the 95% confidence interval around the mean accuracy of the randomized models. As expected, the accuracy of the randomized models is in all cases much below the accuracy of the true (non-randomized) models, and very close to the NOMER%, suggesting a low probability of chance correlations for the true models.

External validation was performed using the 333-compound independent test set. The results are summarized in **Table 2**.

TABLE 1 | Results of the internal validation procedures for the best 11 individual classifiers.

Model	Training set	LGO	Randomization	
	Acc (%)	Average Acc (%)	Confidence interval 95%	
594	84.615	83.740	53.882	61.283
516	88.462	86.712	56.623	63.267
477	84.615	83.835	56.158	64.501
975	87.363	86.374	53.309	62.844
244	90.110	88.712	55.312	62.160
504	85.714	83.765	55.978	61.824
870	86.264	82.753	56.962	65.126
154	86.813	85.168	54.677	62.246
764	84.615	83.080	53.273	62.112
564	85.714	82.636	54.814	62.000
80	86.264	85.378	56.980	61.921

In general, the individual classifiers show an acceptable performance. Due to the unbalanced nature of the test set (31 active compounds and 302 inactive ones) in comparison to the test set (91 active and 91 inactive compounds) some of the differences in the statistical parameters of the training and test sets are to be expected (i.e., decreased sensitivity in the test set, sharp drop in the positive predictivity and concomitant increase in the negative predictivity).

The best individual model included the following features:

Model 594

Class = −0.48333 + 0.38415*SM08_AEA(bo) - 6.50601*SpPosA_A - 0.12786*C-005 + 0.35800*B05[N-N] + 0.13459*nR=Cs + 0.21576*CATS2D_02_DD + 0.25881*nS(=O)2 - 0.33510*B03[O-S] - 0.07816*N-072 + 0.16832*B06[C-S]

Wilks' Lambda:.45705 approx. $F_{(10,\ 171)} = 20.314\ p < 0.0000$. Dragon's nomenclature for the molecular descriptors has been kept in the previous expression. SM08_AEA(bo) corresponds to the spectral moment of order 8 from augmented edge adjacency matrix weighted by bond order; SpPosA_A is the

TABLE 2 | Statistical parameters of the best individual classifiers, for both the training and test sets.

Model	Se	Sp	Acc	F-measure	Positive predictivity	Negative predictivity
Training set						
Model 594	0.88	0.81	0.85	0.31	0.82	0.87
Model 516	0.89	0.88	0.88	0.21	0.88	0.89
Model 477	0.86	0.84	0.85	0.28	0.84	0.85
Model 975	0.89	0.86	0.87	0.25	0.86	0.89
Model 244	0.92	0.88	0.90	0.21	0.88	0.92
Model 504	0.87	0.85	0.86	0.26	0.85	0.87
Model 870	0.89	0.84	0.86	0.28	0.84	0.88
Model 154	0.88	0.86	0.87	0.25	0.86	0.88
Model 764	0.84	0.86	0.85	0.24	0.85	0.84
Model 564	0.85	0.87	0.86	0.23	0.87	0.85
Model 80	0.89	0.84	0.86	0.28	0.84	0.88
Test set						
Model 594	0.84	0.80	0.80	0.32	0.30	0.98
Model 516	0.77	0.82	0.82	0.29	0.31	0.97
Model 477	0.71	0.84	0.83	0.26	0.31	0.97
Model 975	0.87	0.80	0.81	0.32	0.31	0.98
Model 244	0.84	0.77	0.78	0.36	0.28	0.98
Model 504	0.81	0.81	0.81	0.30	0.31	0.98
Model 870	0.81	0.81	0.81	0.31	0.30	0.98
Model 154	0.71	0.82	0.81	0.29	0.29	0.96
Model 764	0.74	0.83	0.83	0.27	0.32	0.97
Model 564	0.77	0.84	0.83	0.27	0.33	0.97
Model 80	0.81	0.75	0.76	0.38	0.25	0.97

The default score cutoff value (0.5) was used to discriminate between active and inactive compounds and estimate the parameters. Note that this score has been later optimized to obtain improved Se/Sp relationships.

normalized spectral positive sum from adjacency matrix; C-005 refers to the frequency of CH3X groups where X indicates an electronegative atom (O, N, S, P, Se, halogens); B05[N-N] indicates the presence/absence of the N – N pair at topological distance 5; nR=Cs refers to the number of aliphatic secondary C(sp2); CATS2D_02_DD is the CATS2D Donor-Donor at lag 02; nS(=O)2 symbolizes the number of sulfones; B03[O-S] indicates the presence/absence of O – S pair at topological distance 3; N-072 refers to frequency of the atom-centered fragment RCO-N< / >N-X=X; B06[C-S] denotes the presence/absence of a C – S pair at topological distance 6. The molecular descriptors associated to presence/absence or frequency of a given feature indicate differences in the frequencies at which such features appear in the active and inactive class of the training set. Those descriptors associated in the model to a positive weighting coefficient (B05[N-N], nR=Cs, nS(=O)2, and B06[C-S]) show that such feature is more frequent in the active compounds than in the inactive ones. In contrast, the descriptors associated to a negative coefficient (SpPosA_A, C-005, and N-072) indicate that such features appear more frequently in the compounds of the inactive class than in the ones of the active class. CATS2D_02_DD is a two-dimensional Chemically Advanced Template Search descriptor similar to a pharmacophore pair (Reutlinger et al., 2013), but considering topological distances between the pharmacophore points instead of geometrical distances. Here, the descriptor suggests that two H-bond donors at a topological distance of two are a desirable feature in falcipain-2 inhibitors.

The physicochemical interpretation of the two descriptors associated to spectral moments of a topological matrix (SM08_AEA(bo) and SpPosA_A) is less immediate.

An augmented edge adjacency matrix aE(w) is a symmetric square matrix that can be derived from an edge-weighted molecular graph, for any weighting scheme w. The elements from such matrix [aEw]ij take values of 1 if i and j are adjacent edges/bonds, values wi if i equals j (that is, for the elements in the diagonal) and values of 0 otherwise (i.e., for non-diagonal elements corresponding to non-adjacent edges; Liu et al., 2018). The kth spectral order μ_k of a topological matrix M can be defined as:

$$\mu_k = \mathrm{tr}(M^k)$$

where k is the power of the matrix and tr is its trace, i.e., the sum of the diagonal elements (Estrada, 1996). The kth spectral moment of the edge adjacency matrix has a simple graph theoretical interpretation (Estrada, 1996): it is the sum of all self-returning walks of length k in the line graph of the molecular graph, beginning and ending with the same vertex. It may then be appreciated that the value of such descriptor would be highly influenced by the presence of ring systems and the nature of such cycles (e.g., fused rings). Since the considered augmented edge matrix is weighted by the bond order, the presence of double and triple bonds and aromatic systems will tend to increase the value of the descriptor. Generally speaking, active examples in our training set tend to display higher values of SM08_AEA(bo).

Regarding SpPosA_A, it denotes the normalized sum of positive eigenvalues of the adjacency matrix. Its value diminishes with increase branching, with greater emphasis in terminal rather than in central branching (Balaban et al., 1991).

The 11 best individual models and a brief description of the descriptors included in them have been listed as **Supplementary Data Sheet 2**.

For a more challenging and realistic simulation, the enrichment behavior of the individual models was studied through a retrospective virtual screen on DUDE-A library, where a small proportion of active compounds (31) was dispersed among a high number (1500) of putative decoys. Initially, we compute the area under the Receiver Operating Characteristic curve (AUC ROC) to assess the classificatory performance of the models. 100, 93.4 and 3.1% of the individual classifiers displayed AUC ROCs above 0.8 for the training set, the test set and the DUD-A library, in that order. 85.8% of the individual models achieved an AUC ROC > 0.90 for the training set, whereas only one of the models (named model 975) got an AUC ROC above 0.9 for the test set, none of the models achieved an AUC ROC above 0.9 for the DUDE-A library. This suggests that our random subspace approach has been successful in finding individual classifiers with good explanatory and predictive power, but also that some degree of overfitting may also be present. Results also suggests that the retrospective screening experiment on DUDE-A is the more challenging tasks for the classifiers. **Table 3** shows the 11 individual classifiers that showed the best performance on the DUDE-A library, along with their AUC ROC, BEDROC, and RIE values.

Whereas, the performance of the best individual classifiers was quite satisfactory, we explored ensemble learning approaches to obtain meta-classifiers with improved accuracy and a more robust behavior. **Figure 2** shows the AUC ROC values (DUDE-A) obtained when systematically combining between the 2 and

TABLE 3 | Values of the AUC ROC, BEDROC, and RIE metrics for the 11 individual classifiers that displayed the best performance on the DUDE-A library.

Model	AUC ROC			BEDROC (α = 20)	RIE 1%
	Training set	Test set	DUDE-A	DUDE-A	DUDE-A
594	0.9162	0.8819	0.8529	0.2565	0.0000
516	0.9396	0.8819	0.8508	0.3150	0.0000
477	0.9123	0.8910	0.8419	0.2647	3.2258
975	0.9475	0.9105	0.8355	0.2191	3.2258
244	0.9492	0.8599	0.8343	0.2597	3.2258
504	0.9343	0.8812	0.8314	0.2355	0.0000
870	0.9291	0.8776	0.8294	0.2195	0.0000
154	0.9275	0.8730	0.8283	0.2769	3.2258
764	0.9195	0.8810	0.8268	0.2361	0.0000
564	0.9271	0.8992	0.8205	0.1673	0.0000
80	0.9233	0.8478	0.8198	0.1969	0.0000

100 individual models that displayed the best performance on the DUDE-A library, using four combination schemes: Minimum score (MIN), average score (AVE), average ranking (RANK), and average voting (VOT). The expectations on the ensembles were confirmed statistically: two combination schemes (minimum of the best 11 models and average ranking of the 4 best models) statistically outperformed the individual models in the DUDE-A database ($p = 0.0003$ and $p = 0.0132$, in that order). The MIN operator consistently outperformed the other combination schemes. When considering the influence of the number of models combined by the MIN operator on the AUC ROC metric, it was observed that above 11 models the AUC ROC did not improve substantially but poorer statistical behavior in terms of the standard deviation of the mean estimation was observed. The enrichment metrics for the best ensembles are shown in **Table 4**. Note that when applied in the screening of the DUDE-B database, the enrichment metrics for the 11-model combination based on the MIN operator (MIN-11) are similar (or in some cases, even better) than when screening DUDE-A database, validating the enrichment power of the best model combination. It may also be observed that best ensemble achieved good to excellent enrichment metrics. For instance, in the DUDE-A library, the RIE metric indicates that among the top 15 ranked compounds, 10 are known active ones.

Based on the previous results, we chose to move to the prospective (real) virtual screening campaign with the combination scheme based on the MIN operator (MIN-11). In our experience, this model combination scheme leads to high-specific model combinations (i.e., small false positive rate), which is a particularly convenient approach in our context (a small academic group from a low- to mid-income country, with limited resources to invest in hit validation); we thus often prefer to reduce the false positive rate even if this means losing sensitivity and sacrificing some active scaffolds. We have chosen to refine the former criteria (prioritizing Sp) by resorting to PPV surface analysis (Alberca et al., 2018). With the help of PPV surfaces, the evolution of the most relevant metric for our purposes, the PPV, i.e., the actual probability that a predicted hit will confirm activity when submitted to experimental testing, can be visually optimized as a function of the (Se/Sp) ratio across a range of Ya values. For this analysis, we have considered that the association between the Se/Sp and the score values of the MIN-11 model ensemble (observed in the retrospective screening campaign on DUDE-A) will hold when performing screens on other libraries (e.g., in a prospective virtual screening application). This is a strong assumption that of course is not necessarily true. However, since the AUC ROC values obtained for the DUDE-A library are unmistakably high (above 0.9 for the best model ensemble) while on the other hand the DUDE-A database Ya ratio (0.02) and size (>1,000 compounds) speak of a controlled statistical behavior (Truchon and Bayly, 2007), we believe it is a reasonable assumption in the present setting.

Using PPV surfaces (**Figure 3**), we chose 0.58 as score threshold to be used in our prospective virtual screening campaign; such score is associated to a Se/Sp ratio of 0.561 for MIN-11, and to a PPV value $\geq$ 20% for a Ya of 0.01. This means that if Ya in the real virtual screen was 0.01, we would have to submit about five predicted hits to experimental testing in order to find one confirmed hit. The virtual screen using the previous score cutoff value resulted in 157 hits, with 72 of them corresponding to approved drugs. Based on the previous analysis and our funding availability, we acquired and submitted four hits (**Figure 4**) to experimental testing: the antibiotic methacycline, the antihypertensives benzthiazide and bendroflumethiazide, and the abandoned drug odanacatib (an inhibitor of the cysteine protease cathepsin K that was pursued as a treatment for osteoporosis and bone metastasis but whose development was abandoned at Phase III long-term clinical trials due to safety issues; Drake et al., 2017).

To evaluate the ability of the selected hits to inhibit falcipain-2, we performed a two-round screening strategy. First, compounds were assayed in single dose (31.25 μM) to discard inactive molecules. Given that all of them were able to reduce to some extent (6–85%) the activity of falcipain-2 in comparison with the DMSO vehicle; we decided to evaluate the four hits in a dose-response manner (375 μM–0.45 pM) under balanced assay conditions to equalize the chances to detect competitive, non-competitive and uncompetitive inhibitors (Copeland, 2003; Yang et al., 2009). At the excitation/emission wavelengths used for AMC recording, compounds showed no significant autofluorescence in the concentration range tested. Prior to the analysis of the complete data, we explored the correlations between inhibition percentages in the primary (31.25 μM) and secondary (23.4 μM) screenings.

Compounds showed consistent results in both screenings (correlation coefficient $r^2 = 0.98$; slope $=$ 0.9732; **Supplementary Data Sheet 3**), with odanacatib and methacycline being the most active. These compounds showed typical progression (**Supplementary Data Sheet 3**) and dose-response curves (**Figure 5**), with measurable IC_{50} and Hill slope values of 0.186 μM and −1.079 for odanacatib, and 106.4 μM and −0.9294 for methacycline. In the same range of concentrations, benzthiazide and bendroflumethiazide showed no dose-dependent inhibition.

We further characterized odanacatib and methacycline in terms of the reversibility and time-dependence of falcipain-2 inhibition. Reversible interaction with falcipain-2 was verified for both compounds by the recovery of enzyme activity after rapid addition of substrate (100-fold dilution) to the pre-incubated mix of enzyme and inhibitor (**Figures 6A,B**). In this experiment, methacycline displayed a linear progress curve (**Figure 6A**) with a stable inhibition value, indicative of rapid onset of steady state (i.e., rapid dissociation of EI complex). In the presence of odanacatib, however, the enzyme took several minutes to recover full activity and to show a permanent inhibition value (concave progress curve), suggesting slow dissociation of inhibitor from the complex with falcipain-2 (**Figure 6B**). Similarly, both inhibitors displayed different kinetic behavior when enzyme was added to a reaction mix previously containing inhibitor and substrate (**Figures 6C,D**). Methacycline displayed a typical linear progress curve (**Figure 6C**), showing a defined (stable) value of inhibition during the whole assay. In contrast, odanacatib showed non-linear kinetics

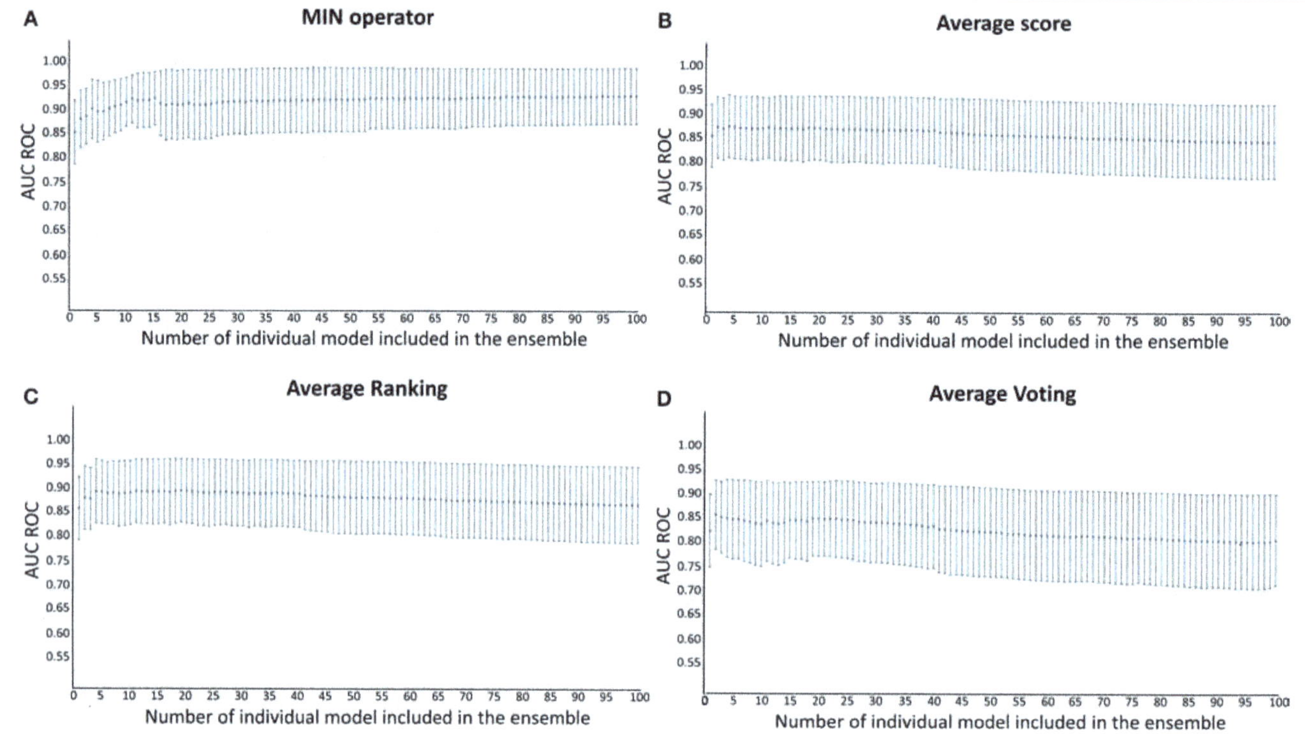

FIGURE 2 | AUC ROC metric vs. the number of combined models in the DUD-E database. **(A)** Minimum score; **(B)** Average score; **(C)** Average ranking; **(D)** Average voting.

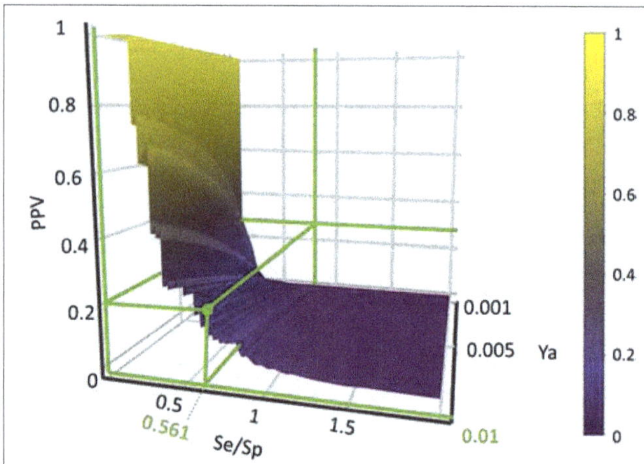

FIGURE 3 | PPV surface for the best 11-model ensemble on the DUDE-A library. The Se/Sp ratio correspondent to the chosen score cut-off value and the associated PPVs within the Ya 0.001–0.010 range are signaled.

(**Figure 6D**) with inhibition progressively increasing over time (time-dependent inhibition). As stable inhibition was observed only after ~15 min, all subsequent kinetic experiments for odanacatib included preincubation ($\geq$ 30 min at 30°C) with the enzyme.

To investigate the mode of inhibition of odanacatib, we first evaluated the impact of substrate concentration on the apparent IC_{50} value over a wide range (0.4–13.2xK_M) of substrate saturation levels. For this, we used a reduced set of three odanacatib concentrations selected to: (i) include IC_{50} value at each substrate condition and (ii) cover the wider inhibition range (~15–80%) in the central stretch of the dose-response curves. As observed in **Figures 7A,B**, apparent IC_{50} values increased linearly with the increment of substrate concentration, indicating a competitive mode of inhibition for odanacatib on the activity of falcipain-2. The global fitting of all the Michaelis curves to the equation of competitive inhibition (**Figure 7C**) allowed us to estimate a Ki value of 98.2 ± 10.2 nM. As this estimation is in the limit of tight-binding inhibition (Ki $\leq 10^{-7}$ M), kinetic data were transformed to fractional velocity vs. inhibitor concentration and re-analyzed by global fitting to the Morrison equation[32]. Ki value for odanacatib determined from this approach (**Figure 7D**)

TABLE 4 | Values of the AUC ROC, BEDROC, and RIE metrics for the best model combination (DUDE-A library).

	AUC ROC		BEDROC (α = 20)		RIE (1%)	
Model	**DUDE A**	**DUDE B**	**DUDE A**	**DUDE B**	**DUDE A**	**DUDE B**
MIN-11	0.9214**	0.8991**	0.6414	0.4252	29.6322	9.0289
M-594	0.8529	0.7415	0.2565	0.2710	0.0000	0.0000

*For comparison purposes, the results of the best individual model (M-594) are also presented, as well as the enrichment metrics for the MIN-11 ensemble on the DUDE-B library. **Statistically significant differences in comparison with the best individual model ($p < 0.01$).*

was 99.88 ± 8.28 nM, very similar to our previous (more approximate) estimation.

For methacycline, which initially showed potency in the high micromolar range, we constructed complete dose-response curves at six fixed substrate concentrations, ranging from 0.2 to 10xK_M. Although substrate concentration was increased 50-fold, only a slight increase (1.42-fold) was observed in the apparent IC_{50} value, suggesting no competition between methacycline and the small peptidic substrate Z-LR-AMC. To directly estimate Ki and α values, Michaelis plots were globally fitted to the model for mixed inhibition. This approach confirmed that methacycline inhibits falcipain-2 activity non-competitively with a Ki value of 84.4 ± 6.5 µM and α =1.42 ± 0.15 (**Figure 8**).

Given that cysteine peptidases require that its catalytic sulfhydryl group be in reduced state to show their maximal enzymatic activity, they are prone to undergo RedOx interferences caused by several classes of thiol-reactive compounds able to simulate genuine inhibition (Thorne et al., 2010). In many cases, this artifactual inhibition can be significantly relieved by simply changing the reduction potential of the activity buffer, thus providing a diagnostic test to detect false-positive RedOx compounds. To establish if this could be the case for methacycline, we further investigated the effect of the strength and concentration of reducing agents (DTT, a strong reducing agent, and cysteine, a weak reducing agent) on the inhibition of falcipain-2 by this molecule. Dose-response curves were very similar regardless of the final concentration of the reducing agent (100-fold range) present in the assay buffer (**Supplementary Data Sheet 3**). These results rule out common types of RedOx interference and suggest that methacycline genuinely inhibits falcipain-2.

Once established that odanacatib and methacycline inhibit the peptidolytic activity of falcipain-2, we assayed whether these molecules could also modulate falcipain-2 proteolytic activity on its natural substrate, human hemoglobin (hHb). To this end, we pre-incubated the enzyme with increasing concentrations of both inhibitors and then added the hHb substrate. E-64, a specific and highly potent irreversible inhibitor of C1A cysteine peptidases, was used as a positive control. After incubation at 37°C for 3 h, reaction mixes were resolved electrophoretically by SDS-PAGE on a 15% acrylamide gel and Coomassie stained. The amount of undegraded hHb, observed as a doublet of around 15 kDa, was estimated densitometrically. As shown in **Supplementary Data Sheet 3**, odanacatib inhibited the hemoglobinase activity of FP2 in a dose-response manner. For methacycline, however, no inhibition was observed in this assay, even at the highest concentration tested (1 mM). Of note, the effective inhibitory concentrations of odanacatib in this assay were in the low-to-middle micromolar range, a significant shift in comparison to the sub-micromolar potency previously observed in the inhibition of Z-LR-AMC hydrolysis. Overall, these observations suggest that (i) the existing differences between the surrogate (peptidic) and the natural (macromolecular) falcipain-2 substrates are somehow important for the inhibitory efficiency of both inhibitory molecules and that, at least, (ii) low-to-middle micromolar compound concentrations would be required to assess their efficacy in a more physiological context (i.e., cellular culture).

To analyze the influence of odanacatib and methacycline in the intraerythrocytic cycle of *P. falciparum*, a synchronized culture of RBCs infected (trophozoite stage) was treated with increasing concentrations of odanacatib (1, 10, or 100 µM) and methacycline (10, 50, or 500 µM). E-64 (1, 5, or 25 µM) was again used as a positive control. After 48 h, the number of infected erythrocytes was evaluated by light microscopy in stained blood smears. Odanacatib (100 µM) significantly reduced the parasitemia (**Figure 9**), with no apparent reduction in the other two concentrations tested. Methacycline significantly reduced the parasitemia at 500 and 50 µM, but not at 10 µM. As expected, E-64 significantly reduced the parasitemia at 5 and 25 µM, but no at 1 µM. Almost no erythrocytes infected at schizont-stage were observed in the treatments (**Supplementary Data Sheet 3**). It is important to mention that at the highest concentrations assayed, methacycline (500 µM) and odanacatib (100 µM) induced cytotoxic effects on RBC, as observed in the hemolysis assay (**Supplementary Data Sheet 3**).

Molecular docking results were in good agreement with the experimental observations. **Figure 10** shows the best result of the docking simulation for odanacatib in the catalytic binding site, that is, the pose that showed lower value of the scoring function. Two hydrogen bonding interactions were found between the compound and GLN36 and ASN173. The docking score was −6.94 kcal/mol, which is lower than the score achieved for E64 in the same conditions (−4.91 kcal/mol). Regarding methacycline, we detected hydrogen bonding interactions between methacycline and the residues of the proposed (non-catalytic) binding pocket. Residues like ASP72, ASN112, PRO111, and ALA110 could be implicated in the stabilization of the complex (docking score of−5.65 kcal/mol). More studies will be performed to evaluate these predictions.

DISCUSSION AND CONCLUSIONS

Using an ensemble learning approximation, we have performed a ligand-based virtual screening campaign to identify new falcipain-2 inhibitors as potential new treatments against malaria. There are some previous reports on the development of ligand-based models to predict the activity of *P. falciparum* cysteine proteases. The approaches used in such studies show considerable differences with the one reported here: they used conformation-dependent descriptors (3D QSAR) to infer regression models; in almost all cases, congeneric series of comparatively narrow chemical diversity have been used to train the models, thus limiting their applicability domain and; the reported models have mostly been used for explanatory rather than predictive purposes. Xue and coworkers realized CoMFA and CoMSIA 3D-QSAR studies on a series of 93 alkoxylated and hydroxylated chalcones (Xue et al., 2004). Potshangbam and coworkers also carried out CoMSIA and CoMFA studies on a series of 54 2-pyrimidinecarbonitrile

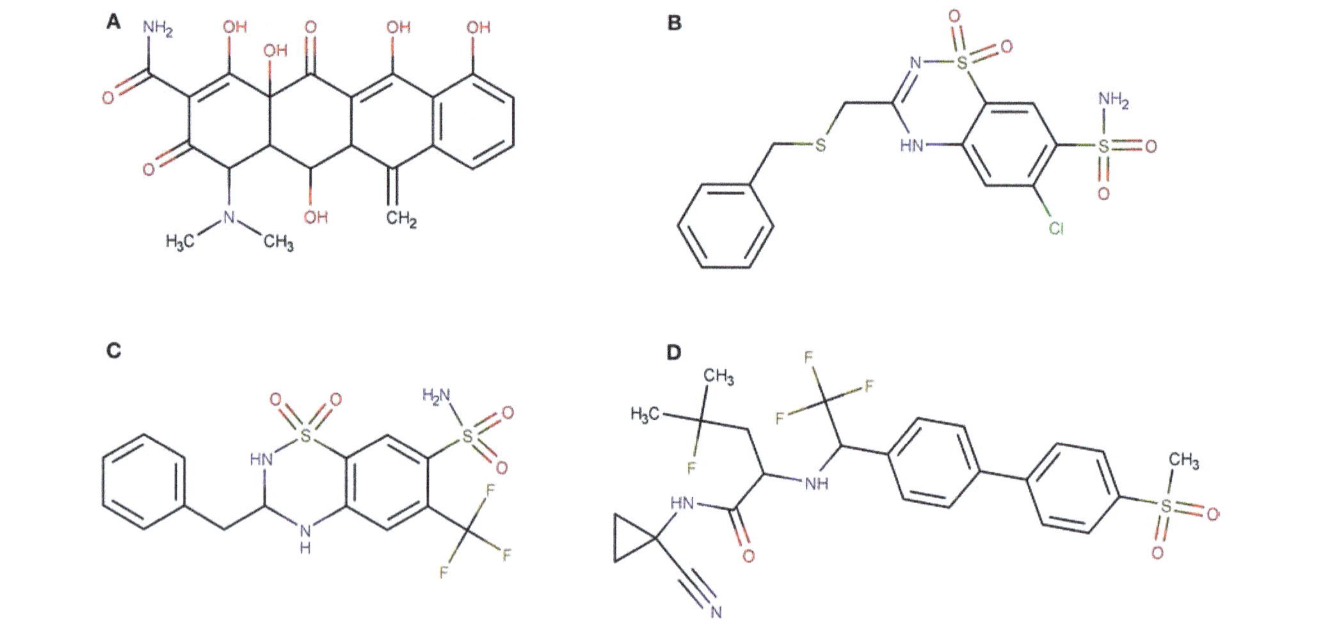

FIGURE 4 | Molecular structures of the hits selected in the prospective virtual screening campaign that were submitted to experimental confirmation. **(A)** methacycline; **(B)** benzthiazide; **(C)** bendroflumethiazide; **(D)** odanacatib.

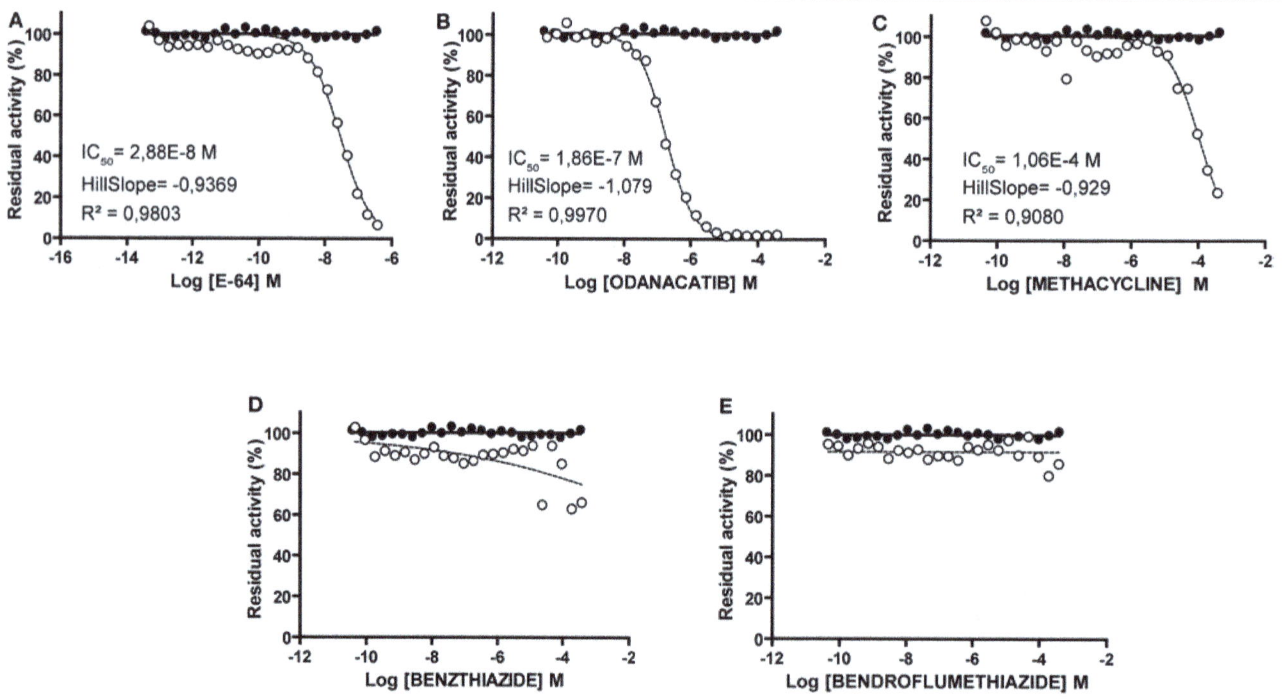

FIGURE 5 | Dose-response curves of identified falcipain-2 inhibitors (open circles). For each compound, dotted line represents the best fit of experimental data to the four-parameter Hill equation. **(A)** E-64. **(B)** Odanacatib. **(C)** Methacycline. **(D)** Benzthiazide. **(E)** Bendroflumethiazide. For those compounds achieving data convergence, the resultant values for the parameters IC50, Hillslope and R2 are indicated. In all cases, equivalent volumes of DMSO vehicle were assayed in parallel (closed circles).

analog inhibitors of falcipain-3 (Potshangbam et al., 2011). Using the same approximations, Wang et al. performed a 3D QSAR study of 247 2-pyrimidinecarbonitrile analog inhibitors of falcipain-3 (Wang et al., 2013). Teixeira and colleagues did a CoMFA and CoMSIA analysis of a series of 39 peptidyl vinyl sulfone derivatives as potential cysteine protease

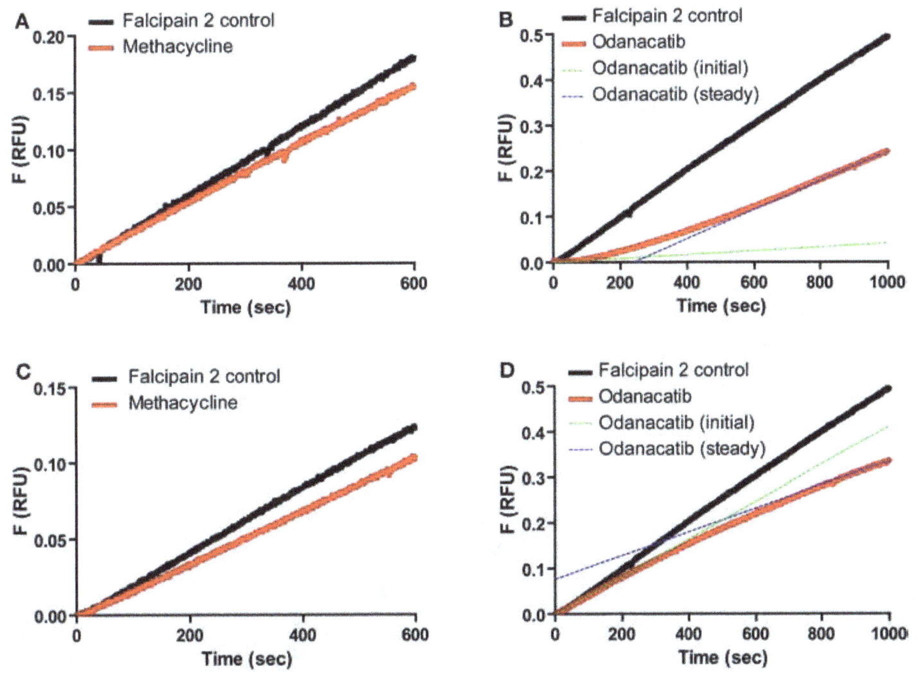

FIGURE 6 | Reversibility and time dependence of the inhibition of falcipain-2 by methacycline and odanacatib. Top panel: Product progress curves for the dissociation of E-I complex by rapid dilution (100-fold) of enzyme-inhibitor mix into substrate solution. **(A)** Methacycline. **(B)** Odanacatib. Bottom Panel: Product progress curves for the formation of E-I complex by rapid addition of enzyme to a substrate-inhibitor mix. **(C)** Methacycline. **(D)** Odanacatib.

inhibitors (Teixeira et al., 2011). Very recently, Allangba et al. derived complexation QSAR models and pharmacophores from a training set of 15 lactone–chalcone and isatin–chalcone hybrid inhibitors with falcipain-2 inhibitory activity (Allangba et al., 2019). The most similar study to our own is possibly the one by Mugumbate and coworkers, who as a part of and hybrid ligand- and structure-based approach, obtained ligand-based models based on Pentacle alignment-independent descriptors, using a training set of nine non-peptide inhibitors of falcipain-2 (Mugumbate et al., 2013). They performed a retrospective pilot screen before using their protocol to explore the ZINC database, retrieving falcipain-2 inhibitors in the low μM range. All in all, the enrichment metrics they computed in their retrospective screen are similar to the ones we obtained here.

Our most predictive model combination was chosen (i.e., trained) based on a retrospective virtual screening campaign (DUDE-A library). The enhanced ability of the selected model-ensemble to retrieve falcipain-2 inhibitors in comparison to our best individual models was checked using a second retrospective virtual screening experiment (DUDE-B library). Four of the hits emerging from our prospective virtual screening experiment were acquired and assayed against the enzyme. Two of them, odanacatib (previously investigated as treatment against osteoporosis and bone metastasis) and methacycline (an antibiotic) confirmed our predictions, reducing the peptidolytic activity of the enzyme. Interestingly, our observed PPV (50%, corresponding to two experimentally confirmed hits out of four assayed compounds) exceeded our theoretic expectations based on PPV surfaces analysis, which suggested a PPV of at least 20% for the chosen score threshold, for a hypothetic yielding of active compounds of 1%.

Both hits displayed different inhibition mechanisms. In agreement with previous reports for the interaction with other Papain-like C1A (Clan CA family) human cathepsins (Gauthier et al., 2008), odanacatib inhibits falcipain-2 in a reversible, competitive and tight-binding (sub-micromomlar) mode. For human cathepsin K, odanacatib inhibition occurs throughout the formation of a covalent but yet reversible thioimidate adduct between the -SH in the catalytic Cys residue and the nitrile warhead (Oballa et al., 2007). This covalent association mechanism results in on- and off-rates of 5.3×10^6 M and 0.0008 s^{-1} ($t_{1/2}$ ~14 min), respectively (Gauthier et al., 2008). These observations are in line with the slow association and dissociation kinetics observed by us for falcipain-2 inhibition, suggesting that a similar chemical inhibition mechanism could be occurring. Other compounds bearing the N-(1-cyanocyclopropyl)-amide inhibitory scaffold present in odanacatib, have been reported as potent (Ki ~1–2 nM) and selective (>15-fold over human cathepsins) falcipain-2 inhibitors (Ang et al., 2011; Nizi et al., 2018).

On the other hand, methacycline acts as a reversible, non-competitive and sub-milimolar inhibitor of falcipain-2. Based on our observations (reproducible, reversible and dose-dependent reduction of enzyme activity, rapid equilibrium onset, Hill slopes ~ −1, inhibitory activity insensitive to the RedOx potential

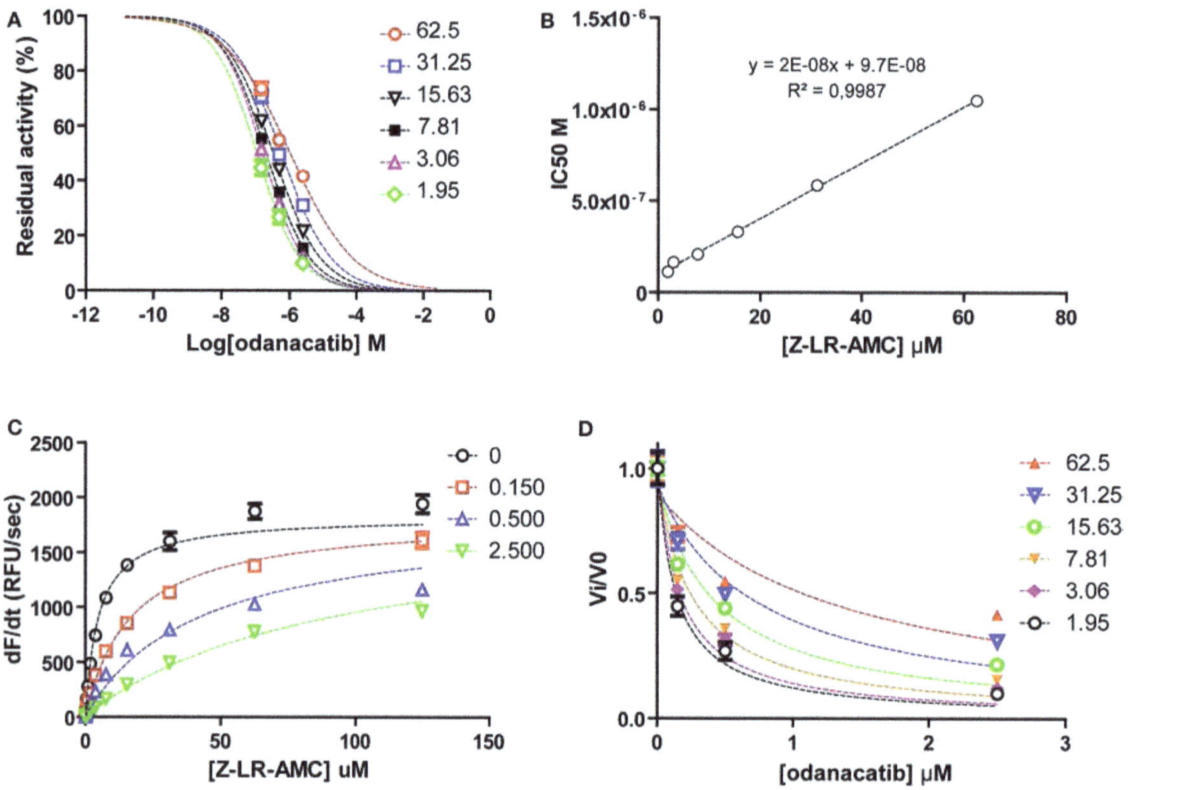

FIGURE 7 | (A) Dose-response curves for odanacatib at fixed substrate concentrations. Dotted lines represent the best fit of experimental data to the four-parameter Hill equation. **(B)** Effect of substrate concentration on the IC50 values of falcipain-2 inhibition by odanacatib. IC50 values increase linearly (>9-fold) with substrate concentration in the range 1.95–62.5 μM. Dotted line represents the best fit of data to linear equation. Y-axis intercept accounts for the Ki value. **(C)** Global fitting of kinetic data to the competitive inhibition model equation. **(D)** Global fit ting of kinetic data to the Morrison equation.

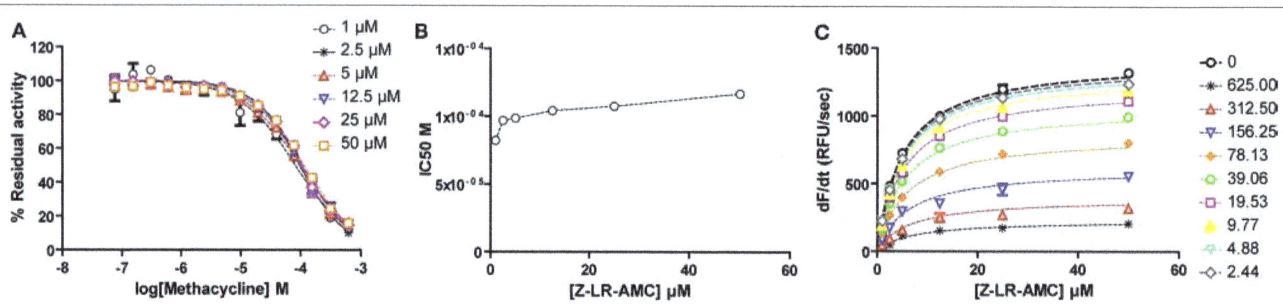

FIGURE 8 | Methacycline is a non-competitive, sub-millimolar inhibitor of falcipain-2. **(A)** Dose-response curves for methacycline at fixed substrate concentrations. Dotted lines represent the best fit of experimental data to the four-parameter Hill equation. **(B)** Half maximal inhibitory concentration of methacycline increases slightly (1.42-fold) with substrate concentration in the range: 1–50 μM. **(C)** Global fitting of kinetic data to the equation of mixed inhibition model.

and no signs of common compound-specific assay interferences such as autofluorescence or aggregate formation), methacycline inhibition seems to occur throughout a genuine mechanism. This may lead to rational optimization efforts to improve affinity. Further studies should be performed to confirm the putative binding pocket suggested by our docking experiments, to move in that direction. To date, only few non-competitive falcipain-2 inhibitors have been reported; including suramin analogs (Marques et al., 2013), heme analogs (Marques et al., 2015), and (E)-chalcones (Bertoldo et al., 2015) reported. Suramin, heme, and their analogs inhibit falcipain-2 with IC_{50} values in the nanomolar range and seem to share a common "non-competitive like" inhibition mechanism that occurs through the formation of a ternary enzyme:inhibitor:substrate complex of stoichiometry 1:1:2. In both cases, the authors argued that the binding of the inhibitor to falcipain-2 reveals a novel regulatory substrate binding site in the enzyme, which allows the subsequent allosteric binding of a second substrate molecule,

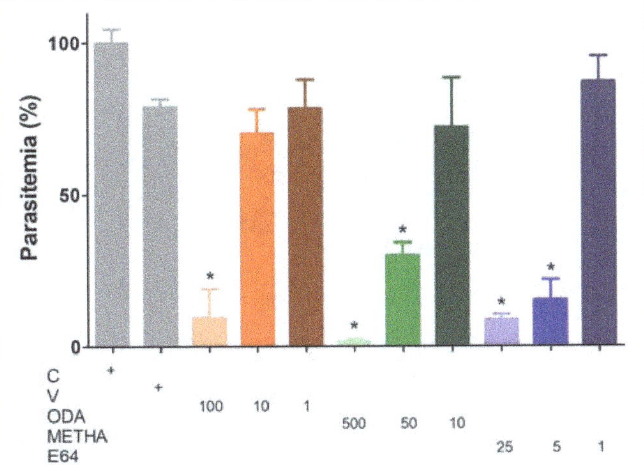

FIGURE 9 | Effect of odanacatib and methacycline on the development of P. falciparum under culture. Cultures of erythrocytes infected (trophozoite stage) at 2% hematocrit and 0.5% parasitemia were incubated with increasing concentrations of odanacatib (ODA; 1, 10, or 100 μM) and methacycline (METHA; 10, 50, or 500 μM). E-64 (1, 5, or 25 μM) was used as positive control of falcipain-2 inhibition. DMSO was used as a vehicle control (V) and RPMI 1640 medium as a control (C). After 48 h, the number of infected erythrocytes (ring, trophozoite, and schizont-stages) was evaluated by light microscopy in stained blood smears. Data are the means ± SD of one experiment performed by triplicate. (*) $p < 0.05$ represents the differences between control and the treatments.

resulting in falcipain-2 inhibition (Marques et al., 2013, 2015). Very similar to what we have found for methacycline, (E)-chalcones 48 (Ki =45 μM, α < 1) and 66 (Ki =7 μM, α = 1) display a classical non-competitive inhibition profile for falcipain-2 with no evidence of substrate inhibition (Bertoldo et al., 2015). None of these inhibitors appear to bind falcipain-2 active site, thus anticipating new routes to overcome the critical issue of selectivity over human cathepsins. In this regard, the identification and targeting of non-active (i.e., allosteric) binding sites within the falcipain-2 molecule seems to be an attractive and effective alternative to traditional active site-directed inhibitors, as recently showed by Pant and coworkers (Pant et al., 2018). Two compounds, rationally designed to target an allosteric site present in the pro-mature domain interface of falcipains-2/-3, were able to bind both pro-enzymes with nanomolar affinities and arrest *P. falciparum* growth, clearly illustrating the potential of this approach.

Of interest, odanacatib inhibits the peptidolytic activity of falcipain-2 much more efficiently than its hemoglobinase activity. Although displaying comparable affinities for the enzyme [K_D^{hHb} =3.3 μM (Hogg et al., 2006); $K_M^{Z-LR-AMC}$ = 4.8 μM], there are important differences between Z-LR-AMC and hHb as falcipain-2 substrates, regarding both their binding modes and their catalytic heterogeneity. In the first case, the small peptidic substrate Z-LR-AMC accommodates completely within falcipain-2 active site and the enzyme-substrate complex relies entirely on active site interactions for its stabilization and catalytic transformation. In addition, Z-LR-AMC substrate comprise a single cleavage site per molecule. These facts seem to make it somehow more vulnerable to the competitive binding of odanacatib to the active site and to the catalytic impairment promoted by the binding of methacycline to a presumptive allosteric site, like the one proposed here. In the case of hHb, it has been shown that interaction with the enzyme depends almost exclusively on a unique falcipain-2 structural motif (the "arm"), located >25 Å away from the active site (Pandey et al., 2005; Wang et al., 2006). In fact, a falcipain-2 mutant lacking most of the arm loop showed no activity or affinity against hHb, although remained fully active against a number of generic peptide and protein substrates (Pandey et al., 2005). Additionally, hHb was able to bind to falcipain-2 molecules with the active site blocked by the irreversible inhibitor E-64, clearly indicating that the recognition of intact hHb is mostly independent of the active site. Considering all these observations, we can hypothesize that the binding of odanacatib to falcipain-2 active site would not be likely to perturb substantially the binding affinity of intact hHb to its exosite and *vice versa*. Thus, with the ability to bind both enzyme forms (falcipain-2 and the falcipain-2-hHb complex) with comparable affinity, odanacatib would probably behave as a non-competitive inhibitor against an exosite-binding substrate such as intact hHb. This has been previously reported for small active site-directed inhibitors of proteases and kinases when acting on their natural macromolecular substrates (Krishnaswamy and Betz, 1997; Pedicord et al., 2004; Blat, 2010). The change in the inhibition modality of odanacatib, however, seems insufficient to explain, *per se*, the magnitude of the drop in its inhibitory potency against the falcipain-2/hHb system. A second line of argument came from the observation that hHb molecule is a catalytically heterogeneous substrate, comprising numerous independent falcipain-2 cleavage sites and whose digestion seems to be a non-ordered process (Subramanian et al., 2009). The occurrence of multiple cleavage events at different sites along the protein sequence leads to the formation of numerous digestion products of lower molecular weight. These digestion products also contain functional falcipain-2 cleavage sites and become new substrates that, after a new round of proteolysis, may generate additional substrate peptides. As the reaction proceeds, this iterative process leads to an increase in the number and the global concentration of peptidyl substrates able to compete for the binding to falcipain-2 active site. This might eventually lead to a partial relief of inhibition by competitive, active site-directed inhibitors, as would be the case of odanacatib.

Considering that falcipain-2 and−3 are the major cysteine proteases required for the intraerythrocytic development of *P. falciparum*, we evaluated the antiparasitic effect of odanacatib and methacycline. The inhibitors of cysteine proteases block the hydrolysis of hemoglobin, causing the development of enlarged, hemoglobin-filled food vacuoles in trophozoites and failure of parasites to complete their development (Marco and Coterón, 2012). The two drugs showed a clear inhibition in a dose-depend manner on the intraerythrocytic cycle of *P. falciparum*. The effective concentrations of odanacatib in *P. falciparum* cultures were in the low-to-middle micromolar range, similar to those observed in the inhibition assay of hemoglobinase activity. This finding is compatible with a hypothetical mode

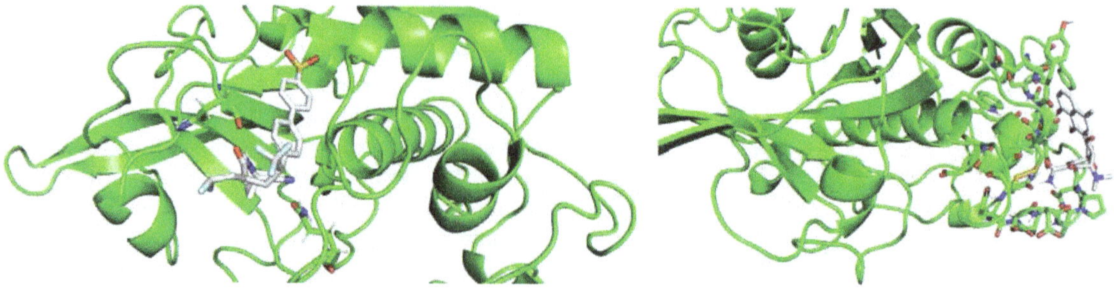

FIGURE 10 | Best poses from the molecular docking experiments for odanacatib **(Left)** and methacycline **(Right)**. Interacting residues are shown in sticks.

of action trough inhibition of falcipain functions within the food vacuole. Although the inhibition of diverse proteases by tetracycline derivatives has previously been reported (Morrison, 1969; Zucker et al., 1985; Sanchez Mejia et al., 2001; Chi et al., 2011), to the best of our knowledge, this is the first report of the inhibition of a C1A cysteine peptidase from a protozoa parasite by an antibiotic of the tetracycline family. The molecular targets for the action of tetracyclines against *Plasmodium* parasites have not been fully elucidated. However, their mode of action seems to include the inhibition of protein synthesis at mitochondrial, plastid and nuclear ribosomes by the association with ribosomal components (Gaillard et al., 2015). Additional mechanisms, such as reduction in *de novo* pyrimidine synthesis and a decrease in the transcription rates of mitochondrial and apicoplast genes, have also been postulated (Briolant et al., 2008; Gaillard et al., 2015). The inclusion of falcipain-2 among the potential targets of tetracycline derivatives adds new possibilities for the development of "two-edged swords" candidate drugs for *P. falciparum*, with potential benefits in terms of potency and delay of resistance appearance (Agarwal et al., 2017). The contribution of this mechanism to the global antimalarial activities of these antibiotics remains to be established in future investigations.

It should also be underlined that odanacatib underwent long-term clinical trials as a treatment of postmenopausal osteoporosis (Bone et al., 2015), which were early stopped due to robust efficacy and a favorable benefit/risk profile. However, its clinical development was dropped due to an increased risk of stroke in the postmenopausal patients on odanacatib vs. a placebo group. Accordingly, our findings on the potential use of the drug against malaria could be considered a drug rescue example, i.e., a proposal on a new medical used of and abandoned or discontinued drug. Do the safety issues of odanacatib pose an inevitable impediment for their potential development as antimalarial treatment? Not necessarily. Although they are indeed a concern, it should be considered that the odanacatib augmented risk of stroke was observed in long-term studies, whereas the drug could possibly be administered in a short-term manner as malaria treatment (for instance, artemisinin-based combination therapies only require a 3-day course to achieve efficacy in cases of uncomplicated *P. falciparum* malaria). Accordingly, the long-term risks of odanacatib use may not have a negative impact on its use as antimalarial. There are well-known examples of drug rescue of discontinued drugs with severe safety issues, that can be re-introduced in a new therapeutic setting with the pertinent precautions. For instance, thalidomide was largely abandoned due to its teratogenic effects, but has been recently relaunched to the market for the treatment of leprosy and multiple myeloma (Teo et al., 2002; Mercurio et al., 2017).

Pharmacokinetics studies reveal that after multiple-dose administration of odanacatib 50 mg (once weekly for 4 weeks), average maximal plasma concentrations of around 400 nM are observed (Chen et al., 2018), although a high fraction of plasma protein bound drug has also been reported (Kassahun et al., 2014). Accordingly, further studies are required to evaluate the dose-compatibility between the previously investigated therapeutic use and the possible antimalarial indication.

AUTHOR CONTRIBUTIONS

All authors listed have made a substantial, direct and intellectual contribution to the work, and approved it for publication.

FUNDING

The authors thank Agencia Nacional de Promoción Científica y Tencológica (PICT 2013-0520, PICT 2017-0643, PICT 2014-0327), University of La

Plata (Incentivos UNLP) and the International Foundation for Science (Grants F/4081-1 and F/4081-2) for funding.

ACKNOWLEDGMENTS

The authors thank CONICET and UNLP. Silvia Repetto for kindly providing us the laboratory for *Plasmodium falciparum* culture. We would like to thank Prof. Luciana Gavernet for her kind advice on the docking simulations. The Titan Xp used for this research was kindly donated by the NVIDIA Corporation.

REFERENCES

Agarwal, D., Gupta, R. D., and Awasthi, S. K. (2017). Are antimalarial hybrid molecules a close reality or a distant dream? *Antimicrob. Agents Chemother.* 61:e00249-e00217. doi: 10.1128/AAC.00249-17

Ajayi, N. A., and Ukwaja, K. N. (2013). Possible artemisinin-based combination therapy-resistant malaria in Nigeria: a report of three cases. *Rev. Soc. Bras. Med. Trop.* 46, 525–527. doi: 10.1590/0037-8682-0098-2013

Alberca, L. N., Sbaraglini, M. L., Balcazar, D., Fraccaroli, L., Carrillo, C., Medeiros, A., et al. (2016). Discovery of novel polyamine analogs with anti-protozoal activity by computer guided drug repositioning. *J. Comput. Aided Mol. Des.* 30, 305–321. doi: 10.1007/s10822-016-9903-6

Alberca, L. N., Sbaraglini, M. L., Morales, J. F., Dietrich, R., Ruiz, M. D., Pino Martínez, A. M., et al. (2018). Cascade ligand- and structure-based virtual screening to identify new trypanocidal compounds inhibiting putrescine uptake. *Front. Cell. Infect. Microbiol.* 8:173. doi: 10.3389/fcimb.2018.00173

Aley, S. B., Sherwood, J. A., Marsh, K., Eidelman, O., and Howard, R. J. (1986). Identification of isolate-specific proteins on sorbitol-enriched *Plasmodium falciparum* infected erythrocytes from Gambian patients. *Parasitology* 92 (Pt 3), 511–525.

Allangba, K. N. P. G., Keita, M., Kre N'Guessan, R., Megnassan, E., Frecer, V., and Miertus, S. (2019). Virtual design of novel *Plasmodium falciparum* cysteine protease falcipain-2 hybrid lactone-chalcone and isatin-chalcone inhibitors probing the S2 active site pocket. *J. Enzyme Inhib. Med. Chem.* 34, 547–561. doi: 10.1080/14756366.2018.1564288

Alvarez, C. L., Schachter, J., de Sa' Pinheiro, A. A., Silva, L., de, S., Verstraeten, S. V., et al. (2014). Regulation of extracellular ATP in human erythrocytes infected with *Plasmodium falciparum*. *PLoS ONE* 9:e96216. doi: 10.1371/journal.pone.0096216

Ang, K. K. H., Ratnam, J., Gut, J., Legac, J., Hansell, E., Mackey, Z. B., et al. (2011). Mining a cathepsin inhibitor library for new antiparasitic drug leads. *PLoS Negl. Trop. Dis.* 5:e1023. doi: 10.1371/journal.pntd.0001023

Balaban, A. T., Ciubotariu, D., and Medeleanu, M. (1991). Topological indices and real number vertex invariants based on graph eigenvalues or eigenvectors. *J. Chem. Inf. Comput. Sci.* 31, 517–523. doi: 10.1021/ci00004a014

Bekono, B. D., Ntie-Kang, F., Owono Owono, L. C., and Megnassan, E. (2018). Targeting cysteine proteases from *Plasmodium falciparum*: a general overview, rational drug design and computational approaches for drug discovery. *Curr. Drug Targets.* 19, 501–526. doi: 10.2174/1389450117666161221122432

Bertoldo, J. B., Chiaradia-Delatorre, L. D., Mascarello, A., Leal, P. C., Cordeiro, M. N., Nunes, R. J., et al. (2015). Synthetic compounds from an in house library as inhibitors of falcipain-2 from *Plasmodium falciparum*. *J. Enzyme Inhib. Med. Chem.* 30, 299–307. doi: 10.3109/14756366.2014.920839

Biot, C., Pradines, B., Sergeant, M. H., Gut, J., Rosenthal, P. J., and Chibale, K. (2007). Design, synthesis, and antimalarial activity of structural chimeras of thiosemicarbazone and ferroquine analogues. *Bioorg. Med. Chem. Lett.* 17, 6434–6438. doi: 10.1016/j.bmcl.2007.10.003

Blat, Y. (2010). Non-competitive inhibition by active site binders. *Chem. Biol. Drug. Des.* 75, 535–540. doi: 10.1111/j.1747-0285.2010.00972.x

Bone, H. G., Dempster, D. W., Eisman, J. A., Greenspan, S. L., McClung, M. R., Nakamura, T., et al. (2015). Odanacatib for the treatment of postmenopausal osteoporosis: development history and design and participant characteristics of LOFT, the Long-Term Odanacatib Fracture Trial. *Osteoporos. Int.* 26, 699–712. doi: 10.1007/s00198-014-2944-6

Briolant, S., Fusaï, T., Rogier, C., and Pradines, B. (2008). Tetracycline antibiotics in malaria. *Open Trop. Med. J.* 1, 31–46. doi: 10.2174/1874315300801010031

Carbonneau, M. A., Granger, E., Raymond, A. J., and Gagnon, G. (2016). Robust multiple-instance learning ensembles using random subspace instance selection. *Pattern Recogn.* 58, 83–99. doi: 10.1016/j.patcog.2016.03.035

Chen, X., Jiang, J., Hu, P., Zajic, S., Liu, W., McCrea, J., et al. (2018). Odanacatib pharmacokinetics comparison between Chinese and non-Chinese postmenopausal women. *Clin. Pharmacol. Drug Dev.* 7, 744–750. doi: 10.1002/cpdd.434

Chi, Z., Liu, R., Yang, H., Shen, H., and Wang, J. (2011). Binding of tetracycline and chlortetracycline to the enzyme trypsin: spectroscopic and molecular modeling investigations. *PLoS ONE* 6:e28361. doi: 10.1371/journal.pone.0028361

Chipeleme, A., Grut, J., Rosenthal, P. J., and Chibale, K. (2007). Synthesis and biological evaluation of phenolic Mannich bases of benzaldehyde and (thio)semicarbazone derivatives against the cysteine protease falcipain-2 and a chloroquine resistant strain of *Plasmodium falciparum*. *Bioorg. Med. Chem.* 15, 273–282. doi: 10.1016/j.bmc.2006.09.055

Chiyanzu, I., Hansell, E., Gut, J., Rosenthal, P. J., McKerrow, J. H., and Chibale, K. (2003). Synthesis and evaluation of isatins and thiosemicarbazone derivatives against cruzain, falcipain-2 and rhodesain. *Bioorg. Med. Chem. Lett.* 13, 3527–3530. doi: 10.1016/S0960-894X(03)00756-X

Conroy, T., Guo, J. T., Elias, N., Cergol, K. M., Gut, J., Legac, J., et al. (2014). Synthesis of gallinamide A analogues as potent falcipain inhibitors and antimalarials. *J. Med. Chem.* 57, 10557–10563. doi: 10.1021/jm501439w

Copeland, R. A. (2003). Mechanistic considerations in high-throughput screening. *Anal. Biochem.* 320, 1–12. doi: 10.1016/S0003-2697(03)00346-4

Copeland, R. A. (2005). Evaluation of enzyme inhibitors in drug discovery. A guide for medicinal chemists and pharmacologists. *Methods Biochem. Anal.* 46, 1–265. doi: 10.1002/9781118540398

Corsello, S. M., Bittker, J. A., Liu, Z., Gould, J., McCarren, P., Hirschman, J. E., et al. (2017). The Drug Repurposing Hub: a next-generation drug library and information resource. *Nat. Med.* 23, 405–408. doi: 10.1038/nm.4306

Desai, P. V., Patny, A., Gut, J., Rosenthal, P. J., Tekwani, B., Srivastava, A., et al. (2006). Identification of novel parasitic cysteine protease inhibitors by use of virtual screening. 2. The available chemical directory. *J. Med. Chem.* 49, 1576–1584. doi: 10.1021/jm0505765

Desai, P. V., Patny, A., Sabnis, Y., Tekwani, B., Gut, J., Rosenthal, P., et al. (2004). Identification of novel parasitic cysteine protease inhibitors using virtual screening. 1. The ChemBridge database. *J. Med. Chem.* 47, 6609–6615. doi: 10.1021/jm0493717

Domínguez, J. N., López, S., Charris, J., Iarruso, L., Lobo, G., Semenov, A., et al. (1997). Synthesis and antimalarial effects of phenothiazine inhibitors of a Plasmodium falciparum cysteine protease. *J. Med. Chem.* 40, 2726–2732. doi: 10.1021/jm970266p

Drake, M. T., Clarke, B. L., Oursler, M. J., and Khosla, S. (2017). Cathepsin K inhibitors for osteoporosis: biology, potential clinical utility, and lessons learned. *Endocr. Rev.* 38, 325–350. doi: 10.1210/er.2015-1114

El Habib Daho, M., and Chikh, M. A. (2015). Combining bootstrapping samples, random subspaces and random forests to build classifiers. *J. Med. Imag. Health Inf.* 5, 539–544. doi: 10.1166/jmihi.2015.1423

Estrada, E. (1996). Spectral moments of the edge adjacency matrix in molecular graphs. 1. Definition and applications to the prediction of physical properties of alkanes. *J. Chem. Inf. Comput. Sci.* 36, 844–849.

Ettari, R., Pinto, A., Tamborini, L., Angelo, I. C., Grasso, S., Zappalà, M., et al. (2014). Synthesis and biological evaluation of papain-family cathepsin L-like cysteine protease inhibitors containing a 1,4-benzodiazepine scaffold as antiprotozoal agents. *ChemMedChem* 9, 1817–1825. doi: 10.1002/cmdc.201402079

Everitt, B. S., Landau, S., Leese, M., and Stahl, D. (2011). *Cluster Analysis, 5th Edn.* West Sussex: Wiley.

Ferreira, L. G., and Andricopulo, A. D. (2016). Drug repositioning approaches to parasitic diseases: a medicinal chemistry perspective. *Drug Discov. Today* 21, 1699–1710. doi: 10.1016/j.drudis.2016.06.021

Fujii, N., Mallari, J. P., Hansell, E. J., Mackey, Z., Doyle, P., Zhou, Y. M., et al. (2005). Discovery of potent thiosemicarbazone inhibitors of rhodesain and cruzain. *Bioorg. Med. Chem. Lett.* 15, 121–123. doi: 10.1016/j.bmcl.2004.10.023

Gaillard, T., Madamet, M., and Pradines, B. (2015). Tetracyclines in malaria. *Malar. J.* 14:445. doi: 10.1186/s12936-015-0980-0

Gantner, M. E., Peroni, R. N., Morales, J. F., Villalba, M. L., Ruiz, M. E., and Talevi, A. (2017). Development and validation of a computational model ensemble for the early detection of BCRP/ABCG2 substrates during the drug design stage. *J. Chem. Inf. Model.* 57, 1868–1880. doi: 10.1021/acs.jcim.7b00016

Gauthier, J. Y., Chauret, N., Cromlish, W., Desmarais, S., Duong, L. T., Falgueyret, J. P., et al. (2008). The discovery of odanacatib (MK-0822), a selective inhibitor of cathepsine K. *Bioorg. Med. Chem. Lett.* 18, 923–928. doi: 10.1016/j.bmcl.2007.12.047

Golbraikh, A., Shen, M., Xiao, Z., Xiao, Y. D., Lee, K. H., and Tropsha, A. (2003). Rational selection of training and test sets for the development of validated QSAR models. *J. Comput. Aided Mol. Des.* 17, 241–253. doi: 10.1023/A:1025386326946

Goud, P. M., Sheri, A., Desai, P. V., Watkins, E. B., Tekwani, B., Sabnis, Y., et al. (2005). Design, synthesis and evaluation of trisubstituted thiazoles targeting Plasmodium falciparum cysteine proteases. *Med. Chem. Res.* 14, 74–105. doi: 10.1007/s00044-005-0126-y

Gramatica, P. (2013). On the development and validation of QSAR models. *Methods Mol. Biol.* 930, 499–526. doi: 10.1007/978-1-62703-059-5_21

Greenbaum, D. C., Mackey, Z., Hansell, E., Doyle, P., Gut, J., Caffrey, C. R., et al. (2004). Synthesis and structure-activity relationships of parasiticidal thiosemicarbazone cysteine protease inhibitors against *Plasmodium falciparum*, *Trypanosoma brucei*, and *Trypanosoma cruzi*. *J. Med. Chem.* 47, 3212–3219. doi: 10.1021/jm030549j

Hans, R. H., Guantai, E. M., Lategan, C., Smith, P. J., Wan, B., Franzblau, S. G., et al. (2010). Synthesis, antimalarial and antitubercular activity of acetylenic chalcones. *Bioorg. Med. Chem. Lett.* 20, 942–944. doi: 10.1016/j.bmcl.2009.12.062

Hogg, T., Nagarajan, K., Herzberg, S., Chen, L., Shen, X., Jiang, H., et al. (2006). Structural and functional characterization of Falcipain-2, a hemoglobinase from the malarial parasite *Plasmodium falciparum*. *J. Biol. Chem.* 281, 25425–25437. doi: 10.1074/jbc.M603776200

Huang, H., Lu, W., Li, X., Cong, X., Ma, H., Liu, X., et al. (2012). Design and synthesis of small molecular dual inhibitor of falcipain-2 and dihydrofolate reductase as antimalarial agent. *Bioorg. Med. Chem. Lett.* 22, 958–962. doi: 10.1016/j.bmcl.2011.12.011

Jadhav, A., Ferreira, R. S., Kulmpp, C., Mott, B. T., Austin, C. P., Inglese, J., et al. (2010). Quantitative analyses of aggregation, autofluorescence, and reactivity artifacts in a screen for inhibitors of a thiol protease. *J. Med. Chem.* 53, 37–51. doi: 10.1021/jm901070c

Jin, G., and Wong, S. T. C. (2015). Toward better drug repositioning: prioritizing and integrating existing methods into efficient pipelines. *Drug Discov. Today* 19, 637–644. doi: 10.1016/j.drudis.2013.11.005

Jin, H., Xu, Z., Cui, K., Zhang, T., Lu, W., and Huang, J. (2014). Dietary flavonoids fisetin and myricetin: dual inhibitors of *Plasmodium falciparum* falcipain-2 and plasmepsin II. *Fitoterapia* 94, 55–61. doi: 10.1016/j.fitote.2014.01.017

Kassahun, K., McIntosh, I., Koeplinger, K., Sun, L., Talaty, J. E., Miller, D. L., et al. (2014). Disposition and metabolism of the cathepsin K inhibitor odanacatib in humans. *Drug. Metab. Dispos.* 42, 818–827. doi: 10.1124/dmd.113.056580

Kerr, I. D., Lee, J. H., Pandey, K. C., Harrison, A., Sajid, M., Rosenthal, P. J., et al. (2009). Structures of falcipain-2 and falcipain-3 bound to small molecule inhibitors: implications for substrate specificity. *J. Med. Chem.* 52, 852–857. doi: 10.1021/jm8013663

Kisinza, W. N., Nkya, T. E., Kabula, B., Overgaard, H. J., Massue, D. J., Mageni, Z., et al. (2017). Multiple insecticide resistance in *Anopheles gambiae* from Tanzania: a major concern for malaria vector control. *Malar. J.* 16, 439. doi: 10.1186/s12936-017-2087-2

Krishnaswamy, S., and Betz, A. (1997). Exosites determine macromolecular substrate recognition by prothrombinase. *Biochemistry* 36, 12080–12086.

Lätti, S., Niinivehmas, S., and Pentikäinen, O. T. (2016). Rocker: Open source, easy-to-use tool for AUC and enrichment calculations and ROC visualization. *J. Cheminform.* 8:45. doi: 10.1186/s13321-016-0158-y

Lauria, A., Tutone, M., and Almerico, A. M. (2011). Virtual lock-and-key approach: the *in silico* revival of Fischer model by means of molecular descriptors. *Eur. J. Med. Chem.* 46, 4274–4280. doi: 10.1016/j.ejmech.2011.06.033

Lauria, A., Tutone, M., Barone, G., and Almerico, A. M. (2014). Multivariate analysis in the identification of biological targets for designed molecular structures: the BIOTA protocol. *Eur. J. Med. Chem.* 75, 106–110. doi: 10.1016/j.ejmech.2014.01.025

Law, V., Knox, C., Djoumbou, Y., Jewison, T., Guo, A. C., Liu, Y., et al. (2014). DrugBank 4.0: shedding new light on drug metabolism. *Nucleic Acids Res.* 42, 1091–1097. doi: 10.1093/nar/gkt1068

Leonard, J. T., and Roy, K. (2006). On selection of training and test sets for the development of predictive QSAR models. *QSAR Comb. Sci.* 25, 235–251. doi: 10.1002/qsar.200510161

Li, H., Huang, J., Chen, L., Liu, X., Chen, T., Zhu, J., et al. (2009). Identification of novel falcipain-2 inhibitors as potential antimalarial agents through structure-based virtual screening. *J.Chem. Eng. Data* 63, 4735–4470. doi: 10.1021/jm801622x

Liu, W., Lu, H., Cao, C., Jiao, Y., and Chen, G. (2018). An improved Quantitative Structure Property Relationship model for predicting thermal conductivity of liquid aliphatic alcohols. *J. Chem. Eng. Data* 63, 4735–4740. doi: 10.1021/acs.jced.8b00764

Luo, W., Lu, W., Cui, K., Liu, Y., Wang, J., and Guo, C. (2012). N1-{4-[(10S)-Dihydroartemisinin-10-oxyl]}phenylmethylene-N2-(2-methylquinoline-4-yl)hydrazine derivatives as antiplasmodial falcipain-2 inhibitors. *Med. Chem. Res.* 21, 3073–3079. doi: 10.1007/s00044-011-9854-3

Marco, M., and Coterón, J. M. (2012). Falcipain inhibition as a promising antimalarial target. *Curr. Top. Med. Chem.* 12, 408–444. doi: 10.2174/156802612799362913

Marques, A. F., Esser, D., Rosenthal, P. J., Kassack, M. U., and Lima, L. M. (2013). Falcipain-2 inhibition by suramin and suramin analogues. *Bioorg. Med. Chem.* 21, 3667–3673. doi: 10.1016/j.bmc.2013.04.047

Marques, A. F., Gomes, P. S., Oliveira, P. L., Rosenthal, P. J., Pascutti, P. G., and Lima, L. M. (2015). Allosteric regulation of the *Plasmodium falciparum* cysteine protease falcipain-2 by heme. *Arch. Biochem. Biophys.* 573, 92–99. doi: 10.1016/j.abb.2015.03.007

Martin, T. M., Harten, P., Young, D. M., Muratov, E. N., Golbraikh, A., Zhu, H., et al. (2012). Does rational selection of training and test sets improve the outcome of QSAR modeling? *J. Chem. Inf. Model.* 52, 2570–2578. doi: 10.1021/ci300338w

Mercurio, A., Adriani, G., Catalano, A., Carocci, A., Rao, L., Lentini, G., et al. (2017). A mini-review on thalidomide: chemistry, mechanisms of action, therapeutic potential and anti-angiogenic properties in multiple myeloma. *Curr. Med. Chem.* 24, 2736–2744. doi: 10.2174/0929867324666170601074646

Micale, N., Kozikowski, A. P., Ettari, R., Grasso, S., Zappalà, M., Jeong, J. J., et al. (2006). Novel peptidomimetic cysteine protease inhibitors as potential antimalarial agents. *J. Med. Chem.* 49, 3064–3067. doi: 10.1021/jm060405f

Min, S. H. (2016). A genetic algorithm-based heterogeneous random subspace ensemble model for bankruptcy prediction. *Int. J. Appl. Eng. Res.* 11, 2927–2931.

Morrison, J. F. (1969). Kinetics of the reversible inhibition of enzyme-catalysed reactions by tight-binding inhibitors. *Biochim. Biophys. Acta* 185, 269–286. doi: 10.1016/0005-2744(69)90420-3

Mugumbate, G., Newton, A. S., Rosenthal, P. J., Gut, J., Moreira, R., Chibale, K., et al. (2013). Novel anti-plasmodial hits identified by virtual screening of the ZINC database. *J. Comput. Aided Mol. Des.* 27, 859–871. doi: 10.1007/s10822-013-9685-z

Mundra, S., and Radhakrishnan, M. (2015a). Insignificant *in vitro* falcipain-2 inhibitory activity of novel 2-(4-(substituted benzoyl) piperazine-1-yl)-N-phenylacetamide derivatives. *J. Pharm. Negative Results* 6, 20–26. doi: 10.4103/0976-9234.157381

Mundra, S., and Radhakrishnan, M. (2015b). Evaluation of novel 1-(4-(substituted)piperazin-1-yl)- 2-(phenylamino)ethanone derivatives as Falcipain-2 inhibitors. *J. Young Pharm.* 7, 96–105. doi: 10.5530/jyp.2015.2.7

Mysinger, M. M., Carchia, M., Irwin, J. J., and Shoichet, B. K. (2012). Directory of useful decoys, enhanced (DUD-E): better ligands and decoys for better benchmarking. *J. Med. Chem.* 55, 6582–6594. doi: 10.1021/jm300687e

Nizi, E., Sferrazza, A., Fabbrini, D., Nardi, V., Andreini, M., Graziani, R., et al. (2018). Peptidomimetic nitrile inhibitors of malarial protease falcipain-2 with high selectivity against human cathepsins. *Bioorg. Med. Chem. Lett.* 28, 1540–1544. doi: 10.1016/j.bmcl.2018.03.069

Novick, P. A., Ortiz, O. F., Poelman, J., Abdulhay, A. Y., and Pande, V. S. (2013). SWEETLEAD: an *in silico* database of approved drugs, regulated chemicals, and herbal isolates for computer-aided drug discovery. *PLoS ONE* 8:e79568. doi: 10.1371/journal.pone.0079568

Oballa, R. M., Truchon, J. F., Baily, C. I., Chauret, N., Day, S., Crane, S., et al. (2007). A generally applicable method for assessing the electrophilicity and reactivity of diverse nitrile-containing compounds. *Bioorg. Med. Chem. Lett.* 17, 998–1002. doi: 10.1016/j.bmcl.2006.11.044

Pandey, K. C., Wang, S. X., Sijwali, P. S., Lau, A. L., McKerrow, J. H., and Rosenthal, P. J. (2005). The *Plasmodium falciparum* cysteine protease falcipain-2 captures its substrate, hemoglobin, via a unique motif. *Proc. Natl. Acad. Sci. U.S.A.* 102, 9138–9143. doi: 10.1073/pnas.0502368102

Pant, A., Kumar, R., Wani, N. A., Verma, S., Sharma, R., Pande, V., et al. (2018). Allosteric site inhibitor disrupting auto-processing of malarial cysteine proteases. *Sci. Rep.* 8, 16193. doi: 10.1038/s41598-018-34564-8

Pedicord, D. L., Seiffert, D., and Blat, Y. (2004). Substrate-dependent modulation of the mechanism of factor XIa inhibition. *Biochemistry* 43, 11883–11888. doi: 10.1021/bi048964g

Perez-Llamas, C., and Lopez-Bigas, N. (2011). Gitools: analysis and visualisation of genomic data using interactive heat-maps. *PLoS ONE* 6:e19541. doi: 10.1371/journal.pone.0019541

Potshangbam, A. M., Tanneeru, K., Reddy, B. M., and Guruprasad, L. (2011). 3D-QSAR and molecular docking studies of 2-pyrimidinecarbonitrile derivatives as inhibitors against falcipain-3. *Bioorg. Med. Chem. Lett.* 21, 7219–7223. doi: 10.1016/j.bmcl.2011.09.107

Pradines, B., Rogier, C., Fusai, T., Mosnier, J., Daries, W., Barret, E., et al. (2001). *In vitro* activities of antibiotics against *Plasmodium falciparum* are inhibited by iron. *Antimicrob. Agents Chemother.* 2001, 45, 1746–1750. doi: 10.1128/AAC.45.6.1746-1750.2001

Praveen Kumar, S., Gut, J., Guedes, R. C., Rosenthal, P. J., Santos, M. M., and Moreira, R. (2011). Design, synthesis and evaluation of 3-methylene-substituted indolinones as antimalarials. *Eur. J. Med. Chem.* 46, 927–933. doi: 10.1016/j.ejmech.2011.01.008

Reutlinger, M., Koch, C. P., Reker,. D., Todoroff, N., Schneider, P., Rodrigues, T., et al. (2013). Chemically Advanced Template Search (CATS) for scaffold-hopping and prospective target prediction for 'orphan' molecules. *Mol. Inform.* 32, 133–138. doi: 10.1002/minf.201200141

Ritchie, H., and Roser, M. (2018). *Causes of Death*. OurWorldInData.org [Online]. Available online at: https://ourworldindata.org/causes-of-death (accessed August, 2018).

Robin, X., Turck, N., Hainard, A., Tiberti, N., Lisacek, F., Sanchez, J. C., et al. (2011). pROC: an open-source package for R and S+ to analyze and compare ROC curves. *BMC Bioinformatics* 12:77. doi: 10.1186/1471-2105-12-77

Roy, K., and Mitra, I. (2011). On various metrics used for validation of predictive QSAR models with applications in virtual screening and focused library design. *Comb Chem. High Throughput Screen* 14, 450–474.

Sanchez Mejia, R. O., Ona, V. O., Li, M., and Friedlander, R. M. (2001). Minocycline reduces traumatic brain injury-mediated caspase-1 activation, Tissue damage, and neurological dysfunction. *Neurosurgery* 48, 1393–1401. doi: 10.1097/00006123-200106000-00051

Satimai, W., Sudathip, P., Vijaykadga, S., Khamsiriwatchara, A., Sawang, S., Potithavoranan, T., et al. (2012). Artemisinin resistance containment project in Thailand. II: responses to mefloquine-artesunate combination therapy among falciparum malaria patients in provinces bordering Cambodia. *Malar. J.* 11:300. doi: 10.1186/1475-2875-11-300

Schmidt, I., Pradel, G., Sologub, L., Golzmann, A., Ngwa, C. J., Kucharski, A., et al. (2016). Bistacrine derivatives as new potent antimalarials. *Bioorg. Med. Chem.* 24, 3636–3642. doi: 10.1016/j.bmc.2016.06.003

Selwyn, M. J. (1965). A simple test for inactivation of an enzyme during assay. *Biochim. Biophys. Acta* 105, 193–195. doi: 10.1016/S0926-6593(65)80190-4

Shah, F., Mukherjee, P., Gut, J., Legac, J., Rosenthal, P. J., Tekwani, B. L., et al. (2011). Identification of novel malarial cysteine protease inhibitors using structure-based virtual screening of a focused cysteine protease inhibitor library. *J. Chem. Inf. Model.* 51, 852–864. doi: 10.1021/ci200029y

Sharma, R. K., Younis, Y., Mugumbate, G., Njoroge, M., Gut, J., Rosenthal, P. J., et al. (2015). Synthesis and structure-activity-relationship studies of thiazolidinediones as antiplasmodial inhibitors of the *Plasmodium falciparum* cysteine protease falcipain-2. *Eur. J. Med. Chem.* 90, 507–518. doi: 10.1016/j.ejmech.2014.11.061

Shenai, B. R., Lee, B. J., Alvarez-Hernandez, A., Chong, P. Y., Emal, C. D., Neitz, R. J., et al. (2003). Structure-activity relationships for inhibition of cysteine protease activity and development of *Plasmodium falciparum* by peptidyl vinyl sulfones. *Antimicrob. Agents Chemother.* 47, 154–160. doi: 10.1128/aac.47.1.154-160.2003

Singh, A. K., Rajendran, V., Pant, A., Ghosh, P. C., Singh, N., Latha, N., et al. (2015). Design, synthesis and biological evaluation of functionalized phthalimides: a new class of antimalarials and inhibitors of falcipain-2, a major hemoglobinase of malaria parasite. *Bioorg. Med. Chem.* 23, 1817–1827. doi: 10.1016/j.bmc.2015.02.029

Stoye, A., Juillard, A., Tang, A. H., Legac, J., Gut, J., White, K. L., et al. (2019). Falcipain inhibitors based on the natural product gallinamide a are potent *in vitro* and *in vivo* antimalarials. *J. Med. Chem.* 62, 5562–5578. doi: 10.1021/acs.jmedchem.9b00504

Subramanian, S., Hardt, M., Choe, Y., Niles, R. K., Johansen, E. B., Legac, J., et al. (2009). Hemoglobin cleavage site-specificity of the *Plasmodium falciparum* cysteine proteases falcipain-2 and falcipain-3. *PLoS ONE* 4:e5156. doi: 10.1371/journal.pone.0005156

Talevi, A. (2018). Drug repositioning: current approaches and their implications in the precision medicine era. *Expert. Rev. Precis. Med. Drug Dev.* 3, 49–61. doi: 10.1080/23808993.2018.1424535

Teixeira, C., Gomes, J. R. B., Couesnon, T., and Gomes, P. (2011). Molecular docking and 3D-quantitative structure activity relationship analyses of peptidyl vinyl sulfones: *Plasmodium falciparum* cysteine proteases inhibitors. *J. Comput. Aided Mol. Des.* 25, 763–775. doi: 10.1007/s10822-011-9459-4

Teo, S., Resztak, K. E., Scheffler, M. A., Kook, K. A., Zeldis, J. B., Stirling, D. I., et al. (2002). Thalidomide in the treatment of leprosy. *Microbes Infect.* 4, 1193–1202. doi: 10.1016/S1286-4579(02)01645-3

Thorne, N., Auld, D. S., and Inglese, J. (2010). Apparent activity in high-throughput screening: origins of compound-dependent assay interference. *Curr. Opin. Chem. Biol.* 14, 315–324. doi: 10.1016/j.cbpa.2010.03.020

Toropova, A. P., and Toropov, A. A. (2017). CORAL: binary classifications (active/inactive) for drug-induced liver injury. *Toxicol. Lett.* 268, 51–57. doi: 10.1016/j.toxlet.2017.01.011

Truchon, J. F., and Bayly, C. L. (2007). Evaluating virtual screening methods: good and bad metrics for the "early recognition" problem. *J. Chem. Inf. Model.* 47, 488–508. doi: 10.1021/ci600426e

Tutone, M., Perricone, U., and Almerico, A. M. (2017). Conf-VLKA: a structure-based revisitation of the Virtual Lock-and-key Approach. *J. Mol. Graph. Model.* 71, 50–57. doi: 10.1016/j.jmgm.2016.11.006.

Valente, C., Guedes, R. C., Moreira, R., Iley, J., Gut, J., and Rosenthal, P. J. (2006). Dipeptide vinyl sultams: synthesis via the Wittig-Horner reaction and activity against papain, falcipain-2 and *Plasmodium falciparum*. *Bioorg. Med. Chem. Lett.* 16, 4115–4119. doi: 10.1016/j.bmcl.2006.04.079

Volkamer, A., Kuhn, D., Rippmann, F., and Rarey, M. (2012). DoGSiteScorer: a web server for automatic binding site prediction, analysis and druggability assessment. *Bioinformatics* 28, 2074–2075. doi: 10.1093/bioinformatics/bts310

Wang, J., Li, F., Li, Y., Yang, Y., Zhang, S., and Yang, L. (2013). Structural features of falcipain-3 inhibitors: an *in silico* study. *Mol. Biosyst.* 9, 2296–2310. doi: 10.1039/c3mb70105k

Wang, L., Zhang, S., Zhu, J., Zhu, L., Liu, X., Shan, L., et al. (2014). Identification of diverse natural products as falcipain-2 inhibitors through structure-based virtual screening. *Bioorg. Med. Chem. Lett.* 24, 1261–1264. doi: 10.1016/j.bmcl.2014.01.074

Wang, S. X., Pandey, K. C., Somoza, J. R., Sijwali, P. S., Kortemme, T., Brinen, L. S., et al. (2006). Structural basis for unique mechanisms of folding and hemoglobin binding by a malarial protease. *Proc. Natl. Acad. Sci. U.S.A.* 103, 11503–11508. doi: 10.1073/pnas.0600489103

Weldon, D. J., Shah, F., Chittiboyina, A. G., Sheri, A., Chada, R. R., Gut, J., et al. (2014). Synthesis, biological evaluation, hydration site thermodynamics, and chemical reactivity analysis of α-keto substituted peptidomimetics for the inhibition of *Plasmodium falciparum*. *Bioorg. Med. Chem. Lett.* 24, 1274–1279. doi: 10.1016/j.bmcl.2014.01.062

World Health Organization (WHO) (2017). *World Malaria Report 2017*. Geneva. Available online at: http://www.who.int/malaria/publications/world-malaria-report-2017/en/ (accessed August 2018).

Xue, C. X., Cui, S. Y., Liu, M. C., Hu, Z. D., and Fan, B. T. (2004). 3D QSAR studies on antimalarial alkoxylated and hydroxylated chalcones by CoMFA and CoMSIA. *Eur. J. Med. Chem.* 39, 745–753. doi: 10.1016/j.ejmech.2004.05.009

Yabuuchi, H., Niijima, S., Takematsu, H., Ida, T., Hirokawa, T., Hara, T., et al. (2011). Analysis of multiple compound–protein interactions reveals novel bioactive molecules. *Mol. Syst. Biol.* 7, 472. doi: 10.1038/msb.2011.5

Yang, J., Copeland, R. A., and Lai, Z. (2009). Defining balanced conditions for inhibitor screening assays that target bisubstrate enzymes. *J. Biomol. Screen.* 14, 111–120. doi: 10.1177/1087057108328763

Yella, J. K., Yaddanapudi, S., Wang, Y., and Jegga, A. G. (2018). Changing trends in computational drug repositioning. *Pharmaceuticals* 11:57. doi: 10.3390/ph11020057

Yu, G., Zhang, G., Domeniconi, C., Yu, Z., and You, J. (2012). Semi-supervised classification based on random subspace dimensionality reduction. *Pattern Recogn.* 45, 1119–1135. doi: 10.1016/j.patcog.2011.08.024

Zhang, Q., and Muegge, I. (2006). Scaffold hopping through virtual screening using 2D and 3D similarity descriptors: ranking, voting, and consensus scoring. *J. Med. Chem.* 49, 1536–1548. doi: 10.1021/jm050468i

Zucker, S., Lysik, R. M., Ramamurthy, N. S., Golub, L. M., Wieman, J. M., and Wilkie, D. P. (1985). Diversity of melanoma plasma membrane proteinases: inhibition of collagenolytic and cytolytic activities by minocycline. *J. Natl. Cancer Inst.* 75, 517–525. doi: 10.1093/jnci/75.3.517

4

A Definition of "Multitargeticity": Identifying Potential Multitarget and Selective Ligands Through a Vector Analysis

Juan Francisco Sánchez-Tejeda[1], *Juan F. Sánchez-Ruiz*[2], *Juan Rodrigo Salazar*[1] *and Marco A. Loza-Mejía*[1*]

[1] *Facultad de Ciencias Químicas, Universidad La Salle, Mexico City, Mexico,* [2] *Ciencia y Estrategia S.A. de C.V., Mexico City, Mexico*

***Correspondence:**
Marco A. Loza-Mejía
marcoantonio.loza@lasalle.mx

The design of multitarget drugs is an essential area of research in Medicinal Chemistry since they have been proposed as potential therapeutics for the management of complex diseases. However, defining a multitarget drug is not an easy task. In this work, we propose a vector analysis for measuring and defining "multitargeticity." We developed terms, such as order and force of a ligand, to finally reach two parameters: multitarget indexes 1 and 2. The combination of these two indexes allows discrimination of multitarget drugs. Several training sets were constructed to test the usefulness of the indexes: an experimental training set, with real affinities, a docking training set, within theoretical values, and an extensive database training set. The indexes proved to be useful, as they were used independently *in silico* and experimental data, identifying actual multitarget compounds and even selective ligands in most of the training sets. We then applied these indexes to evaluate a virtual library of potential ligands for targets related to multiple sclerosis, identifying 10 compounds that are likely leads for the development of multitarget drugs based on their *in silico* behavior. With this work, a new milestone is made in the way of defining multitargeticity and in drug design.

Keywords: multitarget drugs, drug discovery, drug-design, multitarget index, multiple sclerosis, polypharmacology

INTRODUCTION

In the field of polypharmacology, combinatorial therapies and multitarget drugs are the main alternatives for dealing with complex diseases. The first one consists of a combination of multiple single-targeted drugs. On the other hand, multitarget drugs are molecules with the ability to act on different targets at the same time. Designing multitarget drugs is a problematic task; however, it solves several concerns that are seen in combinatorial therapies, such as complex therapeutic regimens, difficulty in including numerous drugs in a single formulation and drug interactions at the different pharmacokinetics levels: absorption, distribution, metabolism, and elimination (Rosini, 2014). In the last two decades, the number of multitarget drugs on the market has been rising. From 2015 to 2017, 21% of the drugs approved by the Food and Drug Administration (FDA) were multitarget drugs (MTD), primarily antineoplastic agents (Ramsay et al., 2018). This trend may indicate that the number of multitarget drugs will continue to rise since they present advantages over single-target drugs. For example, MTDs have higher *in vivo* efficacy, and several *in silico* methods and strategies for designing them are currently being developed (Zhang et al., 2017). A common strategy is to combine two pharmacophores in the same molecule or partially overlap them, allowing binding to two or more targets (Talevi, 2015).

Binding to two or more targets at the same time offers the possibility of treating multifactorial diseases. Neurodegenerative diseases are a potential field for multitarget drugs. For example, ladostigil is a dual cholinesterase–monoamine oxidase-B (MAO-B) inhibitor currently being researched for the treatment of Alzheimer's disease and other neurodegenerative diseases (van der Schyf, 2011). Cancer is another relatively emergent field for multitarget drugs, mainly as more druggable targets are being discovered. The use of multitarget drugs is promising as it lowers the possibility of the disease to evolve into a drug-resistant phenotype (Xie and Bourne, 2015). Currently, several anti-cancer drugs are considered multitarget drugs since they inhibit two or more kinases or receptors (Lu et al., 2012). Another example is in the field of microbiology, in which dual ligands can be used to treat tuberculosis. This dual mechanism of action is useful in treating multidrug-resistant *Mycobacterium tuberculosis* (Chiarelli et al., 2018).

One of the limitations that multitarget drug design faces is data analysis. In some cases, the number of targets or compounds being analyzed can be high. In PubChem, 71,303 molecules have been identified as ligands that have two or more biological targets, and more than 30,000 ligands were found to be active against more than 400 targets (Hu et al., 2014). Quantifying and defining "multitargeticity" may be useful for analyzing these datasets. Additionally, multitarget metrics could help multitarget drug design by providing comparable and workable parameters for drugs and ligands.

To the best of our knowledge, there is no current measurement of "multitargeticity," i.e., how multitargeted a ligand is. Construction of a multitarget parameter should not be based only on the simple average of the *in silico* or experimental data; for example, highly selective ligands to a single target would appear as multitarget drugs, since the average is a measure sensitive to extreme values. With this in mind, our research group suggested the use of a virtual multitarget parameter, which consisted of a weighted average of the docking scores of potential biopesticides (Loza-Mejía et al., 2018). This analysis proved useful for comparing a ligand's "multitargeticity." However, a more rigid index may help even further in multitarget drug design.

Originally, this project started with the purpose of designing dual ligands. We designed 211 ligands, and we wanted a parameter that could summarize or identify the ligands that had the most potency toward the two targets (the nature of the ligands and the targets will be explained later). To analyze the data, we plotted the docking score of the ligands of one target against the docking score of the second one. In this plot (**Figure 1**), a ligand can be described by the coordinates or docking scores of both targets. Since they are coordinates, the ligand describes an *arrow* or vector, starting from the origin. The angle described by the vector is the selectivity; in fact, the formula of the tangent is the formula for selectivity (Equation 1).

$$\tan\alpha = \frac{\textit{Target \#2 ligand's affinity}}{\textit{Target \#1 ligand's affinity}} \tag{1}$$

Moreover, the magnitude of the vector is likely related to how potent the ligand is. Greater affinities reflect greater magnitudes. With the graph (**Figure 1**), there is a sense of what a multitarget drug would be: one that equally distributes its magnitude among the two targets. In other words, a ligand that had the same affinity for both targets. Measuring the multitargeticity of a dual ligand can be as simple as obtaining the tangent of the angle (Equation 1). If the tangent equals 1 ($\alpha = 45°$), then mathematically, the ligand attacks both targets with the same "strength." However, this interpretation was meant for more targets. In these scenarios, a single parameter for defining multitargeticity would not suffice because more angles are involved.

A radial plot was considered to extend the analysis to further dimensions (**Figure 1**). The central idea was kept: **a** multitarget ligand would equally distribute its *strength* among all the targets. In the radial representation, a multitarget drug would appear as a regular polygon, and the area could be considered the magnitude or strength of the ligand. Multitargeticity could be defined by the similarity between the figure described by the ligand and a regular polygon. We calculated some parameters that could be used to describe this relationship and therefore give a quantitative definition of multitargeticity. However, the area and shape are sensible to the order in which the targets are analyzed. A different order would give a completely different value, as shown in **Figure 1**.

The solution was to treat ligands as vectors and extend the analysis to further dimensions, even if it cannot be visualized. With two targets, an ideal multitarget drug is a vector that makes a perfect square in a 2D plane. In 3 dimensions, a cube would be the shape of an ideal multitarget ligand. Therefore, a hypercube is the central analysis of this interpretation. In contrast, a different distribution of affinities would produce the shape of a rectangle, rectangular cuboid, or hyperrectangle, depending on the number of targets analyzed. Measuring the similarity between the hyperrectangle and a hypercube is, in fact, a measure of multitargeticity, which is only a mathematical definition of how much a ligand equally distributes its *strength* among all the targets. With this analysis, another step was made toward defining and measuring multitargeticity.

One of the several complex diseases that can be treated with a multitarget drug approach is multiple sclerosis (MS). MS is a disease that affects the central nervous system. Currently, MS is the neurological disease with the highest incidence; in 2013, ~2.3 million people were estimated to have MS (Browne et al., 2014). The pathophysiology of the disease is based on the demyelination of axons, primarily due to the loss of oligodendrocytes, cells responsible for maintaining the myelin sheaths around them (Dobson and Giovannoni, 2019). Although the exact origin of MS is not known, it is well-established that it causes damage to the myelin sheath. Depending on the type of MS and the damage

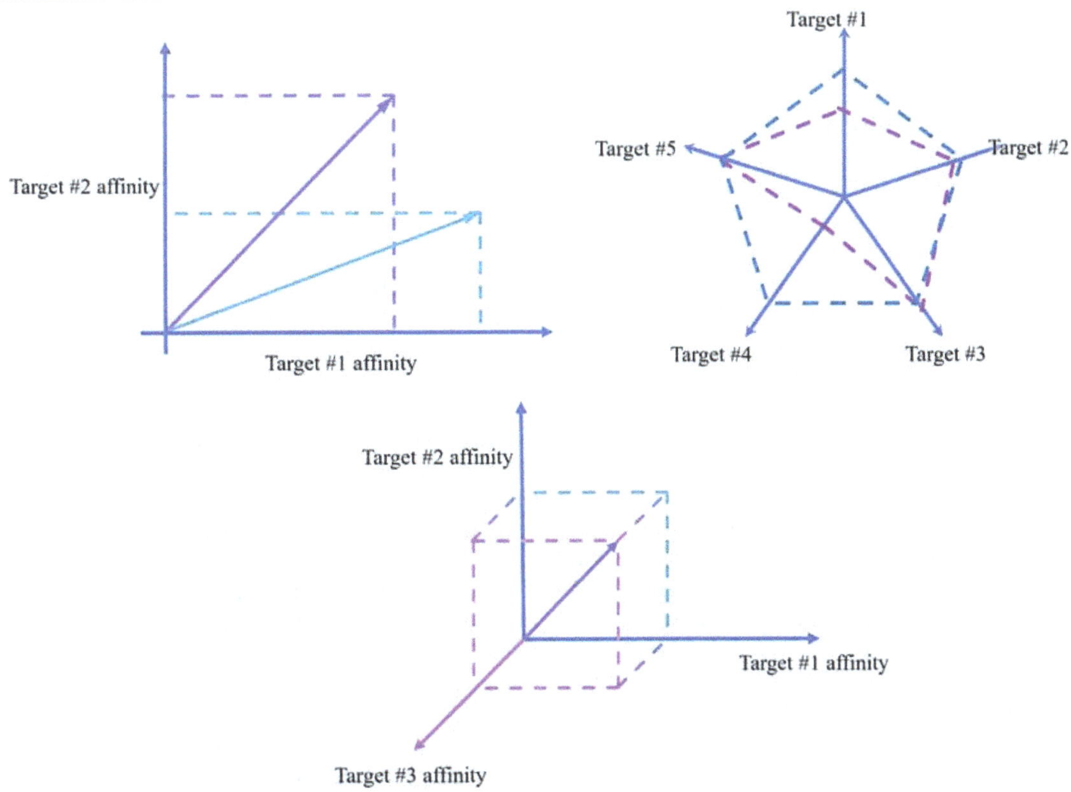

FIGURE 1 | Plotting the ligands' affinities in a dispersion plot describe vectors in a 2D space. For further targets, in a radial plot, an ideal multitarget would describe a regular polygon. Measuring the area of these polygons is influenced by the order in which the targets are plotted. A hypercube is not affected by ordering and therefore makes an ideal representation of what a multitarget ligand would be.

present, the slow transmission of electronic impulses may lead to axon loss, consequently damaging the optic nerve and leading to degeneration of vision, weakness, atrophy, and muscular rigidity, coordination and balance failures, recurrent fatigue, dysphagia, depression, and anxiety, among other symptoms (Huang et al., 2017). PAR-1 and KLK-6 are two molecules of biological interest as possible targets for MS treatment due to their role in oligodendrogliopathy and autoimmune response (Burda et al., 2013). PAR-1 is a protease-activated receptor involved in coagulation, angiogenesis, proinflammatory responses, oligodendrocyte death, and myelination (Macfarlane et al., 2001; Yoon et al., 2015; Pan et al., 2016; Lee et al., 2017). Antagonists of PAR-1 have been shown to reduce the symptoms of experimental autoimmune encephalomyelitis (EAE), which is the most studied animal model for MS (Kim et al., 2015). Kallikrein 6 (KLK-6) is the most abundant serine protease in the central nervous system (CNS) and has proteolytic activity against myelin basic protein (MBP) and amyloid precursor protein, which are part of the myelin sheath and are involved in myelination (Burda et al., 2013; Yoon and Scarisbrick, 2016). KLK-6 is also involved in T-cell survival and apoptotic signalizing (Scarisbrick et al., 2011).

Additionally, recently, a new drug for secondary progressive MS was approved by the FDA: siponimod, which is sold under the trade name Mayzent®. Siponimod is a dual drug itself: it binds to sphingosine-1-phosphate receptor 1 and 5 (S1PR1 and S1PR5) (O'Sullivan et al., 2016). Siponimod reduces oligodendrocyte death and demyelination, acting as an effective neuroprotective agent (Behrangi et al., 2019). S1PR1 is involved in regulating the inflammatory response and therefore is of interest as a third biological target (Chi and Nicol, 2010).

In this work, we present the construction of multitarget indexes as parameters that can define multitargeticity, their evaluation on several datasets, and their use in identifying potential multitarget ligands for PAR-1, KLK-6, and S1PR1.

MATERIALS AND METHODS

Construction of an Experimental Training Set: Multi-Kinase Ligands

We selected 10 known FDA-approved drugs labeled multikinase-directed drugs as models of multitarget drugs (Li et al., 2016). Additionally, two non-multikinase drugs were included as negative controls. The binding affinity (defined in terms of K_i) of each drug to its target was searched in the Binding DB (Gilson et al., 2016). The targets of each ligand were selected according to the FDA approved information. For the negative controls, tyrosine-protein kinase ABL1 was included in the analysis. The K_i was transformed into pM units and linearized. The objective of this analysis was to test if the multitarget index could correctly classify drugs using experimental values. The analysis was done, as stated in section Construction of the Multitarget Index.

Construction of a Docking Training Set: Multi-Kinase Ligands

We selected 10 known FDA-approved drugs labeled multikinase-directed drugs as models of multitarget drugs (Li et al., 2016). The full list of the drugs we considered can be found in the **Supplementary Information**. Three non-multikinase drugs were also included as negative controls. The 13 ligands were docked on the tyrosine-protein kinase KIT (PDB id: 4HVS), vascular endothelial growth factor receptor 2 (PDB id: 3VO3) and platelet-derived growth factor receptor beta (PDB id: 1SHA). The docking studies were carried out in Molegro Virtual Docker version 6.0 using the standard protocol suggested by the manufacturer. All waters, cofactors, and non-active ligands were removed from the workspace. MolDock optimizer was used as the running algorithm with 25 runs per ligand. A sphere with a radius of 15 Å was constructed around the active sites of the three proteins and selected as the search site. The poses with the lowest MolDock score were used for further analysis. The objective of this analysis was to determine if the multitarget index could correctly classify drugs using theoretical values. The data were processed, as stated in section Construction of the Multitarget Index.

Construction of an Experimental Evaluation Set: DUD

We downloaded the database of DUD (Directory of Useful Decoys; Huang et al., 2006), containing the energy scores of nearly 98258 molecules against 40 targets; some targets had a smaller number of calculated energies but were included in the analysis, as this would challenge the indexes. The package was cleaned so that only the negative energies of each ligand were analyzed. The objective of this analysis was to determine if the multitarget index could filter an extensive database. The data were processed, as stated in section Construction of the Multitarget Index.

Virtual Library of Ligands for MS

Selection and Construction of the Virtual Library

For ligand construction, PAR-1 antagonists with demonstrated activity were searched. Vorapaxar is a commercially available platelet antiaggregant whose mechanism of action is PAR-1 antagonism; therefore, it was used as a reference ligand. F16357 and SCH79797 are molecules whose antagonism has been previously studied, and thus, they were used as starting points for the design of multitarget molecules (Manaenko et al., 2013; Readmond and Wu, 2017). Four possible scaffolds were selected for PAR-1 (**Figure 2**), of which scaffolds W and X were obtained by scaffold hopping from F16357 and vorapaxar, respectively, with the help of Mcule (Kiss et al., 2012). F16357 was used as scaffold Y, and scaffold Z was an annular modification of SCH79797.

For the selection of KLK-6 ligands, benzamidine isosteres were designed, because this compound is known to be a serine protease inhibitor (Silva et al., 2017). The selected benzamidine isosteres were aminopyridine (A), aminopyridine with carboxylic acid (B), aminopyridine with alcohol (C), 2-aminopirimidine aminoquinoline (E), aminoisoquinoline (F), aminoquinazoline (G), and benzylamine (H) (**Figure 3**). Currently, there are no

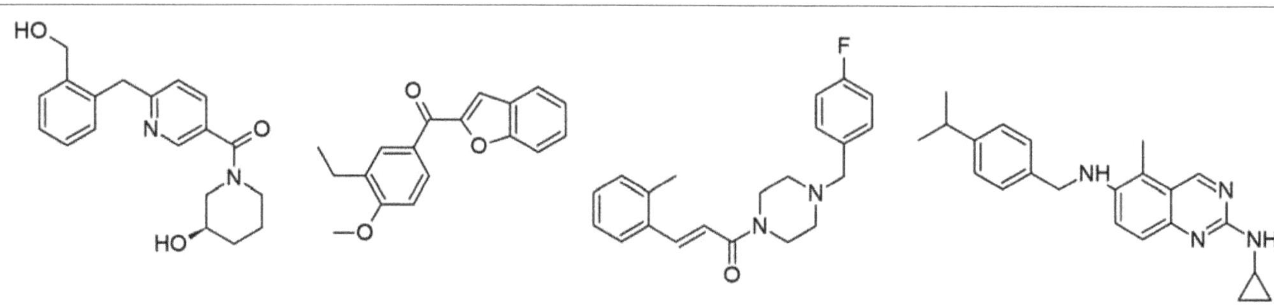

W X Y Z

FIGURE 2 | The four scaffolds used for ligand construction.

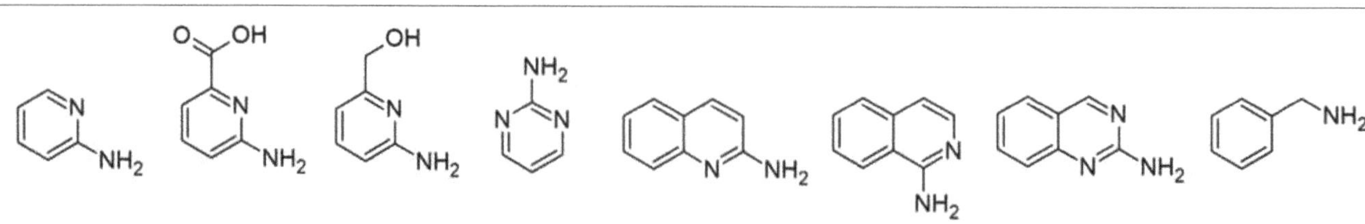

A B C D E F G H

FIGURE 3 | Proposed isosteres that may interact in the active site of KLK-6.

commercially available drugs whose mechanism of action is selective inhibition of KLK-6. However, it was found that 0HM, a benzylamine derivative, was previously determined as a compound with high binding energy to KLK-6 and thus was used as a reference ligand for this enzyme (Liang et al., 2012).

Finally, 211 compounds were constructed from a combination of both types of ligands with the help of Marvin Sketch 16.2.22.0 and saved in *.smiles format. The three-dimensional geometry was optimized with Spartan '14 (1.1.4) using MMFF and HF 6-31 G*.

Molecular Docking

The crystalline structures of PAR-1 complexed with vorapaxar (PDB id: 3VW7), human S1PR1(PDB id: 3V2Y) and human KLK-6 with 0HM (PDB id: 4D8N) were downloaded (Bernett et al., 2002; Hanson et al., 2012; Liang et al., 2012; Zhang et al., 2012). The water molecules and co-crystallized ligands were removed from the work area. The docking procedure was carried out in the same manner used for multikinase ligands.

Cheminformatics Analysis

The smiles codes of the 211 ligands were placed in admetSAR in order to predict some of their pharmacokinetic properties (Cheng et al., 2012). The following probability scores were obtained: permeability of the blood-brain barrier (BBB), human intestinal absorption (HIA), glycoprotein P substrate (PGP-substrate), carcinogen, acute oral toxicity (AOT) and inhibition of hERG (human Ether-à-go-go-Related Gene). A coefficient of +1 was assigned to all values that fulfilled the following conditions: BBB +, HAI +, PGP-non-substrate, non-carcinogen, AOT III, or IV and weak hERG inhibitor. Otherwise, a negative coefficient was assigned in such a way that the desirable properties were considered positive. With these coefficients, an average of the chemoinformatic properties was calculated, which was called Chemoinformatic Score (CIS).

Construction of the Multitarget Index

Vector analysis, mentioned in the introduction, was used as the mathematical basis for the index construction. Besides, vector analysis allowed new interpretations of ligands, concepts, and parameters that may have a significant impact on multitarget drug design.

Order of a Ligand

The core idea of the index is to interpret ligands as vectors. The theoretical affinity or score for a target may be interpreted as a coordinate within this vector. This interpretation treats targets as independent variables that are orthogonal to each other. The ligand (L) is then defined as follows:

$$\vec{L} = (a_1, a_2, \ldots, a_i) \tag{2}$$

where a_i is the affinity for each target. The usefulness is that the number of targets is now coded as the number of coordinates or dimensions. Therefore, the order of a ligand (n) relates to the number of targets being tested: a multitarget of order n.

Force of a Ligand

This parameter corresponds to the norm of the vector, which is a metric that combines all the affinities of the ligands into a single value. It is generally understood as magnitude, meaning that greater values correspond to ligands whose particular affinities are large. It is a useful parameter when trying to compare combined affinities. However, this metric is also sensible to extreme values. The force of each ligand (F) was calculated in the following way:

$$F = ||\vec{L}|| = \sqrt{a_1{}^2 + a_2{}^2 + \ldots + a_n{}^2} \tag{3}$$

Plotting the ligand can enhance the interpretation, as seen in **Figure 1**. However, for more than three coordinates, representations must be truncated into a radial web for better visualization.

Binding Capacity and Total Multitarget Capacity

Because each coordinate is a vector, the cross product of all the targets will give a new vector. This new vector is an indirect measure of the binding capacity of a ligand, which geometrically corresponds to an nth volume (Equation 4). This metric is more sensible than the force because it is a multiplication of affinities, and considerable differences between affinities have greater repercussions. This operation is the same as calculating the geometric mean. We interpreted the metric as the binding capacity, a measure of a ligand's tendency to bind to more targets. Higher binding capacity means it can bind efficiently to more targets.

$$\text{Bc} = \text{geometric mean} = \sqrt[n]{\prod_{i=1}^{n} a_n} \tag{4}$$

The average is interpreted as a ligand's affinity to all the targets. The average simulates a drug that has equal affinities for all the proteins. Therefore, the average (μ) is defined as the total multitarget capacity of the ligand (MTc) (Equation 5). It is only a capacity since it is an idealized value.

$$\text{MTc} = \mu = \frac{1}{n}\sum_{i=n}^{n} a_i \tag{5}$$

Finally, the quotient of the binding capacity and the total multitarget capacity gives a proportion of how much of that multitarget capacity is being used. If the binding capacity equals the total multitarget capacity, then the ligand is a true multitarget ligand. By itself, this quotient is an index of "multitargeticity" that can be expressed in percentage for easier reading and read as "used multitarget capacity" (U_{MTc}).

$$U_{MTc} = \frac{\text{Bc}}{\text{MTc}} \tag{6}$$

Index Standardization, Definition, and Interpretation

Since the idea behind the index is to compare different ligands, it is necessary to standardize the index. The following scheme was proposed: the ligand should be its own reference for standardization. This can be achieved through the following formula, in which the individual contribution of each affinity to the force is calculated.

$$\hat{L_s} = n\left(\frac{\vec{L}}{F}\right)^2 = \left(n\cdot\left[\frac{a_1}{F}\right]^2, n\cdot\left[\frac{a_2}{F}\right]^2, \ldots, n\cdot\left[\frac{a_n}{F}\right]^2\right) \quad (7)$$

where n is the number of targets, F is the norm or force of the ligand, and a is the affinity. This formula also standardizes the mean, or multitarget capacity (MTc) to 1, independently of the number of targets or the type of input used. For simplicity, the new coordinates were renamed "standardized affinities" ($\hat{a}$).

$$\hat{L_s} = (\hat{a_a}, \hat{a_2}, \ldots, \hat{a_n}) \quad (8)$$

This simplifies the standardized, used multitarget capacity (U_{MTc}) to a simple geometric mean ranging from 0 to 1, effectively making it an index or measurement of "multitargeticity." As in linear regression, a quadratic estimator exacerbates the value, making it ideal for a multitarget index (Equation 9).

$$^{1st}MTi = \left(\sqrt[n]{\prod_{i=1}^{n} \hat{a}_n}\right)^2 = \left(\prod_{i=1}^{n} \hat{a}_n\right)^{2/n} \quad (9)$$

The interpretation is the one originally described in the introduction: how similar the hyperrectangle described by the ligand is similar to a hypercube. Alternatively, in a less abstract way, it is an efficiency measurement: how much "multitarget capacity" is being used.

A Second Multitarget Index

A second parameter was calculated; the standard deviation (σ). With this, another index was constructed that could measure the dispersion of the affinities: the bigger the value, the less variation among the targets. Since the standardized affinities' mean equals one, the second multitarget index is defined as follows:

$$^{2nd}MTi = 1 - \sigma \quad (10)$$

As in ^{1st}MTi, the value can be expressed as a percentage (%). This is a more sensitive parameter that ranges from 1 to negative values. This index also encodes selectivity: smaller values, even negative, indicate more selectivity.

Defining of a Multitarget Ligand

With the two indexes, we propose the following values for classifying a ligand as a multitarget:

The ligand is multitarget if $^{1st}MTi \geq 0.84$ and $^{2nd}MTi \geq 0.60$

These values correspond to an ~20% deviation from the mean affinity. It is worth mentioning that, although this gives a quantitative definition of multitargeticity, ligands that do not fulfill the criteria should not be discarded. These indexes quantify the dispersion and variation of the affinities and do not indicate in any way the potency.

Multitarget Potency and Selectivity

Equally low affinities will give high MT indexes values. For this reason, a final critical parameter was introduced: the multitarget potency. This value is the product of the force times, both multitarget indexes (Equation 11), which is the equivalent of calculating how much of that force is due to the multitargeticity of the ligand.

$$P_{MT} = \frac{F}{\sqrt{n}} \cdot {}^{1st}MTi \cdot {}^{2nd}MTi \quad (11)$$

We propose the multitarget potency as a metric for drug design since the highest values of potency represent a possible multitarget hit or even multitarget lead. In the same line of thought, the next parameter that we propose is an attempt to identify selective ligands. The selectivity is calculated as follows:

$$S = \frac{F}{\sqrt{n}} \cdot (1 - {}^{1st}MTi)(1 - {}^{2nd}MTi) \quad (12)$$

Both parameters maintain the desired properties (higher values indicate higher potency and selectivity) and are useful for identifying possible multitarget and selective ligands. These metrics, as with any other, have their benefits and drawbacks and will be discussed further on.

RESULTS AND DISCUSSIONS

Performance of the MT Indexes in the Experimental Training Set

With the criteria set on point 2.5.6, of the 10 approved multikinase drugs analyzed (imatinib, sunitinib, dasatinib, afatinib, bosutinib, lapatinib, nintedanib, pazopanib, sorafenib, vandetanib), only afatanib was not classified as a multitarget ligand. Although it is biologically active in both of its targets, the epidermal growth factor receptor (EGFR) and the receptor tyrosine-protein kinase erbB-2 (HER2 or erbB2), it has a considerable preference over EGFR ($K_i = 0.1$ vs. $K_i = 5$ [nM]).

The two negative controls did not fulfill the criteria to be cataloged as multitarget drugs. In fact, the epidermal growth factor receptor (EGFR) is the main and only target for gefitinib and erlotinib (Wishart et al., 2018). The indexes can reliably classify and discriminate multitarget molecules in experimental values, giving strength to the analysis.

The multitarget potency, the critical parameter proposed, supports the findings, making dasatinib the most potent multitarget drug of the analyzed set ($P_{MT} = 16.4$). Sunitinib was de 2nd most potent multitarget ($P_{MT} = 14.6$); although it had better indexes, the total strength was reduced since it had more targets tested, and the affinities were not as strong as dasatinib (**Figure 4**). In contrast, gefitinib was the least potent ($P_{MT} = 14.6$), but it was also the 2nd most selective ligand of the dataset ($S_{gefitinib} = 2.7$ vs. $S_{dasatinin} = 1.3$ and $S_{sunitinib} = 0.2$), being afatinib the first ($S_{afatinib} = 2.9$).

*All P_{MT} and S values are dimensionless.

Performance of the MT Indexes in the Docking Training Set

With the criteria set on point 2.5.6, of the ten known approved multikinase drugs tested, only sorafenib was not classified as a multitarget ligand. By contrast, the three negative controls were classified as multitarget ligands according to the index. The apparent discrepancy between these results and the experimental ones is explained by considering that all the 13 ligands were docked in the same three targets, indistinctively if they were active or not, while in the experimental analysis, the preferred targets were analyzed according to each ligand. Sorafenib had larger calculated affinities than most of the ligands but was further apart from each other, which lead to it nor being classified as multitarget. The performance of sunitinib and dasatinib is observed in **Figure 5**, and the results agree with the experimental set. The only difference is that sunitinib is, in this case, the most potent multitarget ligand.

The analysis still proves useful once the ligands are arranged in order of highest to lowest multitarget potency, or the force of each ligand is compared. It is important to emphasize that the purpose of the index is not to reclassify drugs but instead to provide useful metrics for analyzing data and aiding in the drug design process, especially in the design of multitarget drugs. In this case, seven multitarget ligands would be discovered or tested

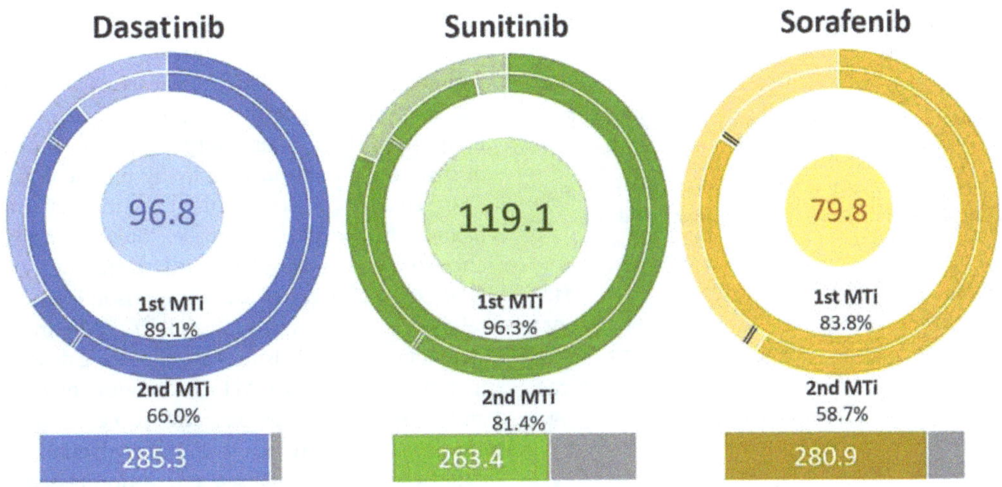

FIGURE 4 | Dasatinib had 3 targets ($n = 3$) tested and greater affinities toward those, while sunitinib had order $n = 5$ and gefitinib $n = 4$. That is why, although sunitinib has better MTi values, dasatinib has more multitarget potency (the number inside the circle). All the values are presented as % (or times 100). The threshold for considering a ligand multitarget is viewed as a cut in the circles. The inner and outer rings are the 1st and 2nd MT indexes, respectively.

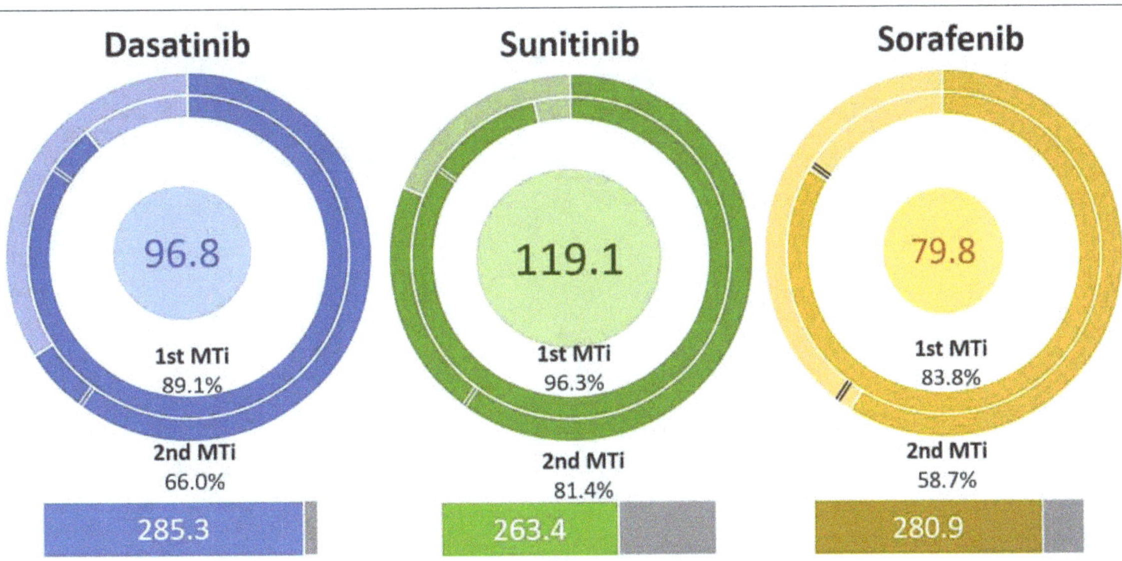

FIGURE 5 | Comparing with **Figure 4**, the multitarget tendency of sunitinib and dasatinib remains similar. The difference in the calculated affinities gives the change in the potency. Sorafenib is an example of how the MT indexes affect the strength of the ligand, since that strength is unevenly distributed. The inner circle is the MT potency. The inner and outer rings are the 1st and 2nd MT index, respectively. The inferior rectangle is the force of the ligand.

before encountering a non-multitarget drug previously classified as an MT drug. The multitarget indexes are useful when they are used with the force of the ligand. The top 7 ligands are indeed classified as multitarget ligands and are approved by the FDA as multikinase drugs, and a summary of the performance can be reviewed in **Table 1**.

Since this is an *in silico* evaluation, the scoring is affected by the computational limitations of the docking procedures. These limitations should be taken into consideration when applying the metrics previously described. These are virtual metrics and are sensible to the *in silico* scoring functions, which themselves do not reflect the *in vivo* effect. Furthermore, the indexes and metrics should be tested with experimental values to prove the strength, robustness, and validity of this classification. As mentioned above, the criteria for classifying a ligand as a multitarget can be modified, but the measure of multitargeticity persists.

TABLE 1 | Sunitinib, imatinib, and sorafenib are approved multitarget drugs by the FDA.

Name	4HVS MolDock score	3VO3 MolDock score	1SHA MolDock score	F	1stMT index (%)	2ndMT index (%)	P_{MT}
Sunitinib	−166.0	−131.5	−156.6	263.4	96.3	81.4	**119.1**
Imatinib	−193.9	−130.7	−163.2	285.1	90.4	69.1	**102.8**
Idelalisib	−138.7	−104.8	−129.5	216.8	94.7	77.9	**92.4**
Sorafenib	−201.6	−119.8	−154.8	280.9	83.8	58.7	**79.8**
Letrozole	−137.9	−98.4	−114.8	204.6	92.7	72.4	**79.3**

*Sorafenib did classify as a multitarget drug. However, the multitarget potency of sunitinib and imatinib compared to letrozole and idelasib (negative controls in purple) is greater. The rest of the molecules can be found in the **Supplementary Information**. The bold values indicate the main or critical parameter(s) being evaluated.*

DUD Database

From the 98258 ligands analyzed, 5561 molecules were found to be multitarget. This corresponds to about 5.7% of all the analyzed ligands. The orders of the ligands varied widely, ranging from 9 to 40. A total of 912 ligands were found to be multitarget of order 24. The distribution can be seen in **Graph 1**. The multitarget index filtered the ligands, meaning it does not classify every ligand as multitarget, and only a subset is eligible according to the criteria. It is important to notice that the chemical structures in this dataset were diverse. In these cases, the MT indexes gain strength as they "clean" the database and facilitating further research.

The most potent multitarget ligands were an unnamed compound of the ZINC database, which could be further tested to determine if its potential multitargeticity is only theoretical. This is the purpose of the indexes, to be useful in drug design and in identifying potential multitarget ligands. The selectivity was also used to identify the most selective ligands. In the DUD database, the third most selective ligand corresponded to hepsulfam, with the following MT indexes: 6.6% (1st) and −272.1% (2nd). A comparison is made in **Figure 6**. The selectivity was toward catechol-O-methyltransferase (COMT). Hepsulfam is an alkylsulfonate alkylating drug-like busulfan used in cancer therapy. COMT is a modulator of the dopaminergic and adrenergic response, and it can influence nausea and vomiting (Gan and Habib, 2016). Hepsulfam binding to COMT could explain mild nausea and vomiting seen in clinical trials, contrasting serious nausea present in other types of anticancer drugs (Ravdin et al., 1991).

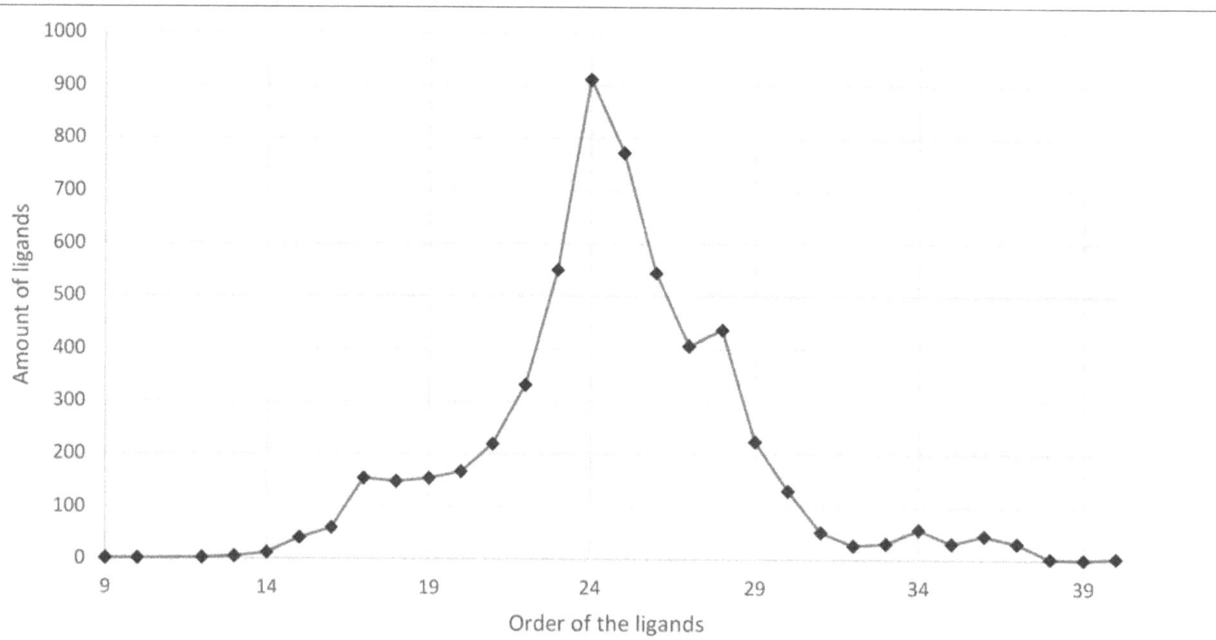

Graph 1 | Distribution of how many orders of ligands were among the 5561 ligands identifies as multitarget.

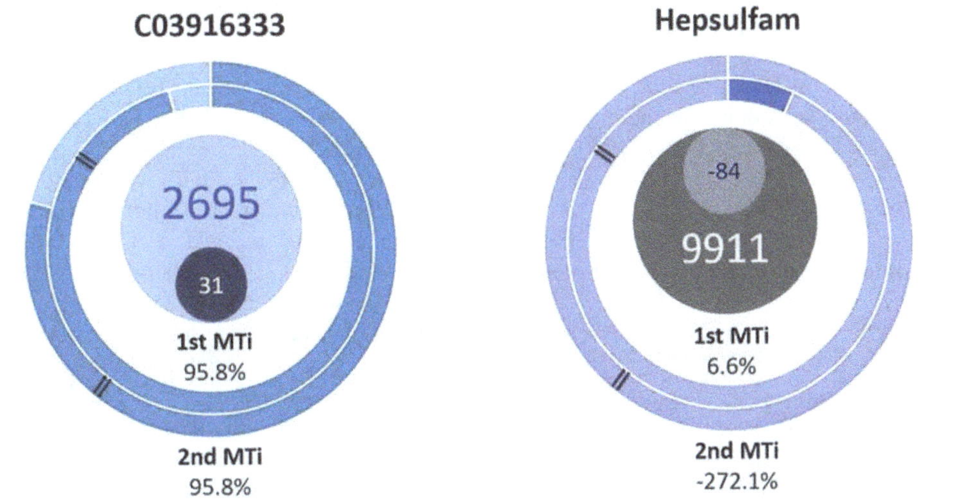

FIGURE 6 | Multitarget parameters of the most potent multitarget ligand and hepsulfam, the 3rd most selective. The darker circle represents the selectivity, while the lighter represents de potency. Hepsulfam had a negative MT potency.

Advantages and Limitations of the Multitarget Indexes

The usefulness of using a multitarget index varies highly according to the necessities of each research group. As a first instance, the multitarget indexes give an initial quantitative and workable definition for what a multitarget drug is. They define and measure multitargeticity. The primary purpose of the analysis is in drug design for identification of *in silico* and potential *in vivo* multitarget drugs. In a sense, these indexes could be useful in identifying multitarget hits and leads in the drug discovery process. Second, because it is an index, it can be useful in data analysis when comparing several ligands or targets at the same time. Moreover, the analysis assumes that the targets are independent of each other, which provides freedom regarding the number of studied targets.

The index is also modifiable and perfectible in several ways. For example, if highlighting a particular target is desired, then coefficients can be introduced so that the affinities are weighted. More calculations may be performed on the affinities in previous steps without changing the procedure or interpretation of the index, such as introducing ligand efficiency metrics. The multitarget indexes do not only identify multitarget ligands but are useful when selectivity is desired, making them not only applicable in multitarget drug design but also in designing selective single-target drugs and in the drug discovery process in general. Finally, the analysis can be further perfected with more statistical rigor, more meaningful parameters, and an *in vitro* and *in vivo* extensions.

Like all other metrics, it has limitations that skew or simplify the underlying mechanisms. For example, equal affinities may not necessarily imply multitarget *in vivo* effectiveness, since there are more variables to consider.

Various suppositions are needed in order to treat ligands as vectors. The most obvious one is that indexes do not consider how the ligand binds the target or the mechanism of action. Second, it is assumed the affinities are calculated or measured under the same conditions. Third, although the coordinates can be any type of input, the final MT index value changes if the units of the affinities introduced are different; therefore, MT index values can only be compared if the data is processed the same way and is in the same units.

The performance of the MT indexes in all the training sets shows that they correctly classify drugs using experimental values, identify potential multitarget ligands *in silico*, and can filter an extensive database, making them valuable for the intended purposes.

MT Indexes in the Virtual Library of Candidates for MS

With the known limitations and advantages, the MT indexes were used to analyze the experimental set. The 214 docked ligands were submitted to the analysis previously described and ranked in descending order of multitarget potency. Of the 211 designed compounds, 45 were derivatives from scaffold W, 34 from scaffold X, 29 from scaffold Y, and 103 from scaffold Z. Scaffold Z was present in 9 out of the top 10 most potent multitarget ligands. Benzamidine isostere A was present in 5 of them, hinting that an aminopyridine fragment may be ideal for a multitarget effect.

In most cases, a linker of 1 carbon atom and an ester group were found in the most potent ligands. More linkers diminished the MT index value, increasing the selectivity toward KLK-6, the only exception to this rule was the top, most potent molecule with four linkers. The reference molecules and their multitarget parameters can be seen in **Table 2**. In **Table 3**, the top 5 most potent multitarget ligands from the experimental set are presented.

In multitarget drug design, the multitarget potency combines the two indexes and the force. For choosing candidates, the force against the 2nd MT index can be plotted, and the regions divided into quadrants. The most favorable zone would be the upper left since it would group the most potent and most specific multitarget ligands (**Graph 2**).

Chemoinformatic Analysis

With the help of the chemoinformatic score (CIS), the ligands were classified into three arbitrary categories: preferred (CIS> 0.75), sufficient (0.75> CIS> 0.5) and risky (CIS <0.5). In total, nine ligands (4.23%) entered the preferred classification. Of these, eight belonged to scaffold X, and 1 to scaffold Z. Overall, 165 ligands (77.46%) fit into the sufficient category, and 39 (18.31%) were classified as risky (see **Table 4**).

From the 45 scaffold W ligands, 14 (31.11%) were considered risky, while 31 ligands (68.89%) were considered sufficient; none reached a CIS> 0.75. From scaffold X, 11 ligands (32.35%) obtained a risky score, 15 ligands (44.11%) were sufficient, and 8 (23.23%) were preferred. Scaffold Y had seven ligands (24.14%) classified as risky, and 22 ligands (75.86%) classified as sufficient. Finally, seven ligands (6.80%) of scaffold Z were considered risky, while 95 ligands (92.22%) were considered sufficient, and only 1 (~1%) was preferred. These results can be seen in **Table 5**.

TABLE 2 | Summary of the multitarget metrics of the reference ligands.

Name	KLK-6 MolDock Score	PAR-1 MolDock Score	S1RP1 MolDock Score	F	1stMT index (%)	2ndMT index (%)	P_{MT}
Vorapaxar	−183.0	−147.7	−128.2	267.9	91.7	70.2	**99.6**
Siponimod	−143.9	−184.2	−155.8	280.9	95.7	78.8	**122.3**
OHM	−185.5	−140.5	−148.2	275.9	94.1	74.5	**111.8**

The bold values indicate the main or critical parameter(s) being evaluated.

TABLE 3 | Summary of the top 5 ligands which had the highest potency.

Name	KLK-6 MolDock score	PAR-1 MolDock score	S1RP1 MolDock score	F	1stMT index (%)	2ndMT index (%)	P_{MT}
$Z_{b0}A_{d4}$	−210.2	−174.8	−177.9	326.2	97.2	82.6	261.9
$Z_{b0}C_{o11}$	−193.4	−161.3	−188.9	314.8	97.5	84.8	260.5
$Z_{c0}B_{o11}$	−190.1	−160.9	−176.8	305.4	98.2	86.6	259.5
$Z_{d0}A_{p2}$	−167.1	−153.4	−165.5	280.8	99.4	92.6	258.5
$Z_{b0}A_{d1}$	−202.5	−164.5	−183.8	319.1	97.2	83.2	257.9

TABLE 4 | Distribution of the chemoinformatic score among the ligands with the 4 scaffolds.

	Preferred (CIS>0.75)	Sufficient (0.75>CIS>0.5)	Risky (CIS<0.5)	Total
Scaffold W	-	31 (68.9%)	14 (31.1%)	45
Scaffold X	8 (23.2%)	15 (44.1%)	11 (32.3%)	34
Scaffold Y	-	22 (75.8%)	7 (24.1%)	29
Scaffold Z	1 (~1%)	95 (92.2%)	7 (6.8%)	103
Total	9	163	39	211

Ligands with scaffold X were the most preferred in terms of pharmacokinetics theoretical properties.

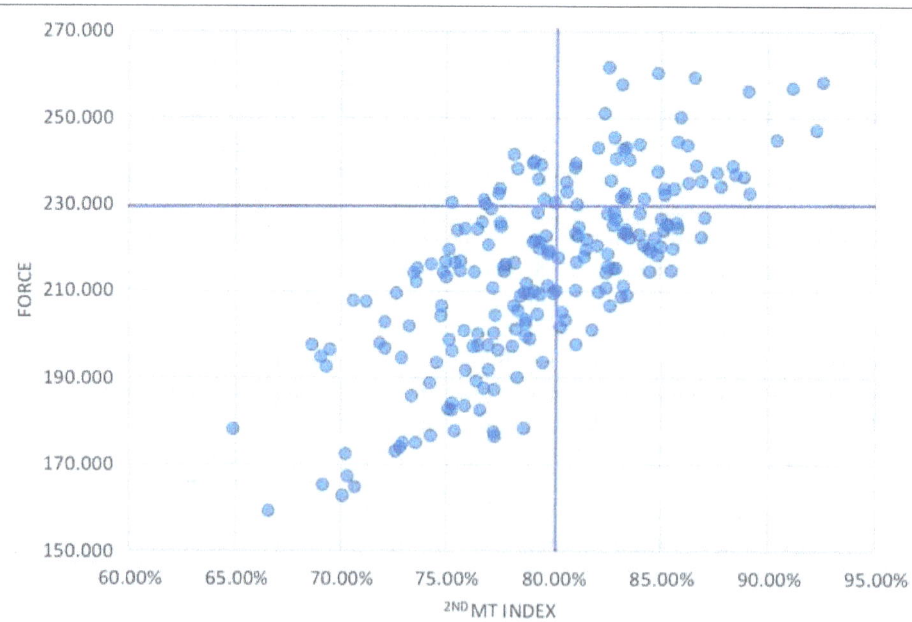

Graph 2 | When plotted, the upper left quadrant is the most valuable or with the most potentially multitarget ligands.

TABLE 5 | Distribution of the chemoinformatic score among benzamidine isosteres.

	Preferred (CIS>0.75)	Sufficient (0.75>CIS>0.5)	Risky (CIS<0.5)	Total
Isostere A	8 (5.9%)	114 (83.8%)	14 (10.3%)	136
Isostere B	-	2 (15.4%)	11(84.6%)	13
Isostere C	-	7 (53.8%)	6 (46.1%)	13
Isostere D	-	6 (66.6%)	3 (33.3%)	9
Isostere E	-	10 (100%)	-	10
Isostere F	-	9 (100%)	-	9
Isostere G	1 (10%)	7 (70%)	2 (20%)	10
Isostere H	-	9 (81.8%)	2 (18.2%)	11

A considerable proportion of ligands with isosteres B and C were classified as risky, while ligands with isostere A had more preferred CIS.

TABLE 6 | Summary of the top 5 ligands which had the highest combined values of Potency and CIS.

Name	F	1st MTi (%)	2nd MTi (%)	P	CIS	Final value
$X_{b0}G_0$	**294.1**	96.9	82.7	235.8	0.81	**10.5**
$Z_{b0}A_{s0}$	**314.3**	95.8	79.4	239.3	0.78	**10.4**
$X_{b0}A_{s0}$	**269.4**	97.8	85.7	225.9	0.82	**10.4**
$X_{b0}A_{m1}$	**273.4**	97.2	84.0	223.3	0.82	**10.3**
$X_{b0}A_{m0}$	**261.1**	98.2	86.9	222.7	0.80	**10.1**

The bold values indicate the main or critical parameter(s) being evaluated.

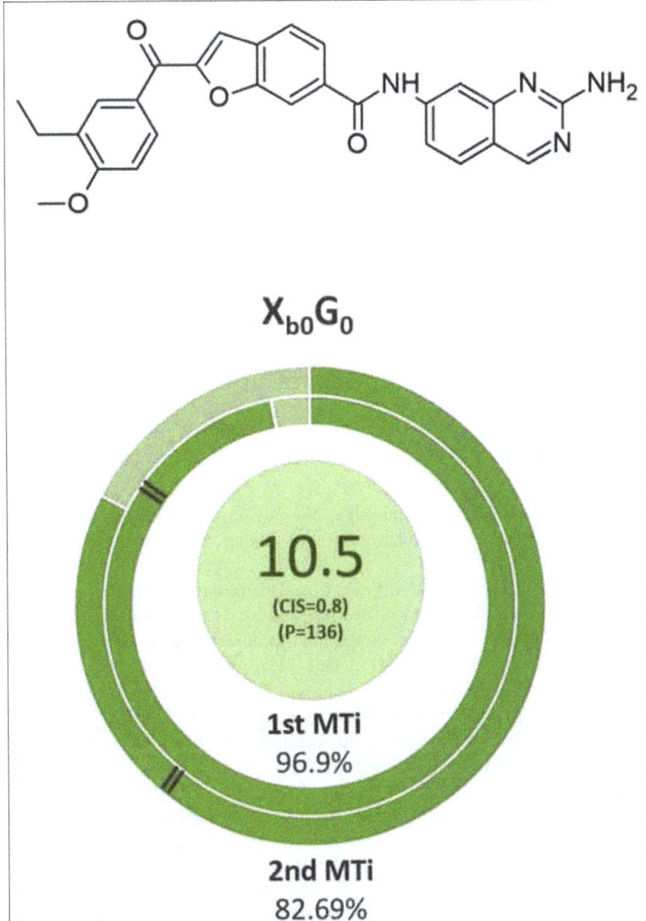

FIGURE 7 | Ligand Xb0G0 had the highest combined multitarget theoretical affinity and *in silico* ADME profile. The parameters of the MT indexes analysis. The final score is the combination of the MT potency and CIS (in parenthesis).

These results show that scaffold Z has the most balanced theoretical pharmacological properties. However, scaffold X also presented desirable properties in the CIS; scaffold X is pharmacokinetically desired. It is also worth mentioning that the aminopyridine derivatives with carboxylic acids (B) and alcohols (C) presented a risky CIS in the chemoinformatic analysis. Therefore, ligands with these isosteres are not considered candidates for therapeutic applications.

Pharmacokinetic and Pharmacodynamic Viable Candidates

For determining possible final candidates, the CIS score and multitarget potency were combined with the geometric mean. The final table (**Table 6**) groups the ligands that combine the highest potency and CIS values, meaning they are the most likely to have a biological effect while remaining relatively safe. This is a theoretical approach; therefore, the top molecules are potential multitarget alternative candidates to treat MS. The ligands with the highest combined score shared scaffold X in most of the cases (10 out of the 20 top ligands), with scaffold Z being the second most shared among the top 20. In 9 out of the top 10 ligands, isostere A was present in the ligand structure. It is also noted that a small linker is optimal for joining these two fragments. From these results, it is assumed that isostere A, as well as scaffolds X and Z, contribute to theoretical multitarget effects. However, scaffold X ligands do not have as much multitargeticity nor force as ligands with scaffold Z but remain the safest and more pharmacokinetically favorable. The applied multitarget metrics simplified the analysis and criteria for determining viable candidates. In **Figure 7**, the most viable candidate is presented.

CONCLUSIONS

As multitarget drugs are designed and tested, methods for effectively comparing and optimizing ligands are required. We present a new interpretation of ligands as vectors; new multitarget definitions and metrics, such as order of a ligand, the force of a ligand, binding capacity and multitarget capacity; and two multitarget indexes representing multitarget potency and selectivity, all of which might prove useful in drug design. The training sets allowed the identification of the advantages and disadvantages of using these metrics in multitarget drug discovery. The data analyzed through the MT indexes served to identify pharmacokinetically and pharmacodynamically viable multitarget therapeutic candidates for MS. The indexes were also useful for identifying selective ligands. The definitions, metrics, and analysis proposed here may provide a guide toward the definition of "multitargeticity."

AUTHOR CONTRIBUTIONS

All authors have contributed significantly to this work, in the design of the model, performance of the computational experiments, analysis of the generated data, and writing the paper. All authors read, edited, and approved the final manuscript.

ACKNOWLEDGMENTS

The authors wish to thank Universidad La Salle for funding through project NEC-07/18.

REFERENCES

Behrangi, N., Fischbach, F., and Kipp, M. (2019). Mechanism of siponimod: anti-inflammatory and neuroprotective mode of action. *Cells* 8:24. doi: 10.3390/cells8010024

Bernett, M. J., Blaber, S. I., Scarisbrick, I. A., Dhanarajan, P., Thompson, S. M., and Blaber, M. (2002). Crystal structure and biochemical characterization of human kallikrein 6 reveal that a trypsin-like kallikrein is expressed in the central nervous system. *J. Biol. Chem.* 277, 24562–24570. doi: 10.1074/jbc.M202392200

Browne, P., Chandraratna, D., Angood, C., Tremlett, H., Baker, C., Taylor, B. V., et al. (2014). Atlas of multiple sclerosis 2013: a growing global problem with widespread inequity. *Neurology* 83, 1022–1024. doi: 10.1212/WNL.0000000000000768

Burda, J. E., Radulovic, M., Yoon, H., and Scarisbrick, I. A. (2013). Critical role for PAR1 in kallikrein 6-mediated oligodendrogliopathy. *Glia* 61, 1456–1470. doi: 10.1002/glia.22534

Cheng, F., Li, W., Zhou, Y., Shen, J., Wu, Z., Liu, G., et al. (2012). admetSAR: a comprehensive source and free tool for assessment of chemical ADMET properties. *J. Chem. Inf. Model.* 52, 3099–3105. doi: 10.1021/ci300367a

Chi, X. X., and Nicol, G. D. (2010). The sphingosine 1-phosphate receptor, S1PR1, plays a prominent but not exclusive role in enhancing the excitability of sensory neurons. *J. Neurophysiol.* 104, 2741–2748. doi: 10.1152/jn.00709.2010

Chiarelli, L. R., Mori, G., Orena, B. S., Esposito, M., Lane, T., de Jesus Lopes Ribeiro, A. L., et al. (2018). A multitarget approach to drug discovery inhibiting *Mycobacterium tuberculosis* PyrG and PanK. *Sci. Rep.* 8:3187. doi: 10.1038/s41598-018-21614-4

Dobson, R., and Giovannoni, G. (2019). Multiple sclerosis - a review. *Eur. J. Neurol.* 26, 27–40. doi: 10.1111/ene.13819

Gan, T. J., and Habib, A. S. (2016). *Postoperative Nausea and Vomiting: A Practical Guide.* Cambridge, UK: Cambridge University Press. doi: 10.1017/CBO9781316135853

Gilson, M. K., Liu, T., Baitaluk, M., Nicola, G., Hwang, L., and Chong, J. (2016). BindingDB in 2015: a public database for medicinal chemistry, computational chemistry and systems pharmacology. *Nucleic Acids Res.* 44, D1045–D1053. doi: 10.1093/nar/gkv1072

Hanson, M. A., Roth, C. B., Jo, E., Griffith, M. T., Scott, F. L., Reinhart, G., et al. (2012). Crystal structure of a lipid G protein–coupled receptor. *Science* 335, 851–855. doi: 10.1126/science.1215904

Hu, Y., Gupta-Ostermann, D., and Bajorath, J. (2014). Exploring compound promiscuity patterns and multi-target activity spaces. *Comput. Struct. Biotechnol. J.* 9:e201401003. doi: 10.5936/csbj.201401003

Huang, N., Shoichet, B. K., and Irwin, J. J. (2006). Benchmarking sets for molecular docking. *J. Med. Chem.* 49, 6789–6801. doi: 10.1021/jm0608356

Huang, W.-J., Chen, W.-W., and Zhang, X. (2017). Multiple sclerosis: pathology, diagnosis and treatments. *Exp. Ther. Med.* 13, 3163–3166. doi: 10.3892/etm.2017.4410

Kim, H. N., Kim, Y. R., Ahn, S. M., Lee, S. K., Shin, H. K., and Choi, B. T. (2015). Protease activated receptor-1 antagonist ameliorates the clinical symptoms of experimental autoimmune encephalomyelitis via inhibiting breakdown of blood-brain barrier. *J. Neurochem.* 135, 577–588. doi: 10.1111/jnc.13285

Kiss, R., Sandor, M., and Szalai, F. A. (2012). http://Mcule.com: a public web service for drug discovery. *J. Cheminform.* 4:P17. doi: 10.1186/1758-2946-4-S1-P17

Lee, P. R., Johnson, T. P., Gnanapavan, S., Giovannoni, G., Wang, T., Steiner, J. P., et al. (2017). Protease-activated receptor-1 activation by granzyme B causes neurotoxicity that is augmented by interleukin-1β. *J. Neuroinflamm.* 14:131. doi: 10.1186/s12974-017-0901-y

Li, Y. H., Wang, P. P., Li, X. X., Yu, C. Y., Yang, H., Zhou, J., et al. (2016). The human kinome targeted by fda approved multi-target drugs and combination products: a comparative study from the drug-target interaction network perspective. *PLoS ONE* 11:e0165737. doi: 10.1371/journal.pone.0165737

Liang, G., Chen, X., Aldous, S., Pu, S.-F., Mehdi, S., Powers, E., et al. (2012). Human kallikrein 6 inhibitors with a para-amidobenzylanmine P1 group identified through virtual screening. *Bioorg. Med. Chem. Lett.* 22, 2450–2455. doi: 10.1016/j.bmcl.2012.02.014

Loza-Mejía, M., Salazar, J., and Sánchez-Tejeda, J. (2018). *In Silico* studies on compounds derived from calceolaria: phenylethanoid glycosides as potential multitarget inhibitors for the development of pesticides. *Biomolecules* 8:121. doi: 10.3390/biom8040121

Lu, J.-J., Pan, W., Hu, Y.-J., and Wang, Y.-T. (2012). Multi-target drugs: the trend of drug research and development. *PLoS ONE* 7:e40262. doi: 10.1371/journal.pone.0040262

Macfarlane, S. R., Seatter, M. J., Kanke, T., Hunter, G. D., and Plevin, R. (2001). Proteinase-activated receptors. *Pharmacol. Rev.* 53, 245–282.

Manaenko, A., Sun, X., Kim, C. H., Yan, J., Ma, Q., and Zhang, J. H. (2013). PAR-1 antagonist SCH79797 ameliorates apoptosis following surgical brain injury through inhibition of ASK1-JNK in rats. *Neurobiol. Dis.* 50, 13–20. doi: 10.1016/j.nbd.2012.09.004

O'Sullivan, C., Schubart, A., Mir, A. K., and Dev, K. K. (2016). The dual S1PR1/S1PR5 drug BAF312 (Siponimod) attenuates demyelination in organotypic slice cultures. *J. Neuroinflamm.* 13:31. doi: 10.1186/s12974-016-0494-x

Pan, H., Boucher, M., and Kaunelis, D. (2016). *PAR-1 Antagonists: An Emerging Antiplatelet Drug Class. CADTH Issues in Emerging Health Technologies.* Canadian Agency for Drugs and Technologies in Health. Retrieved from http://www.ncbi.nlm.nih.gov/pubmed/27809429

Ramsay, R. R., Popovic-Nikolic, M. R., Nikolic, K., Uliassi, E., and Bolognesi, M. L. (2018). A perspective on multi-target drug discovery and design for complex diseases. *Clin. Transl. Med.* 7:3. doi: 10.1186/s40169-017-0181-2

Ravdin, P. M., Havlin, K. A., Marshall, M. V., Brown, T. D., Koeller, J. M., Kuhn, J. G., et al. (1991). A phase I clinical and pharmacokinetic trial of hepsulfam. *Cancer Res.* 51(23 Pt 1), 6268–6272.

Readmond, C., and Wu, C. (2017). Investigating detailed interactions between novel PAR1 antagonist F16357 and the receptor using docking and molecular dynamic simulations. *J. Mol. Graph. Model.* 77, 205–217. doi: 10.1016/j.jmgm.2017.08.019

Rosini, M. (2014). Polypharmacology: the rise of multitarget drugs over combination therapies. *Future Med. Chem.* 6, 485–487. doi: 10.4155/fmc.14.25

Scarisbrick, I. A., Epstein, B., Cloud, B. A., Yoon, H., Wu, J., Renner, D. N., et al. (2011). Functional role of kallikrein 6 in regulating immune cell survival. *PLoS ONE* 6:e18376. doi: 10.1371/journal.pone.0018376

Silva, R. N., Oliveira, L. C. G., Parise, C. B., Oliveira, J. R., Severino, B., Corvino, A., et al. (2017). Activity of human kallikrein-related peptidase 6 (KLK6) on substrates containing sequences of basic amino acids. Is it a processing protease? *Biochim. Biophys. Acta Proteins Proteom.* 1865, 558–564. doi: 10.1016/j.bbapap.2017.02.017

Talevi, A. (2015). Multi-target pharmacology: possibilities and limitations of the "skeleton key approach" from a medicinal chemist perspective. *Front. Pharmacol.* 6:205. doi: 10.3389/fphar.2015.00205

van der Schyf, C. J. (2011). The use of multi-target drugs in the treatment of neurodegenerative diseases. *Expert Rev. Clin. Pharmacol.* 4, 293–298. doi: 10.1586/ecp.11.13

Wishart, D. S., Feunang, Y. D., Guo, A. C., Lo, E. J., Marcu, A., Grant, J. R., et al. (2018). DrugBank 5.0: a major update to the DrugBank database for 2018. *Nucleic Acids Res.* 46, D1074–D1082. doi: 10.1093/nar/gkx1037

Xie, L., and Bourne, P. E. (2015). Developing multi-target therapeutics to fine-tune the evolutionary dynamics of the cancer ecosystem. *Front. Pharmacol.* 6:209. doi: 10.3389/fphar.2015.00209

Yoon, H., Radulovic, M., Drucker, K. L., Wu, J., and Scarisbrick, I. A. (2015). The thrombin receptor is a critical extracellular switch controlling myelination. *Glia* 63, 846–859. doi: 10.1002/glia.22788

Yoon, H., and Scarisbrick, I. A. (2016). Kallikrein-related peptidase 6 exacerbates disease in an autoimmune model of multiple sclerosis. *Biol. Chem.* 397, 1277–1286. doi: 10.1515/hsz-2016-0239

Zhang, C., Srinivasan, Y., Arlow, D. H., Fung, J. J., Palmer, D., Zheng, Y., et al. (2012). High-resolution crystal structure of human protease-activated receptor 1. *Nature* 492, 387–392. doi: 10.1038/nature 11701

Zhang, W., Pei, J., and Lai, L. (2017). Computational multitarget drug design. *J. Chem. Inf. Model.* 57, 403–412. doi: 10.1021/acs.jcim. 6b00491

5

Pushing the Ligand Efficiency Metrics: Relative Group Contribution (RGC) Model as a Helpful Strategy to Promote a Fragment "Rescue" Effect

***Andrés Felipe Vásquez*[1,2] *and Andrés González Barrios*[1*]**

[1] Grupo de Diseño de Productos y Procesos (GDPP), School of Chemical Engineering, Universidad de los Andes, Bogotá, Colombia, [2] Laboratorio de Fisiología Molecular, Instituto Nacional de Salud, Bogotá, Colombia

***Correspondence:**
Andrés González Barrios
andgonza@uniandes.edu.co

The ligand efficiency (LE) indexes have long been used as decision-making criteria in drug discovery and development. However, in the context of fragment-based drug design (FBDD), these metrics often exhibit a strong emphasis toward the selection of highly efficient "core" fragments for potential optimization, which are not usually considered as parts of a larger molecule with a size typical for a drug. In this study, we present a relative group contribution (RGC) model intended to predict the efficiency of a drug-sized compound in terms of its component fragments. This model could be useful not only in rapidly predicting all the possible combinations of promising fragments from an earlier hit discovery stage, but also in enabling a relatively low-LE fragment to become part of a drug-sized compound as long as it is "rescued" by other high-LE fragments.

Keywords: ligand efficiency metrics, fragment-based screening, property-based design, drug discovery, protein-ligand interactions, structure-activity relationship, fragment library

INTRODUCTION

Ligand efficiency metrics have been applied as a decision-making strategy nearly universally accepted during the last two decades (Hopkins et al., 2014). They are intended to compare the quality of hits and leads during hit to lead and lead optimization phases of drug discovery (Cavalluzzi et al., 2017). Among these metrics, the ligand efficiency (LE), firstly described by Hopkins et al. (2004), continues to be the most widely used index to discriminate between promising molecules and those which are not (Reynolds, 2015). LE is defined by the following formula:

$$LE = \frac{\Delta G}{N} \tag{1}$$

where $\Delta G = -RTInK_d$, N (also known as HAC or heavy atom count) represents the number of heavy, non-hydrogen atoms, and K_d corresponds to the equilibrium dissociation constant.

As shown in Equation (1), LE normalizes the potency by size, specifically representing the average contribution ΔG (Gibbs free energy) per heavy atom. LE is typically used in FBDD as cut-off criterion to retrieve just high-LE fragments in a screening process (Murray and Verdonk, 2006; Schultes et al., 2010). Intriguingly, because LE usually considers fragments as independent chemical entities, some other metrics have emerged to consider the change in affinity as a fragment is developed into a larger, high-affinity drug-sized compound. One prime example is the group efficiency (GE), described in 2008 (Verdonk and Rees, 2008), which allows measuring the contribution to the binding efficiency of a particular group of atoms added to an existing lead molecule:

$$GE = \frac{\Delta\Delta G}{\Delta N} \tag{2}$$

where $\Delta\Delta G = \Delta G(B)\text{-}\Delta G(A)$ and $\Delta N = (N(B)\text{-}N(A)$; in other words, $\Delta\Delta G$ is equal to the difference between the Gibbs free energy of the existing molecule (or fragment) "A" and the new combined molecule "B" and ΔN corresponds to the difference between the number of non-hydrogen atoms of molecules "A" and "B." However, GE is based on a pairwise comparison of structurally closely related compounds and, hence, it is frequently applied for optimization of a high-efficient fragment (Hopkins et al., 2014). Therefore, a rapid and simple method for comparing efficiency of different fragments as part of a whole, including if they are dissimilar to each other (or if they occupy different pockets in the target molecule), needs to be developed.

Several independent studies in the past two decades have indicated an overemphasis on potency by the pharmaceutical industry (Albert et al., 2007; Hopkins et al., 2014). Still, other factors such as chemical novelty (Medina-Franco et al., 2014), selectivity fine-tuning (Costantino and Barlocco, 2018), structural alerts avoidance (Jasial et al., 2017), and synthetic accessibility (Fukunishi et al., 2014) are increasingly playing a key role in drug design. Considering these non-mutually exclusive events, we hypothesize that fragments that not necessarily exhibit a high efficiency level during a screening procedure, either virtual or experimental, would still have the possibility of taking part in a complete drug-sized compound.

In this study, we propose that a relative group contribution (RGC) model based on the efficiency of its component fragments may estimate the efficiency of a drug-sized compound. This model calculates the minimum efficiency required for unknown fragments by considering the efficiency of those already known, which facilitates a rapid elucidation of the best combinations of fragments. Likewise, this model facilitates that fragments with a relatively low efficiency may not necessarily be eliminated at an early stage of the screening process and, consequently, may become eventually represented as chemical moieties within the final candidate compound -a phenomenon herein referred to as fragment "rescue" effect.

THEORETICAL FRAMEWORK OF THE RGC MODEL

The proposed model is based on three main assumptions:

1. The efficiency of an entire molecule may be estimated as the weighted root mean square (WMRS) of the efficiency of its component fragments. The rational for using this type of mean is intended to (1) cope with the negative values of ΔG and (2) consider effectively the potentially different number of non-hydrogen atoms (N) for each component fragment.
2. The efficiency of each fragment (regarded as the entire ratio and not just the quotient) is, in principle, dependent on each other, excepting in cases of two fragments when the N for them is equal to each other (and then their weight is equivalent), or in cases when three or more fragments are involved.
3. The efficiency of each fragment is directly calculated from the ΔG resulting in its direct interaction with a specific location (i.e., binding site or pocket) in a particular receptor.

Our hypothesis assumes, according to its first principle, that the WRMS of the LEs of the fragments composing an entire molecule ($\overline{LE_q}$) corresponds to the actual LE of this latter (LE_T) (A comprehensive list of mathematical terms is shown in **Supplementary Material**). Because this mean is intended to be proportionally similar to the real, total LE of an entire molecule (LE_T), we refer herein to it as the apparent total LE (LE_T^{app}):

$$\overline{LE_q} = LE_T^{app} \approx LE_T \tag{3}$$

For clarity of the RGC concept, we consider first the LE_T^{app} as a simple arithmetic mean:

$$LE_T^{app} = \frac{1}{x}(LE_1 + LE_2 + LE_3 + \ldots + LE_x) \tag{4}$$

where LE_i corresponds to the LE of the component fragments (LE_1, LE_2, etc.), and x refers to the number of fragments composing the molecule. Therefore, once LE is expressed in terms of the Equation (1):

$$LE_T^{app} = \frac{1}{x}\left(\frac{\Delta G_1}{N_1} + \frac{\Delta G_2}{N_2} + \frac{\Delta G_3}{N_3} + \ldots + \frac{\Delta G_x}{N_x}\right) \cong \frac{\Delta G_T}{xN_T} \tag{5}$$

where ΔG_i is the change in Gibbs free energy for each composing fragment (ΔG_1, ΔG_2, etc.) up to a maximum number of fragments x and N_i correspond to the number of non-hydrogen atoms of each fragment. Similarly, ΔG_T and N_T represent the change in Gibbs free energy and number of non-hydrogen atoms for the entire molecule, respectively. Should be remembered that (5) is based on an arithmetic mean and hence it assumes that N is equal among all composing fragments, so that it would just be applicable in this specific scenario.

If we consider the Equation (5) for a molecule composed by a single fragment:

$$LE_T^{app} = \frac{1}{x}\sum_{i=1}^{x}\left(\frac{\Delta G}{N}\right)_i = LE_1 \tag{6}$$

we can observe that LE_T^{app} correspond to the LE value of the unique component fragment, namely LE1, which supports a scenario where the component fragment is also the entire "final" molecule. However, expressing (5) for a molecule composed by two fragments:

$$LE_T^{app} = \frac{1}{x}\sum_{i=1}^{x}\left(\frac{\Delta G}{N}\right)_i = \frac{1}{2}\sum_{i=1}^{2}\left(\frac{\Delta G}{N}\right)_i = \frac{1}{2}(LE_1 + LE_2) \tag{7}$$

we could notice that, in contrast to the one-fragment case, the existence of more than one compound allows for the solution of the equation in terms of a particular fragment:

$$LE_2 = 2LE_T^{app} - LE_1 \tag{8}$$

The last equation poses a simple but important principle: Starting from an "ideal" LE_T^{app}, a particular low-LE fragment can be successfully chosen or "rescued" by one or more high-LE fragments. Now, if we consider a three-fragment case:

$$LE_T^{app} = \frac{1}{x}\sum_{i=1}^{x}\left(\frac{\Delta G}{N}\right)_i = \frac{1}{3}\sum_{i=1}^{3}\left(\frac{\Delta G}{N}\right)_i = \frac{1}{3}(LE_1 + LE_2 + LE_3) \quad (9)$$

Interestingly, for this case, even if we assume in this example that we know LE_1, it is still possible to consider a LE value for the unknown fragments LE_2 and LE_3 grouping them together into a single term:

$$LE_T^{app} = \frac{1}{3}(LE_1 + 2LE_\delta) \quad (10)$$

where the LE delta (LE_δ) corresponds to a transient, "ideal" value intended to be equal for all the fragments which individual LE is still unknown. Therefore, as we will discuss below, this value will be modified as long as new LE values are known for fragments, independently of their position.

Likewise, assuming also that we just know LE_1, we could express LE_T^{app} for the two-fragment case:

$$LE_T^{app} = \frac{1}{2}(LE_1 + LE_\delta) \quad (11)$$

which would indicate that:

$$LE_\delta = LE_2 \quad (12)$$

This result suggests, as we also discuss below, that a LE_δ is expected to equal the LE value of a last fragment to be known (LE_u), independently of the number of fragments and their position. This behavior corresponds to a subtractive average (SA). Remarkably, although the nature of LE_δ is somewhat similar to the cumulative average (CA) or moving average (MA), the number of fragments with unknown LE is continuously decreasing and LE_δ does not "run" within a predetermined window size.

Finally, assuming also that we just know LE_1, we could express LE_T^{app} for the one-fragment case:

$$LE_T^{app} = [\,LE_1 + 0\,(LE_\delta)] = LE_1 \quad (13)$$

indicating that LE_δ can only be calculated if there are at least two starting fragments and, more importantly, it is especially useful in cases of three or more of them.

At this point, think of the LE_T^{app} as a whole for an undetermined series of fragments:

$$LE_T^{app} = \frac{1}{x}(LE_1 + \ldots + LE_x) \quad (14)$$

If we assume again that we just know LE_1, it is possible to rearrange LE_T^{app} using LE_δ:

$$LE_T^{app} = \frac{1}{x}[LE_1 + (x-1)\,LE_\delta] \quad (15)$$

where (x-1) corresponds to the coefficient of the LE_δ value independently of the number of starting fragments as shown in Equations (10, 11, 13). Hence, if we resolve for LE_δ:

$$LE_\delta = \frac{1}{x-1}(xLE_T^{app} - LE_1) \quad (16)$$

Now, if we take into account that the number 1 in this equation actually corresponds to the number of known LE values of fragments or a, we can observe that:

$$if\ (x - a) \to 1,\ then\ LE_\delta \to LE_u \quad (17)$$

What means that the more (x-a) tends to 1, the more LE_δ tends to LE_u, just as we saw previously in Equation (12). Finally, considering the formula for LE_δ in terms of an undetermined number of fragments with different known and unknown LE values:

$$LE_\delta = \frac{1}{x-a}\left[\sum_{i=1}^{x}\left(\frac{\Delta G}{N}\right)_i - \sum_{j=0}^{a}\left(\frac{\Delta G}{N}\right)_j\right] \quad (18)$$

$$if\ and\ only\ if \begin{cases} 1 \le x < \infty \\ x \in \mathbb{N} \\ 0 \le a < x \\ a \in \mathbb{Z}_0^+ \end{cases}$$

where the first summation term indicates the "ideal" sum of LE values for the existing fragments (LE_i) as if they would have the same value, and the second summation term refers to the "real" sum of all fragments which LE value is already known (LE_j). On the other hand, if a = o, LE_0 would not proceed as a real value (and by extension the second summation term). Therefore, in this specific case a consequence would be that:

$$LE_\delta = LE_T^{app} \quad (19)$$

Now, after having explained the basic concepts of RGC and LE_δ, we could express LE_T^{app} in terms of the WMRS according to our hypothesis:

$$LE_T^{app} = \sqrt{\sum_{i=1}^{x} LE_i^2 w_i / \sum_{i=1}^{x} w_i} = \sqrt{\sum_{i=1}^{x}\left(\frac{\Delta G}{N}\right)_i^2 w_i / \sum_{i=1}^{x} w_i} \quad (20)$$

where LE_i corresponds to the LE of each component fragment, w_i refers to the weight of each fragment (depending on the N of each one) and x refers to the number of fragments.

Likewise, our formula for LE_δ would be:

$$LE_\delta = \frac{1}{\sqrt{w_\delta(x-a)}}\left[\sqrt{\sum_{i=1}^{x}\left(\frac{\Delta G}{N}\right)_i^2 w_i - \sum_{j=0}^{a}\left(\frac{\Delta G}{N}\right)_j^2 w_j}\right] \quad (21)$$

$$if\ and\ only\ if \begin{cases} 1 \le x < \infty \\ x \in \mathbb{N} \\ 0 \le a < x \\ a \in \mathbb{Z}_0^+ \end{cases}$$

The additional term in this equation, namely W_δ, corresponds to the "ideal" weight of all fragments with unknown LE value, as if they would have the same value. Just as with LE_δ, this parameter is expected to change with every new LE value of fragment known, until the value (weight) corresponding to the last fragment with unknown LE value is adopted.

FRAGMENT SELECTION AND LE_T PREDICTION BY THE RGC MODEL

As presented in a hypothetical example (**Figure 1**), three central premises may be elucidated for the RGC model by selecting hit compounds, starting from a cut-off LE value:

1. A low-efficiency fragment (i.e., with a LE $< LE_T^{app}$) can be rescued IF there exists high-efficiency fragments (i.e., with a LE $> LE_T^{app}$) in ALL the other positions (i.e., binding sites or pockets) of the target molecule, usually a protein. If this condition is not satisfied, the fragment could be automatically rejected from the set of possible combinations of fragments for an entire molecule.
2. If there are no high-efficiency fragments in all the other positions simultaneously, a molecular fragment with low-efficiency fragment can still be rescued IF at least one fragment in any other position with an efficiency high enough to reach exists, in average with the first, the LE_T^{app}. This implies, therefore, that once a fragment is rescued by one or more high-efficiency fragments in other positions, any fragment in subsequent unexplored positions is just required to have a mid-efficiency (with a LE $\cong LE_\delta$ ideal) as a minimum. Additionally, each time LE_δ changes, a differential "pushing" over the LE of unknown fragments occurs in terms of ΔG and/or N, which could be potentially modified to achieve an acceptable LE value and could therefore be selected.
3. Even if a low-efficiency fragment is not rescued after implementing the strategies stated in Equation (1, 2), a potential rescue could still take place exploring a more diverse library sample of fragments, assuming that (1) you are dealing with a number of fragments well-below under the maximum theoretical chemical space for them (a population of about 10^7 molecules) and (2) the fragment is not an outlier compared to other fragments intended to combine.

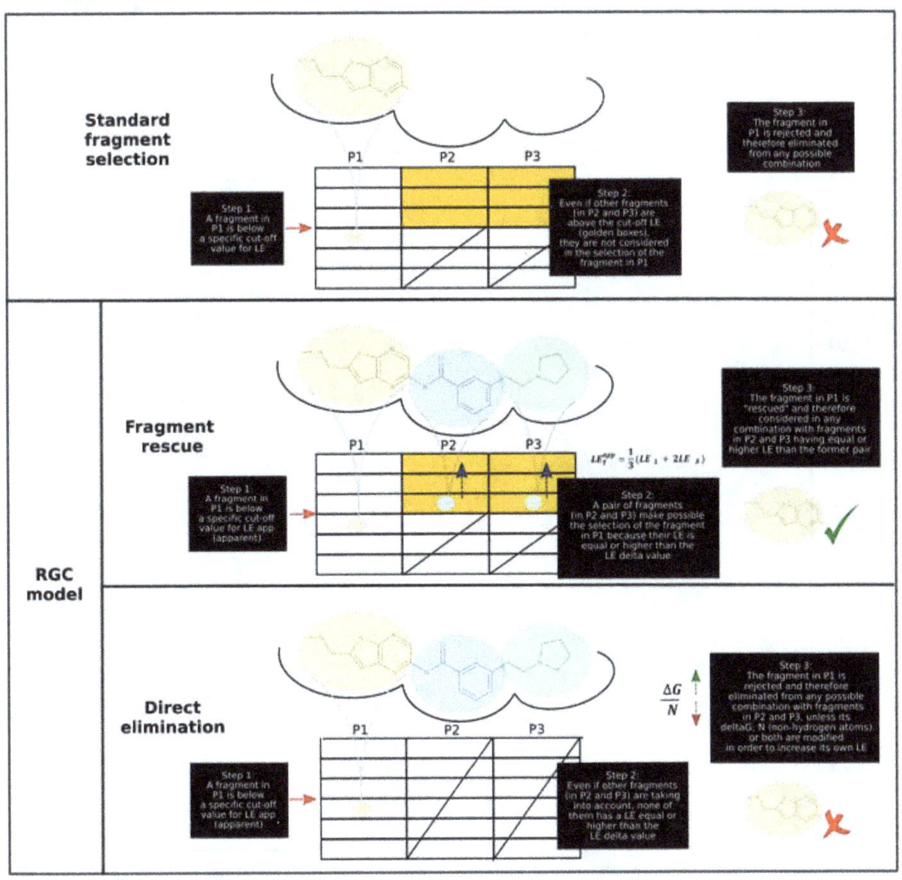

FIGURE 1 | Application of RGC model to a hypothetical fragment-based drug design (FBDD) campaign. (**Upper**) In the "standard" or classical screening approach, a fragment is selected (i.e., can be part of a final drug-size compound) depending exclusively upon their own LE. If this parameter is not equal or greater than a pre-established cut-off value, the fragment is rejected. (**Lower**) According to the RGC model, a fragment is selected depending on the fragments on the other positions. Based on the presence of high-LE fragments in alternative positions (illustrated by yellow boxes), a low-LE fragment may become either rescued or rapidly discarded (using the dynamic LE_δ value in both cases).

In addition, and according to our preliminary results, we found that LE_T^{app} values predicted by this model were consistent with the LE_T values calculated experimentally from a set of 16 drug-sized molecules taken from scientific literature (**Figure 2**, **Table 1S**).

DISCUSSION

The present study pretends to propose the RGC model as an innovative and effective approach to apply in drug design. This model and, especially, the fragment "rescue" effect that is conceptually implicit, offer an alternative for the long-standing FBDD paradigm of designing compounds merely based on the intrinsic binding energy of fragments, facilitating the introduction of other decision–making criteria that are becoming increasingly common.

If the principles of the RGC model are considered together, it is possible to elucidate two major advantages. First, we count on a limited amount of data and in order to more clearly reveal any trends, LE_T^{app} appears to increase as much as the LE_T, and there appears to be no dramatic shift toward higher efficiencies for particular fragments or protein targets. Secondly, since a particular fragment could be directly rejected early in the process and there are many fragments by pocket in a typical FBDD campaign, this model might dramatically reduce the computational and synthetic costs, respectively (which is especially true in cases of three or more pockets).

The RGC model is, however, not free of inherent shortcomings. As a LE-derived metric, all fragments are assumed to maintain equal orientations both individually and as part of a larger chemical compound (Zartler and Shapiro, 2008), and phenomena such as hot spots (Zerbe et al., 2012; Rathi et al., 2017) or synergy (also called "super-additivity") (Hebeisen et al., 2008; Nazaré et al., 2012) are not directly considered. Likewise, because its average-based nature, ΔG of each fragment is normalized not only at the number of non-hydrogen atoms but also on the number of component fragments. Therefore, the less accurate (or more extreme) ΔG values for fragments in each position are, the greater the difference expected between the LE_T^{app} and the LE_T. However, we believe that the impact of these hurdles could be minimized, improving the confidence of any potential fragment "rescue," if additional energy terms derived from rigid body barrier (ΔG_{rigid}), linker binding ($\Delta G_{binding}$) or strain (ΔG_{strain}) (Murray and Verdonk, 2006; Cherry and Mitchell, 2008) are included and the ΔG values are both accurate and above a reasonable cut-off value.

A final examination about the implications of this work leads us to assert that the fragment "rescue" phenomenon is far from being new: it has already occurred and continues to

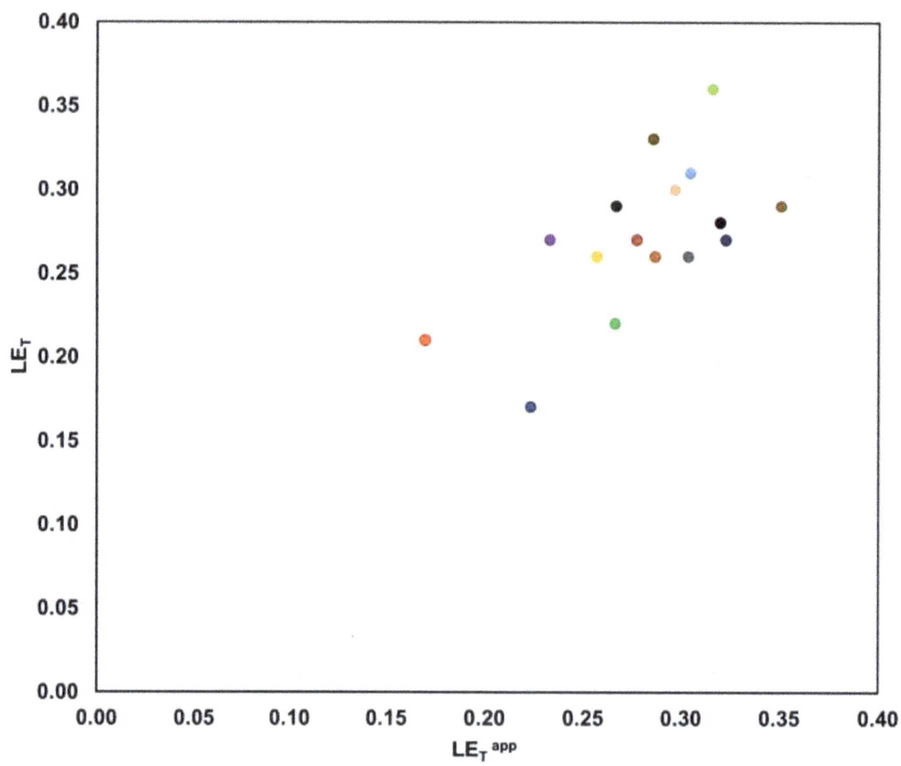

FIGURE 2 | Preliminary comparison between LE_T^{app} and LE_T for a set of 16 drug-sized literature compounds developed during FBDD studies. All compounds were elaborated using a linking strategy (on two fragments) for 10 different protein targets [●/● LDHA ● Replication Protein A (RPA) ●/● Blood coagulation factor Xa ● Bcl-2 ● DOT1L ● Hsp90 ●/● Pantothenate synthetase (PtS) ● Blood coagulation factor XIa ● CK2 ● BACE1 ● Endothiapepsin (Epn) ● Bcl-x_L ● PKM2].

occur, but usually during a lead optimization instead an earlier hit discovery phase. The rationale for this statement lies in two central facts. First, we currently know that the LE value of a compound tends to decrease during optimization process (Bembenek et al., 2009), while both its lipophilicity and its MW (and, hence, the number of non-hydrogen atoms -N) tends to increase (Ferenczy and Keseru, 2016). Second, the energy of supramolecular interactions is widely known to be largely different depending on the chemical moiety involved and, thus, ionic and hydrogen bonds are expected to account for a larger part of the drug-receptor binding energy (i.e., its ΔG) compared with hydrophobic interactions (Ermondi and Caron, 2006). Therefore, it is decidedly inviting to believe that, in many drug discovery initiatives, both the increase in LE and the decrease in MW and lipophilicity observed during lead optimization-could be explained by the addition of large and hydrophobic chemical moieties such as those cyclic aliphatic, which have a much smaller ΔG/N ratio compared to other fragments. Interestingly, these aliphatic moieties have been recently suggested by some authors to be more "developable" compared its aromatic analogs, which could be an additional factor behind this phenomenon (Lovering et al., 2009).

The RGC model presented in this study is based on the assumption that the LE of a drug-sized molecule may be estimated using the relative contribution of each component fragment. We believe this model could serve as a complementary benchmark for medicinal chemists in experimental or virtual fragment-based screening campaigns. Likewise, we consider that the RGC model could be implemented with other metrics based on either LE or a potency/size ratio and could be eventually adjusted to consider not only "linking" but also "growing" or "merging" as alternative fragment elaboration strategies.

AUTHOR CONTRIBUTIONS

AV planned and performed the entire *in silico* work presented in this study, contributed to the analysis and interpretation of data, and assisted the writing, editing, and submission of this manuscript. AG made substantial contributions to the data analysis, critical revision for important intellectual content, and document editing. All authors have read and approved the final manuscript.

FUNDING

We acknowledge funds from the Colombian Department of Science, Technology and Innovation COLCIENCIAS Grant No. 727.

ACKNOWLEDGMENTS

The authors gratefully acknowledge Professor Marco de Vivo from Istituto Italiano di Tecnologia (IIT), in Genoa (Italy) for helpful discussions and recommendations.

REFERENCES

Albert, J. S., Blomberg, N., Breeze, A., Brown, A., Burrows, J., Edwards, P., et al. (2007). An integrated approach to fragment-based lead generation: philosophy, strategy and case studies from AstraZeneca's Drug Discovery Programmes. *Curr. Top. Med. Chem.* 7, 1600–1629. doi: 10.2174/156802607782341091

Bembenek, S. D., Tounge, B. A., and Reynolds, C. H. (2009). Ligand efficiency and fragment-based drug discovery. *Drug Discov. Today* 14, 278–283. doi: 10.1016/j.drudis.2008.11.007

Cavalluzzi, M. M., Mangiatordi, G. F., Nicolotti, O., and Lentini, G. (2017). Ligand efficiency metrics in drug discovery: the pros and cons from a practical perspective. *Expert Opin. Drug Discov.* 12, 1087–1104. doi: 10.1080/17460441.2017.1365056

Cherry, M., and Mitchell, T. (2008). "Introduction to fragment-based drug discovery," in *Fragment-Based Drug Discovery*, eds E. R. Zartler and M. J. Shapiro, 1-32. doi: 10.1002/9780470721551.ch1

Costantino, L., and Barlocco, D. (2018). "Designing Approaches to Multitarget Drugs," in *Drug Selectivity: An Evolving Concept in Medicinal Chemistry*, 161–205.

Ermondi, G., and Caron, G. (2006). Recognition forces in ligand-protein complexes: blending information from different sources. *Biochem. Pharmacol.* 72, 1633–1645. doi: 10.1016/j.bcp.2006.05.022

Ferenczy, G. G., and Keseru, G. M. (2016). "Ligand efficiency metrics and their use in fragment optimizations," in *Fragment-Based Drug Discovery Lessons and Outlook*, eds D. A. Erlanson and W. Jahnke (Wiley-VCH Verlag GmbH & Co. KGaA), 75–98. doi: 10.1002/9783527683604.ch04

Fukunishi, Y., Kurosawa, T., Mikami, Y., and Nakamura, H. (2014). Prediction of synthetic accessibility based on commercially available compound databases. *J. Chem. Inf. Model.* 54, 3259–3267. doi: 10.1021/ci500568d

Hebeisen, P., Kuhn, B., Kohler, P., Gubler, M., Huber, W., Kitas, E., et al. (2008). Allosteric FBPase inhibitors gain 10(5) times in potency when simultaneously binding two neighboring AMP sites. *Bioorganic Med. Chem. Lett.* 18, 4708–4712. doi: 10.1016/j.bmcl.2008.06.103

Hopkins, A. L., Groom, C. R., and Alex, A. (2004). Ligand efficiency: a useful metric for lead selection. *Drug Discov. Today* 9, 430–431. doi: 10.1016/S1359-6446(04)03069-7

Hopkins, A. L., Keser,ü, G. M., Leeson, P. D., Rees, D. C., and Reynolds, C. H. (2014). The role of ligand efficiency metrics in drug discovery. *Nat. Rev. Drug Discov.* 13, 105–121. doi: 10.1038/nrd4163

Jasial, S., Hu, Y., and Bajorath, J. (2017). How frequently are pan-assay interference compounds active? Large-scale analysis of screening data reveals diverse activity profiles, low global hit frequency, and many consistently inactive compounds. *J. Med. Chem.* 60, 3879–3886. doi: 10.1021/acs.jmedchem.7b00154

Lovering, F., Bikker, J., and Humblet, C. (2009). Escape from flatland: increasing saturation as an approach to improving clinical success. *J. Med. Chem.* 52, 6752–6756. doi: 10.1021/jm901241e

Medina-Franco, J. L., Martinez-Mayorga, K., and Meurice, N. (2014). Balancing novelty with confined chemical space in modern drug discovery. *Expert Opin. Drug Discov.* 9, 151–165. doi: 10.1517/17460441.2014.872624

Murray, C. W., and Verdonk, M. L. (2006). "Entropic consequences of linking ligands," in *Fragment-Based Approaches in Drug Discovery*, eds R. Mannhold, H. Kubinyi, G. Folkers, W. Jahnke, and D. A. Erlanson (Weinheim: Wiley-VCG Verlag GmbH & Co. KGaA), 55–66. doi: 10.1002/3527608761.ch3

Nazaré, M., Matter, H., Will, D. W., Wagner, M., Urmann, M., Czech, J., et al. (2012). Fragment deconstruction of small, potent factor xa inhibitors: exploring the superadditivity energetics of fragment linking in protein-ligand complexes. *Angew. Chemie Int. Ed.* 51, 905–911. doi: 10.1002/anie.201107091

Rathi, P. C., Ludlow, R. F., Hall, R. J., Murray, C. W., Mortenson, P. N., and Verdonk, M. L. (2017). Predicting "Hot" and "Warm" Spots for Fragment Binding. *J. Med. Chem.* 60, 4036–4046. doi: 10.1021/acs.jmedchem.7b00366

Reynolds, C. H. (2015). Ligand efficiency metrics: why all the fuss? *Future Med. Chem.* 7, 1363–1365. doi: 10.4155/fmc.15.70

Schultes, S., De Graaf, C., Haaksma, E. E. J., De Esch, I. J. P., Leurs, R., and Krämer, O. (2010). Ligand efficiency as a guide in fragment hit selection and optimization. *Drug Discov. Today Technol.* 7, 157–162. doi: 10.1016/j.ddtec.2010.11.003

Verdonk, M. L., and Rees, D. C. (2008). Group efficiency: a guideline for hits-to-leads chemistry. *Chem. Med. Chem.* 3, 1179–1180. doi: 10.1002/cmdc.200800132

Zartler, E. R., and Shapiro, M. J. (eds.). (2008). "Designing a fragment process to fit your needs," in *Fragment-Based Drug Discovery* (John Wiley & Sons, Ltd.), 15–37. doi: 10.1002/9780470721551.ch2

Zerbe, B. S., Hall, D. R., Vajda, S., Whitty, A., and Kozakov, D. (2012). Relationship between hot spot residues and ligand binding hot spots in protein-protein interfaces. *J. Chem. Inf. Model.* 52, 2236–2244. doi: 10.1021/ci300175u

6

Teaching an Old Dog New Tricks: Strategies that Improve Early Recognition in Similarity-Based Virtual Screening

Ruifeng Liu[1,2]*, *Mohamed Diwan M. AbdulHameed*[1,2] *and Anders Wallqvist*[1]*

[1] *Department of Defense Biotechnology High Performance Computing Software Applications Institute, Telemedicine and Advanced Technology Research Center, U.S. Army Medical Research and Development Command, Fort Detrick, MD, United States,* [2] *The Henry M. Jackson Foundation for the Advancement of Military Medicine, Inc., Bethesda, MD, United States*

***Correspondence:**
Ruifeng Liu
rliu@bhsai.org
Anders Wallqvist
sven.a.wallqvist.civ@mail.mil

High throughput screening (HTS) is an important component of lead discovery, with virtual screening playing an increasingly important role. Both methods typically suffer from lack of sensitivity and specificity against their true biological targets. With ever-increasing screening libraries and virtual compound collections, it is now feasible to conduct follow-up experimental testing on only a small fraction of hits. In this context, advances in virtual screening that achieve enrichment of true actives among top-ranked compounds ("early recognition") and, hence, reduce the number of hits to test, are highly desirable. The standard ligand-based virtual screening method for large compound libraries uses a molecular similarity search method that ranks the likelihood of a compound to be active against a drug target by its highest Tanimoto similarity to known active compounds. This approach assumes that the distributions of Tanimoto similarity values to all active compounds are identical (i.e., same mean and standard deviation)—an assumption shown to be invalid (Baldi and Nasr, 2010). Here, we introduce two methods that improve early recognition of actives by exploiting similarity information of all molecules. The first method ranks a compound by its highest z-score instead of its highest Tanimoto similarity, and the second by an aggregated score calculated from its Tanimoto similarity values to all known actives and inactives (or a large number of structurally diverse molecules when information on inactives is unavailable). Our evaluations, which use datasets of over 20 HTS campaigns downloaded from PubChem, indicate that compared to the conventional approach, both methods achieve a ~10% higher Boltzmann-enhanced discrimination of receiver operating characteristic (BEDROC) score—a metric of early recognition. Given the increasing use of virtual screening in early lead discovery, these methods provide straightforward means to enhance early recognition.

Keywords: lead discovery, virtual screening, early recognition, Tanimoto similarity, z-score, BEDROC, ROCS

INTRODUCTION

Lead discovery by high throughput screening (HTS) is often described as a process akin to finding a needle in a haystack (Aherne et al., 2002). Given the significant achievements in automation, major pharmaceutical companies now routinely screen hundreds of thousands of samples to identify compounds that are active against specific drug targets. However, the number of chemicals available for bioactivity testing has increased exponentially over the past decade. For instance, as of 2015, the number of structurally unique chemicals registered in PubChem was more than 60 million (Kim et al., 2016), and in 2018, the total number of organic and inorganic substances disclosed in the literature was estimated to be 154 million[1]. Thus, despite the increased screening capacity, it remains impractical to assay a significant fraction of all available chemicals. Consequently, virtual screening is becoming increasingly important to prioritize and select compounds (Kar and Roy, 2013). The most widely used virtual screening methods are based on molecular similarity searches (Kristensen et al., 2013). These approaches typically rank molecules in a chemical library based on their structural similarity to a set of molecules known to be active against a desired target. Chemicals ranked high on the list can then be acquired and tested for the desired activity or property.

The most commonly used metric to compare the performance of different virtual screening methods is the area under the receiver operating characteristic curve (ROC_AUC) (Triballeau et al., 2005). This is useful for comparing overall performance of methods for ranking a database (Truchon and Bayly, 2007; Zhao et al., 2009). However, the ROC_AUC is inappropriate for virtual screening when the goal is to create a smaller subset enriched with the maximum number of actives (Truchon and Bayly, 2007). The distinction is critical, especially when the chemical libraries are large and only a small fraction of compounds can be tested. Truchon and Bayly (2007) illustrated the difference using three basic cases: (1) half of the actives ranked at the top of a rank-ordered list and the other half at the bottom; (2) all actives randomly distributed across ranks; and (3) all actives ranked in the middle of the list. In all three cases, the ROC_AUC value is 0.5 and, therefore, according to this metric, all three virtual screening methods that generated the three rank-ordered lists perform equally. However, because only a small fraction of chemicals in a large library can be tested, "early recognition" of actives is practically important. That is, case 1 is preferable to case 2 or 3, and case 2 could be considered more desirable than case 3.

Many metrics have been proposed to address early recognition. Examples include the partial area under the ROC curve (McClish, 1989), enrichment factor (Halgren et al., 2004), area under the accumulation curve (Kairys et al., 2006), robust initial enhancement (Sheridan et al., 2001), Boltzmann-enhanced discrimination of the receiver operating characteristic (BEDROC) (Truchon and Bayly, 2007), and predictiveness curve (Empereur-Mot et al., 2015). Although no metric is perfect, perhaps the most frequently adopted is BEDROC, which employs an adjustable parameter, α, to define "early detection." Truchon and Bayly suggest setting this parameter to 20.0, which dictates that 80% of the maximum contribution to BEDROC comes from the top 8% of the ranked list. A comparatively higher BEDROC score between two virtual screening methods indicates an enhanced ability to enrich the list of top-ranking compounds with active molecules.

Using both AUC_ROC and BEDROC, Nasr et al. (2009) carried out a large-scale study of the performance of 14 similarity search methods, including eight parameter-free methods (no parameters to be learned from training data) and six with one or two parameters to be learned from training data. Consistent with previous results, they found that the best parameter-free method is the Max-Sim method, which ranks molecules based on their maximum Tanimoto coefficient (TC, also commonly referred to as Tanimoto similarity) to the active query molecules. Among the six methods that require parameters to be fit to the data, the exponential Tanimoto discriminant (ETD) method was the best performer overall. This method is defined by the following equations.

$$S(B) = \frac{\sum_{i=1}^{m} S(A_i, B)}{\sum_{j=1}^{n} S(I_j, B)} \tag{1}$$

$$S(A, B) = \left[\lambda^{TC_{AB}} (1 - \lambda)^{1 - TC_{AB}}\right]^{\frac{1}{k}} \tag{2}$$

$$TC_{AB} = \frac{A \cap B}{A \cup B} \tag{3}$$

Here, $S(B)$ denotes the aggregated score for molecule B, m, and n, respectively denote the numbers of active and inactive query molecules, A_i denotes the ith active query molecule, I_j denotes the jth inactive molecule, TC_{AB} denotes the TC between molecules A and B, λ, and k denote parameters to be learned from the data. The higher the aggregated score, the more likely it is that molecule B is active. Nasr et al. (2009) provided neither recommended default parameter values for λ and k, nor values learned from any of their datasets.

In this article, we introduce two parameter-free similarity search methods that improve the early recognition of actives over the Max-Sim method. Using HTS data, we demonstrate that, on average, the BEDROC values derived from both methods are about 10% higher than those derived from the Max-Sim scoring method.

METHODS AND MATERIALS

Rank by Z-Scores

In a Max-Sim similarity search, we first calculate all TCs between the compounds in a chemical library and active query molecules. The library compounds are then ranked based on their highest TCs. The underlying assumption is that the higher the TC, the more likely a compound is to be active. This assumption is valid for searches with a single active query molecule, and for searches with multiple active query molecules if the distributions of TCs are identical (i.e., have the same mean and standard deviation irrespective of the query molecules). Although it has been standard practice for many years to conduct Max-Sim similarity searches, no study had examined the statistical distribution of

[1] https://www.cas.org/about/cas-content (accessed July 5, 2019).

TCs until 2010, when Baldi and Nasr (2010) investigated in detail the significance of Tanimoto similarity. They showed that the statistical distribution of TCs is not invariant, but depends on the number of fingerprint features present in a query molecule. This finding and its implications, however, are largely overlooked by the cheminformatics community, perhaps due to the reasonably good performance of the Max-Sim method and the extremely low mean TCs for any query molecule. As an example, **Figure 1** shows the means and standard deviations of the TCs of 10,000 chemicals randomly selected from the U.S. National Cancer Institute (NCI) chemical library calculated with respect to each of three drugs approved by the U.S. Food and Drug Administration. All of the means and standard deviations are close to zero, suggesting that most NCI compounds do not have the same activity as that of the approved drugs. The small mean TCs may obscure an important fact—that the values are not identical and could be significantly different. For instance, the mean TC of scopolamine is 43% higher than that of pemirolast. To appreciate the implications of the difference, let us assume that a molecule has TCs of 0.80 and 0.70 calculated with respect to scopolamine and pemirolast, respectively. Based on the Max-Sim method, one would expect the molecule to have activities more similar to those of scopolamine. However, because of the difference in the means and standard deviations, the z-scores of the molecule calculated with respect to scopolamine and pemirolast are 17.3 and 22.8, respectively, suggesting that the molecule is more likely to have activities similar to those of pemirolast than to those of scopolamine. If we consider that there are differences in mean TCs and standard deviations, then ranking molecules by the maximum z-score is statistically preferable in a similarity search. Accordingly, we designate this approach as the maxZ method.

Rank by Aggregated Similarity

In the past two decades, HTS has contributed to the discovery of numerous structurally novel active compounds against many important drug targets. As these compounds are identified from large experimentally tested screening libraries, they are classified as either active or inactive based on predefined activity criteria. In follow-up studies based on virtual screening by similarity search methods, only active compounds are used as queries. As noted in the Introduction, Nasr et al. (2009) developed the ETD method, which exploits information of both active and inactive compounds. They found that ETD performed best among 14 parameterized and non-parameterized TC-based similarity search methods. An undesirable feature of this method, however, is that it requires two parameters that may not be universally applicable, but still need to be fit for each individual dataset. Here, we propose an aggregated similarity (AS) method that does not require any parameter fitting based on individual datasets. We define the AS method by the following equation:

$$AS\,(X) = \frac{\sum_{i=1}^{m} e^{-\frac{1-TC(A_i,X)}{\alpha+TC(A_i,X)}}}{\sum_{j=1}^{n} e^{-\frac{1-TC(I_j,X)}{\alpha+TC(I_j,X)}}} \quad (4)$$

where, X denotes a compound in a chemical library, m and n, respectively denote the number of active and inactive molecules, $TC(A_i, X)$ denotes the TC between the ith active molecule and X, $TC(I_j, X)$ denotes the TC between the jth inactive molecule and X, and α is set to 10^{-6}—a small number to avoid division by zero when TC equals zero. Possible $AS(X)$ values range from zero to infinity, where zero indicates that molecule X shares no fingerprint features with any of the active query molecules, i.e., all $TC\,(A_i, X) = 0$, and infinity indicates that molecule X shares no fingerprint features with any of the inactive query molecules. In reality, because the number of inactive molecules is large (i.e., a positive is like a needle in a haystack and, therefore, most molecules can be classified as inactives), the probability of X sharing no fingerprint features with any of the inactive query molecules is zero, unless a very small number of inactive query molecules is used (even though a large number of them should be available).

One problem with using information on inactive compounds is that the results of large-scale screening campaigns are not equally reliable for active and inactive compounds. This is because such campaigns are typically executed in multiple confirmatory steps focusing on active compounds. The first step involves an initial primary screening of a large number of samples at a single concentration with few or no replicates. Samples deemed to meet the primary activity criteria are then selected and retested in multiple replicates, usually with counter-assays to affirm activity. Samples that satisfy the retesting criteria may be further tested at multiple concentrations to determine potency. One consequence of this screening protocol is that the activities of a positive compound are more reliable because they are reassessed in multiple tests, whereas compounds fail to meet primary active criteria are not retested to confirm inactivity. As a result, the set of inactive molecules is likely to contain false negatives. A more obvious problem with the AS method is that it cannot be applied to cases where information on inactives is unavailable. As a means to overcome this challenge, we suggest that a set of structurally diverse compounds can be used as putative inactive compounds. This is because compounds that are truly active against the most valuable drug targets are rare (i.e., needles in a haystack). Therefore, within a structurally diverse set of compounds, the number of compounds that are active against a drug target should be small. Here, we tested the validity of this hypothesis by using 10,000 structurally diverse compounds as putative inactives. We selected these compounds by clustering ~275,000 compounds of the NCI virtual screening library (Shiryaev et al., 2011) into 10,000 clusters based on the TC (a measure of molecular similarity), and selecting the cluster centers as structurally diverse compounds to represent coverage of the chemical space of the full dataset. In doing so, we considered a singleton as a cluster of size one.

Datasets

We evaluated the performance of the similarity search methods using HTS data generated from the National Center for Advancing Translational Sciences of the National Institutes of Health. We downloaded the data in two batches. The first batch consisted of the results of ~8,000 samples screened against 10 toxicity-related targets using 12 different assays, with two different assays deployed for two of the 10 targets. Thus, roughly

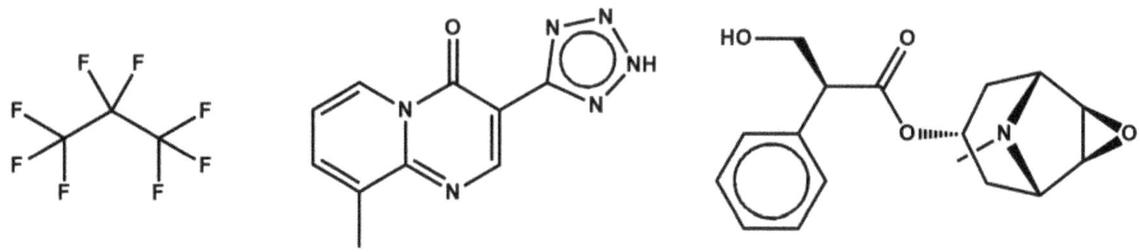

FIGURE 1 | Examples of means and standard deviations (STD) of the Tanimoto coefficients (TCs) of 10,000 compounds randomly selected from the National Cancer Institute's virtual screening library calculated with respect to three drugs approved by the Food and Drug Administration.

the same 8,000 samples were tested in 12 assays, generating 12 molecular activity datasets. As these datasets were used in the Tox21 Data Challenge for molecular activity predictions (Huang and Xia, 2017), we downloaded them from Tox21 Data Challenge web site[2]. Because the datasets were relatively small (consisting of ~7,000 structurally unique compounds), we used them to evaluate maxZ scoring methods based on two-dimensional (2-D) molecular fingerprints and three-dimensional (3-D) molecular shapes.

A library consisting of 8,000 samples can hardly be considered a "large" library for HTS. Therefore, we used a second batch of data that consisted of results for a few thousand to a few hundred thousand samples screened against 12 different molecular targets. We downloaded these data from the PubChem web site (https://pubchem.ncbi.nlm.nih.gov/) using their assay IDs as queries. **Table 1** shows the assay IDs of these datasets together with the Tox21 Challenge datasets. Details of the datasets, including the molecular targets, specific assays, number of samples screened, and number of samples deemed active, can be found from PubChem using the respective assay IDs as queries.

Because some samples were prepared from the same parent chemicals, we first cleaned the data before using them to evaluate the performance of the similarity search methods. We first removed counter-ions in salts and retained the largest component in samples consisting of non-bonded (i.e., disconnected) components. We then standardized the structures by neutralizing acids and bases (protonating acids and de-protonating bases) and generating a canonical SMILES from the standardized structure for each sample. For the results of each dataset, we applied a first-pass filter on canonical SMILES and retained only the first sample entry of a structurally unique parent compound. **Table 1** summarizes the resulting number of structurally unique parent compounds tested and the number of structurally unique actives from each assay.

In addition to the 24 HTS datasets, we also evaluated performance of the methods on 40 datasets in the Directory of Useful Decoys (DUD) (Huang et al., 2006) and an enhanced version of DUD consisting of 102 datasets called DUDE datasets (Mysinger et al., 2012). Each of these datasets consists of compounds known active on a protein target and many compounds of similar physicochemical properties as the actives but of very different molecular structures as the actives. These datasets are designed for evaluating the performance of docking-based virtual screening methods. We expect them to be less challenging than the HTS datasets for 2-D molecular similarity search methods, because in these datasets the actives and decoys are well-separated in molecular structure space and, therefore, any fingerprint-based similarity search methods are expected to perform well on these datasets.

Evaluation Protocol

To evaluate the performance of the methods, for each dataset we randomly selected 100 actives as the queries, and combined the other actives with the other compounds tested. We then calculated the maximum TC for each of these compounds with respect to the queries, as well as the maximum z-score and AS score. For these calculations, we used the extended connectivity fingerprint (Rogers and Hahn, 2010) with a maximum diameter of four chemical bonds (ECFP_4) and a fixed fingerprint length of 2,048 bits. We calculated ROC_AUC and BEDROC values for the Max-Sim, maxZ, and AS methods. For all BEDROC calculations, we used the default parameter setting of $\alpha = 20.0$, i.e., corresponding to 80% of the maximum contribution to BEDROC coming from the top 8% of the list of ranked molecules. To ensure statistical significance of the findings, we repeated the calculations nine times, using 100 randomly selected actives as queries each time. We compared the performance of the methods based on the resulting mean ROC_AUC and BEDROC values.

RESULTS

Performance of the maxZ Method

Table 2 shows a summary of the mean ROC_AUC and BEDROC values derived from the Max-Sim and maxZ methods for the 24

[2] https://tripod.nih.gov/tox21/challenge/data.jsp (accessed July 5, 2019).

TABLE 1 | PubChem datasets used in this study to evaluate performance of similarity search methods.

Dataset[a]	PubChem Assay ID[b]	Samples[c]	Unique structures[d]	Unique actives[e]
AHR	743122	8169	6318	723
AR	743040	9362	7009	290
ARE	743219	7167	5643	889
AR-lbd	743053	8599	6524	233
Aromatase	743139	7226	5601	273
ATAD5	720516	9091	6825	253
ER	743079	7697	5993	716
ER-lbd	743077	8753	6727	324
HSE	743228	8150	6253	337
MMP	720637	7320	5625	885
P53	720552	8634	6544	410
PPARg	743140	8184	6232	174
4-MU	589	59070	58199	6146
ALDH1A1	1030	220365	215450	15847
BRCA1	624202	377534	373883	3938
DNApb	485314	337903	333082	4466
ERK	1454	133383	130623	532
GCN5L2	504327	387577	379179	741
hERG	588834	5363	4568	553
Lucif	411	72335	70939	1558
MiRNAs	2289	336623	332205	3265
Mitoch	485298	322909	320471	734
NPC1	485313	321376	319001	7532
PR901	1347036	9523	7177	111

[a] *All datasets are derived from quantitative high throughput screening conducted at the National Center for Advancing Translational Sciences to ascertain chemical activities against different molecular targets. The first 12 datasets were used in the 2014 Tox21 Data Challenge.*
[b] *The datasets can be accessed from the PubChem website using the assay IDs as queries.*
[c] *Total number of samples screened in each dataset.*
[d] *Number of structurally unique parent molecules (non-salts, non-mixtures) derived from retaining the largest chemical structure in each sample and performing structure standardization.*
[e] *Number of structurally unique active parent molecules.*
Dataset names: AHR, activators of aryl hydrocarbon receptor; AR, activators of androgen receptor; AR-lbd, activators of androgen receptor ligand binding domain; Aromatase, aromatase inhibitors; ER, estrogen receptor activators; ER-lbd, activators of estrogen receptor ligand binding domain; PPARg, activators of peroxisome proliferator-activated receptor gamma; ARE, activators of antioxidant response element; ATAD5, ATPase family AAA domain-containing protein 5; HSE, activators of heat shock response signaling pathway; MMP, disruptors of mitochondrial membrane potential; p53, activators of p53 signaling pathway; hERG, blockers of hERG potassium channel; PR901, agonists of progesterone receptor; 4-MU, spectroscopic response at the 4-methylumbelliferone region as a counter assay for fluorescence detection; Lucif, inhibitors of Luciferase; ERK, inhibitors of mitogen-activated protein kinase 1; ALDH1A1, inhibitors of aldehyde dehydrogenase 1 family, member A1; NPC1, promoters of Niemann-Pick C1 protein precursor; Mitoch, inhibitors of mitochondrial division; MiRNAs, modulators of miRNAs; DNApb, inhibitors of DNA polymerase beta; BRCA1, activators of BRCA1 expression; GCN5L2, inhibitors of histone acetyltransferase KAT2A.

datasets. The mean ROC_AUC values derived from the Max-Sim method and those derived from the maxZ method were similar, with the latter only 3.7% higher than the former. In contrast, the mean difference in BEDROC values between the maxZ and Max-Sim methods was as high as 15%. However, the result for one dataset, NPC1, was an outlier, as the difference was as high as 170%, and the mean difference in BEDROC values decreased to 8.7% when it was excluded. Nonetheless, the maxZ method still outperformed the Max-Sim method, as the ROC_AUC and BEDROC values derived from maxZ were smaller than those derived from Max-Sim in only two of the 24 datasets. Although the differences between the maxZ and Max-Sim results were small for some datasets, for those showing a considerable difference, maxZ performed significantly better. For instance, the ROC_AUC values derived from maxZ were at least 5% higher than those derived from Max-Sim in 8 of the 24 datasets, whereas Max-Sim performed better than maxZ by 5% or more in only two datasets. This difference was even more pronounced for BEDROC values, as maxZ outperformed Max-Sim by 5% or more in 15 of the 24 datasets, whereas the opposite was true in only one dataset. Overall, the ROC_AUC values show that the maxZ method performs only slightly better than the Max-Sim method for ranking all samples in the dataset, whereas the BEDROC values indicate that the maxZ method performs markedly better than the Max-Sim method in the early recognition of active compounds.

A popular 3-D equivalent of 2-D fingerprint-based molecular similarity search is the Rapid Overlay of Chemical Structures (ROCS) method (OpenEye Scientific Software, Santa Fe, NM) (Fontaine et al., 2007), which calculates the Tanimoto similarity between 3-D molecular shapes and pharmacophore features. Because of the similarity between 2-D fingerprint-based and

TABLE 2 | Mean and standard deviation of ROC_AUC and BEDROC values derived from a similarity search using the rank by maximum similarity (Max-Sim) and maximum z-score (maxZ) approaches over 10 runs, each with 100 randomly selected actives as queries.

	ROC_AUC					BEDROC				
	Max-Sim		maxZ			Max-Sim		maxZ		
Dataset	Mean	Std	Mean	Std	%Diff[a]	Mean	Std	Mean	Std	%Diff[b]
AHR	0.754	0.011	0.759	0.012	0.7	0.402	0.016	0.365	0.019	−9.3
AR	0.740	0.009	0.748	0.009	1.0	0.482	0.019	0.509	0.014	5.6
ARE	0.539	0.008	0.544	0.009	1.0	0.225	0.014	0.266	0.018	17.9
AR-lbd	0.815	0.011	0.811	0.011	−0.5	0.607	0.023	0.610	0.028	0.6
Aromatase	0.662	0.017	0.686	0.016	3.6	0.263	0.026	0.291	0.019	10.7
ATAD5	0.713	0.022	0.724	0.018	1.6	0.303	0.025	0.313	0.020	3.4
ER	0.665	0.005	0.667	0.009	0.4	0.380	0.009	0.395	0.012	3.8
ER-lbd	0.715	0.011	0.726	0.010	1.5	0.381	0.026	0.382	0.025	0.0
HSE	0.579	0.027	0.595	0.027	2.8	0.186	0.020	0.205	0.023	10.3
MMP	0.694	0.009	0.704	0.018	1.4	0.414	0.024	0.469	0.025	13.2
P53	0.611	0.013	0.649	0.013	6.1	0.251	0.016	0.265	0.012	5.8
PPARg	0.681	0.018	0.686	0.027	0.7	0.274	0.031	0.277	0.030	1.0
4-MU	0.565	0.007	0.604	0.007	7.0	0.272	0.010	0.316	0.009	16.1
ALDH1A1	0.506	0.004	0.513	0.009	1.3	0.104	0.007	0.111	0.007	6.8
BRCA1	0.667	0.006	0.694	0.004	4.2	0.147	0.006	0.155	0.006	5.5
DNApb	0.591	0.011	0.633	0.012	7.1	0.137	0.006	0.163	0.012	18.9
ERK	0.647	0.021	0.698	0.017	8.0	0.235	0.017	0.250	0.016	6.3
GCN5L2	0.541	0.014	0.651	0.016	20.5	0.179	0.015	0.245	0.015	36.9
hERG	0.745	0.009	0.732	0.013	−1.8	0.460	0.009	0.447	0.012	−2.7
Lucif	0.707	0.008	0.737	0.010	4.1	0.255	0.010	0.268	0.012	4.9
MiRNAs	0.574	0.004	0.609	0.010	6.1	0.128	0.004	0.144	0.008	12.0
Mitoch	0.510	0.006	0.546	0.007	7.0	0.079	0.007	0.101	0.006	28.9
NPC1	0.653	0.007	0.696	0.007	6.5	0.079	0.007	0.213	0.006	170.0
PR901	0.931	0.013	0.945	0.013	1.5	0.800	0.025	0.822	0.022	2.8
Mean					**3.8**					**15.4**

[a] *Percent difference between mean ROC_AUC values for Max-Sim and maxZ methods.*
[b] *Percent difference between mean BEDROC values for Max-Sim and maxZ methods.*

3-D ROCS-based similarity searches, we hypothesized that the maxZ method would also improve early recognition for ROCS-based 3-D similarity searches. To test this hypothesis, we generated up to 15 low-energy conformers for each molecule in the 12 datasets used in the 2014 Tox21 Data Challenge, using Omega version 3.0.1.2 (OpenEye Scientific Software) with default parameters (Hawkins et al., 2010). We then conducted ROCS-based similarity searches for each dataset using randomly selected 10% actives as active queries. Each query molecule was represented by up to 15 of its lowest-energy conformers. We calculated the Tanimoto combo similarity (commonly called the combo score, which is the sum of the shape TC and color force field TCs) pairwise between the conformers of each active query and each conformer of the other compounds using ROCS version 3.2.2.2 with default parameters. The maximum Tanimoto combo score between a query molecule and a non-query molecule is designated as the Tanimoto combo score of the non-query molecule. We then calculated the ROC_AUC and BEDROC values using the maximum Tanimoto combo scores and the maximum z-scores calculated from the Tanimoto combo scores. We repeated this calculation nine more times, each with 10% of the actives randomly selected as active query molecules. **Table 3** shows the means and standard deviations of the ROC_AUC and BEDROC values. The results were similar to those of 2-D fingerprint-based similarity searches, i.e., the ROC_AUC values derived from the maxZ method were a few percentage points higher than those derived from the Max-Sim method, but the difference between BEDROC values was 12,6% on average. Thus, sorting the samples by the maximum z-values of the combo scores led to a substantial improvement in early recognition.

We evaluated the maxZ method for 3-D similarity search of the Tox21 Challenge datasets only, because the datasets were small (7,009 structurally unique compounds in the largest) and the computations could be completed within a reasonable amount of time. Most of the other datasets are much larger, with up to a few hundred thousand structurally unique compounds. We did not evaluate the performance of the maxZ method on these datasets, because the ROCS calculations would have required substantially more computing resources.

TABLE 3 | Mean and standard deviation of ROC_AUC and BEDROC values derived from a ROCS-based 3-D molecular similarity search using the rank by maximum similarity (Max-Sim) and maximum z-score (maxZ) methods.

	ROC_AUC					BEDROC				
	Max-Sim		maxZ			Max-Sim		maxZ		
Dataset	Mean	Std	Mean	Std	%Diff[a]	Mean	Std	Mean	Std	%Diff[b]
AHR	0.588	0.004	0.603	0.004	2.5	0.112	0.003	0.126	0.003	12.7
AR	0.729	0.007	0.749	0.015	2.7	0.201	0.010	0.234	0.013	16.2
ARE	0.547	0.004	0.560	0.005	2.5	0.090	0.003	0.101	0.002	12.6
AR-lbd	0.645	0.020	0.661	0.023	2.4	0.168	0.014	0.208	0.012	23.3
Aromatase	0.562	0.011	0.579	0.013	3.1	0.068	0.005	0.080	0.004	17.2
ATAD5	0.663	0.010	0.686	0.012	3.5	0.164	0.009	0.183	0.009	11.5
ER	0.685	0.007	0.703	0.009	2.6	0.168	0.007	0.184	0.005	10.1
ER-lbd	0.679	0.007	0.697	0.008	2.8	0.181	0.006	0.201	0.006	11.0
HSE	0.526	0.011	0.538	0.012	2.3	0.078	0.005	0.085	0.005	8.7
MMP	0.553	0.002	0.568	0.003	2.6	0.119	0.003	0.127	0.001	7.0
P53	0.575	0.009	0.590	0.011	2.5	0.091	0.006	0.101	0.004	11.2
PPARg	0.569	0.016	0.592	0.020	3.9	0.104	0.010	0.114	0.008	9.7
Mean					**2.8**					**12.6**

[a] *Percent difference between mean ROC_AUC values for Max-Sim and maxZ methods.*
[b] *Percent difference between mean BEDROC values for Max-Sim and maxZ methods.*

Performance of the AS Method

Table 4 shows the ROC_AUC and BEDROC values calculated from the Max-Sim and AS methods for the 12 Tox21 Challenges datasets. We calculated the AS score using a negative set (inactives) of 1,000 randomly selected compounds from the set of all screening negatives. We used the rest of the actives and inactives in each dataset as test data to evaluate the performance of each similarity search method. Both ROC_AUC and BEDROC values calculated from AS scores were significantly higher than the corresponding values obtained using the Max-Sim method, confirming that exploiting the available information on inactives improves the performance of both virtual screening methods. Note that the improvement of BEDROC values is significantly greater than that of ROC_AUC values, suggesting that the performance gains are mainly due to early recognition of actives in the AS method.

As noted in section Rank by Aggregated Similarity, because drug discovery involves rigorous confirmation of the activities of actives, but rarely any investments in efforts to confirm inactivity, information on inactive compounds is usually less reliable than that on active compounds. In addition, for some projects, active queries are not derived from screening of chemical libraries and, hence, there is no information on inactive compounds. However, because the number of compounds that are active against any drug target can be assumed to be miniscule compared to the number of all available compounds, we hypothesized that a large number of structurally diverse compounds should be able to serve as putative inactive compounds for the AS method. To test this hypothesis, we repeated the evaluation above, using 10,000 structurally diverse compounds selected from the NCI library. **Table 5** shows that the replacement of inactive compounds by structurally diverse compounds led to a significant performance deterioration of the AS method, especially in terms of ROC_AUC values, which were only 2.6% higher on average than those of the Max-Sim method. However, the overall mean BEDROC value was still 14.6% higher than that of the Max-Sim method, indicating that early recognition improved even when inactive compounds from screening were unavailable.

To assess the validity of the findings on the 12 Tox21 Challenge datasets for a wider range of datasets with the number of chemicals ranging from a few thousand to few hundred thousand, we conducted virtual screening using the AS method and the same 10,000 structurally diverse NCI compounds as putative inactive compounds. The results were comparable to those obtained from the Tox21 Challenge datasets, indicating that the method is applicable to a wide range of HTS datasets (**Table 6**).

Performance of the maxZ and AS Methods on the DUD and DUDE Datasets

Because most DUD and DUDE datasets contain <100 actives, we performed evaluations on these datasets by randomly selecting 10% of the actives as queries. We used the remaining actives and all decoys as test sets to evaluate the performance of the methods. As these datasets do not contain any experimentally determined inactives, we used the same set of 10,000 structurally diverse NCI compounds as putative inactives in testing the performance of the AS method. **Table S1** shows detailed results obtained from the 40 DUD and 102 DUDE datasets and **Table 7** summarizes these results.

The most obvious difference between the summary results in **Table 7** and the results in **Table 2** was that the ROC_AUC and BEDROC values of the HTS datasets derived from the Max-Sim method were significantly lower than the corresponding values of the DUD and DUDE datasets. The mean ROC_AUC

TABLE 4 | Mean and standard deviation of ROC_AUC and BEDROC values derived from a fingerprint-based similarity search using the rank by maximum similarity (Max-Sim) and rank by aggregated score (AS) methods.

	ROC_AUC					BEDROC				
	Max-Sim		AS			Max-Sim		AS		
Dataset	Mean	Std	Mean	Std	%Diff[a]	Mean	Std	Mean	Std	%Diff[b]
AHR	0.734	0.010	0.829	0.010	13.0	0.385	0.016	0.534	0.018	38.6
AR	0.749	0.013	0.809	0.013	8.0	0.443	0.020	0.618	0.019	39.7
ARE	0.537	0.008	0.650	0.011	21.0	0.264	0.021	0.404	0.015	53.2
AR-lbd	0.795	0.017	0.823	0.014	3.5	0.574	0.026	0.605	0.022	5.5
Aromatase	0.615	0.016	0.727	0.021	18.2	0.219	0.029	0.323	0.019	47.3
ATAD5	0.652	0.018	0.717	0.018	9.9	0.273	0.023	0.303	0.024	11.0
ER	0.602	0.024	0.683	0.024	13.6	0.234	0.016	0.439	0.039	87.7
ER-lbd	0.689	0.014	0.713	0.011	3.6	0.374	0.027	0.386	0.017	3.3
HSE	0.557	0.009	0.650	0.012	16.8	0.122	0.010	0.210	0.024	71.8
MMP	0.663	0.011	0.760	0.007	14.6	0.398	0.030	0.565	0.026	41.9
P53	0.588	0.020	0.723	0.013	23.0	0.224	0.017	0.262	0.020	16.9
PPARg	0.678	0.029	0.744	0.025	9.7	0.262	0.036	0.279	0.036	6.3
Mean					**12.9**					**35.3**

[a] *Percent difference between mean ROC_AUC values for Max-Sim and AS methods.*
[b] *Percent difference between mean BEDROC values for Max-Sim and AS methods.*

TABLE 5 | Mean and standard deviation of ROC_AUC and BEDROC values derived from a fingerprint-based similarity search using the rank by maximum similarity (Max-Sim) and rank by aggregated score (AS) methods, using 10,000 structurally diverse compounds as inactive compounds.

	ROC_AUC					BEDROC				
	Max-Sim		AS			Max-Sim		AS		
Dataset	Mean	Std	Mean	Std	%Diff[a]	Mean	Std	Mean	Std	%Diff[b]
AHR	0.730	0.010	0.758	0.009	3.8	0.337	0.023	0.407	0.017	20.8
AR	0.754	0.012	0.768	0.011	1.9	0.436	0.024	0.596	0.017	36.8
ARE	0.535	0.007	0.549	0.009	2.6	0.224	0.021	0.258	0.024	15.2
AR-lbd	0.790	0.018	0.807	0.021	2.2	0.550	0.020	0.614	0.030	11.6
Aromatase	0.621	0.024	0.663	0.023	6.7	0.202	0.040	0.289	0.036	43.2
ATAD5	0.653	0.024	0.666	0.025	2.0	0.268	0.021	0.281	0.023	4.9
ER	0.600	0.009	0.567	0.014	−5.5	0.197	0.010	0.136	0.021	−30.8
ER-lbd	0.683	0.018	0.712	0.017	4.2	0.366	0.030	0.461	0.019	25.8
HSE	0.553	0.013	0.576	0.016	4.2	0.118	0.018	0.147	0.026	24.4
MMP	0.651	0.016	0.689	0.012	5.9	0.336	0.029	0.454	0.019	35.0
P53	0.573	0.018	0.594	0.020	3.6	0.203	0.026	0.202	0.020	−0.2
PPARg	0.689	0.023	0.689	0.022	0.0	0.278	0.024	0.245	0.043	−12.0
Mean					**2.6**					**14.6**

[a] *Percent difference between mean ROC_AUC values for the Max-Sim and AS methods.*
[b] *Percent difference between mean BEDROC values for the Max-Sim and AS methods.*

values of the DUD and DUDE datasets were 0.90 and 0.96, respectively, and the corresponding mean BEDROC values were 0.76 and 0.90. These values were significantly higher than the corresponding mean ROC_AUC and BEDROC values of 0.66 and 0.29 for the 24 HTS datasets. These results corroborate our expectation that, because the actives and decoys are well-separated in molecular structure space, the DUD and DUDE datasets present much less of a challenge than do the HTS datasets for similarity search methods. Because the Max-Sim method achieved near perfect performance for these datasets, as indicated by an average ROC_AUC value of 0.96 and an average BEDROC value of 0.90 for the DUDE datasets, any improvement beyond the Max-Sim results will necessarily be small given the little room left for improvement. Indeed, **Table 7** shows that on average, the ROC_AUC or BEDROC values derived from the maxZ or AS method were only about 1%

TABLE 6 | Mean and standard deviation of ROC_AUC and BEDROC values derived from a fingerprint-based similarity search using the rank by maximum similarity (Max-Sim) and rank by aggregated score (AS) methods, using 10,000 structurally diverse compounds as inactive compounds.

	ROC_AUC					BEDROC				
	Max-Sim		AS			Max-Sim		AS		
Dataset	**Mean**	**Std**	**Mean**	**Std**	**%Diff[a]**	**Mean**	**Std**	**Mean**	**Std**	**%Diff[b]**
4-MU	0.513	0.007	0.525	0.016	2.3	0.143	0.012	0.175	0.014	22.1
ALDH1A1	0.510	0.004	0.519	0.004	1.8	0.142	0.004	0.144	0.003	1.0
BRCA1	0.643	0.008	0.657	0.008	2.3	0.143	0.008	0.146	0.009	2.1
DNApb	0.527	0.010	0.588	0.009	11.7	0.111	0.007	0.173	0.007	55.5
ERK	0.624	0.011	0.672	0.008	7.6	0.247	0.014	0.299	0.011	21.3
GCN5L2	0.542	0.015	0.542	0.017	−0.1	0.132	0.009	0.133	0.012	0.9
hERG	0.725	0.011	0.794	0.006	9.6	0.411	0.032	0.522	0.024	27.2
Lucif	0.735	0.009	0.782	0.006	6.3	0.285	0.015	0.335	0.010	17.5
MiRNAs	0.613	0.006	0.635	0.006	3.6	0.143	0.006	0.153	0.007	7.0
Mitoch	0.512	0.008	0.513	0.007	0.1	0.082	0.008	0.097	0.008	18.4
NPC1	0.681	0.005	0.705	0.007	3.6	0.222	0.005	0.242	0.008	9.0
PR901	0.896	0.019	0.901	0.020	0.5	0.718	0.030	0.757	0.037	5.5
Mean					**4.1**					**15.6**

[a]*Percent difference between mean ROC_AUC values for the Max-Sim and AS methods.*
[b]*Percent difference between mean BEDROC values for the Max-Sim and AS methods.*

TABLE 7 | Summary of the performance of similarity search methods on 40 DUD[a] and 102 DUDE[b] datasets.

Metric	Mean Max-Sim value[c]	Mean%diff[d]	Diff ≥ 0%[e]	Diff < 0%[f]	Diff ≥ 1%[g]	Diff < −1%[h]
MaxZ vs. Max-Sim method on 40 DUD datasets						
ROC_AUC	0.91	1.0	30	10	13	0
BEDROC	0.79	1.7	30	10	16	1
AS vs. Max-Sim method on 40 DUD datasets						
ROC_AUC	0.90	1.2	28	12	15	3
BEDROC	0.76	1.1	25	15	16	10
MaxZ vs. Max-Sim method on 102 DUDE datasets						
ROC_AUC	0.96	0.5	90	12	18	0
BEDROC	0.90	0.7	87	15	28	2
AS vs. Max-Sim method on 102 DUD datasets						
ROC_AUC	0.96	0.2	55	47	13	3
BEDROC	0.90	0.2	58	44	27	20

[a]*DUD: Directory of Useful Decoys, http://dud.docking.org/.*
[b]*DUDE: Database of Useful Decoys: Enhanced, http://dude.docking.org/.*
[c]*Mean ROC_AUC or BEDROC value calculated from the Max-Sim method over 40 DUD or 102 DUDE datasets.*
[d]*Mean percentage difference between ROC_AUC or BEDROC values derived from the maxZ or AS methods and the Max-Sim method.*
[e]*Number of datasets for which ROC_AUC or BEDROC values calculated from the maxZ or AS methods were higher than or equal to the corresponding values calculated from the Max-Sim method, i.e., the number of datasets on which the maxZ or AS method performed comparable to or better than the Max-Sim method did.*
[f]*Number of datasets for which ROC_AUC or BEDROC values calculated from the maxZ or AS methods were lower than the corresponding values calculated from the Max-Sim method, i.e., the number of datasets on which the maxZ or AS method performed worse than the Max-Sim method.*
[g]*Number of datasets for which ROC_AUC or BEDROC values calculated from the maxZ or AS methods were at least 1% higher than the corresponding values calculated from the Max-Sim method.*
[h]*Number of datasets for which ROC_AUC or BEDROC values calculated from the Max-Sim method was more than 1% higher than the corresponding values calculated from the maxZ or AS methods.*

higher and <1% higher than the corresponding values of the Max-Sim method for the DUD and DUDE datasets, respectively. Nevertheless, **Table 7** shows that the number of datasets for which the maxZ and AS methods performed better than the Max-Sim method by more than 1% was significantly higher than that for which the Max-Sim method performed better by more than 1%. Thus, for these datasets, the maxS and AS methods still outperformed the Max-Sim method (albeit with a smaller effect size) even though the Max-Sim method already achieved near perfect performance.

DISCUSSION

Fingerprint-based molecular similarity search is one of the most important tools for virtual screening of large chemical libraries. Over the years, many similarity search methods have been investigated, but the simple, parameter-free, rank-by-maximum Tanimoto similarity approach remains a popular method. It achieves robust performance based on the Tanimoto similarity of each compound in a compound library to its closest query molecule and disregarding its similarity to all other query molecules. In addition, it compares the values of Tanimoto similarity to different query molecules directly. This is theoretically correct only if the distribution of similarity values to all other query molecules is identical, an assumption that has been shown to be invalid (Baldi and Nasr, 2010).

In this study, we proposed and evaluated two parameter-free similarity search methods. The AS method considers information on the similarity to all query molecules, whereas the maxZ method converts the Tanimoto similarity into a z-score for a statistically sound, direct comparison. The results of our evaluations using over 20 HTS datasets indicated that neither method achieved significantly higher ROC_AUC values over the standard Max-Sim method. However, BEDROC values derived from both methods were ~10% higher than those of the Max-Sim method. Thus, although our methods perform comparably to the standard similarity search method when judged by ranking all compounds in a screening library, they perform better on early recognition by placing more actives at the top of a ranked list. This is an important trait for virtual screening of large chemical libraries, considering that follow-up experimental testing is feasible for only a small fraction of chemicals.

A conventional similarity search calculates TCs between all query molecules and all library molecules, and these values are sufficient for converting TCs to z-scores. As such, the additional computational cost to perform a similarity search using the maxZ method is minimal. Conversely, the AS method is notably slower than the Max-Sim method. However, with the ever-increasing power and decreasing cost of computing hardware, the method can become competitive based on its performance. Thus, when early recognition is among the objectives of virtual screening, the two methods provide alternatives to the standard Max-Sim method.

AUTHOR CONTRIBUTIONS

All authors contributed to the conception of the ideas and planned computational evaluations. RL performed the evaluations and wrote the first draft of the manuscript. AW supervised the project and contributed to the final manuscript.

FUNDING

The research was supported by the U.S. Army Medical Research and Development Command (Ft. Detrick, MD) as part of the U.S. Army's Network Science Initiative, and by the Defense Threat Reduction Agency (Grant No. CBCall14-CBS-05-2-0007).

ACKNOWLEDGMENTS

The authors gratefully acknowledge the assistance of Dr. Tatsuya Oyama in editing the manuscript. The opinions and assertions contained herein are the private views of the authors and are not to be construed as official or as reflecting the views of the U.S. Army, the U.S. Department of Defense, or The Henry M. Jackson Foundation for Advancement of Military Medicine, Inc.

REFERENCES

Aherne, G. W., McDonald, E., and Workman, P. (2002). Finding the needle in the haystack: why high-throughput screening is good for your health. *Breast Cancer Res.* 4, 148–154. doi: 10.1186/bcr440

Baldi, P., and Nasr, R. (2010). When is chemical similarity significant? The statistical distribution of chemical similarity scores and its extreme values. *J. Chem. Inf. Model.* 50, 1205–1222. doi: 10.1021/ci100010v

Empereur-Mot, C., Guillemain, H., Latouche, A., Zagury, J. F., Viallon, V., and Montes, M. (2015). Predictiveness curves in virtual screening. *J. Cheminform.* 7:52. doi: 10.1186/s13321-015-0100-8

Fontaine, F., Bolton, E., Borodina, Y., and Bryant, S. H. (2007). Fast 3D shape screening of large chemical databases through alignment-recycling. *Chem. Cent. J.* 1:12. doi: 10.1186/1752-153X-1-12

Halgren, T. A., Murphy, R. B., Friesner, R. A., Beard, H. S., Frye, L. L., Pollard, W. T., et al. (2004). Glide: a new approach for rapid, accurate docking and scoring. 2. Enrichment factors in database screening. *J. Med. Chem.* 47, 1750–1759. doi: 10.1021/jm030644s

Hawkins, P. C., Skillman, A. G., Warren, G. L., Ellingson, B. A., and Stahl, M. T. (2010). Conformer generation with OMEGA: algorithm and validation using high quality structures from the Protein Databank and Cambridge Structural Database. *J. Chem. Inf. Model.* 50, 572–584. doi: 10.1021/ci100031x

Huang, N., Shoichet, B. K., and Irwin, J. J. (2006). Benchmarking sets for molecular docking. *J. Med. Chem.* 49, 6789–6801. doi: 10.1021/jm0608356

Huang, R., and Xia, M. (2017). Editorial: Tox21 Challenge to build predictive models of nuclear receptor and stress response pathways as mediated by exposure to environmental toxicants and drugs. *Front. Environ. Sci.* 5:3. doi: 10.3389/fenvs.2017.00003

Kairys, V., Fernandes, M. X., and Gilson, M. K. (2006). Screening drug-like compounds by docking to homology models: a systematic study. *J. Chem. Inf. Model.* 46, 365–379. doi: 10.1021/ci050238c

Kar, S., and Roy, K. (2013). How far can virtual screening take us in drug discovery? *Expert Opin. Drug Discov.* 8, 245–261. doi: 10.1517/17460441.2013.761204

Kim, S., Thiessen, P. A., Bolton, E. E., Chen, J., Fu, G., Gindulyte, A., et al. (2016). PubChem substance and compound databases. *Nucleic Acids Res.* 44, D1202–D1213. doi: 10.1093/nar/gkv951

Kristensen, T. G., Nielsen, J., and Pedersen, C. N. (2013). Methods for similarity-based virtual screening. *Comput. Struct. Biotechnol. J.* 5:e201302009. doi: 10.5936/csbj.201302009

McClish, D. K. (1989). Analyzing a portion of the ROC curve. *Med. Decis. Making* 9, 190–195. doi: 10.1177/0272989X8900900307

Mysinger, M. M., Carchia, M., Irwin, J. J., and Shoichet, B. K. (2012). Directory of useful decoys, enhanced (DUD-E): better ligands and decoys for better benchmarking. *J. Med. Chem.* 55, 6582–6594. doi: 10.1021/jm300687e

Nasr, R. J., Swamidass, S. J., and Baldi, P. F. (2009). Large scale study of multiple-molecule queries. *J. Cheminform.* 1:7. doi: 10.1186/1758-2946-1-7

Rogers, D., and Hahn, M. (2010). Extended-connectivity fingerprints. *J. Chem. Inf. Model.* 50, 742–754. doi: 10.1021/ci100050t

Sheridan, R. P., Singh, S. B., Fluder, E. M., and Kearsley, S. K. (2001). Protocols for bridging the peptide to nonpeptide gap in topological similarity searches. *J. Chem. Inf. Comput. Sci.* 41, 1395–1406. doi: 10.1021/ci0100144

Shiryaev, S. A., Cheltsov, A. V., Gawlik, K., Ratnikov, B. I., and Strongin, A. Y. (2011). Virtual ligand screening of the National Cancer Institute (NCI) compound library leads to the allosteric inhibitory scaffolds of the West Nile Virus NS3 proteinase. *Assay Drug Dev. Technol.* 9, 69–78. doi: 10.1089/adt.2010.0309

Triballeau, N., Acher, F., Brabet, I., Pin, J. P., and Bertrand, H. O. (2005). Virtual screening workflow development guided by the "receiver operating characteristic" curve approach. Application to high-throughput docking on metabotropic glutamate receptor subtype 4. *J. Med. Chem.* 48, 2534–2547. doi: 10.1021/jm049092j

Truchon, J. F., and Bayly, C. I. (2007). Evaluating virtual screening methods: good and bad metrics for the "early recognition" problem. *J. Chem. Inf. Model.* 47, 488–508. doi: 10.1021/ci600426e

Zhao, W., Hevener, K. E., White, S. W., Lee, R. E., and Boyett, J. M. (2009). A statistical framework to evaluate virtual screening. *BMC Bioinformatics* 10:225. doi: 10.1186/1471-2105-10-225

7

Computational Insight into the Small Molecule Intervening PD-L1 Dimerization and the Potential Structure-Activity Relationship

Danfeng Shi [1], Xiaoli An [1], Qifeng Bai [2], Zhitong Bing [2,3], Shuangyan Zhou [1,4], Huanxiang Liu [4] and Xiaojun Yao [1,5]**

[1] State Key Laboratory of Applied Organic Chemistry, Department of Chemistry, Lanzhou University, Lanzhou, China, [2] School of Basic Medical Science, Lanzhou University, Lanzhou, China, [3] Institute of Modern Physics of Chinese Academy of Sciences, Lanzhou, China, [4] School of Pharmacy, Lanzhou University, Lanzhou, China, [5] State Key Laboratory of Quality Research in Chinese Medicine, Macau Institute for Applied Research in Medicine and Health, Macau University of Science and Technology, Macau, China

***Correspondence:**
Huanxiang Liu
hxliu@lzu.edu.cn
Xiaojun Yao
xjyao@lzu.edu.cn

Recently, small-molecule compounds have been reported to block the PD-1/PD-L1 interaction by inducing the dimerization of PD-L1. All these inhibitors had a common scaffold and interacted with the cavity formed by two PD-L1 monomers. This special interactive mode provided clues for the structure-based drug design, however, also showed limitations for the discovery of small-molecule inhibitors with new scaffolds. In this study, we revealed the structure-activity relationship of the current small-molecule inhibitors targeting dimerization of PD-L1 by predicting their binding and unbinding mechanism via conventional molecular dynamics and metadynamics simulation. During the binding process, the representative inhibitors (BMS-8 and BMS-1166) tended to have a more stable binding mode with one PD-L1 monomer than the other and the small-molecule inducing PD-L1 dimerization was further stabilized by the non-polar interaction of Ile54, Tyr56, Met115, Ala121, and Tyr123 on both monomers and the water bridges involved in $_{A}$Lys124. The unbinding process prediction showed that the PD-L1 dimerization kept stable upon the dissociation of ligands. It's indicated that the formation and stability of the small-molecule inducing PD-L1 dimerization was the key factor for the inhibitory activities of these ligands. The contact analysis, R-group based quantitative structure-activity relationship (QSAR) analysis and molecular docking further suggested that each attachment point on the core scaffold of ligands had a specific preference for pharmacophore elements when improving the inhibitory activities by structural modifications. Taken together, the results in this study could guide the structural optimization and the further discovery of novel small-molecule inhibitors targeting PD-L1.

Keywords: PD-L1, small-molecule inhibitors, molecular dynamics simulation, metadynamics simulation, R-group QSAR

INTRODUCTION

The blockage of the protein-protein interaction (PPI) between programmed cell death protein 1 (PD-1) and programmed cell death 1 ligand 1 (PD-L1) can reactivate the effector functions of T cell and eliminate tumor phenotypes with significant PD-L1 expression (Gatalica et al., 2014; Patel and Kurzrock, 2015; Sharma and Allison, 2015a,b). The crystal structures of PD-1/PD-L1 complex revealed the interface and hot-spot domains for both proteins (Zak et al., 2015; Pascolutti et al., 2016), which provided the structural basis for drug design. Ligands such as monoclonal antibodies (mAbs) (Lee et al., 2016, 2017; Liu K. et al., 2016; Tan et al., 2017; Zhang et al., 2017a,b), peptides (Chang et al., 2015; Magiera-Mularz et al., 2017), and small-molecule compounds (Abdel-Magid, 2015; Zak et al., 2016; Skalniak et al., 2017) had been discovered to interact with the PPI interface of PD-1 or PD-L1, showed obvious inhibitory activities against PD-1/PD-L1 signaling pathways. As the small-molecule inhibitors have better characteristic on aspects like production cost, drug-like property, immunogenic side effects, and half-life period (Liu K. et al., 2016) than peptides and monoclonal antibodies, the development of small-molecule inhibitor tended to be more promising. The crystal structures of small-molecule complex provided a good chance for the drug design of anti-cancer immunotherapy targeting on PD-1/PD-L1 immune checkpoint.

According the patents by Bristol-Myers Squibb (BMS) company, the compounds with (2-methyl-3-biphenylyl)methanol scaffold were privileged for inducing the dimerization of PD-L1 and interacted with the hydrophobic tunnel formed by two PD-L1 monomers (Zak et al., 2016; Guzik et al., 2017). Previously, George F. Gao's group resolved a dimeric interface of PD-L1 formed by B, C″, D, and E strands on each monomer, which was proved to be either a functional unit in immunological synapse formation or a revolution relics of B7 family (Tan et al., 2016). The crystal lattice analysis by Zak et al. also didn't suggest the spontaneous dimerization of PD-L1 (Zak et al., 2015), indicating that the interfacial interaction between two PD-L1 monomers was quite weak for dimerization process. As for the small molecule intervening PD-L1 dimerization, the interacting interface analysis showed that these ligands interacted with the G, F, C, C′ strands of PD-L1 in a competitive manner vs. PD-1 like mAbs or peptide inhibitors (Sharpe et al., 2011; Liu A. et al., 2016). Specially, the dimerized crystal structures tend to be a common pharmacodynamic characteristics for BMS small-molecule analogs despite of inhibitory activity difference from millimole to nanomole level (Abdel-Magid, 2015; Zak et al., 2016; Skalniak et al., 2017; Perry et al., 2019). Considering the potential relationship between the inhibitory activities of BMS small-molecule inhibitors and the stabilities of the dimerized complex systems, the dimerization process and the structure-activity relationship of small-molecule inhibitors need to be further elucidated. Besides, the broad, scattered and hydrophobic interface on PD-L1 makes it difficult for the discovery of novel small molecule ligands and also results in the strong hydrophobicity of BMS small-molecule inhibitors (Zarganes-Tzitzikas et al., 2016). Therefore, an understanding of the inhibitory mechanism of small-molecule ligands targeting PD-L1 such as key residues at the binding site, effect of the solvation and binding or unbinding process of small molecule inhibitors would help in the discovery of novel inhibitors and structural optimization of reported small-molecule inhibitors.

TABLE 1 | The details of conventional molecular dynamics simulations.

	Dimer systems	Monomer systems	
	PD-L1 dimer	PD-L1 (Conformation A)	PD-L1 (Conformation B)
BMS-8	150 ns	150 ns × 2	150 ns × 2
BMS-1166	150 ns	150 ns × 2	150 ns × 2

In this study, we aimed to reveal the detailed molecular mechanism of BMS small-molecule inhibitors from the formation and disassociation of PD-L1 dimers by multiple molecular modeling methods. Two representative compounds (BMS-8 and BMS-1166) with known inhibitory activities and complex crystal structures were selected to perform molecular dynamics simulations. During the formation process, both monomer and dimer systems of PD-L1 in complex with small-molecule ligands were applied to evaluate the stabilities of binding modes between ligands and PD-L1. The binding free energy calculation by MM-PBSA and MM-GBSA (Genheden and Ryde, 2015; Chen et al., 2018; Sun et al., 2018) were also used to analyze the energy contribution of the interfacial residues on PD-L1 dimers. During the disassociation process, metadynamics simulations (Bernardi et al., 2015) with specific collective variables (CVs) were performed to explore the key transition states along unbinding pathways. Based on the results of molecular modeling, an interplay mechanism of BMS small-molecule ligands with PD-L1 was proposed. Finally, R-group based QSAR analysis (Holliday et al., 2003; Hirons et al., 2005) and molecular docking were constructed on the reported BMS small-molecule inhibitors. The results of this study would provide a good guidance for the discovery of novel small-molecule inhibitors and structural modification of BMS small-molecule inhibitors targeting PD-L1.

METHODS AND MATERIALS

The Conventional Molecular Dynamics Simulations

The complex crystal structures of BMS-8 and BMS-1166 were used to perform conventional molecular dynamics simulations. The Cartesian coordinates of the heavy atoms of PD-L1 (sequence 18–132) and small-molecule ligands were derived from the PDB database with accession number of 5J8O (Zak et al., 2016) and 5NIX (Skalniak et al., 2017). In order to eliminate the electrostatic effect of terminal residues, both monomers were capped with ACE and NME at two ends. The simulation details of the monomer systems and dimer systems were shown in **Table 1**. All the complex systems were firstly prepared through structural inspection and optimization in Schrödinger 2015 software suite (Schrödinger, LLC: New York, NY, 2015). Then, the complex proteins were solvated in a rectangular box of TIP3P waters and neutralized with Na^+ ions. The periodic boundary conditions were setup with all the solvents at least 10 Å away from the complex. Then, the solvated systems were parameterized using the AMBER FF14SB force field (Case et al., 2014). The molecular dynamics simulations were performed in four steps. Firstly, energy minimization was performed to remove the local atomic collision in the systems. The energy minimization was conducted by both descent steepest method and conjugated gradient method with 5,000 steps. Then, the temperature of each system was gradually upgraded from 0 to 300 K in the NVT ensemble with all the solute atoms constrained with a force constant of 2.0 kcal $mol^{-1}·Å^{-2}$. After that, each system was equilibrated with the force constant decreasing from 2.0 to 0 kcal $mol^{-1}·Å^{-2}$ in a period of 1 ns. Finally, a production run of 150 ns was performed for each system in the NPT ensemble at 300 K and 1.0 atm condition. The snapshots for all the trajectories were saved every 2 ps.

The Binding Free Energy Calculation

For dimer systems of BMS-8 and BMS1166, two PD-L1 monomers were selected as the receptor, while small-molecule inhibitors were selected as the ligand. Both MM-PBSA and MM-GBSA methods were performed to calculate the binding free energy of BMS inhibitors according to the equation below:

$$\Delta G = < G_{Complex} - G_{Receptor} - G_{Ligand} > \quad (1)$$

Where < > represents the average value for all the snapshots used for MM-PBSA and MM-GBSA calculation. Different energy

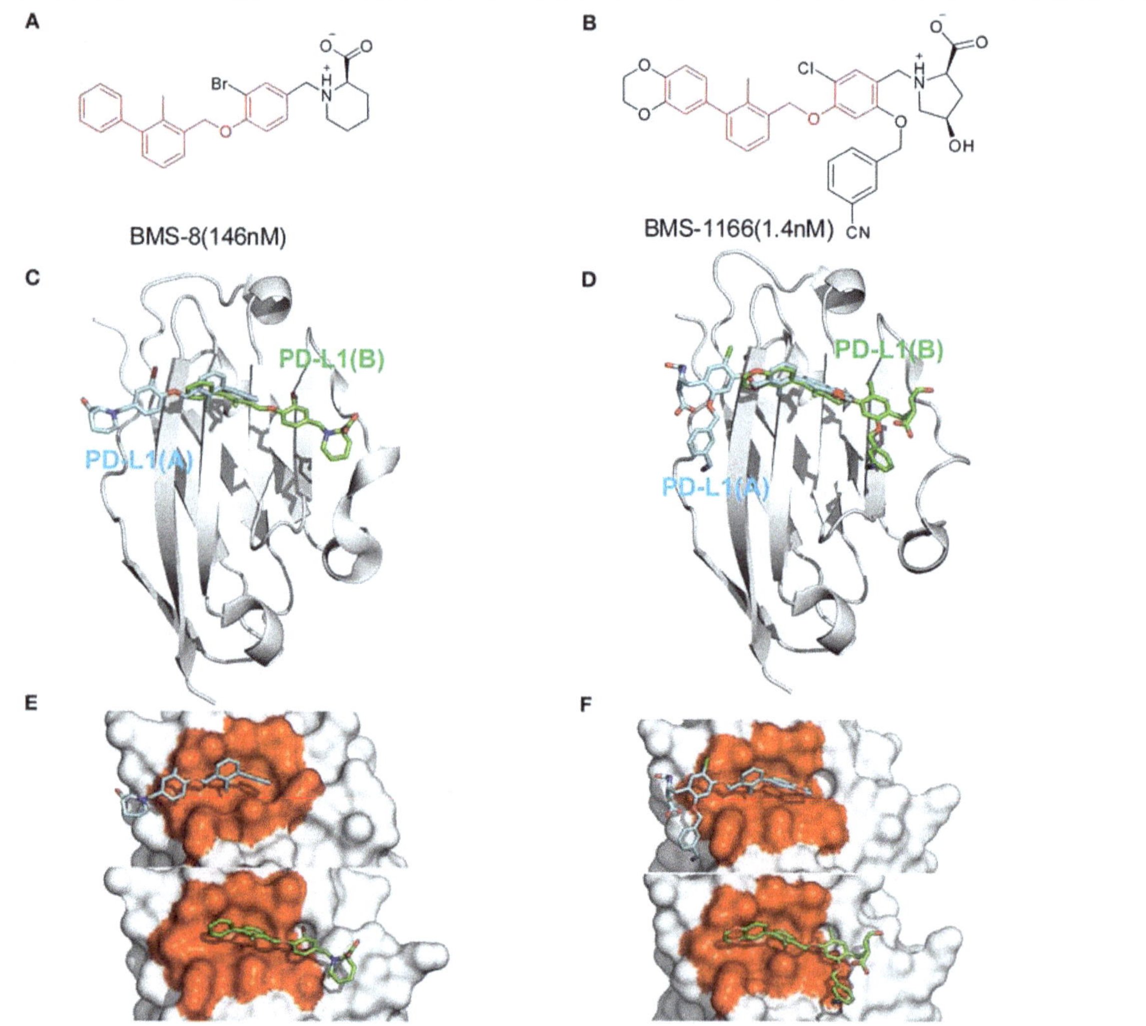

FIGURE 1 | The structural information of BMS-8 and BMS-1166. **(A,B)** The chemical formulas of BMS-8 and BMS-1166. The core scaffold is colored in red. **(C,D)** The conformational superposition of BMS-8 and BMS-1166 interacting with the monomer conformation A, B of PD-L1. **(E,F)** The surface of PD-L1 (A) and PD-L1 (B) interacting with BMS-8 and BMS-1166. The binding pockets formed by I54, V55, Y56, M115, I116, S117, A121, D122, and Y123 were colored in red.

terms can be estimated as follows:

$$\Delta G = \Delta H - T\Delta S \quad (2)$$

$$\Delta H = \Delta E_{gas} + \Delta E_{sol} = \Delta E_{polar} + \Delta E_{nonpolar} \quad (3)$$

$$\Delta E_{gas} = \Delta E_{int} + \Delta E_{ele} + \Delta E_{vdW} \quad (4)$$

$$\Delta H_{sol} = \Delta E_{ele,\ sol} + \Delta E_{nonpl,sol} \quad (5)$$

$$\Delta E_{nonpl,sol} = \gamma * \Delta SASA \quad (6)$$

500 snapshots were extracted from the last 20 ns trajectories and used for MM-PBSA and MM-GBSA calculation. The parameter settings during MM-PBSA and MM-GBSA calculation were referred to the previous works published by our group (Xue et al., 2013). Then, the per-residue based decomposition was performed to identify the key residues in both dimer systems. Finally, the contribution of entropy change ($-T\Delta S$) was calculated by 100 snapshots from the last 20 ns trajectory.

The Calculation of Water Occupancies

The water molecules on the surface affected the conformational stability of proteins (Bellissent-Funel et al., 2016). By calculating the water occupancies on the surface of protein complex, water sites with a higher probability of finding a water molecule could be identified (Gauto et al., 2013). The water molecules at those sites were involved in the water bridges between protein and ligand and could enhance the stability of protein complex thermodynamically (Romero et al., 2016). To evaluate the effects of the water-mediated complex stability upon the binding of BMS inhibitors, the water occupancies and the water bridges were calculated over the last 20 ns trajectories for each dimer system using the "cpptraj" module of the AMBER14. All the

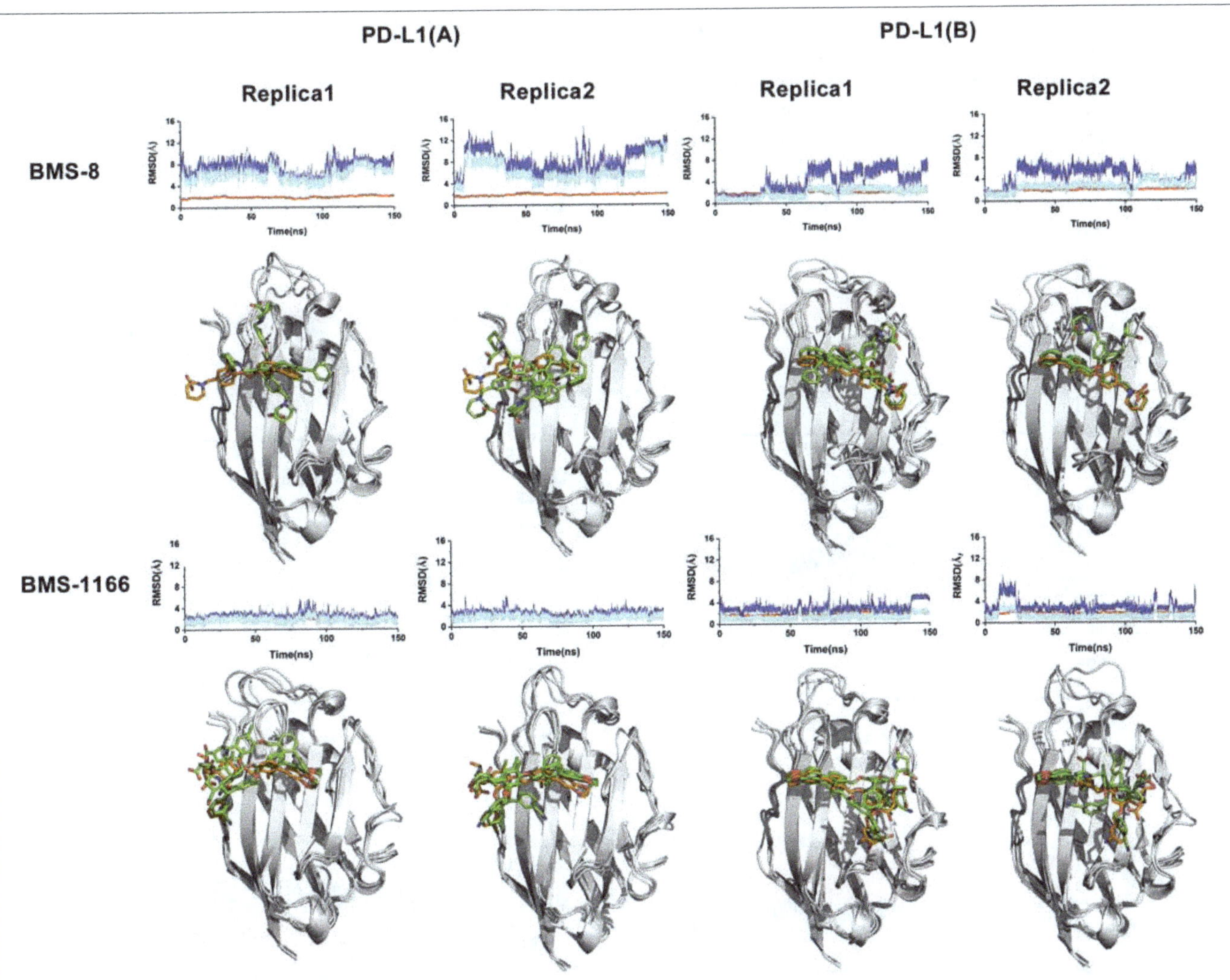

FIGURE 2 | The stability evaluation of the monomer systems. The RMSDs of the heavy atoms of PD-L1 monomer, ligands (BMS-8, BMS-1166) and the core scaffold of the ligand are shown in red, blue, and cyan lines, respectively. The representative conformations of three clusters for every monomer system was shown below the corresponding system. PD-L1 is shown in gray cartoon while the initial conformation of ligand is shown in orange sticks and the dynamics conformations of ligand is shown in green sticks.

trajectories were first imaged and fit to the first frame by the root mean square deviation (RMSD) of the heavy atoms of PD-L1 dimers. Then, the water occupancies were calculated using the "grid" command with a 0.5 Å *0.5 Å * 0.5 Å spacing over the whole box. And the water occupancies for both dimer systems were represented in the Chimera software (Pettersen et al., 2004).

Metadynamics Simulations

Metadynamics simulations have been widely used to predict the unbinding pathways and dissociation energy barrier of ligands for ligand-target systems (Cavalli et al., 2015). The sampling process of metadynamics simulations had an advantage of not requiring an initial estimate of the energy landscape to explore by periodically adding history-dependent biasing potential on selected collective variables (CVs) (Masetti et al., 2009; Barducci et al., 2011; Casasnovas et al., 2017; Sun et al., 2017). In this study, CV1 was selected as the distance between the mass center of the heavy atoms on ligand and the mass center of heavy atoms on key residues including Ile54, Tyr56, Met115, Ala121, Tyr123 in both chains; CV2 was selected as the angle between the C_α atom of Tyr56 and two carbon atoms that were the furthest away from each other on the core scaffold. The metadynamics simulations were performed for both dimer systems. The prepared topology files and coordinate files by AMBER ff14SB force field were further applied in the NAMD2.9 software (Kalé et al., 1999) implemented by PLUMED code (Bonomi et al., 2009). The initial structures were minimized for 5,000 steps with all the atoms on protein and ligand restrained with 5 kcal $mol^{-1}\cdot Å^{-2}$ and all restraints released therewith. Then the temperature of systems were upgraded to 300 K in 30,000 steps. Afterward, all the systems were submitted to two short time NVT simulations (100,000 steps) to equilibrate the systems with restraining force constant of 5 kcal $mol^{-1}\cdot Å^{-2}$ and all restraints released therewith. Finally, the equilibrated structures restarted from the NVT simulation were used for metadynamics simulations.

$$V(s,t) = \sum_{k\tau < t} W(k\tau)\; exp(-\sum_{i=1}^{d} \frac{\left(s_i - s_i(q(k\tau))\right)^2}{2\sigma_i^2}) \quad (7)$$

$$W(k\tau) = W_0\; exp(-\frac{V(s(q(k\tau)), k\tau)}{K_B \Delta T}) \quad (8)$$

$$\gamma = \frac{T + \Delta T}{T} \quad (9)$$

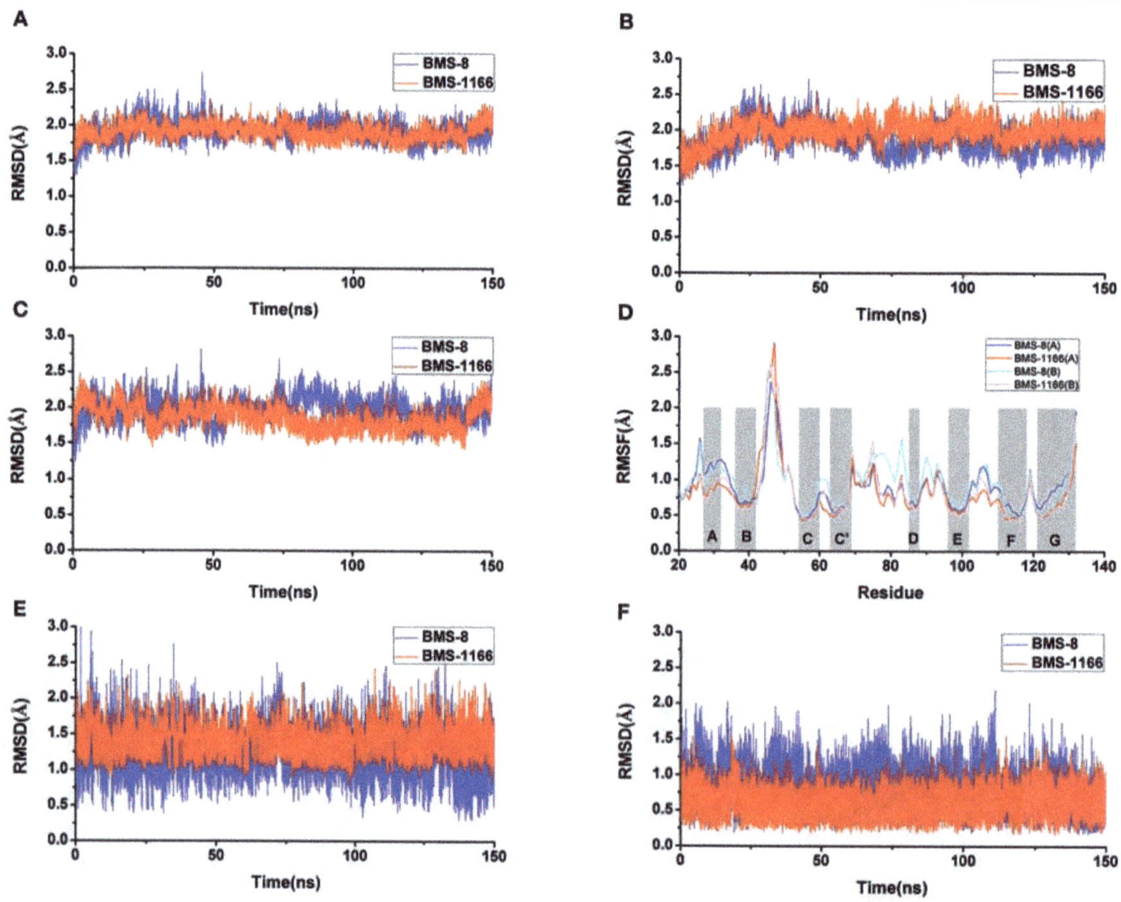

FIGURE 3 | The RMSDs and RMSFs of the heavy atoms in dimer systems. **(A)** RMSD of complex, **(B)** RMSD of PD-L1 at conformation A, **(C)** RMSD of PD-L1 at conformation B, **(D)** RMSF of residues on PD-L1 at conformation A, B, **(E)** RMSD of the ligand, and **(F)** RMSD of the core scaffold.

Metadynamics could reconstruct the free-energy surface as a function of specific collective variables (CVs). The general formalism of history-dependent Gaussian potential was shown as Equation (7). V represents the sum of the history-dependent Gaussian potential along the specific reactive coordinate (s_i) during time span ($k\tau$). In this study, the deposition time (τ) was set as 1 ps to give enough dissociation time for ligands without adding biasing potential on the dissociation boundary. The Gaussian width (σ) of CV1 and CV2 were set to 0.8 Å and 0.02 rad, respectively. As for the well-tempered metadynamics, the height of the Gaussian potential (W) is affected by a parameter ΔT as Equation (8). The initial hill height (W_0) of Gaussian potential was set to 0.6 kcal/mol·ps and the bias-factor (γ) was set to 10 with a temperature (T) of 300 K to control the decrease rate of the biasing potential as Equation (9).

R-Group QSAR Model and Molecular Docking of BMS Small-Molecule Inhibitors

The pharma R-group quantitative structure-activity relationship (RQSAR) models tended to be an effective approach for the SAR evaluation of the congeneric series of compounds (Adhikari et al., 2015). It was more suggestive than other approaches for the structural modification of small-molecule inhibitors by identifying the core scaffold and evaluating the effective pharma element at different attachment points (Kolarevic et al., 2018; Ts Mavrova et al., 2018). A total of 110 BMS small-molecule inhibitors with 2-methyl-3-(phenoxymethyl)-1,1'-biphenyl scaffold were collected from the patents of BMS company (Abdel-Magid, 2015; **Table S1**). All these small molecules had seven attachment points and diverse substitution groups, which were suitable to perform R-group QSAR analysis in the Canvas software of Schrödinger Suite (Duan et al., 2010; Sastry et al., 2010). The linear relationship between the substitutions and the activities (–log IC_{50}) was analyzed and the importance of six key pharmacophore elements including hydrogen bond acceptor (A), hydrogen bond donor (D), hydrophobic group (H), negative ionic group (N), positive ionic group (P), and aromatic ring (A) were evaluated at each attachment point. During the process, the error and the importance were both set as 0.30. Eight representative small-molecule inhibitors (NO. of compound:4, 101, 102, 103, 104, 108, 109, 110) with substitutions on R1, R2, or R3 were selected to perform molecular docking to further study the binding modes. In order the compare the effect of R-groups, the core scaffold atoms with SMILES of "cOCc(c1C)cccc1c" were constrained with RMSD of 0.5 angstrom while other atoms were selected flexible. The standard precision (SP) docking score was used to evaluate the binding poses. The molecular docking was performed in Schrödinger 2015 software suite (Schrödinger, LLC: New York, NY, 2015).

Residue-Ligand Contact Analysis

In this study, we performed residue-ligand contact analysis to detect the surrounding residues around different substituent groups of BMS-8 and BMS-1166. It is assumed that the contacts exist between two groups as long as their distance was below a cutoff of 3.5 Å. The occupancy of each contact was calculated by the existence frequency in the 5,000 snapshots of the last 50 ns trajectories.

TABLE 2 | The binding free energies of BMS-8 and BMS-1166 evaluated by MM-PBSA, MM-GBSA, and metadynamics simulations.

Contribution[a]	BMS-8	BMS-1166	$\Delta\Delta E$ ($\Delta E_{BMS-1166} - \Delta E_{BMS-8}$)
$\Delta E_{ele,gas}$	−29.29 ± 6.14	−72.23 ± 12.05	−42.94 ± 13.52
$\Delta E_{vdw,gas}$	−63.45 ± 2.77	−81.60 ± 3.72	−18.15 ± 4.64
$\Delta E_{nonpl,sol}$	−6.62 ± 0.18	−9.17 ± 0.19	−2.55 ± 0.26
$\Delta E_{polar,sol,PB}$	49.89 ± 7.19	105.28 ± 10.16	55.39 ± 12.45
$\Delta E_{sol,PB}$	43.27 ± 7.07	96.11 ± 10.11	52.84 ± 12.34
$\Delta E_{polar,sol,GB}$	45.04 ± 5.85	93.32 ± 9.91	48.28 ± 11.51
$\Delta E_{sol,GB}$	38.42 ± 5.75	84.15 ± 9.88	45.73 ± 11.43
ΔH_{PB}	−49.49 ± 3.71	−57.72 ± 4.64	−8.23 ± 5.94
ΔH_{GB}	−54.32 ± 3.14	−69.69 ± 3.32	−15.37 ± 4.57
$-T\Delta S$	24.72 ± 5.75	27.02 ± 5.89	2.30 ± 8.23
ΔG_{PB}	−24.77 ± 6.84	−30.70 ± 7.50	−5.93 ± 10.15
ΔG_{GB}	−29.60 ± 6.55	−42.67 ± 6.76	−13.07 ± 9.41
ΔE_{CV1}[b]	−16.23	−28.79	−12.56
ΔE_{CV2}[c]	−15.51	−27.89	−12.38
ΔE_{exp}[d]	−9.32	−12.07	−2.75

[a] *The unit for the free energy contributions are shown in kcal/mol.*

[b,c] *ΔE_{CV1} and ΔE_{CV2} were estimated by the history-dependent free energy surfaces along CV1 and CV2.*

[d] *The experimental affinities for BMS-8 and BMS-1166 were extracted from the reference and calculated by using the equation as follows: $\Delta G = -RT \ln(1/IC_{50})$ at 298.15 K.*

RESULTS AND DISCUSSION

The Conformational Stabilities Between PD-L1 Monomer and BMS Small-Molecule Inhibitors

In order to explore the interactive process of BMS small-molecule inhibitors, we constructed two kinds of ligand-bound PD-L1 monomer systems as shown in **Figure 1** and used molecular dynamics simulations to evaluate the stabilities of both binding modes by two replicas. As shown in **Figure 2**, the stabilities of both binding modes were evaluated by the RMSD of the heavy atoms of receptor, ligand and the core scaffold of ligands in two replicas. The core scaffold of BMS-8 tended to have a more stable contact with the conformation B than conformation A of PD-L1 according to the comparison of RMSD and the representative conformations of both binding modes. The detailed docking interactions diagram in **Figures S1, S2** showed that the π-π stacking interaction between the biphenyl moiety and $_A$Tyr56 tended to be easily affected by the conformation of $_A$Tyr56 and unstable among three clusters, while the hydrophobic interaction between biphenyl moiety and residues on conformation B of PD-L1 tended to be stable among all three clusters. As for BMS-1166, both binding modes seemed to be quite stable, which probably accounting for the best inhibitory activities of BMS-1166 among

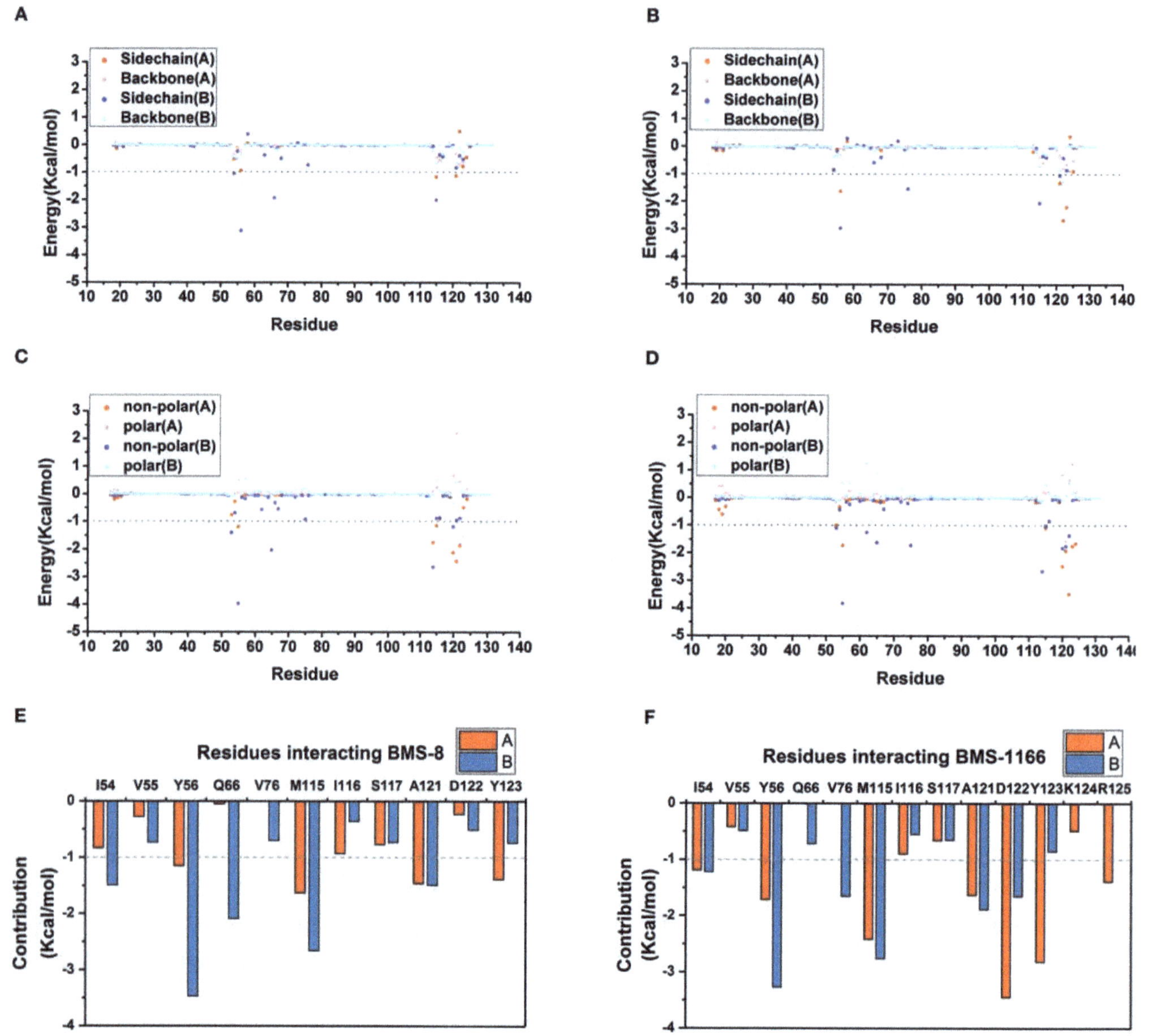

FIGURE 4 | The residue energy decomposition of the key residues for BMS-8 **(A,C,E)** and BMS-1166 **(B,D,F)** dimer systems. **(A,B)** The energy contribution of sidechain and backbone, **(C,D)** the energy contribution of polar and non-polar interaction, **(E,F)** the total energy contribution for each residue. The cutoff value of the energy contribution for key residues were set as −1 kcal/mol.

TABLE 3 | The hydrogen bond analysis of the BMS-8 and BMS-1166 dimer systems.

Acceptor	DonorH	Donor	Occupancy[a] (%)	Distance (Å)[b]	Angle (°)[c]
$_B$Gln66@OE1	BMS-8@H1	BMS-8@N1	57.21	2.90	162.74
$_A$Asp122@OD2	BMS-1166@H1	BMS-1116@O5	63.54	2.71	161.10
$_A$Asp122@OD1	BMS-1166@H1	BMS-1116@O5	47.58	2.93	151.41
$_A$Asp122@OD1	BMS-1166@H20	BMS-1116@N2	41.43	2.93	144.20
$_A$Asp122@OD2	BMS-1166@H20	BMS-1116@N2	29.74	3.01	140.98
$_A$Asp122@OD1	BMS-1166@H19	BMS-1116@N2	21.02	2.90	139.00
BMS-1166@N1	$_A$Arg125@H	$_A$Arg125@N	81.70	3.08	149.17
BMS-1166@O5	$_A$Thr20@HG1	$_A$Thr20@OG1	36.64	2.95	154.22

[a] *The occupancy of hydrogen bonds were analyzed through the last 20 ns trajectories and only hydrogen bonds with an occupancy more than 0.20 were extracted and shown.*
[b,c] *The hydrogen bonds were determined by an acceptor-donor atom distance of <3.5 Å and acceptor H-donor angle of >120°.*

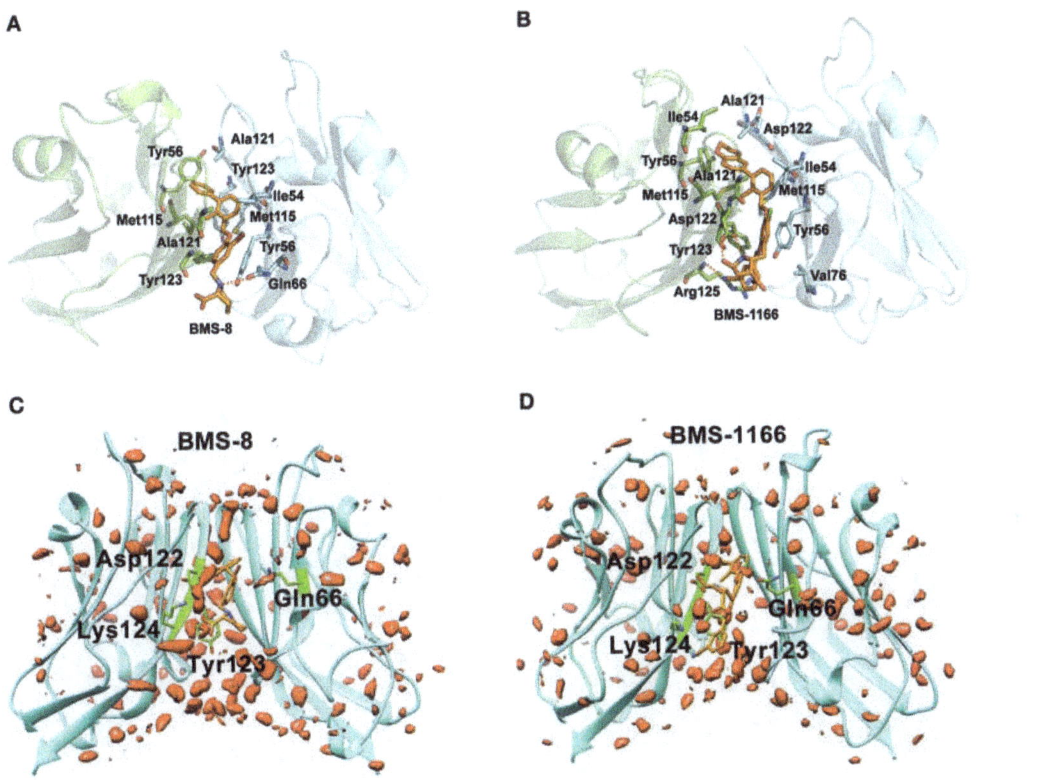

FIGURE 5 | The binding modes and water occupancies in dimer systems. **(A,B)** The binding modes of BMS-8 and BMS-1166. The key residues were shown in green and cyan sticks and the ligand was shown in orange sticks. The hydrogen bonds were shown in red dash. **(C,D)** The water occupancies in BMS-8 and BMS-1166 dimer systems. The PD-L1 dimer is shown in cyan cartoon and the residues involved in water bridges are shown in green sticks. The water distributions are shown in red solid surface and the small molecule ligands are shown in orange sticks.

TABLE 4 | The water bridge with occupancies higher than 20.00% in the BMS-8 and BMS-1166 dimer systems.

Residues involving in water bridge	BMS-8 (%)	BMS-1166 (%)
$_A$Thr20	–	32.42
$_A$Asp122	25.04	–
$_A$Lys124	91.57	94.15
$_A$Arg125	–	22.63
$_B$Gln66	58.62	32.93
$_B$Lys75	–	22.58
$_B$Val76	–	50.13
$_B$Asp122	–	29.66
$_A$Phe19, $_A$Ala121, $_A$Asp122	–	23.52
$_A$Asp122, $_A$Tyr123, $_A$Lys124	38.90	65.18

the small-molecule inhibitors of BMS. The detailed docking interactions diagram in **Figures S3, S4** showed that the biphenyl moiety had less conformational fluctuation and more stable hydrophobic interactions among the clusters of conformation A and B of PD-L1. The stabilities of the monomer complex of PD-L1 and ligand was affected by the hydrophobic interactions and turned out to be associated with the inhibitory activities of BMS small-molecule inhibitors.

The Interaction Stabilities Between PD-L1 Dimer and BMS Small-Molecule Inhibitors

The conformational stabilities of the dimer systems were evaluated by root mean square deviation (RMSD) and mean square root fluctuation (RMSF) as shown in **Figure 3**. The RMSDs of the complex, two PD-L1 monomers in complex systems showed that both dimer and monomers of PD-L1 had strong structural stabilities upon ligand binding. The conformational fluctuation of PD-L1 indicated that PD-L1 showed more flexibilities upon BMS-8 binding than BMS-1166. The comparison of the RMSDs of the core scaffold of two ligands showed that BMS-1166 had a more stable binding modes than BMS-8. The binding free energies were also calculated to evaluate the affinities of dimer systems. As shown in **Table 2**, the energy items of $\Delta\Delta G_{PB}$, $\Delta\Delta G_{GB,}$ and $\Delta\Delta E_{exp}$ by MM-PBSA and MM-GBSA methods could properly evaluate the difference of affinities of BMS-8 and BMS-1166, which showed the fact that the affinities between small-molecule inhibitors and PD-L1 dimer could reflect the inhibitory activities relatively. BMS-1166 had a stronger enthalpy contribution ($\Delta\Delta H_{PB}$, $\Delta\Delta H_{GB}$) and a worse entropy contribution ($-T\Delta\Delta S$) than BMS-8, which were consistent with the stability difference of BMS-8 and BMS-1166 dimer complex.

The key residues on two PD-L1 monomers interacting with ligands were recognized by per-residue energy decomposition.

The energy contribution for each residue were decomposed into the sidechain part and the backbone part, the non-polar part and the polar part as shown in **Figures 4A–D**. It could be seen that BMS-8 and BMS-1166 mainly formed non-polar interactions with the sidechain of the residues on PD-L1. With a cutoff value of −1.0 kcal/mol, the key residues in BMS-8 dimer system included $_{A}$Tyr56, $_{A}$Met115, $_{A}$Ala121, $_{A}$Tyr123 and $_{B}$Ile54, $_{B}$Tyr56, $_{B}$Gln66, $_{B}$Met115, $_{B}$Ala121 as shown in **Figure 4E**, while the key residues in BMS-1166 dimer system included $_{A}$Ile54, $_{A}$Tyr56, $_{A}$Met115, $_{A}$Ala121, $_{A}$Asp122, $_{A}$Tyr123, $_{A}$Arg125 and $_{B}$Ile54, $_{B}$Tyr56, $_{B}$Val76, $_{B}$Met115, $_{B}$Ala121, $_{B}$Asp122 as shown in **Figure 4F**. Taken together, the interaction residues on conformation A and conformation B of PD-L1 were symmetrical both including Ile54, Tyr56, Met115, Ala121, and Tyr123. The hydrogen bond analysis in **Table 3**, **Figures 5A,B** showed that the protonated tertiary ammonium in BMS-8 formed a hydrogen bond with the side-chain oxygen of $_{B}$Gln66 with an occupancy of 57.21%, while the BMS-1166 dimer system also formed hydrogen bond between the ammonium group on BMS-1166 and the carboxyl group of $_{A}$Asp122. The binding mode analysis of substitute groups on BMS-8 and BMS-1166 with the interfacial residues

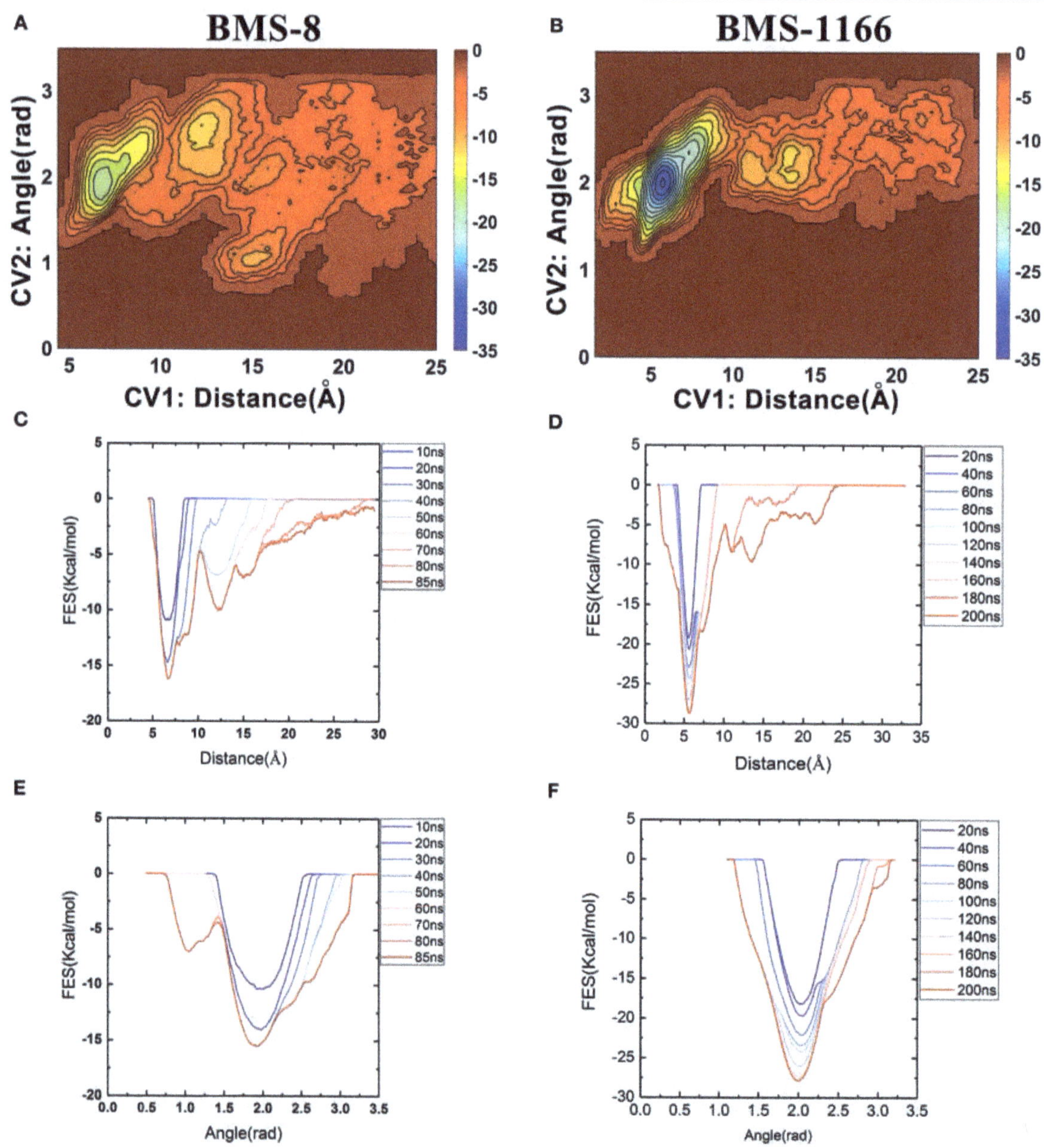

FIGURE 6 | The energy change during the unbinding process. **(A,B)** The free energy landscapes for the unbinding process of BMS-8 and BMS-1166. **(C–F)** The convergence of sampling process during the unbinding process of BMS-8 and BMS-1166. The history-dependent free energy surfaces along CV1 **(C,D)** and CV2 **(E,F)** are estimated by a segmented accumulation of simulation time. The unit for the free energy is kcal/mol.

on PD-L1 indicated that the interaction with the peripheral residues including $_{A}$Ile54, $_{A}$Arg125, $_{B}$Val76, and $_{B}$Asp122 could significantly enhance the inhibitory activities of BMS small-molecule inhibitors.

In order to analyze the effect of solvent on PD-L1 dimer complex, water occupancies and water bridges involved in receptor-ligand interaction were both calculated. As shown in **Table 4**, the residues or residue pairs involved in water bridges with an occupancy higher than 20% were extracted from both dimer systems. It can be seen in **Figure 5** that three water bridges involved in $_{A}$Asp122, $_{A}$Tyr123, $_{A}$Lys124, and $_{B}$Gln66 were stable in both dimer systems. Both ligands formed a strong water bridge with $_{A}$Lys124 with an occupancy higher than 90%, which indicated that $_{A}$Lys124 had a significant effect on the stabilities of the ligand conformations.

The Disassociation Process of BMS Small-Molecule Inhibitors

The free energy landscape of the unbinding processes of both BMS small-molecule inhibitors were constructed by CV1 and CV2. The distribution of minima in the landscapes showed that the most stable conformational state in the unbinding

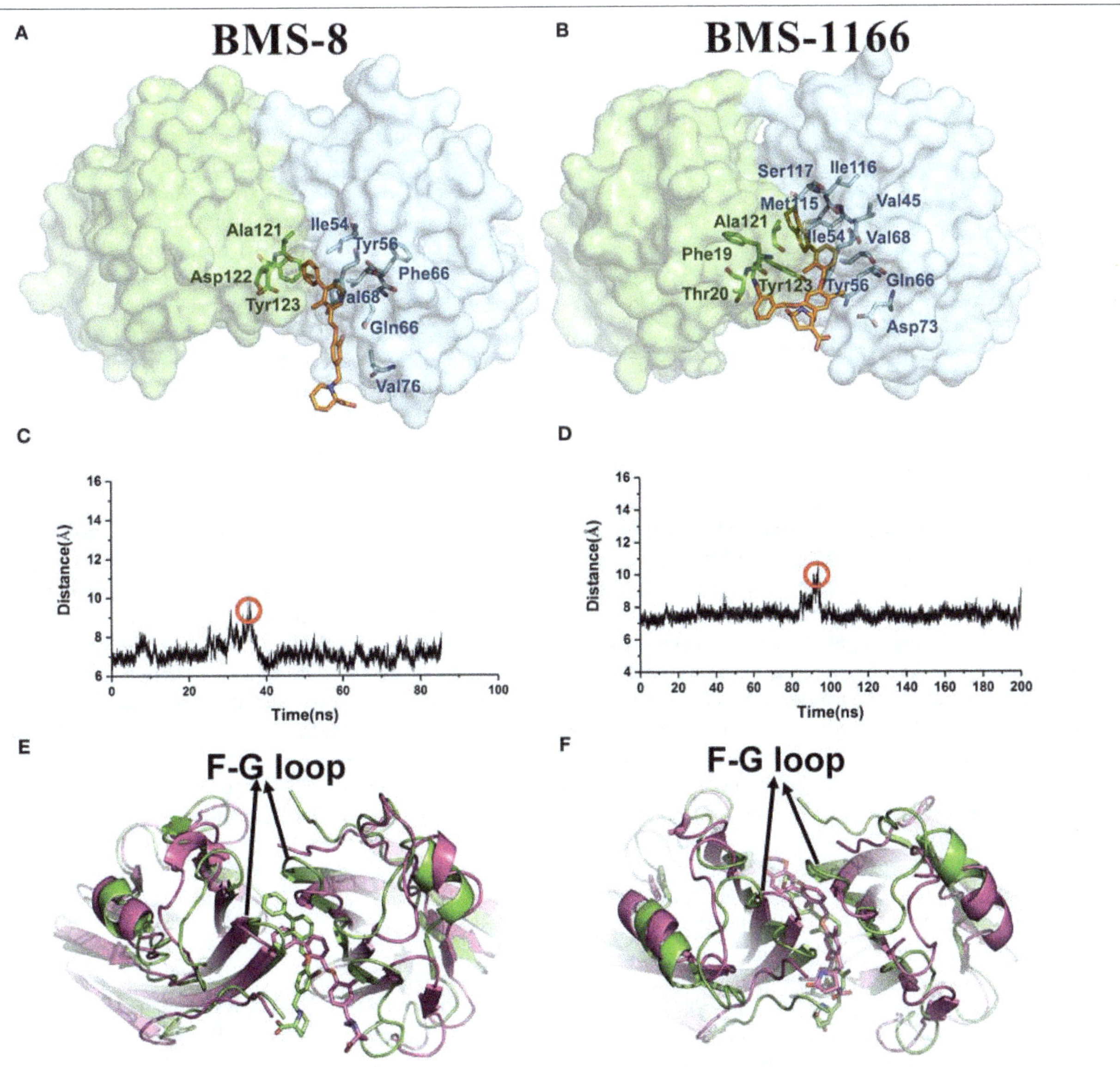

FIGURE 7 | The conformational change during the unbinding process. **(A,B)** The key transition conformational states of BMS-8 and BMS-1166 during the unbinding process with CV1 value of 12.54 Å and 10.95 Å, respectively. The chain A and chain B of PD-L1 dimers are shown in green and cyan surface, respectively. The key residues (green or cyan) and ligands (orange) are shown in sticks. **(C,D)** The distance between Ile54, Tyr56, Met115, Ala121, and Tyr123 on conformation A and conformation B of PD-L1 during the unbinding process of BMS-8 and BMS-1166. **(E,F)** The extracted conformational state (green cartoon) of each complex with the largest distance between two PD-L1 monomers was overlapped with the original crystal structures (magenta cartoon).

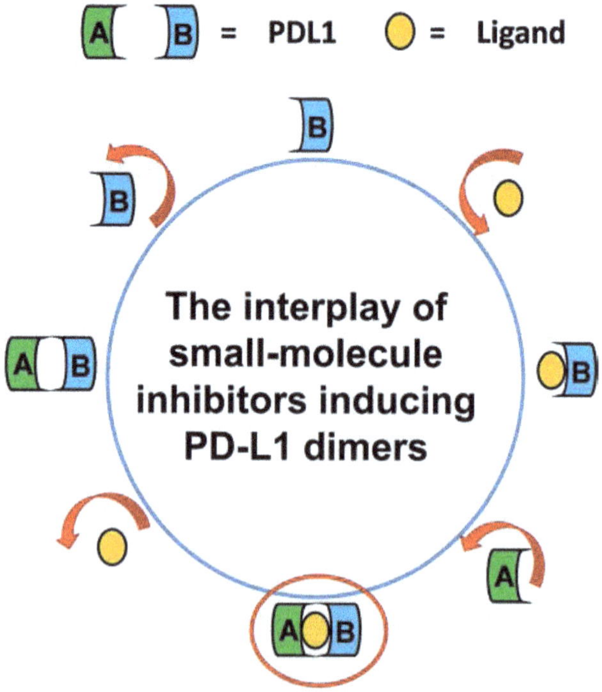

FIGURE 8 | The complete binding and unbinding mechanism of BMS small-molecule inhibitors. The conformation A and conformation B of PD-L1 monomer, the small-molecule ligand are represented by green, light blue, orange objects, respectively.

process was corresponding to the conformational states of the initial crystal structures as shown in **Figures 6A,B**. During the unbinding process, there were four different transition states for BMS-8 and three transition states for BMS-1166. In order to test the convergence of unbinding process, the free energies along both CVs were estimated. It can be seen that the free energy surface of CV1 (**Figures 6C,D**) and CV2 (**Figures 6E,F**) gradually came to a convergence along with the accumulation of time. As CV1 represented the distance between the ligand and the binding site of PD-L1 dimer and depicted the unbinding process better than CV2, the corresponding minimum points along CV1 were extracted from the unbinding trajectories. In BMS-8 complex systems, the minima along CV1 were 6.75 Å (−16.34 kcal/mol), 12.54 Å (−10.12 kcal/mol), and 14.97 Å (−7.31 kcal/mol). In BMS-1166 complex systems, the minima along CV1 were 5.67 Å (−28.79 kcal/mol), 10.95 Å (−8.50 kcal/mol), and 13.46 Å (−9.74 kcal/mol). The ultimate unbinding energy barriers of both small-molecule ligands estimated by CV1 and CV2 were shown in **Table 1** and **Figure 6**, which were in good consistency with the inhibitory activities. Considering the difference between the binding free energies predicted by different methods, MM-PBSA and MM-GBSA calculated the binding free energies using implicit water models while metadynamics simulation considered the explicit water interaction between protein and ligand. Therefore, the results from metadynamics simulation tended to be more approximate to the experimental results.

From the free energy estimation of different conformational states, it can be seen that the conformational states of the crystal structures were much more stable than the other transition conformational states along the unbinding process. Therefore, the dissociation of small-molecule ligands of the initial conformational states tended to be the most important intermediate process for the unbinding of small-molecule ligands, which were corresponding to the minima of CV1 at 12.54 Å in BMS-8 dimer systems and the minima of CV1 at 10.95 Å in BMS-202 dimer systems. The corresponding transition states were extracted from the trajectories as shown in **Figures 7A,B**. The binding poses of BMS small-molecule ligands at the transition states were quite distinct from each other, which was probably owing to the difference of substituent groups. A common feature for both systems was that the ligands at transition states significantly lost the interaction with the chain A while the interaction with chain B were still compact and involved with a series of residues especially in BMS-1166 dimer systems. During the unbinding process, the core scaffold of ligands gradually divorced from the location of $_{A}$Tyr56 and got away from the pocket formed by PD-L1 dimer. In order to monitor the conformational change of the pocket formed by PD-L1 monomers, the distance between chain A and chain B were calculated by the distance between Ile54, Tyr56, Met115, Ala121, Tyr123 on each chain as shown in **Figures 7C–F**. The conformational fluctuation of PD-L1 monomers was reflected by the conformational change of the F-G loops on both PD-L1 monomers. It can be seen that the pockets in BMS-8 and BMS-1166 complex systems were quite stable with occasionally occurring conformational fluctuations. According to unbinding processes of BMS ligands, it can be seen that the dimer of PD-L1 had a large tendency to keep stable although accompanied with subtle conformational fluctuation of PD-L1 dimer.

Taken together, the most possible deduction for the interaction mechanism of BMS small-molecule inhibitors with PD-L1 was depicted as shown in **Figure 8**. Firstly, all BMS small-molecule inhibitors with different activities tended to interacted with a monomer conformation B of PD-L1. As the PD-L1 dimer complex had strong conformational stability, the PD-L1 monomer complex further interacted with the other monomer of PD-L1 to form PD-L1 dimer complex. According to the results of metadynamics simulation, a complete dissociation for BMS inhibitors would probably be like that the small-molecule ligand was firstly unbound from the PD-L1 dimer and the rest receptor part was further depolymerized into monomer.

The R-Group QSAR Model of BMS Small-Molecule Inhibitors

110 BMS small-molecule inhibitors with 2-methyl-3-(phenoxymethyl)-1,1′-biphenyl scaffolds were tested with diverse inhibitory activities with IC_{50} ranging from 9.492 μM to 1.4 nM. As shown in **Figure 9A**, there were 7 different of attachment points from R1 to R7 and the substituent groups of R6 and R7 had a relatively larger proportion than other

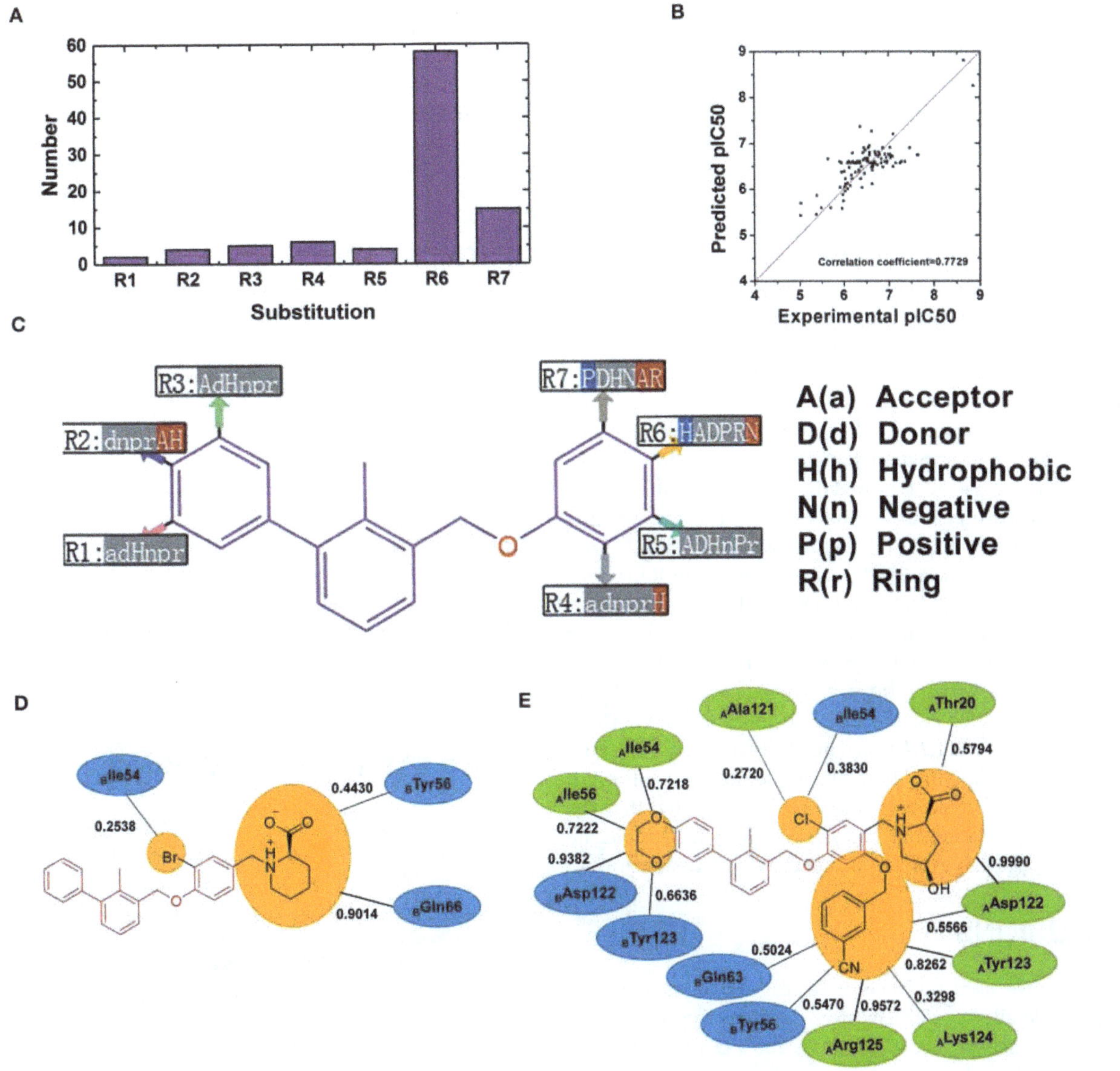

FIGURE 9 | The R-group based QSAR for BMS small-molecule inhibitors. **(A)** The number of substituent groups at seven attachment points of BMS small molecule inhibitors. **(B)** The correlation validation between the predicted pIC50 and experimental pIC50. **(C)** R-group QSAR model for the BMS small molecule inhibitors. The case-insensitive alphabets A(a), D(d), H(h), N(n), P(p), and R(r), respectively represent the hydrogen bond acceptor, the hydrogen bond donor, the hydrophobic, the negative ionic, the positive ionic, aromatic ring. The significantly increase effect is colored in red while the significantly decrease effect is colored in blue. **(D,E)** The interacting residues of different substituent groups of BMS-8 and BMS-1166. The occupancies of the contact between each residues and substituent group were listed along with the black solid.

attachment points. As shown in **Figure 9B**, the correlation coefficient between the predicted pIC_{50} and the experimental pIC_{50} was 0.7729. According to the evaluation of six key pharmacophore elements in **Figure 9C**, the substituent groups at R2, R4, R6, and R7 had obvious effect on the affinity of BMS small-molecule inhibitors. The substituent groups at R2, R4, R6, R7 of BMS-8 and BMS-116 as well as the interaction residues were recognized by the contact analysis as shown in **Figures 9D,E**. The contact analysis of BMS-1166 showed that the 1,4-benzodioxinyl group at R2 mainly was involved in the interaction with $_{A}$Ile54, $_{A}$Tyr56, $_{B}$Asp122, $_{B}$Tyr123. The hydrogen bond acceptor and hydrophobic groups at R2 were favorable for BMS inhibitors such as the 2, 3-dihydro-1, 4-benzodioxinyl group on BMS-114, BMS-200, BMS-1001, and BMS-1166. The analysis of effect of solvent in dimer systems showed that the substituent groups at R4, R5, R6, and R7 were exposed to solvent environment. The hydrophobic groups at R4 were favorable for BMS inhibitors, which corresponded to the fact that the bromine atom on BMS-8 and the chlorine atom on BMS-1166 had a close contact with $_{B}$Ile54. The hydrophobic group at R6 was adverse while the negative ionic group was favorable. The substituent group at R6 of BMS-8 mainly interacted with $_B$Tyr56 and $_B$Gln66, however, that of BMS-1166 mainly interacted with $_A$Thr20 and $_A$Asp122. Nevertheless, the substituent group at R6 of BMS-8 and BMS-1166 both formed hydrogen bonding with PD-L1. The positive ionic at R7 was adverse while the hydrogen bond acceptor and aromatic ring were favorable. The substituent group at R7 of BMS-1166 formed interaction with $_A$Asp122, $_A$Tyr123, $_A$Lys124, $_A$Arg125, $_B$Tyr56, and $_B$Gln63. The comparison of the contact residues between BMS-8 and BMS-1166 indicated that the substituent group at R2 and R7 strongly strengthened the interactions with the conformation A of PD-L1, which was consistent with the stability of the monomer complex of conformation A and BMS-1166.

The further molecular docking study of eight representative small-molecule inhibitors showed that the docking scores had a good linear correlation with the experimental inhibitory activities (**Figure S5**). The further residue contribution comparison (**Figure S6**) and conformational analysis (**Figure S7**) of the residues within 5 angstroms showed that the residues interacting with R-group substituents had an obvious effect on the docking scores including $_B$Asp122 (interacting with R1 to R3) and $_A$Asp122, $_A$Lys124, $_B$Tyr56, $_B$Gln66 (interacting with R4 to R7). The binding mode analysis of novel series of [1,2,4]triazolo[4,3-a]pyridines designed by Qin et al. also revealed the retaining hydrophobic interaction with Tyr56, Met115, and Ala121 on both chain of PD-L1 and extra π-π stacking with the $_B$Tyr56 and π-anion interactions with $_A$Asp122 (Qin et al., 2019). These interacting modes of [1,2,4]triazolo[4,3-a]pyridines inhibitors were consistent with the binding mode analysis of eight representative small-molecule inhibitors. It's suggested that the structure-activity relationship analysis of BMS small-molecule inhibitors was applicable for the further structure modifications.

CONCLUSIONS

In this study, we used multiple molecular modeling methods to study the detailed molecular mechanism of the interaction between BMS small-molecule inhibitors and PD-L1. A detailed mechanism of the interaction process between small-molecule inhibitors and PD-L1 was proposed and validated by molecular dynamics simulations.

The BMS small-molecule inhibitors tended to interact with one PD-L1 monomer first and further formed dimer with the other monomer for an advantage of stability. The results of binding free energy and water occupancy calculation revealed the key stability factors for ligand-induced PD-L1 dimers including the hydrophobic contribution of Ile54, Tyr56, Met115, Ala121, and Tyr123 on both monomers and the water bridges involved in $_A$Lys124. The unbinding pathway prediction also indicated that the tunnel formed by PD-L1 dimers tended to be stable upon the getting away of BMS-inhibitors. The R-group QSAR model suggested that the substituents at R2, R4, R6, and R7 had a significant effect on the inhibition activities of BMS inhibitors. The structural modification with these substituent positions tended to be an effective way to improve the inhibition activities of BMS inhibitors. Taken together, this study would provide a comprehensive view of the inhibition mechanism for BMS small-molecule inhibitors and guide the further development of more potential small-molecule inhibitors targeting PD-L1.

AUTHOR CONTRIBUTIONS

DS, HL, and XY designed the research. DS and XY were responsible for the writing and revising of the manuscript. XA, QB, SZ, and ZB were responsible the main data analysis in the manuscript.

FUNDING

This work was supported by the National Natural Science Foundation of China (Grant Nos. 21475054 and 2175060).

SUPPLEMENTARY MATERIAL

Figure S1 | The interactions diagrams between the monomer conformation A of PD-L1 (the initial crystal structure and three respective dynamics structures) and BMS-8 in the monomer system of replica 2.

Figure S2 | The interaction diagrams between the monomer conformation B of PD-L1 (the initial crystal structure and three respective dynamics structures) and BMS-8 in the monomer system of replica 2.

Figure S3 | The interaction diagrams between the monomer conformation A of PD-L1 (the initial crystal structure and three respective dynamics structures) and BMS-1166 in the monomer system of replica 2.

Figure S4 | The interaction diagrams between the monomer conformation B of PD-L1 (the initial crystal structure and three respective dynamics structures) and BMS-1166 in the monomer system of replica 2.

Figure S5 | The linear correlation between experimental pIC50 and the absolute values of the docking scores.

Figure S6 | The distance and residue contribution analysis of the binding poses of eight representative small-molecule inhibitors. **(A)** The respective and average distance between the small-molecule inhibitor and the residues on PD-L1 dimer. **(B)** The respective energy contribution of residues on PD-L1 dimer when interacting with the small-molecule inhibitor.

Figure S7 | The binding pose analysis of eight representative small-molecule inhibitors. **(A)** The surrounding residues of the substituent groups at R1 to R3 for eight representative small-molecule inhibitors. **(B–I)** The surrounding residues of the substituent groups at R4 to R7 for small-molecule inhibitor with NO. of 4, 101, 102, 103, 104, 108, 119, 110, respectively.

Table S1 | The detailed structural and activity information for 110 BMS small-molecule inhibitors.

REFERENCES

Abdel-Magid, A. F. (2015). Inhibitors of the PD-1/PD-L1 pathway can mobilize the immune system: an innovative potential therapy for cancer and chronic infections. *ACS Med. Chem. Lett.* 6, 489–490. doi: 10.1021/acsmedchemlett.5b00148

Adhikari, N., Halder, A. K., Saha, A., Das Saha, K., and Jha, T. (2015). Structural findings of phenylindoles as cytotoxic antimitotic agents in human breast cancer cell lines through multiple validated QSAR studies. *Toxicol. In Vitro* 29, 1392–1404. doi: 10.1016/j.tiv.2015.05.017

Barducci, A., Bonomi, M., and Parrinello, M. (2011). Metadynamics. *Wiley Interdiscip. Rev. Comput. Mol.* 1, 826–843. doi: 10.1002/wcms.31

Bellissent-Funel, M. C., Hassanali, A., Havenith, M., Henchman, R., Pohl, P., Sterpone, F., et al. (2016). Water determines the structure and dynamics of proteins. *Chem. Rev.* 116, 7673–7697. doi: 10.1021/acs.chemrev.5b00664

Bernardi, R. C., Melo, M. C., and Schulten, K. (2015). Enhanced sampling techniques in molecular dynamics simulations of biological systems. *Biochim. Biophys. Acta. Gen. Sub.* 1850, 872–877. doi: 10.1016/j.bbagen.2014.10.019

Bonomi, M., Branduardi, D., Bussi, G., Camilloni, C., Provasi, D., Raiteri, P., et al. (2009). PLUMED: a portable plugin for free-energy calculations with molecular dynamics. *Comput. Phys. Commun.* 180, 1961–1972. doi: 10.1016/j.cpc.2009.05.011

Casasnovas, R., Limongelli, V., Tiwary, P., Carloni, P., and Parrinello, M. (2017). Unbinding kinetics of a p38 MAP kinase type II inhibitor from metadynamics simulations. *J. Am. Chem. Soc.* 139, 4780–4788. doi: 10.1021/jacs.6b12950

Case, D., Babin, V., Berryman, J., Betz, R., Cai, Q., Cerutti, D., et al. (2014). *AMBER 14.* San Francisco, CA: University of California.

Cavalli, A., Spitaleri, A., Saladino, G., and Gervasio, F. L. (2015). Investigating drug-target association and dissociation mechanisms using metadynamics-based algorithms. *Acc. Chem. Res.* 48, 277–285. doi: 10.1021/ar500356n

Chang, H. N., Liu, B. Y., Qi, Y. K., Zhou, Y., Chen, Y. P., Pan, K. M., et al. (2015). Blocking of the PD-1/PD-L1 interaction by a D-peptide antagonist for cancer immunotherapy. *Angew. Chem. Int. Edit.* 54, 11760–11764. doi: 10.1002/anie.201506225

Chen, F., Sun, H., Wang, J., Zhu, F., Liu, H., Wang, Z., et al. (2018). Assessing the performance of MM/PBSA and MM/GBSA methods. 8. Predicting binding free energies and poses of protein-RNA complexes. *RNA* 24, 1183–1194. doi: 10.1261/rna.065896.118

Duan, J., Dixon, S. L., Lowrie, J. F., and Sherman, W. (2010). Analysis and comparison of 2D fingerprints: insights into database screening performance using eight fingerprint methods. *J. Mol. Graph. Model.* 29, 157–170. doi: 10.1016/j.jmgm.2010.05.008

Gatalica, Z., Snyder, C., Maney, T., Ghazalpour, A., Holterman, D. A., Xiao, N., et al. (2014). Programmed cell death 1 (PD-1) and its ligand (PD-L1) in common cancers and their correlation with molecular cancer type. *Cancer Epidem. Biomar.* 23, 2965–2970. doi: 10.1158/1055-9965.EPI-14-0654

Gauto, D. F., Petruk, A. A., Modenutti, C. P., Blanco, J. I., Di Lella, S., and Marti, M. A. (2013). Solvent structure improves docking prediction in lectin-carbohydrate complexes. *Glycobiology* 23, 241–258. doi: 10.1093/glycob/cws147

Genheden, S., and Ryde, U. (2015). The MM/PBSA and MM/GBSA methods to estimate ligand-binding affinities. *Expert Opin. Drug Discov.* 10, 449–461. doi: 10.1517/17460441.2015.1032936

Guzik, K., Zak, K. M., Grudnik, P., Magiera, K., Musielak, B., Törner, R., et al. (2017). Small-molecule inhibitors of the Programmed Cell Death-1/Programmed Death-ligand 1 (PD-1/PD-L1) interaction via transiently-induced protein states and dimerization of PD-L1. *J. Med. Chem.* 60, 5857–5867. doi: 10.1021/acs.jmedchem.7b00293

Hirons, L., Holliday, J. D., Jelfs, S. P., Willett, P., and Gedeck, P. (2005). Use of the R-group descriptor for alignment-free QSAR. *QSAR Comb. Sci.* 24, 611–619. doi: 10.1002/qsar.200510102

Holliday, J., Jelfs, S., Willett, P., and Gedeck, P. (2003). Calculation of intersubstituent similarity using R-group descriptors. *J. Chem. Inf. Comput. Sci.* 43, 406–411. doi: 10.1021/ci025589v

Kalé, L., Skeel, R., Bhandarkar, M., Brunner, R., Gursoy, A., Krawetz, N., et al. (1999). NAMD2: greater scalability for parallel molecular dynamics. *J. Comput. Phys.* 151, 283–312. doi: 10.1006/jcph.1999.6201

Kolarevic, A., Ilic, B. S., Anastassova, N., Mavrova, A. T., Yancheva, D., Kocic, G., et al. (2018). Benzimidazoles as novel deoxyribonuclease I inhibitors. *J. Cell. Biochem.* 119, 8937–8948. doi: 10.1002/jcb.27147

Lee, H. T., Lee, J. Y., Lim, H., Lee, S. H., Moon, Y. J., Pyo, H. J., et al. (2017). Molecular mechanism of PD-1/PD-L1 blockade via anti-PD-L1 antibodies atezolizumab and durvalumab. *Sci. Rep.* 7:5532. doi: 10.1038/s41598-017-06002-8

Lee, J. Y., Lee, H. T., Shin, W., Chae, J., Choi, J., Kim, S. H., et al. (2016). Structural basis of checkpoint blockade by monoclonal antibodies in cancer immunotherapy. *Nat. Commun.* 7:13354. doi: 10.1038/ncomms13354

Liu, A., Dong, L., Wei, X. L., Yang, X. H., Xiao, J. H., and Liu, Z. Q. (2016). Development of amino- and dimethylcarbamate-substituted resorcinol as programmed cell death-1 (PD-1) inhibitor. *Eur. J. Pharm. Sci.* 88, 50–58. doi: 10.1016/j.ejps.2016.03.023

Liu, K., Tan, S., Chai, Y., Chen, D., Song, H., Zhang, C. W., et al. (2016). Structural basis of anti-PD-L1 monoclonal antibody avelumab for tumor therapy. *Cell Res.* 27, 151–153. doi: 10.1038/cr.2016.102

Magiera-Mularz, K., Skalniak, L., Zak, K. M., Musielak, B., Rudzinska-Szostak, E., Berlicki, Ł., et al. (2017). Bioactive macrocyclic inhibitors of the PD-1/PD-L1 immune checkpoint. *Angew. Chem. Int. Ed.* 129, 13920–13923. doi: 10.1002/ange.201707707

Masetti, M., Cavalli, A., Recanatini, M., and Gervasio, F. L. (2009). Exploring complex protein–ligand recognition mechanisms with coarse metadynamics. *J. Phys. Chem. B* 113, 4807–4816. doi: 10.1021/jp803936q

Pascolutti, R., Sun, X., Kao, J., Maute, R. L., Ring, A. M., Bowman, G. R., et al. (2016). Structure and dynamics of PD-L1 and an ultra-high-affinity PD-1 receptor mutant. *Structure* 24, 1719–1728. doi: 10.1016/j.str.2016.06.026

Patel, S. P., and Kurzrock, R. (2015). PD-L1 expression as a predictive biomarker in cancer immunotherapy. *Mol. Cancer Ther.* 14, 847–856. doi: 10.1158/1535-7163.MCT-14-0983

Perry, E., Mills, J. J., Zhao, B., Wang, F., Sun, Q., Christov, P. P., et al. (2019). Fragment-based screening of programmed death ligand 1 (PD-L1). *Bioorg. Med. Chem. Lett.* 29, 786–790. doi: 10.1016/j.bmcl.2019.01.028

Pettersen, E. F., Goddard, T. D., Huang, C. C., Couch, G. S., Greenblatt, D. M., Meng, E. C., et al. (2004). UCSF chimera—a visualization system for exploratory research and analysis. *J. Comput. Chem.* 25, 1605–1612. doi: 10.1002/jcc.20084

Qin, M., Cao, Q., Zheng, S., Tian, Y., Zhang, H., Xie, J., et al. (2019). Discovery of [1,2,4]Triazolo[4,3-a]pyridines as potent inhibitors targeting the programmed cell death-1/programmed cell death-ligand 1 interaction. *J. Med. Chem.* 62, 4703–4715. doi: 10.1021/acs.jmedchem.9b00312

Romero, J. M., Trujillo, M., Estrin, D. A., Rabinovich, G. A., and Di Lella, S. (2016). Impact of human galectin-1 binding to saccharide ligands on dimer dissociation kinetics and structure. *Glycobiology* 26, 1317–1327. doi: 10.1093/glycob/cww052

Sastry, M., Lowrie, J. F., Dixon, S. L., and Sherman, W. (2010). Large-scale systematic analysis of 2D fingerprint methods and parameters to improve virtual screening enrichments. *J. Chem. Inf. Model.* 50, 771–784. doi: 10.1021/ci100062n

Sharma, P., and Allison, J. P. (2015a). The future of immune checkpoint therapy. *Science* 348, 56–61. doi: 10.1126/science.aaa8172

Sharma, P., and Allison, J. P. (2015b). Immune checkpoint targeting in cancer therapy: toward combination strategies with curative potential. *Cell* 161, 205–214. doi: 10.1016/j.cell.2015.03.030

Sharpe, A. H., Butte, M. J., and Oyama, S. (2011). *Modulators of Immunoinhibitory Receptor pd-1, and Methods of Use Thereof.* U.S. Patent Application.

Skalniak, L., Zak, K. M., Guzik, K., Magiera, K., Musielak, B., Pachota, M., et al. (2017). Small-molecule inhibitors of PD-1/PD-L1 immune checkpoint alleviate the PD-L1-induced exhaustion of T-cells. *Oncotarget* 8, 72167–72181. doi: 10.18632/oncotarget.20050

Sun, H., Duan, L., Chen, F., Liu, H., Wang, Z., Pan, P., et al. (2018). Assessing the performance of MM/PBSA and MM/GBSA methods. 7. Entropy effects on the performance of end-point binding free energy calculation approaches. *Phys. Chem. Chem. Phys.* 20, 14450-14460. doi: 10.1039/c7cp07623a

Sun, H., Li, Y., Shen, M., Li, D., Kang, Y., and Hou, T. (2017). Characterizing drug-target residence time with metadynamics: how to achieve dissociation rate efficiently without losing accuracy against time-consuming approaches. *J. Chem. Inf. Model.* 57, 1895–1906. doi: 10.1021/acs.jcim.7b00075

Tan, S., Chen, D., Liu, K., He, M., Song, H., Shi, Y., et al. (2016). Crystal clear: visualizing the intervention mechanism of the PD-1/PD-L1 interaction by two cancer therapeutic monoclonal antibodies. *Protein Cell* 7, 866–877. doi: 10.1007/s13238-016-0337-7

Tan, S., Liu, K., Chai, Y., Zhang, C. W., Gao, S., Gao, G. F., et al. (2017). Distinct PD-L1 binding characteristics of therapeutic monoclonal antibody durvalumab. *Protein Cell* 9, 135–139. doi: 10.1007/s13238-017-0412-8

Ts Mavrova, A., Dimov, S., Yancheva, D., Kolarevic, A., Ilic, B. S., Kocic, G., et al. (2018). Synthesis and DNase I inhibitory properties of some 5,6,7,8-tetrahydrobenzo[4,5]thieno[2,3-d]pyrimidines. *Bioorg. Chem.* 80, 693–705. doi: 10.1016/j.bioorg.2018.07.009

Xue, W., Jin, X., Ning, L., Wang, M., Liu, H., and Yao, X. (2013). Exploring the molecular mechanism of cross-resistance to HIV-1 integrase strand transfer inhibitors by molecular dynamics simulation and residue interaction network analysis. *J. Chem. Inf. Model.* 53, 210–222. doi: 10.1021/ci300541c

Zak, K. M., Grudnik, P., Guzik, K., Zieba, B. J., Musielak, B., Dömling, A., et al. (2016). Structural basis for small molecule targeting of the programmed death ligand 1 (PD-L1). *Oncotarget* 7, 30323–30335. doi: 10.18632/oncotarget.8730

Zak, K. M., Kitel, R., Przetocka, S., Golik, P., Guzik, K., Musielak, B., et al. (2015). Structure of the complex of human programmed death 1, PD-1, and its ligand PD-L1. *Structure* 23, 2341–2348. doi: 10.1016/j.str.2015.09.010

Zarganes-Tzitzikas, T., Konstantinidou, M., Gao, Y., Krzemien, D., Zak, K., Dubin, G., et al. (2016). Inhibitors of programmed cell death 1 (PD-1): a patent review (2010-2015). *Expert Opin. Ther. Pat.* 26, 973–977. doi: 10.1080/13543776.2016.1206527

Zhang, F., Qi, X., Wang, X., Wei, D., Wu, J., Feng, L., et al. (2017a). Structural basis of the therapeutic anti-PD-L1 antibody atezolizumab. *Oncotarget* 8, 90215–90224. doi: 10.18632/oncotarget.21652

Zhang, F., Wei, H., Wang, X., Bai, Y., Wang, P., Wu, J., et al. (2017b). Structural basis of a novel PD-L1 nanobody for immune checkpoint blockade. *Cancer Discov.* 3:17004. doi: 10.1038/celldisc.2017.4

8

Structure-Based Virtual Screening: From Classical to Artificial Intelligence

Eduardo Habib Bechelane Maia[1,2*], *Letícia Cristina Assis*[1], *Tiago Alves de Oliveira*[2], *Alisson Marques da Silva*[2] *and Alex Gutterres Taranto*[1]

[1] *Laboratory of Pharmaceutical Medicinal Chemistry, Federal University of São João Del Rei, Divinópolis, Brazil,* [2] *Federal Center for Technological Education of Minas Gerais—CEFET-MG, Belo Horizonte, Brazil*

Correspondence:
Eduardo Habib Bechelane Maia
habib@cefetmg.br

The drug development process is a major challenge in the pharmaceutical industry since it takes a substantial amount of time and money to move through all the phases of developing of a new drug. One extensively used method to minimize the cost and time for the drug development process is computer-aided drug design (CADD). CADD allows better focusing on experiments, which can reduce the time and cost involved in researching new drugs. In this context, structure-based virtual screening (SBVS) is robust and useful and is one of the most promising *in silico* techniques for drug design. SBVS attempts to predict the best interaction mode between two molecules to form a stable complex, and it uses scoring functions to estimate the force of non-covalent interactions between a ligand and molecular target. Thus, scoring functions are the main reason for the success or failure of SBVS software. Many software programs are used to perform SBVS, and since they use different algorithms, it is possible to obtain different results from different software using the same input. In the last decade, a new technique of SBVS called consensus virtual screening (CVS) has been used in some studies to increase the accuracy of SBVS and to reduce the false positives obtained in these experiments. An indispensable condition to be able to utilize SBVS is the availability of a 3D structure of the target protein. Some virtual databases, such as the Protein Data Bank, have been created to store the 3D structures of molecules. However, sometimes it is not possible to experimentally obtain the 3D structure. In this situation, the homology modeling methodology allows the prediction of the 3D structure of a protein from its amino acid sequence. This review presents an overview of the challenges involved in the use of CADD to perform SBVS, the areas where CADD tools support SBVS, a comparison between the most commonly used tools, and the techniques currently used in an attempt to reduce the time and cost in the drug development process. Finally, the final considerations demonstrate the importance of using SBVS in the drug development process.

Keywords: SBVS, homology modeling, consensus virtual screening, scoring functions, computer-aided drug design

INTRODUCTION

In the past, the discovery of new drugs was made through random screening and empirical observations of the effects of natural products for known diseases.

This random screening process, although inefficient, led to the identification of several important compounds until the 1980s. Currently, this process is improved by high-throughput screening (HTS), which is suitable for automating the screening process of many thousands of compounds against a molecular target or cellular assay very quickly. The milestone of HTS was used in the identification of cyclosporine A as a immunosuppressant (von Wartburg and Traber, 1988). Subsequently, several drugs such as nevirapine (Merluzzi et al., 1990), gefitinib (Ward et al., 1994), and maraviroc (Wood and Armour, 2005) have reached the market. Notably, gefitinib was discovered by computational methods through a collection of 1500 compounds by ALLADIN (Martin, 1992) software. In addition, computational methods have been used to search successful compounds against malaria disease (Nunes et al., 2019). The structures of these molecules are in **Figure 1**.

Alternatively, the increased cost and evolution of medicines available in the last century have led to an improvement in the quality of life of the world population. However, while the average quality of life has been improved, a third of the population is still without access to essential medicines, which means that more than 2 billion people cannot afford to buy basic medicines (Leisinger et al., 2012). This problem is even worse in some places in Africa and Asia, where more than 50% of the people face problems obtaining medicines (Leisinger et al., 2012). Moreover, throughout the world, more than 18 million deaths that occur every year could be avoided, as well as tens of millions of deaths related to poverty and lack of access to essential medicines (Sridhar, 2008). The price of many medicines is inaccessible to limited-income populations and middle-income countries (Stevens and Huys, 2017).

While there is a need to increase the population's access to medicines, the pharmaceutical industry is facing unprecedented challenges in its business model (Paul et al., 2010). The current process of developing new drugs began to mature only in the second half of the twentieth century. The process evolved from observations made in the correlation of certain physical-chemical properties of organic molecules with biological potency. Optimization of these compounds by the incorporation of more favorable substituents resulted in more potent drugs. X-ray crystallography and nuclear magnetic resonance (NMR) techniques have provided information on the structures of enzymes and drug receptors. Many drugs, such as angiotensin-converting-enzyme (ACE) inhibitors, have been introduced to the clinical practice from this structural information.

The drug development process aims to identify bioactive compounds to assist in the treatment of diseases. In summary (**Figure 2**), the process starts with the identification of molecular targets for a given compound (natural or synthetic) and is followed by their validation. Then, virtual screening (VS) can be used to assist in hit identification (identification of active drug candidates) and lead optimization (biologically active compounds are transformed into appropriate drugs by improving their physicochemical properties). Finally these optimized leads will undergo preclinical and clinical trials to ultimately be approved by regulatory bodies (Lima et al., 2016).

In general, this process is time-consuming, laborious and expensive. The development of a new drug has an average cost between 1 and 2 billion USD and could take 10–17 years (Leelananda and Lindert, 2016), since it has to move through all phases for new drug development, from target discovery to drug registration. Even so, Arrowsmith (2012) showed that the probability of a drug candidate reaching the market after entering Phase I clinical trials fell from 10% in the 2002–2004 period to approximately 5% between 2006 and 2008, which represents a 50% decrease in just 4 years.

Thus, researchers are constantly investing in the development of new methods to increase the efficiency of the drug discovery process (Hillisch et al., 2004). The computer-aided drug design (CADD) approach, which employs molecular modeling techniques, has been used by researchers to increase the efficacy in the development of new drugs since it uses *in silico* simulations. Molecular modeling allows the analysis of many molecules in a short period of time, demonstrating how they interact with targets of pharmacological interest even before their synthesis. The technique allows the simulation and prediction of several essential factors, such as toxicity, activity, bioavailability and efficacy, even before the compound undergoes *in vitro* testing, thus allowing better planning and direction of the research (Ferreira et al., 2011). Better planning of the research means, in this case, fewer *in vitro* and *in vivo* experiments. Therefore, it reduces the run time and overall research costs.

In this context, virtual screening (VS) is a promising *in silico* technique used in the drug discovery process. An indispensable condition in performing virtual screening is the availability of a 3D structure of the target protein (Cavasotto, 2011). Therefore, some virtual databases were created to store 3D structures of molecules. Virtual screening is now widely applied in the development of new drugs and has already contributed to compounds on the market. Examples of drugs that came to the market with the assistance of VS include captopril (antihypertensive drug), saquinavir, ritonavir, and indinavir (three drugs for the treatment of human immunodeficiency virus), tirofiban (fibrinogen antagonist), dorzolamide (used to treat glaucoma), zanamivir (a selective antiviral for influenza virus), aliskiren (antihypertensive drug), boceprevir (protease inhibitor used for the treatment of hepatitis C), nolatrexed (in phase III clinical trial for the treatment of liver cancer) (Talele et al., 2010; Sliwoski et al., 2013; Devi et al., 2015; Nunes et al., 2019). The structures of these molecules are in **Figures 3, 4**.

This review will present an overview of the challenges involved in the development of new drugs. Section Computer-aided drug design (CADD) will describe CADD while section 3 will demonstrate how VS has been used as an agent in the process of developing of new drugs. Section Virtual screening (VS), in turn, will explain the main scoring functions used in recent scientific research. Section Consensus docking will explain consensus docking, which is a relatively unexplored

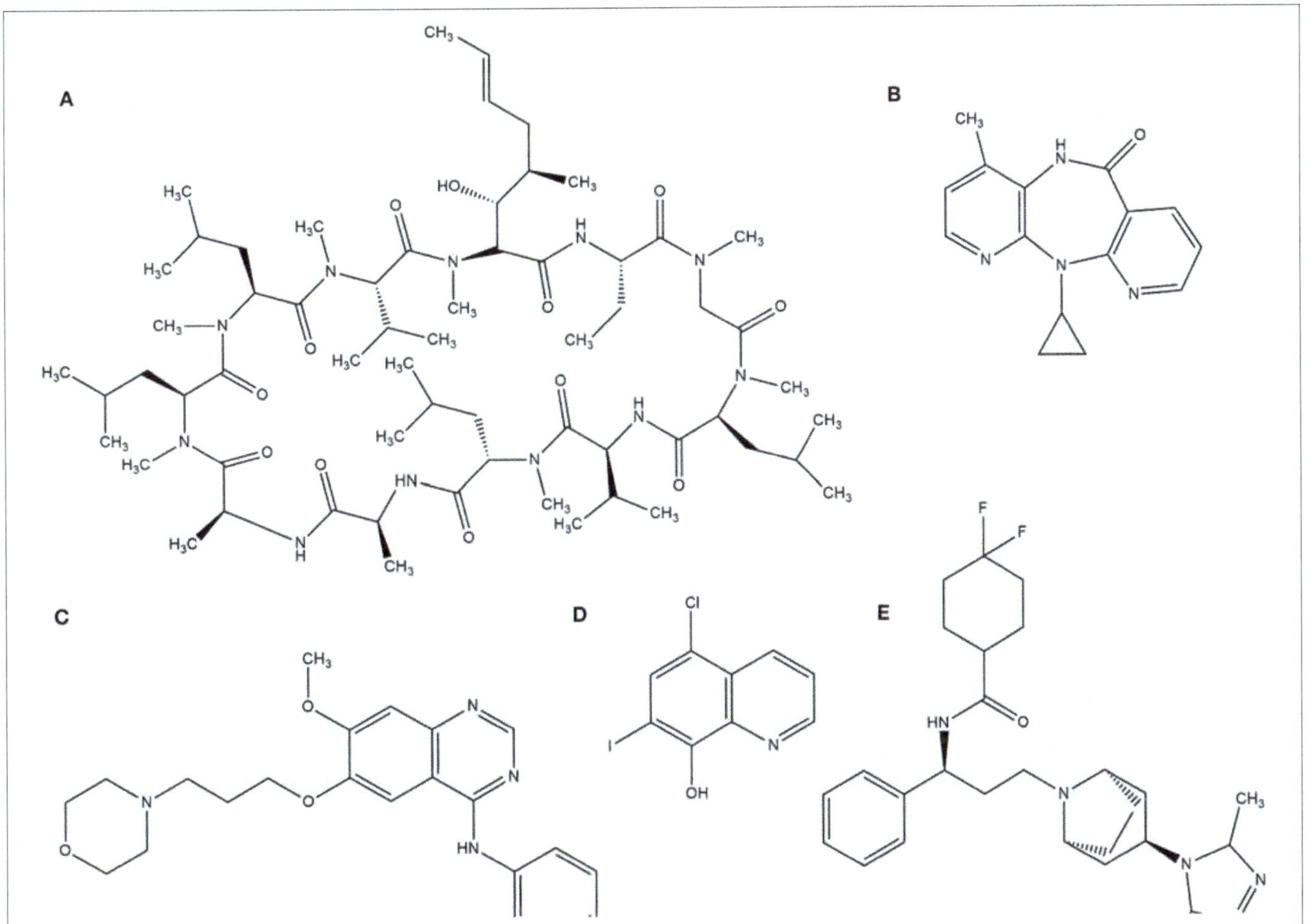

FIGURE 1 | Examples of structures identified by HTS. **(A)** cyclosporine A, **(B)** Neviparine, **(C)** Gefitinib, **(D)** Clioquinol, and **(E)** Maraviroc.

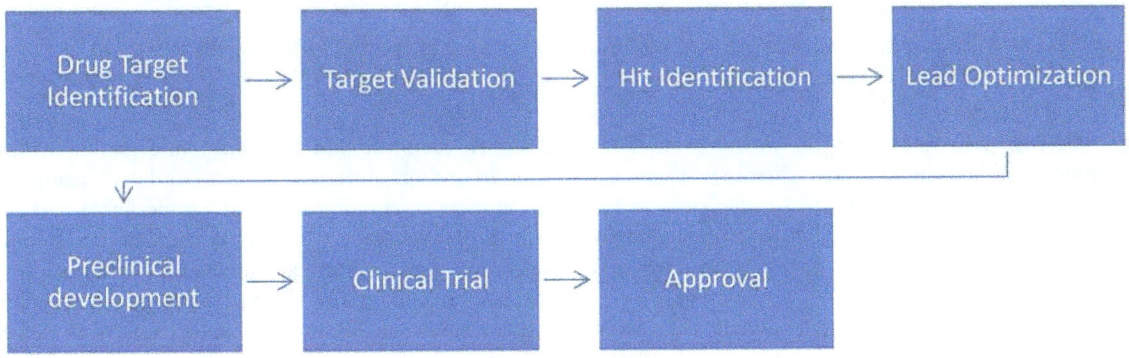

FIGURE 2 | Drug development timeline.

topic in the virtual screening process. Section Virtual Databases will list the main virtual databases used in this task. Section Virtual screening algorithms presents the main VS algorithms used. Section Methods of evaluating the quality of a simulation will present some evaluation methods used to verify if the quality of the performed model/simulation is good. Section VS software programs, in turn, will present the main VS software currently used. Section Final considerations will present final considerations.

COMPUTER-AIDED DRUG DESIGN (CADD)

One approach used to increase the effectiveness in the development of new drugs is the use of computer-aided

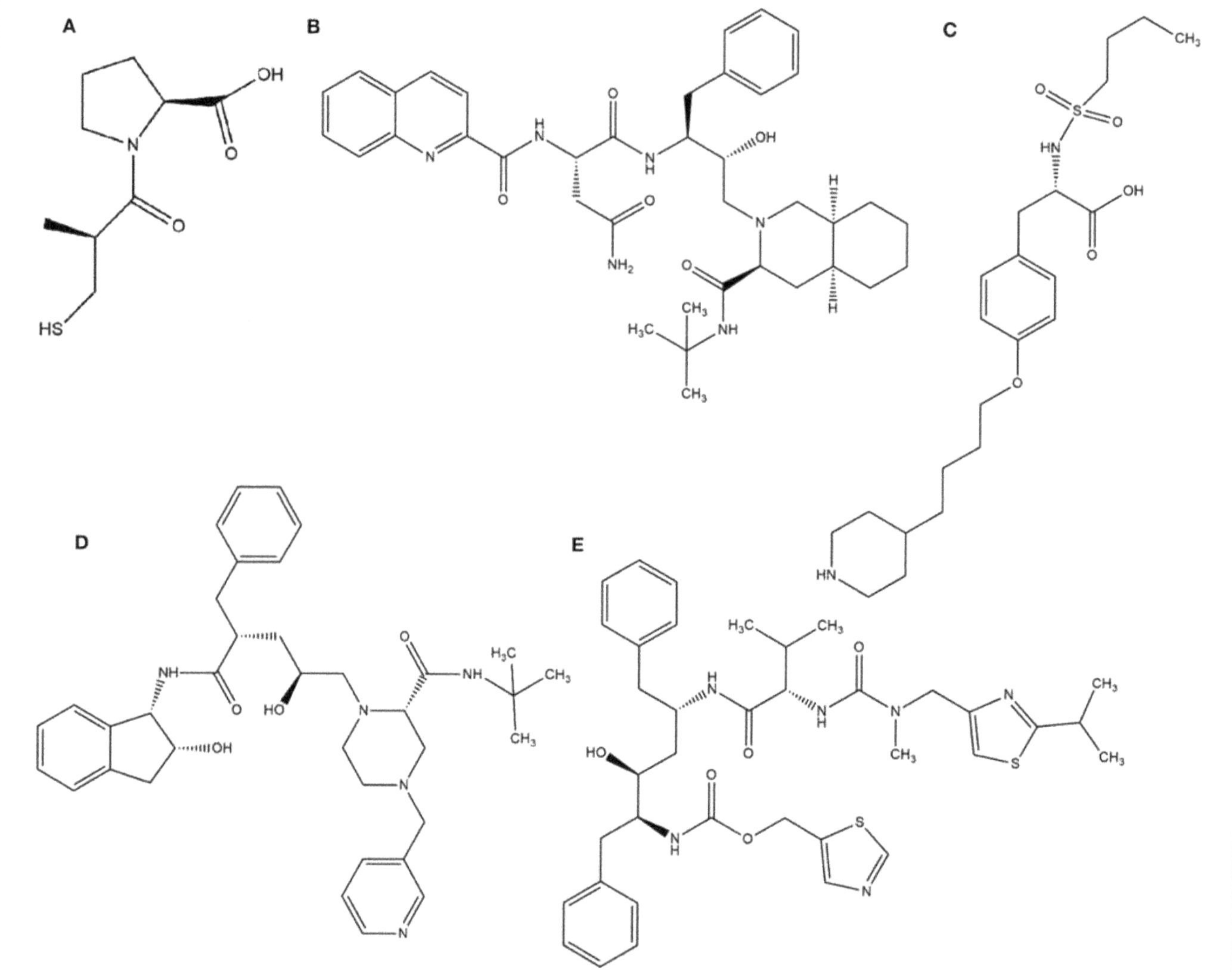

FIGURE 3 | Drugs that came to the market with the assistance of VS: **(A)** Captopril, **(B)** Saquinavir, **(C)** Tirofiban, **(D)** Indinavir, **(E)** Ritonavir.

drug design (CADD, well known as an *in silico* method) techniques, which uses a computational chemistry approach for the drug discovery process. CADD is a cyclic process for developing new drugs, in which all stages of design and analysis are performed by computer programs, operated by medicinal chemists (Oglic et al., 2018).

Strategies for CADD may vary, depending on what information about the target and ligand are available. In the early stage of the drug development process, it is normal for little or no information to exist about the target, ligands, or their structures. CADD techniques are able to obtain this information, such as which proteins can be targeted in pathogenesis and what are the possible active ligands that can inhibit these proteins. Kapetanovic (2008) briefly notes that CADD comprises (i) making the drug discovery and development process faster with the contribution of *in silico* simulations; (ii) optimizing and identifying new drugs using the computational approach to discover chemical and biological information about possible ligands and/or molecular targets; and (iii) using simulations to eliminate compounds with undesirable properties and selecting candidates with more chances for success. Recent software uses empirical molecular mechanics, quantum mechanics and, more recently, statistical mechanics. This last advancement allows the explicit effects of solvents to be incorporated (Das and Saha, 2017).

CADD gained prominence, as it allows obtaining information about the specific properties of a molecule, which can influence its interaction with the receptor. Thus, it has been considered a useful tool in rational planning and the discovery of new bioactive compounds. Alternatively, CADD simulations require a high computational cost, taking up to weeks if long jobs are used for molecular dynamics simulations. Therefore, it is a continuous challenge to find viable solutions that reduce the simulation runtime and simultaneously increase the accuracy of the

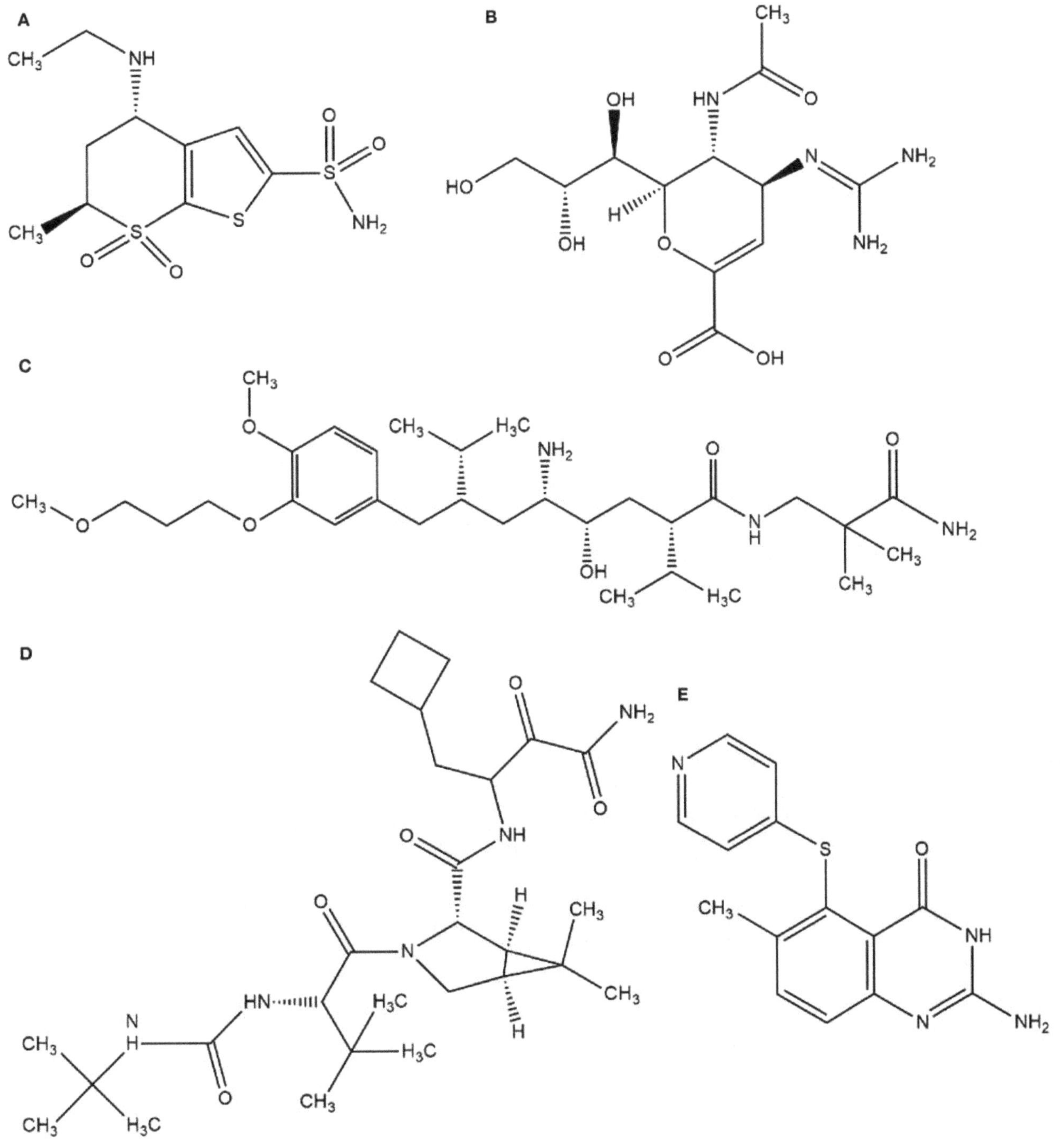

FIGURE 4 | Drugs that came to the market with the assistance of VS. **(A)** Dorzolamide, **(B)** Zanamivir, **(C)** Aliskiren, **(D)** Boceprevir, **(E)** Nolatrexid.

simulations (Ripphausen et al., 2011). In this context, VS is a promising approach.

VIRTUAL SCREENING (VS)

Popular VS techniques originated in the 1980s, but the first publication about VS appeared in 1997 (Horvath, 1997). In recent times, the use of VS techniques has been shown to be an excellent alternative to high throughput screening, especially in terms of cost-effectiveness and probability of finding the most appropriate result through a large virtual database (Surabhi and Singh, 2018).

VS is an *in silico* technique used in the drug discovery process. During VS, large databases of known 3D structures are automatically evaluated using computational methods (Maia et al., 2017). VS works like a funnel, by selecting

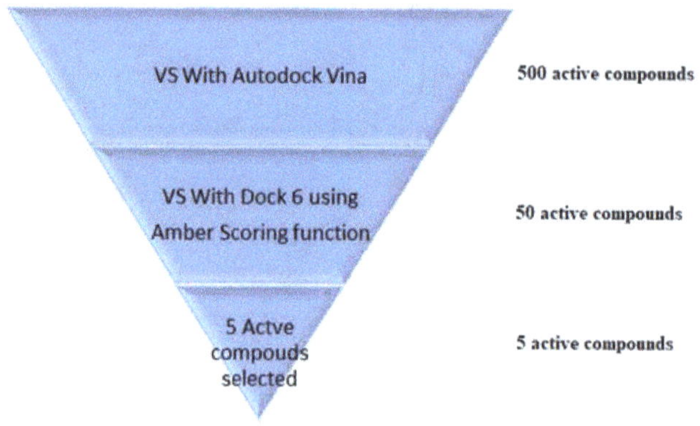

FIGURE 5 | VS scheme.

more promising molecules for *in vitro* assays to be performed. In the example shown in **Figure 5**, it is assumed that a virtual screening will be performed on 500 possible active ligands for a target. Then, VS with AutoDock Vina (Trott and Olson, 2009) was carried out and the top 50 ligands were selected. Then, a VS using DOCK 6 (Allen et al., 2015) with the Amber scoring function was performed. DOCK 6 with Amber scoring function takes longer, because it performs molecular dynamics, but it promises better results. Finally, after VS with DOCK 6, the top 5 active compounds are selected to be purchased and then tested *in vitro*. With the use of VS, it is expected that those identified molecules are more susceptible to binding to the molecular target, which is typically a protein or enzyme receptor. Therefore, VS assists in identifying the most promising hits able to bind to the target protein or enzyme receptor, and only the most promising molecules are synthesized. In addition, VS identifies compounds that may be toxic or have unfavorable pharmacodynamic (for example, potency, affinity, selectivity) and pharmacokinetic (for example, absorption, metabolism, bioavailability) properties. Thus, VS techniques play a prominent role among strategies for the identification of new bioactive substances (Berman et al., 2013).

VS for drug discovery is becoming an essential tool to assist in fast and cost-effective lead discovery and drug optimization (Maia et al., 2017). This technique can aid in the discovery of bioactive molecules, since they allow the selection of compounds in a structure database that are most likely to show biological activity against a target of interest. After identification, these bioactive molecules undergo biological assays. In addition, there are VS techniques using machine learning methods that predict compounds with specific pharmacodynamic, pharmacokinetic or toxicological properties based on their structural and physicochemical properties that are derived from the ligand structure (Ma et al., 2009). Hence, VS tools play a prominent role among the strategies used for the identification of new bioactive substances, since they increase the speed of the drug discovery process as long as they automatically evaluate large compound libraries through computational simulations (Maithri and Narendra, 2016).

Structure based virtual screening (SBVS) is a robust, useful and promising *in silico* technique for drug design (Lionta et al., 2014). Therefore, this review will address SBVS, although there are other types of VS such as ligand-based virtual screening (Banegas-Luna et al., 2018) and fragment-based virtual screening (Wang et al., 2015).

4-Structure-Based Virtual Screening (SBVS)

Structure-based virtual screening (SBVS), also known as target-based virtual screening (TBVS), attempts to predict the best interaction between ligands against a molecular target to form a complex. As a result, the ligands are ranked according to their affinity to the target, and the most promising compounds are shown at the top of the list. SBVS methods require that the 3D structure of the target protein be known so that the interactions between the target and each chemical compound can be predicted *in silico* (Liu et al., 2018). In this strategy, the compounds are selected from a database and classified according to their affinity for the receptor site.

Among the techniques of SBVS, molecular docking is noteworthy due to its low computational cost and good results achieved (Meng et al., 2011). This technique emerged in the 1980s, when Kuntz et al. (1982) designed and tested a set of algorithms that could explore the geometrically feasible alignments of a ligand and target. However, although the approach was promising, it was only in the 1990s that it became widely used after there was an improvement in the techniques used in conjunction with an increase in the computational power and a greater access to the structural data of target molecules. During the execution of SBVS, the evaluated molecules are sorted according to their affinity to the receptor site. Hence, it is possible to identify ligands that are more likely to present some pharmacological activity with the molecular target. Score functions are used to verify the likelihood of a binding site describing the affinity between the ligand and target. In this process, a reliable scoring function is the critical component of the docking process (Leelananda and Lindert, 2016).

The use of SBVS has advantages and disadvantages. Among the advantages are the following:

I There is a decrease in the time and cost involved in the screening of millions of small molecules.
II There is no need for the physical existence of the molecule, so it can be tested computationally even before being synthesized.
III There are several tools available to assist SBVS.

The disadvantages can be highlighted as the following:

I Some tools work best in specific cases, but not in more general cases (Lionta et al., 2014).
II It is difficult to accurately predict the correct binding position and classification of compounds due to the difficulty of parameterizing the complexity of ligand-receptor binding interactions.
III It can generate false positives and false negatives.

Despite the disadvantages noted above, many studies using SBVS have been developed in recent years (Carregal et al., 2017; Mugumbate et al., 2017; Wójcikowski et al., 2017; Carpenter et al., 2018; Dutkiewicz and Mikstacka, 2018; Surabhi and Singh, 2018; Nunes et al., 2019), which shows that although SBVS has disadvantages, it is still wide used for developing drugs due to the reduction of time and cost. However, docking protocols are essential for achieving accurate SBVS. These protocols are composed of two main components: the search algorithm and the score function.

Search Algorithms

Search algorithms are used to systematically search for ligand orientations and conformations at the binding site. A good docking protocol will achieve the most viable ligand conformations, in addition the most realistic position of the ligand at the binding site.

Thus, the search algorithm explores different positions of ligands at the active binding site using translational and rotational degrees of freedom in the case of rigid docking, while flexible docking adds conformational degrees of freedom to translations and rotations of the ligands. To predict the correct conformation of ligands, search algorithms adopt various techniques, such as checking the chemistry and geometry of the atoms involved [DOCK 6 (Allen et al., 2015), FLEXX (Rarey et al., 1996)], genetic algorithm [GOLD (Verdonk et al., 2003)] and incremental construction (Friesner et al., 2004). Algorithms that consider ligand flexibility can be divided into three types: systematic, stochastic and deterministic (Ruiz-Tagle et al., 2018). Some software uses more than one of these approaches to obtain better results.

Systematic search algorithms exploit the degrees of freedom of the molecules, usually through their incremental construction at the binding site. Increasing the degree of freedom (rotatable bonds) increases the number of evaluations needed to be performed by the algorithm. Increasing the degree of freedom (rotary links) increases the number of evaluations required to be performed by the algorithm, causing an increase in the time required for its execution. To reduce the time it takes to execute, termination criteria are inserted that prevent the algorithm from trying solutions that are in the space known to lead to wrong solutions. DOCK 6 (Allen et al., 2015), FLEXX (Rarey et al., 1996), and Glide (Friesner et al., 2004) are examples of software that uses systematic search algorithms.

Stochastic search algorithms perform random changes in the spatial conformation of the ligand, usually changing one system degree of freedom at a time, which leads to the exploration of several possible conformations (Ruiz-Tagle et al., 2018). The main problem of stochastic algorithms is the uncertainty of converging to a good solution. For this reason, to minimize this problem, several independent executions of stochastic algorithms are usually performed. Examples of stochastic research algorithms are Monte Carlo (MC) methods used by Glide (Friesner et al., 2004) and MOE (Vilar et al., 2008) and genetic algorithms used by GOLD (Verdonk et al., 2003) and AutoDock4 (Morris et al., 2009).

During the execution of a deterministic search algorithm, the initial state is responsible for determining the movement that can be made to generate the next state, which generally must be equal to or less in the energy from the initial state. One problem with deterministic algorithms is that they are often trapped in local minima because they cannot cross barriers; there are approaches, such as increasing the simulation temperature, that can be implemented to circumvent this problem. Energy minimization methods are an example of deterministic algorithms. Molecular dynamics (MD) is also an example of a deterministic search algorithm and is used by DOCK 6 (Allen et al., 2015). However, MD computational demands are very high, and while MD promises to have better results and ensures full-system flexibility, the runtime becomes a limiting factor for simulations because structure databases can have millions of ligands and targets.

Scoring Functions

Molecular docking software uses scoring functions to estimate the force of non-covalent interactions between a ligand and molecular target using mathematical methods. A scoring function is one of the most important components in SBVS (Huang et al., 2010) as it is primarily responsible for predicting the binding affinity between a target and its ligand candidate. Thus, the scoring functions are the main reason for the success or failure of docking tools (ten Brink and Exner, 2009). Therefore, despite the wide use, the estimation of the interaction force between a ligand and molecular target remains a major challenge in VS. **Figure 6** illustrates docking using Autodock Vina between cyclooxygenase-2 (PDB ID: 4PH9) and two ligands (a) an inactive ligand and (b) celecoxib (an anti-inflammatory). Compared to the inactive ligand, celecoxib is observed to have much more interactions with the protein, which causes celecoxib to form a more stable binding in the VS. This result causes the AutoDock Vina scoring function to see a binding energy of −10.4 kcal/mol for celecoxib and −5.4 kcal/mol for the inactive compound. The ligand with the highest binding affinity to the target can be selected for further testing. Therefore, in this case celecoxib would be chosen.

In general, there are three important applications of scoring functions in molecular docking. First, they can be used to determine the ligand binding site and the conformation between a target and ligand. This approach can be used to search for allosteric sites. Second, they can be used to predict the binding affinity between a protein and ligand. Third, they can also be used in lead optimization (Li et al., 2013).

Most authors define the scoring functions as three types (Huang et al., 2010; Ferreira et al., 2015; Haga et al., 2016): force field (FF), empirical and knowledge-based. Liu and Wang (2015) define two more types of scoring functions as: machine-learning-based and hybrid methods.

The force field scoring functions are based on the intermolecular interactions between the ligand and target atoms, such as the van der Waals, electrostatic and bond stretching/bending/torsional force interactions, obtained from experimental data and in accordance with the principles of

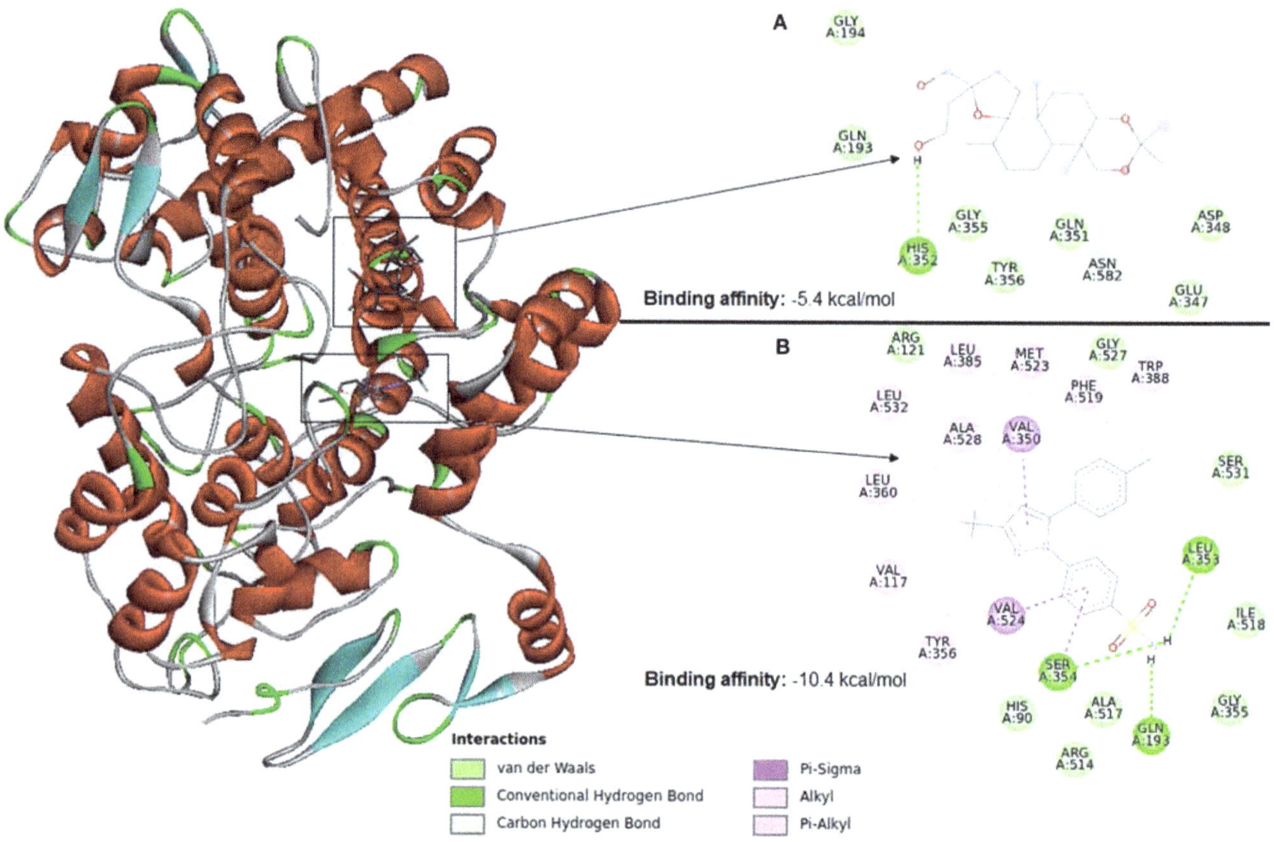

FIGURE 6 | Identification of a ligand candidate by using a typical scoring function. The hydrogens were omitted for better visualization. **(A)** Inactive ligand, **(B)** celecoxib.

molecular mechanics (Ferreira et al., 2015). Some published force-field scoring functions include the ones described in Li et al. (2015), Goldscore (Verdonk et al., 2003), and Sybyl/D-Score (Ash et al., 1997).

Empirical scoring functions estimate the binding free energy based on weighted structural parameters by adjusting the scoring functions to experimentally determine the binding constants of a set of complexes (Ferreira et al., 2015). To create an empirical scoring function, a set of data from protein-binding complexes whose affinities are known is initially used for training. A linear regression is then performed as a way of predicting the values of some variables (Huang et al., 2010). The weight constants generated by the empirical function are used as coefficients to adjust the equation terms. Each term of the function describes a type of physical event involved in the formation of the ligand-receptor complex. Thus, hydrogen bonding, ionic bonding, non-polar interactions, desolvation and entropic effects are considered. Some popular empirical, scoring functions include Glide-Score (Friesner et al., 2004), Sybyl-X/F-score (Certara, 2016) and DOCK 6 empirical force field (Allen et al., 2015).

In the knowledge-based scoring functions, the binding affinity is calculated by summing the binding interactions of the atoms of a protein and the molecular target (Ferreira et al., 2015). These functions consider statistical observations performed on large databases (Ferreira et al., 2015). The method uses pairwise energy potentials extracted from known ligand-receptor complexes to obtain a general scoring function. These methods assume that intermolecular interactions occurring near certain types of atoms or functional groups that occur more frequently are more likely to contribute favorably to the binding affinity. The final score is given as a sum of the score of all individual interactions. One example of software that uses a knowledge-based scoring function is ParaDockS (Meier et al., 2010).

In addition, machine-learning-based methods (Liu and Wang, 2015) have been considered as a fourth type of scoring function. Machine learning-based methods have gained attention for their reliable prediction (Pereira et al., 2016; Chen et al., 2018). Many researchers have used machine learning to improve SBVS algorithms, but we do not know any drugs developed after combining SBVS with machine learning. However, some researchers applied machine learning techniques to discover a new antibiotic capable of inhibiting the growth of *E. coli* bacteria (Stokes et al., 2020). These techniques have been used in quantitative structure-activity relationship (QSAR) analysis to predict various physical-chemical (for example, hydrophobicity, and stereochemistry of the molecule), biological (for example, activity and selectivity), and pharmaceutical (for example, absorption, and metabolism) properties of small molecule compounds. In these types of scoring functions, modern QSAR analyses can be applied to derive statistical models that calculate protein-ligand binding scores. Some scoring functions of this type are NNScore 2.0 (Durrant and McCammon, 2011), RF-Score-VS (Wójcikowski et al., 2017), SFCscoreRF (Zilian and Sotriffer, 2013), SVR-KB (Li et al., 2011), SVR-EP (Li et al., 2011), ID-Score (Li et al., 2013) and CScore (Ouyang et al., 2011).

There are some hybridized scoring functions that cannot easily be classified into any of the categories listed above because they combine two or more of the previously defined scoring function types [force field (FF), empirical, knowledge based and machine-learning-based] into one scoring function. Therefore, they are called hybrid scoring functions. In general, the hybrid scoring function is a linear combination of the two or more scoring function components derived from a multiple linear regression fitting procedure (Tanchuk et al., 2016). For example, the GalaxyDock score function is a hybrid of physics-based, empirical, and knowledge-based score terms that has the advantages of each component. As a result, the performance was improved in decoy pose discrimination tests (Baek et al., 2017). A few recently published examples of this type of scoring function include the hybrid scoring function developed by Tanchuk et al. (Tanchuk et al., 2016), which combines force field machine learning scoring functions; SMoG2016 (Geng et al., 2019), which combines knowledge-based and an empirical scoring functions; GalaxyDock BP2 (Baek et al., 2017), which combines force field, empirical, and knowledge-based scoring functions and iScore (Geng et al., 2019), which combines empirical and force-field scoring functions.

Consensus Docking

In the last decade, a new technique of VS called consensus docking (CD) has been used in some studies (Park et al., 2014; Tuccinardi et al., 2014; Chermak et al., 2016; Poli et al., 2016; Aliebrahimi et al., 2017) to increase the accuracy of VS studies and to reduce the false positives obtained in VS experiments (Aliebrahimi et al., 2017).

This technique is a combination of two different approaches, in which the resultant combination is better than a single approach alone. However, Poli et al. (2016) reported that there are few studies that evaluate the possibility of combining the results from different VS methods to achieve higher success rates in VS studies.

Houston and Walkinshaw (2013) described the main reason for using this combination: the individual program may present incorrect results and these errors are mostly random. Therefore, even when two programs present different results, the combination of these results may, in principle, be much closer to the correct answer than even the best program alone. Houston and Walkinshaw also suggest that CD approaches using two different docking programs improve the precision of the predicted binding mode for any VS study. The same study also verified that a greater level of consensus in a given pose indicates a greater reliability in this result. Finally, the results presented by the authors suggest that the CD approach works as well as the best VS approaches available in the literature.

Park et al. (2014) use an approach in which they used a combination of the programs AutoDock 4.2 (Morris et al., 2009) and FlexX (Rarey et al., 1996) programs. These programs were chosen because both use different types of score functions (force field in AutoDock and empirical in FlexX). In this study, they achieved superior performance with the application of consensus docking than using each of the programs alone.

Alternatively, when using two different VS programs, there is extra time to run the two different tools and combine the results. However, Houston and Walkinshaw (2013) showed that the increased runtime may be advantageous; using AutoDock Vina (Trott and Olson, 2009) in a VS approach along with AutoDock4 (Morris et al., 2009) increased the final runtime by ~10%. This combination is interesting given the potential gains from its use.

Therefore, the use of consensus docking is a recent technique, and although there are few papers in the literature on the subject, it seems to be a promising approach for further VS studies.

VIRTUAL DATABASES

An indispensable condition in performing VS is the availability of a 3D structure of the target protein (Cavasotto, 2011) and ligands to be docked. Some databases were created to store 3D structures of molecules. Some of the free databases include Protein Data Bank (PDB) (Berman et al., 2013), PubChem (Kim et al., 2016), ChEMBL (Bento et al., 2014), ChemSpider (Pence and Williams, 2010), Zinc (Sterling and Irwin, 2015), Brazilian Malaria Molecular Targets (BraMMT) (Nunes et al., 2019), Drugbank (Wishart et al., 2018), and Our Own Molecular Targets (OOMT) (Carregal et al., 2013). In addition, there are some commercially available databases such as the MDL Drug Data Report[1] Below we are going to present a brief explanation of each of these databases:

- Protein Data Bank (PDB) (Berman et al., 2013): PDB is the public database where three-dimensional structures of proteins, nucleic acids, and complex molecules have been deposited since 1971. The worldwide PDB organization ensures that PDB files are publicly available to the global community. It is widely used by the academic community and has grown consistently in recent years. In the last 10 years, the number of 3D structures of the PDB increased from 48,169 at the end of 2008 to 147,604 in the end of 2018, an increase of nearly 207%. This implies that in the last 10 years, almost 9,943 new structures have been added to the PDB every year, just over 27 structures per day, on average. The pace of this growth has increased. At the beginning of this decade approximately 25 new entries were added per day on average. In 2018, over 31 new structures were added per day, an average daily growth of 24% compared to 2010.
- PubChem (Kim et al., 2016): PubChem is a public database, aggregating information from smaller, more specific databases. It has more than 97 million compounds available.

[1] http://accelrys.com/products/collaborative-science/databases/bioactivity-databases/mddr.html

- ChEMBL (Bento et al., 2014): ChEMBL is a database of bioactive molecules with medicinal properties maintained by the European Institute of Bioinformatics (EBI) of the European Molecular Biology Laboratory (EMBL). Currently, it has almost 2.3 million compounds and 15.2 million known biological activities.
- Zinc (Sterling and Irwin, 2015): Zinc is a free database of commercially available compounds for VS. Zinc has more than 230 million commercially available compounds in the 3D format. Zinc is maintained by Irwin and Shoichet Laboratories of the Department of Pharmaceutical Chemistry at the University of California, San Francisco (UCSF).
- NatProDB (Paixão and Pita, 2016): The State University of Feira de Santana has made NatProDB available. This database stores 3D structures of the semiarid biome. The pharmacological profile of compounds from the semiarid flora have not yet been studied, which has motivated our research group to deepen the research by their molecular targets (Taranto et al., 2015).
- Our Own Molecular Target (OOMT) (Carregal et al., 2013): OOMT is a special molecular target database because it has the biological assay for all its molecular targets, and includes specific targets for cancer, dengue, and malaria. OOMT was created by a group of researchers from Federal University of São João del-Rei (UFSJ).
- Brazilian Malaria Molecular Targets (BraMMT) (Nunes et al., 2019): The BRAMMT database comprises thirty-five molecular targets for *Plasmodium falciparum* retrieved from the PDB database. This database allows *in silico* virtual high throughput screening (vHTS) experiments against a pool of *P. falciparum* molecular targets.
- Drugbank (Wishart et al., 2018): DrugBank is a database that contains comprehensive molecular information about drugs, their mechanisms, their interactions, and their targets. The database contains more than 11,900 drug entries, including nearly 2,538 FDA-approved small molecule drugs, 1,670 biotechnology (protein / peptide) drugs approved by the FDA, 129 nutraceuticals and nearly 6,000 investigational drugs.

Commercially available Databases:

- MDL Drug Data Report (MDDR) (Sci Tegic Accelrys Inc, 2019): MDDR is a commercial database built from patent databases, publications and congresses. It has more than 260,000 biologically relevant compounds and approximately 10,000 compounds are added every year.
- ChemSpider (Pence and Williams, 2010): ChemSpider is a database of chemical substances owned by the Royal Society of Chemistry. It has more than 71 million chemical structures from over 250 data sources. ChemSpider allows downloading up to 1000 structures per day. Previous contact is needed for the download of more structures, and ChemSpider is therefore not a totally free database.

VIRTUAL SCREENING ALGORITHMS

In VS, we are targeting proteins in the human body to find novel ligands that will bind to them. VS can be divided into two classes: structure-based and ligand-based. In structure-based virtual screening, a 3D structure of the target protein is known, and the goal is to identify ligands from a database of candidates that will have better affinity with the 3D structure of the target. VS can be performed using molecular docking, a computational process where ligands are moved in 3D space to find a configuration of the target and ligand that maximizes the scoring function. The ligands in the database are ranked according to their maximum score, and the best ones can be investigated further, e.g., by examining the mode and type of interaction that occurs. Additionally, VS techniques can be divided according to the algorithms used as follows:

- Machine Learning-based Algorithms
    - Artificial neural networks (ANNs) (Ashtawy and Mahapatra, 2018);
    - Support vector machines (Sengupta and Bandyopadhyay, 2014);
    - Bayesian techniques (Abdo et al., 2010);
    - Decision tree (Ho, 1998);
    - k-nearest neighbors (kNN) (Peterson et al., 2009);
    - Kohonen's SOMs and counterpropagation ANNs (Schneider et al., 2009);
    - Ensemble methods using machine learning (Korkmaz et al., 2015);
- Evolutionary Algorithms
    - Genetic algorithms (Xia et al., 2017);
    - Differential evolution (Friesner et al., 2004), Gold (Verdonk et al., 2003), Surflex (Spitzer and Jain, 2012) and FlexX (Hui-fang et al., 2010);
    - Ant colony optimization (Korb et al., 2009);
    - Tabu search (Baxter et al., 1998);
    - Particle swarm optimization (Gowthaman et al., 2015) and PSOVina (Ng et al., 2015);
- Local search such as Autodock Vina (Trott and Olson, 2009), SwissDock/EADock (Grosdidier et al., 2011) and GlamDock (Tietze and Apostolakis, 2007);
- Exhaustive search such as eHiTS (Zsoldos et al., 2007);
- Linear programming methods such as Simplex Method (Ruiz-Carmona et al., 2014);
- Systematic methods such as incremental construction used by FlexX (Rarey et al., 1996), Surflex (Spitzer and Jain, 2012), and Sybyl-X (Certara, 2016);
- Statistical methods
    - Monte Carlo (Harrison, 2010);
    - Simulated annealing (SA) (Doucet and Pelletier, 2007), Hatmal and Taha (Hatmal and Taha, 2017);
    - Conformational space annealing (CSA) (Shin et al., 2011);
- Similarity-based algorithms
    - Based on substructures (Tresadern et al., 2009);
    - Pharmacochemical (Cruz-Monteagudo et al., 2014);
    - Overlapping volumes (Leach et al., 2010);
    - Molecular interaction fields (MIFs) (Willett, 2006);

- Hybrid approach (Morris et al., 2009; Haga et al., 2016);

After performing a VS simulation, it is necessary to verify whether the quality of the generated protein-ligand complexes can represent a complex that could be reproduced in experiments. There are several methods that can perform this assessment, which will be explained in the next section.

METHODS OF EVALUATING THE QUALITY OF A SIMULATION

To verify the quality of a docking approach, some methods are used to evaluate generated complexes and to verify if the protein generated by the docking can reproduce the experimental data results of the ligand-receptor complex. The most common evaluation methods are root mean square deviation (RMSD) (Hawkins et al., 2008), receiver operating characteristic (ROC), area under the curve ROC (AUC-ROC) (Flach and Wu, 2005; Trott and Olson, 2009) enrichment factors (EFs) (Truchon and Bayly, 2007) and Boltzmann-enhanced discrimination of ROC (BEDROC) (Truchon and Bayly, 2007).

Root-Mean-Square Deviation (RMSD)

One of the aspects evaluated in docking programs is the accuracy of the generated geometry (Jain, 2008). Docking programs attempt to reproduce the conformation of the ligand-receptor complex in a crystallographic structure. The metric root-mean-square deviation (RMSD) of atomic coordinates after the ideal superposition of rigid bodies of two structures is popular. Its popularity is because it allows the quantification of the differences between two structures, and these can be structures with the same and different amino acid sequences (Sargsyan et al., 2017). RMSD is widely used to evaluate the quality of a docking process performed by a program (Ding et al., 2016). The RMSD between two structures can be calculated according to the following equation (Sargsyan et al., 2017):

$$RMSD\,(A, B) = \frac{1}{N}\sum_{i=1}^{n} d_i^2$$

where d is the distance between atom i in the two structures and N is the total number of equivalent atoms. Since the calculation of RMSD requires the same number of atoms in both structures, it is often used in the calculation of only the heavy atoms or backbone of each amino acid residue.

Using the RMSD calculation, it is possible to evaluate if a program was able to reliably reproduce a known crystallographic conformation, as well as their respective intramolecular interactions. To verify if a given program can accomplish this task, ligand-targets complexes are subjected to a redocking process. After redocking, the overlap of the crystallographic ligand with the conformation of the ligand obtained with the docking program is then performed. Then, the RMSD calculation is used to check the average distance between the corresponding atoms (usually backbone atoms).

Generally, the RMSD threshold value is 2.0 Å (Jain, 2008; Meier et al., 2010; Gowthaman et al., 2015). However, for ligands with several dihedral angles, an RMSD value of 2.5 Å is considered acceptable (De Magalhães et al., 2004). In the case of binding a large ligand, some authors generally relax this criterion (Méndez et al., 2003; Verschueren et al., 2013). For a model generated by homology modeling, evaluating the RMSD value is important, although visual inspection of the generated model is also essential.

However, RMSD has some important limitations:

- RMSD can only compare structures with the same number of atoms;
- A small perturbation in just one part of the structure can create large RMSD values, suggesting that the two structures are very different, although they are not (Carugo, 2007);
- It has also been observed that RMSD values depend on the resolution of structures that are compared (Carugo, 2003);
- RMSD does not distinguish between a structure with some very rigid regions and some very flexible regions from a molecule in which all regions are semiflexible (Sargsyan et al., 2017);

Comparing the RMSD value of large structures may be significantly distorted from the commonly used 2Å threshold (Méndez et al., 2003). Despite these limitations, RMSD remains one of the most commonly used metrics to quantify differences between structures (Sargsyan et al., 2017).

Figure 7 shows the visualization of the FCP ligand superposed with its conformation after redocking to a protein (PDB ID: 1VZK, A Thiophene Based Diamidine Forms a "Super" AT Binding Minor Groove Agent). The RMSD between the crystallographic ligand and the same ligand after the redocking using DOCK6 is 0.97 Å. In the figure below, red represents the crystallographic ligand FCP and yellow represents FCP ligand after redocking using DOCK 6.

ROC Curve and AUC

One of the great challenges of VS methods is the ability to differentiate true positive compounds (TPCs) against the target from false positive compounds (FPCs) (Awuni and Mu, 2015). Thus, it is important that VS tools have ways to assist their users in distinguishing TPCs from FPCs. The ROC curve and the area under the ROC curve (AUC-ROC) (Lätti et al., 2016) are widely used methodologies for this purpose.

TPC and decoys are used to create a ROC curve and AUC-ROC. TPCs are those with known biological activity for the molecular target of interest. Some databases, such as ChEMBL (Gaulton et al., 2012; Bento et al., 2014), allows users to search for these compounds. Alternatively, decoys are compounds that, although possessing physical properties similar to a TPC (such as molecular mass, number of rotatable bonds, and logP), have different chemical structures that make them inactive. They are generated from random molecular modifications in the structure of a TPC (Huang et al., 2006). Some databases, such as DUD-E (Mysinger et al., 2012) and Zinc (Sterling and Irwin, 2015), provide decoys for compounds of interest. DUD-E generates 50 different decoys for each TPC. The idea of using DUD-E decoys in VS is that the result of VS is more reliable if the program can

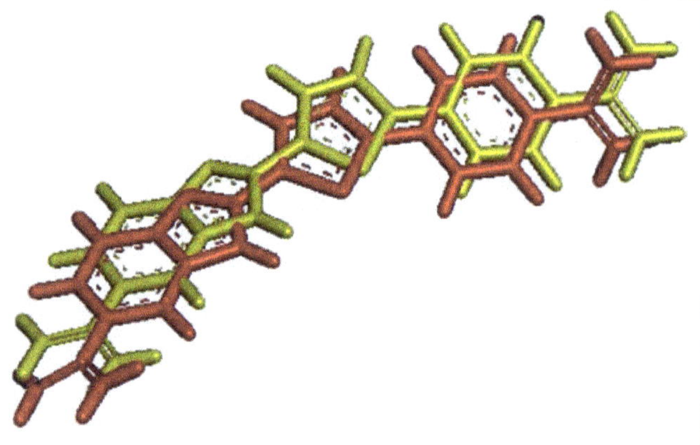

FIGURE 7 | RMSD between the ligand FCP with a protein (PDB ID: 1VZK) after redocking using DOCK6.

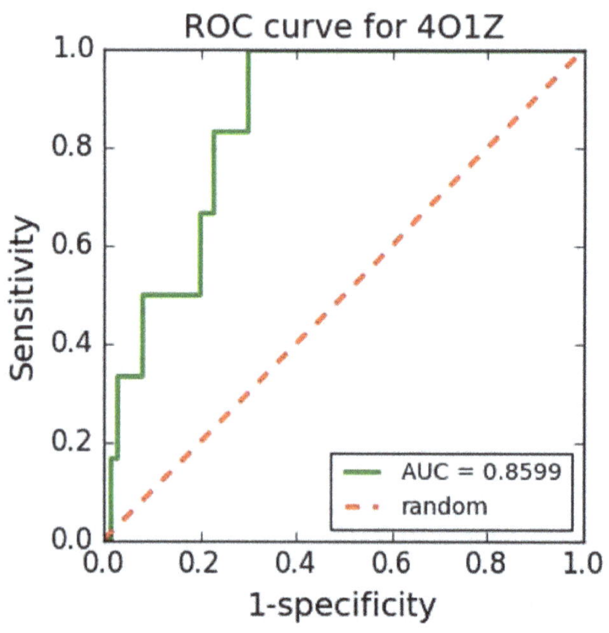

FIGURE 8 | ROC curve example.

separate TPCs from FPCs generated by DUD-E because FPCs have many TPC-like physical properties but are known to be inactive. A small number (>2) of known TPCs have to be used to calculate an AUC-ROC (Lätti et al., 2016).

After generating decoys, a VS process is performed using known TPCs and decoys against a target of interest (Yuriev and Ramsland, 2013). For each ligand-target complex, an affinity energy is then calculated. TPCs are expected to have lower affinity energy than inactive compounds. The ROC curve plots the distribution of true and false results on a graph, while AUC-ROC allows the evaluation of the probability of a result to be false. Hence, AUC-ROC reflects the probability of recovering an active compound preferentially to inactive compounds (Triballeau et al., 2005; Zhao et al., 2009), allowing verification of the sensitivity of a VS experiment in relation to its specificity. The larger the area under the curve, the better the ability to have a TPC and fewer FPC.

The AUC value can vary between 0 and 1. Hamza (Hamza et al., 2012) showed a practical way of interpreting the AUC values:

- AUC between 0.90 and 1.00: Excellent
- AUC between 0.80 and 0.90: Good
- AUC between 0.70 and 0.80: Fair
- AUC between 0.60 and 0.70: Poor
- AUC between 0.50 and 0.60: Failure

Therefore, the closer the AUC is to 1, the greater the ability of the VS tool to separate between TPCs and FPCs. AUC-ROC values close to 0.5 indicate a random process (Ogrizek et al., 2015). Acceptable values should be >0.7.

Figure 8 shows an example of an ROC curve generated in a VS performed with cyclooxygenase-1 complexed with meloxicam (PDB ID: 4O1Z) protein using five TPCs and 250 decoys. The VS tool was able to distinguish well between TPCs and FPCs with the generated ROC curve and its respective AUC, which was 0.8628.

Boltzmann-Enhanced Discrimination of ROC (BEDROC)

There is much criticism in the use of the ROC curve as a method to measure virtual screening performance because it does not highlight the best ranked active compounds that would be used in *in vitro* experiments, which is called early recognition. Thus, Tuchon and Bayly (Truchon and Bayly, 2007) proposed Boltzmann-Enhanced Discrimination of ROC (BEDROC), which uses exponential weighting to give early rankings of active compounds more weight than late rankings of active compounds. However, Nicholls (Nicholls, 2008) say that AUC-ROC and BEDROC correlate when considering virtual screening simulations, and therefore, the ROC curve is a sufficient metric for performance measurements.

Enrichment Factors (EFs)

The enrichment factor (EF) consists of the number of active compounds found in a fraction of $0 < \chi < 1$ in relation to the number of active compounds that would be found after a random search (Truchon and Bayly, 2007). EFs are often calculated against a given percentage of the database. For example, EF10% represents the value obtained when 10% of the database is screened. EFs can be defined by the following formula (1):

$$EF = \frac{\sum_1^n \delta_i}{\chi^n} \quad \text{where } \delta_i = \begin{cases} 1, & r_i \leq \chi N \\ 0, & r_i > \chi N \end{cases} \tag{1}$$

r_i is the rank of the *i*th active compound in the list, N is the total number of compounds and n is the number corresponding to the selected compounds. The maximum value of EF is $1 / \chi$ if $x \geq n / N$ and N / n if $\chi < n / N$. The minimum value for EF is 0.

TABLE 1 | Virtual screening software.

Software	License	Platform	Protein flexibility	Docking algorithm	Scoring function
AutoDock4 (Morris et al., 2009)	Free for academic use	Windows, Linux and Mac	Yes	Genetic algorithm Simulated annealing	Hybrid (Force-field and empirical)
Autodock Vina (Trott and Olson, 2009)	Open- source	Windows, Linux and Mac	Yes	Genetic algorithm Simulated annealing Local search Particle swarm optimization	Hybrid (Empirical and knowledge-based)
DOCK 6 (Allen et al., 2015)	Free for academic use	Windows, Linux and Mac	Yes	Shape fitting (sphere sets) Lowest energy binding	Force-Field Empirical
SwissDock/EADock DSS (Grosdidier et al., 2011)	Free for academic use	Web	No	Stochastic (Tabu search based) Local search Combination of broad and local search of the conformational space	Force-field
eHiTS (Zsoldos et al., 2007)	Freeware for academic use	Unix	No	Exhaustive search	Hybrid (Empirical and knowledge-based)
FITTED (Corbeil et al., 2007, 2008)	Commercial	Linux, Windows and Mac	Yes	Genetic algorithm	Force-field
FlexX (Rarey et al., 1996)	Commercial	Windows and Linux	No	Incremental construction	Empirical
FLIPDock (Zhao and Sanner, 2007)	Freeware for academic Use	Linux e Windows	Yes	Genetic algorithm	Force-field
Fred (McGann, 2011)	Free for academic use	Windows, Linux and Mac	No	Exhaustive search algorithm	Hybrid
GalaxyDock2 (Shin et al., 2013)	Freeware	Linux	Yes	Conformational analysis Genetic algorithm	Force-field
GeauxDock (Fang et al., 2016)	Open-source	Linux	Yes	Monte Carlo	Hybrid (Empirical and knowledge-based)
GlamDock (Tietze and Apostolakis, 2007)	Freeware	Windows, Linux and Mac	No	Monte Carlo Simulated annealing Local search Conformational analysis	Empirical
Glide (Friesner et al., 2004)	Commercial	Windows, Linux	Yes	Conformational analysis Monte Carlo sampling	Empirical
GOLD (Verdonk et al., 2003)	Commercial	Linux and Windows	Yes	Genetic algorithm	Force-field
ICM (Abagyan et al., 1994)	Commercial	Windows, Linux and Mac	Yes	Monte Carlo minimization	Force-field
iGEMDOCK/GEMDOCK (Hsu et al., 2011)	Freeware	Windows and Linux	Yes	Genetic algorithm	Empirical
LigandFit (Montes et al., 2007)	Commercial	Linux	Yes	Monte Carlo	Force-field
LigDockCSA (Shin et al., 2011)	–	–	Yes	Conformational space annealing Global optimization	Hybrid (Empirical and Force-field)
MOE (Vilar et al., 2008)	Commercial	Windows, Linux and Mac	Yes	Conformational analysis	Empirical, Force-field
ParaDockS (Meier et al., 2010)	Freeware	Linux	No	Genetic algorithm	Hybrid (Knowledge-based and empirical)
rDOCK (Ruiz-Carmona et al., 2014)	Open-source	Linux	Yes	Genetic algorithm, Monte CarloSimplex minimization	Hybrid (Empirical and force-field)
SLIDE (Schnecke and Kuhn, 2000)	Free for academic use	Linux	Yes	Conformational analysis	Empirical
Surflex (Spitzer and Jain, 2012)	Commercial	Windows, Linux and Mac	Yes	Incremental xonstruction	Empirical
Sybyl-X (Certara, 2016)	Commercial	Windows	Yes	Incremental construction	Force field
vLifeDock (Chopade, 2015)	Commercial	Windows, Linux and Mac	Yes	Genetic algorithm	Empirical

EF is quite simple, but it has some disadvantages. The EF, in addition to depending on the value set for χ, depends on the number of true positives and true negatives, which makes it another measure of experiment performance rather than measuring method performance (Nicholls, 2011). Another disadvantage of EF is that it weighs active compounds equally within the cutoff, so it is not possible to distinguish the best ranking algorithm in which all active compounds are ranked at the beginning of the ordered list of a worse algorithm and they are sorted immediately before the cutoff value [saturation effect (Lopes et al., 2017)].

The relative enrichment factor (REF) proposed by von Korff et al. (2009) eliminates the problem associated with the saturation effect by normalizing the EF by the maximum possible enrichment. Consequently, REF has well-defined boundaries and is less subject to the saturation effect.

VS SOFTWARE PROGRAMS

There are several VS software programs using different docking algorithms that make a VS process easier for the researchers to execute by avoiding the need to have advanced knowledge of computer science and on how to implement the algorithms used in this task. In this regard, VS software can act as a possible cost reducer, since they function as filters that select from a database with thousands of molecules that are more likely to present biological activity against a target of interest. VS programs measure the affinity energy of a small molecule (ligand) to a molecular target of interest to determine the interaction energy of the resulting complex (Carregal et al., 2017).

Table 1 summarizes the main characteristics of the most used software in VS. The first column contains the software used and its reference. The second column contains the type of software license: free for academic use, freeware, open-source, or commercial. The free for academic use license indicates that the software in question can be used for teaching and research in the academic world without a fee. However, it implies that the software has restrictions for commercial use. A freeware license indicates that the software is free. Thus, users can use it without a fee, and all the functions of the program are available to be used without any restrictions. An open-source license indicates that the software source code is accessible so users can study, change, and distribute the software to anyone and for any purpose. Software developed under a commercial license indicates that it is designed and developed for a commercial purpose. Thus, in general, it is necessary to pay some licensing fee for its use. The third column indicates on which platforms the software can be used (Windows, Linux, or Mac). The next column indicates whether or not the software may consider protein flexibility during anchoring. The docking algorithm column lists the algorithms used by the software to perform the docking. The sixth column, called the scoring function, indicates which scoring functions are used by the software.

FINAL CONSIDERATIONS

CADD has been used to improve the drug development process. In the past, the discovery of new drugs was often conducted through the empirical observation of the effect of natural products in known diseases. Thus, several possible drug candidates were tested without efficacy, and thereby wasted resources. The use of CADD allows for improving the development of new biologically active compounds and decreasing the time and cost for the development of a new drug. Thus, the emergence of SBVS has improved the drug discovery process and was established as one of the most promising *in silico* techniques for drug design.

This review verified that CADD approaches can contribute to many stages of the drug discovery process, notably to perform a search for active compounds by VS.

The use of techniques, such as SBVS, has limitations, such as the possibility of generating false positives and correct ranking of ligands docked. Moreover, there are several CADD methods and it is possible to obtain different results for the same input in different software. However, reducing the time and cost of the new drug development process as well as the constant improvement of existing docking tools indicates that CADD techniques will be one of the most promising techniques in the drug discovery process over the next years.

In the last decade, many studies have applied artificial intelligence in CADD to obtain more accurate models. Thus, most studies and future innovations will benefit from the application of AI in CADD.

Finally, the use of CADD tools requires a variety of expertise of researchers to perform all of the steps of the process, such as selecting and preparing targets and ligands, analyzing the results and having broad knowledge of computation, chemistry and biology. Thus, the researcher's background is important for the selection of new hits and to enrich high throughput experiments.

AUTHOR CONTRIBUTIONS

All authors of this review have made a great contribution to the work. All authors wrote the paper and approved the final version.

FUNDING

Funding sources for this project include FAPEMIG (APQ-02742-17 and APQ-00557-14), CNPq (449984/2014-1), CNPq Universal (426261/2018-6), and UFSJ/PPGBiotec. AT and LA are grateful to CNPq (305117/2017-3) and CAPES for their research fellowships.

ACKNOWLEDGMENTS

The authors would like to thank the Federal Univesity of São João del-Rei (UFSJ) and the Federal Center for Technological Education of Minas Gerais (CEFET-MG) for providing the physical infrastructure.

REFERENCES

Abagyan, R., Totrov, M., and Kuznetsov, D. (1994). ICM - a new method for protein modeling and design: applications to docking and structure prediction from distorted native conformation. *J. Comput. Chem.* 15, 488–506. doi: 10.1002/jcc.540150503

Abdo, A., Chen, B., Mueller, C., Salim, N., and Willett, P. (2010). Ligand-based virtual screening using bayesian networks. *J. Chem. Inf. Model.* 50, 1012–1020. doi: 10.1021/ci100090p

Aliebrahimi, S., Montasser Kouhsari, S., Ostad, S. N., Arab, S. S., and Karami, L. (2017). Identification of phytochemicals targeting c-Met kinase domain using consensus docking and molecular dynamics simulation studies. *Cell Biochem. Biophys.* 76, 135–145. doi: 10.1007/s12013-017-0821-6

Allen, W. J., Balius, T. E., Mukherjee, S., Brozell, S. R., Moustakas, D. T., Lang, P. T., et al. (2015). DOCK 6: impact of new features and current docking performance. *J. Comput. Chem.* 36, 1132–1156. doi: 10.1002/jcc.23905

Arrowsmith, J. (2012). A decade of change. *Nat. Rev. Drug Discov.* 11, 17–18. doi: 10.1038/nrd3630

Ash, S., Cline, M. A., Homer, R. W., Hurst, T., and Smith, G. B. (1997). SYBYL line notation (SLN): a versatile language for chemical structure representation. *J. Chem. Inf. Model.* 37, 71–79. doi: 10.1021/ci960109j

Ashtawy, H. M., and Mahapatra, N. R. (2018). Task-specific scoring functions for predicting ligand binding poses and affinity and for screening enrichment. *J. Chem. Inf. Model.* 58, 119–133. doi: 10.1021/acs.jcim.7b00309

Awuni, Y., and Mu, Y. (2015). Reduction of false positives in structure-based virtual screening when receptor plasticity is considered. *Molecules* 20, 5152–5164. doi: 10.3390/molecules20035152

Baek, M., Shin, W-H., Chung, H. W., and Seok, C. (2017). GalaxyDock BP2 score: a hybrid scoring function for accurate protein–ligand docking. *J. Comput. Aided. Mol. Des.* 31, 653–666. doi: 10.1007/s10822-017-0030-9

Banegas-Luna, A.-J., Cerón-Carrasco, J. P., and Pérez-Sánchez, H. (2018). A review of ligand-based virtual screening web tools and screening algorithms in large molecular databases in the age of big data. *Future Med. Chem.* 10, 2641–2658. doi: 10.4155/fmc-2018-0076

Baxter, C. A., Murray, C. W., Clark, D. E., Westhead, D. R., and Eldridge, M. D. (1998). Flexible docking using Tabu search and an empirical estimate of binding affinity. *Proteins Struct. Funct. Genet.* 33, 367–382. doi: 10.1002/(SICI)1097-0134(19981115)33:3<367::AID-PROT6>3.0.CO;2-W

Bento, A. P., Gaulton, A., Hersey, A., Bellis, L. J., Chambers, J., Davies, M., et al. (2014). The ChEMBL bioactivity database: an update. *Nucleic Acids Res.* 42, D1083–D1090. doi: 10.1093/nar/gkt1031

Berman, H. M., Kleywegt, G. J., Nakamura, H., and Markley, J. L. (2013). The future of the protein data bank. *Biopolymers* 99, 218–222. doi: 10.1002/bip.22132

Carpenter, K. A., Cohen, D. S., Jarrell, J. T., and Huang, X. (2018). Deep learning and virtual drug screening. *Future Med. Chem.* 10, 2557–2567. doi: 10.4155/fmc-2018-0314

Carregal, A. P., Maciel, F. V., Carregal, J. B., dos Reis Santos, B., da Silva, A. M., and Taranto, A. G. (2017). Docking-based virtual screening of Brazilian natural compounds using the OOMT as the pharmacological target database. *J. Mol. Model.* 23:111. doi: 10.1007/s00894-017-3253-8

Carregal, A. P. Jr., Comar, M., and Taranto, A. G. (2013). Our own molecular targets data bank (OOMT). *Biochem. Biotechnol. Reports* 2, 14–16. doi: 10.5433/2316-5200.2013v2n2espp14

Carugo, O. (2003). How root-mean-square distance (r.m.s.d.) values depend on the resolution of protein structures that are compared. *J. Appl. Crystallogr.* 36, 125–128. doi: 10.1107/S0021889802020502

Carugo, O. (2007). Statistical validation of the root-mean-square-distance, a measure of protein structural proximity. *Protein Eng. Des. Sel.* 20, 33–37. doi: 10.1093/protein/gzl051

Cavasotto, C. N. (2011). Homology models in docking and high-throughput docking. *Curr. Top. Med. Chem.* 11, 1528–1534. doi: 10.2174/156802611795860951

Certara (2016). *SYBYL-X Suite 2.1.* Available online at: https://support.certara.com/software/molecular-modeling-and-simulation/sybyl-x/ (accessed August 23, 2017).

Chen, R., Liu, X., Jin, S., Lin, J., and Liu, J. (2018). Machine learning for drug-target interaction prediction. *Molecules* 23:2205. doi: 10.3390/molecules23092208

Chermak, E., De Donato, R., Lensink, M. F., Petta, A., Serra, L., Scarano, V., et al. (2016). Introducing a clustering step in a consensus approach for the scoring of protein-protein docking models. *PLoS ONE* 11:e0166460. doi: 10.1371/journal.pone.0166460

Chopade, A. R. (2015). Molecular docking studies of phytocompounds from phyllanthus species as potential chronic pain modulators. *Sci. Pharm.* 83, 243–267. doi: 10.3797/scipharm.1408-10

Corbeil, C. R., Englebienne, P., and Moitessier, N. (2007). Docking ligands into flexible and solvated macromolecules. 1. development and validation of FITTED 1.0. *J. Chem. Inf. Model.* 47, 435–449. doi: 10.1021/ci6002637

Corbeil, C. R., Englebienne, P., Yannopoulos, C. G., Chan, L., Das, S. K., Bilimoria, D., et al. (2008). Docking ligands into flexible and solvated macromolecules 2 development and application of F ITTED 1. 5 to the virtual screening of potential HCV polymerase inhibitors. *J. Chem. Inf. Model.*, 902–909. doi: 10.1021/ci700398h

Cruz-Monteagudo, M., Medina-Franco, J. L., Pérez-Castillo, Y., Nicolotti, O., Cordeiro, M. N. D. S., and Borges, F. (2014). Activity cliffs in drug discovery: Dr Jekyll or Mr Hyde? *Drug Discov. Today* 19, 1069–1080. doi: 10.1016/j.drudis.2014.02.003

Das, P. S., and Saha, P. (2017). A review on computer aided drug design in drug discovery. *World J. Pharm. Pharm. Sci.* 6, 279–291. doi: 10.20959/wjpps20177-9450

De Magalhães, C. S., Barbosa, H. J. C., and Dardenne, L. E. (2004). "Selection-insertion schemes in genetic algorithms for the flexible ligand docking problem," In: *Genetic and Evolutionary Computation - GECCO 2004. GECCO 2004. Lecture Notes in Computer Science*, ed K. Deb (Berlin, Heidelberg: Springer), 368–379. doi: 10.1007/978-3-540-24854-5_38

Devi, R. V., Sathya, S. S., and Coumar, M. S. (2015). Evolutionary algorithms for *de novo* drug design - a survey. *Appl. Soft Comput. J.* 27, 543–552. doi: 10.1016/j.asoc.2014.09.042

Ding, Y., Fang, Y., Moreno, J., Ramanujam, J., Jarrell, M., and Brylinski, M. (2016). Assessing the similarity of ligand binding conformations with the contact mode score. *Comput. Biol. Chem.* 64, 403–413. doi: 10.1016/j.compbiolchem.2016.08.007

Doucet, N., and Pelletier, J. N. (2007). Simulated annealing exploration of an active-site tyrosine in TEM-1β-lactamase suggests the existence of alternate conformations. *Proteins Struct. Funct. Bioinforma.* 69, 340–348. doi: 10.1002/prot.21485

Durrant, J. D., and McCammon, J. A. (2011). NNScore 2.0: a neural-network receptor-ligand scoring function. *J. Chem. Inf. Model.* 51, 2897–2903. doi: 10.1021/ci2003889

Dutkiewicz, Z., and Mikstacka, R. (2018). Structure-based drug design for cytochrome P450 family 1 inhibitors. *Bioinorg. Chem. Appl.* 2018:3924608. doi: 10.1155/2018/3924608

Fang, Y., Ding, Y., Feinstein, W. P., Koppelman, D. M., Moreno, J., Jarrell, M., et al. (2016). Geauxdock: accelerating structure-based virtual screening with heterogeneous computing. *PLoS ONE* 11:e0158898. doi: 10.1371/journal.pone.0158898

Ferreira, L., dos Santos, R., Oliva, G., and Andricopulo, A. (2015). Molecular docking and structure-based drug design strategies. *Molecules* 20, 13384–13421. doi: 10.3390/molecules200713384

Ferreira, R. S., Glaucius, O., and Andricopulo, A. D. (2011). Integração das técnicas de triagem virtual e triagem biológica automatizada em alta escala: oportunidades e desafios em P&D de fármacos. *Quim. Nova* 34, 1770–1778. doi: 10.1590/S0100-40422011001000010

Flach, P. A., and Wu, S. (2005). Repairing concavities in ROC curves. *IJCAI Int. Joint Conf. Arti. Intell.* 702–707. doi: 10.5555/1642293.1642406

Friesner, R. A., Banks, J. L., Murphy, R. B., Halgren, T. A., Klicic, J. J., Mainz, D. T., et al. (2004). Glide: a new approach for rapid, accurate docking and scoring. 1. method and assessment of docking accuracy. *J. Med. Chem.* 47, 1739–1749. doi: 10.1021/jm0306430

Gaulton, A., Bellis, L. J., Bento, A. P., Chambers, J., Davies, M., Hersey, A., et al. (2012). ChEMBL: a large-scale bioactivity database for drug discovery. *Nucleic Acids Res.* 40, D1100–D1107. doi: 10.1093/nar/gkr777

Geng, C., Jung, Y., Renaud, N., Honavar, V., Bonvin, A. M. J. J., and Xue, L. C. (2019). iScore: a novel graph kernel-based function for scoring protein-protein docking models. *Bioinformatics* 36, 112–121. doi: 10.1101/498584

Gowthaman, R., Lyskov, S., and Karanicolas, J. (2015). DARC 2.0: improved docking and virtual screening at protein interaction sites. *PLoS ONE* 10:e0131612. doi: 10.1371/journal.pone.0131612

Grosdidier, A., Zoete, V., and Michielin, O. (2011). SwissDock, a protein-small molecule docking web service based on EADock DSS. *Nucleic Acids Res.* 39, 270–277. doi: 10.1093/nar/gkr366

Haga, J. H., Ichikawa, K., and Date, S. (2016). Virtual screening techniques and current computational infrastructures. *Curr. Pharm. Des.* 22, 3576–3584. doi: 10.2174/1381612822666160414142530

Hamza, A., Wei, N-N., and Zhan, C-G. (2012). Ligand-based virtual screening approach using a new scoring function. *J. Chem. Inf. Model.* 52, 963–974. doi: 10.1021/ci200617d

Harrison, R. L. (2010). Introduction to monte carlo simulation. *AIP Conf. Proc.* 1204, 17–21. doi: 10.1063/1.3295638

Hatmal, M. M., and Taha, M. O. (2017). Simulated annealing molecular dynamics and ligand–receptor contacts analysis for pharmacophore modeling. *Future Med. Chem.* 9, 1141–1159. doi: 10.4155/fmc-2017-0061

Hawkins, P. C. D., Warren, G. L., Skillman, A. G., and Nicholls, A. (2008). How to do an evaluation: pitfalls and traps. *J. Comput. Aided. Mol. Des.* 22, 179–190. doi: 10.1007/s10822-007-9166-3

Hillisch, A., Pineda, L. F., and Hilgenfeld, R. (2004). Utility of homology models in the drug discovery process. *Drug Discov. Today* 9, 659–669. doi: 10.1016/S1359-6446(04)03196-4

Ho, T. K. (1998). The random subspace method for constructing decision forests. *IEEE Trans. Pattern Anal. Mach. Intell.* 20, 832–844. doi: 10.1109/34.709601

Horvath, D. (1997). A virtual screening approach applied to the search for trypanothione reductase inhibitors. *J. Med. Chem.* 2623, 2412–2423. doi: 10.1021/jm9603781

Houston, D. R., and Walkinshaw, M. D. (2013). Consensus docking: improving the reliability of docking in a virtual screening context. *J. Chem. Inf. Model.* 53, 384–390. doi: 10.1021/ci300399w

Hsu, K-C., Chen, Y-F., Lin, S-R., and Yang, J-M. (2011). iGEMDOCK: a graphical environment of enhancing GEMDOCK using pharmacological interactions and post-screening analysis. *BMC Bioinformatics* 12(Suppl. 1):S33. doi: 10.1186/1471-2105-12-S1-S33

Huang, N., Shoichet, B. K., and Irwin, J. J. (2006). Benchmarking sets for molecular docking. *J. Med. Chem.* 49, 6789–6801. doi: 10.1021/jm0608356

Huang, S-Y., Grinter, S. Z., and Zou, X. (2010). Scoring functions and their evaluation methods for protein–ligand docking: recent advances and future directions. *Phys. Chem. Chem. Phys.* 12, 12899–12908. doi: 10.1039/c0cp00151a

Hui-fang, L., Qing, S., Jian, Z., and Wei, F. (2010). Evaluation of various inverse docking schemes in multiple targets identification. *J. Mol. Graph. Model.* 29, 326–330. doi: 10.1016/j.jmgm.2010.09.004

Jain, A. N. (2008). Bias, reporting, and sharing: computational evaluations of docking methods. *J. Comput. Aided. Mol. Des.* 22, 201–212. doi: 10.1007/s10822-007-9151-x

Kapetanovic, I. M. (2008). Computer aided darug discovery and development: *in silico*-chemico-biological approach. *Chem. Biol. Interact.* 171, 165–176. doi: 10.1016/j.cbi.2006.12.006

Kim, S., Thiessen, P. A., Bolton, E. E., Chen, J., Fu, G., Gindulyte, A., et al. (2016). PubChem substance and compound databases. *Nucleic Acids Res.* 44, D1202–D1213. doi: 10.1093/nar/gkv951

Korb, O., Stutzle, T., and Exner, T. E. (2009). PLANTS: application of ant colony optimization to structure-based drug design. *Theor. Comput. Sci.* 49, 84–96. doi: 10.1007/11839088_22

Korkmaz, S., Zararsiz, G., and Goksuluk, D. (2015). MLViS: a web tool for machine learning-based virtual screening in early-phase of drug discovery and development. *PLoS ONE* 10:e0124600. doi: 10.1371/journal.pone.0124600

Kuntz, I. D., Blaney, J. M., Oatley, S. J., Langridge, R., and Ferrin, T. E. (1982). A geometric approach to macromolecule-ligand interactions. *J. Mol. Biol.* 161, 269–288. doi: 10.1016/0022-2836(82)90153-X

Lätti, S., Niinivehmas, S., and Pentikäinen, O. T. (2016). Rocker: open source, easy-to-use tool for AUC and enrichment calculations and ROC visualization. *J. Cheminform.* 8:45. doi: 10.1186/s13321-016-0158-y

Leach, A. R., Gillet, V. J., Lewis, R. A., and Taylor, R. (2010). Three-dimensional pharmacophore methods in drug discovery. *J. Med. Chem.* 53, 539–558. doi: 10.1021/jm900817u

Leelananda, S. P., and Lindert, S. (2016). Computational methods in drug discovery. *Beilstein J. Org. Chem.* 12, 2694–2718. doi: 10.3762/bjoc.12.267

Leisinger, K. M., Garabedian, L. F., and Wagner, A. K. (2012). Improving access to medicines in low and middle income countries: corporate responsibilities in context. *South. Med Rev.* 5, 3–8.

Li, G. B., Yang, L. L., Wang, W. J., Li, L. L., and Yang, S. Y. (2013). ID-score: a new empirical scoring function based on a comprehensive set of descriptors related to protein-ligand interactions. *J. Chem. Inf. Model.* 53, 592–600. doi: 10.1021/ci300493w

Li, L., Wang, B., and Meroueh, S. O. (2011). Support vector regression scoring of receptor-ligand complexes for rank-ordering and virtual screening of chemical libraries. *J. Chem. Inf. Model.* 51, 2132–2138. doi: 10.1021/ci200078f

Li, Z., Gu, J., Zhuang, H., Kang, L., Zhao, X., and Guo, Q. (2015). Adaptive molecular docking method based on information entropy genetic algorithm. *Appl. Soft Comput.* 26, 299–302. doi: 10.1016/j.asoc.2014.10.008

Lima, A. N., Philot, E. A., Trossini, G. H. G., Scott, L. P. B., Maltarollo, V. G., and Honorio, K. M. (2016). Use of machine learning approaches for novel drug discovery. *Expert Opin. Drug Discov.* 11, 225–239. doi: 10.1517/17460441.2016.1146250

Lionta, E., Spyrou, G., Vassilatis, D., and Cournia, Z. (2014). Structure-based virtual screening for drug discovery: principles, applications and recent advances. *Curr. Top. Med. Chem.* 14, 1923–1938. doi: 10.2174/1568026614666140929124445

Liu, J., and Wang, R. (2015). On classification of current scoring functions. *J. Chem. Inf. Model.* 55, 475–482. doi: 10.1021/ci500731a

Liu, S., Alnammi, M., Ericksen, S. S., Voter, A. F., Ananiev, G. E., Keck, J. L., et al. (2018). Practical model selection for prospective virtual screening. *J. Chem. Inf. Model. 59, 282–293.* doi: 10.1101/337956

Lopes, J. C. D., Dos Santos, F. M., Martins-José, A., Augustyns, K., and De Winter, H. (2017). The power metric: a new statistically robust enrichment-type metric for virtual screening applications with early recovery capability. *J. Cheminform.* 9:7. doi: 10.1186/s13321-016-0189-4

Ma, X., Jia, J., Zhu, F., Xue, Y., Li, Z., and Chen, Y. (2009). Comparative analysis of machine learning methods in ligand-based virtual screening of large compound libraries. *Comb. Chem. High Throughput Screen.* 12, 344–357. doi: 10.2174/138620709788167944

Maia, E. H. B., Campos, V. A., dos Reis Santos, B., Costa, M. S., Lima, I. G., Greco, S. J., et al. (2017). Octopus: a platform for the virtual high-throughput screening of a pool of compounds against a set of molecular targets. *J. Mol. Model.* 23:26. doi: 10.1007/s00894-016-3184-9

Maithri, G, Manasa, B, Vani, S. S., Narendra, A, and Harshita, T (2016). Computational drug design and molecular dynamic studies-a review. *Int. J. Biomed. Data Min.* 6:123. doi: 10.4172/2090-4924.1000123

Martin, Y. C. (1992). 3D database searching in drug design. *J. Med. Chem.* 35, 2145–2154. doi: 10.1021/jm00090a001

McGann, M. (2011). FRED pose prediction and virtual screening accuracy. *J. Chem. Inf. Model.* 51, 578–596. doi: 10.1021/ci100436p

Meier, R., Pippel, M., Brandt, F., Sippl, W., and Baldauf, C. (2010). ParaDockS: a framework for molecular docking with population-based metaheuristics. *J. Chem. Inf. Model.* 50, 879–889. doi: 10.1021/ci900467x

Méndez, R., Leplae, R., De Maria, L., and Wodak, S. J. (2003). Assessment of blind predictions of protein-protein interactions: current status of docking methods. *Proteins Struct. Funct. Genet.* 52, 51–67. doi: 10.1002/prot.10393

Meng, X-Y., Zhang, H-X., Mezei, M., and Cui, M. (2011). Molecular docking: a powerful approach for structure-based drug discovery. *Curr. Comput. Aided. Drug Des.* 7, 146–157. doi: 10.2174/157340911795677602

Merluzzi, V., Hargrave, K., Labadia, M., Grozinger, K., Skoog, M., Wu, J., et al. (1990). Inhibition of HIV-1 replication by a nonnucleoside reverse transcriptase inhibitor. *Science* 250, 1411–1413. doi: 10.1126/science.1701568

Montes, M., Miteva, M. A., and Villoutreix, B. O. (2007). Structure-based virtual ligand screening with LigandFit: pose prediction and enrichment of compound collections. *Proteins Struct. Funct. Bioinforma* 68, 712–725. doi: 10.1002/prot.21405

Morris, G. M., Huey, R., Lindstrom, W., Sanner, M. F., Belew, R. K., Goodsell, D. S., et al. (2009). AutoDock4 and AutoDockTools4: automated docking with selective receptor flexibility. *J. Comput. Chem.* 30, 2785–2791. doi: 10.1002/jcc.21256

Mugumbate, G., Mendes, V., Blaszczyk, M., Sabbah, M., Papadatos, G., Lelievre, J., et al. (2017). Target identification of *Mycobacterium tuberculosis* phenotypic hits using a concerted chemogenomic, biophysical, and structural approach. *Front. Pharmacol.* 8:681. doi: 10.3389/fphar.2017.00681

Mysinger, M. M., Carchia, M., Irwin, J. J., and Shoichet, B. K. (2012). Directory of useful decoys, enhanced (DUD-E): better ligands and decoys for better benchmarking. *J. Med. Chem.* 55, 6582–6594. doi: 10.1021/jm300687e

Ng, M. C. K., Fong, S., and Siu, S. W. I. (2015). PSOVina: the hybrid particle swarm optimization algorithm for protein-ligand docking. *J. Bioinform. Comput. Biol.* 13:1541007. doi: 10.1142/S0219720015410073

Nicholls, A. (2008). What do we know and when do we know it? *J. Comput. Aided. Mol. Des.* 22, 239–255. doi: 10.1007/s10822-008-9170-2

Nicholls, A. (2011). What do we know?: Simple statistical techniques that help. *Chemoinform. Comput. Chem. Biol.* 672, 531–581. doi: 10.1007/978-1-60761-839-3_22

Nunes, R. R., da Fonseca, A. L., Pinto, A. C. D. S., Maia, E. H. B., da Silva, A. M., Varotti, F. de P., et al. (2019). Brazilian malaria molecular targets (BraMMT): selected receptors for virtual high-throughput screening experiments. *Mem. Inst. Oswaldo Cruz.* 114, 1–10. doi: 10.1590/0074-02760180465

Oglic, D., Oatley, S. A., Macdonald, S. J. F., Mcinally, T., Garnett, R., Hirst, J. D., et al. (2018). Active search for computer-aided drug design. *Mol. Inform.* 37:1700130. doi: 10.1002/minf.201700130

Ogrizek, M., Turk, S., Lešnik, S., Sosic, I., Hodošcek, M., Mirković, B., et al. (2015). Molecular dynamics to enhance structure-based virtual screening on cathepsin B. *J. Comput. Aided. Mol. Des.* 29, 707–712. doi: 10.1007/s10822-015-9847-2

Ouyang, X., Handoko, S. D., and Kwoh, C. K. (2011). Cscore : a simple yet effective scoring function for protein – ligand binding affinity prediction using modified cmac learning architecture. *J. Bioinform. Comput. Biol.* 9(Suppl. 1), 1–14. doi: 10.1142/S021972001100577X

Paixão, V. G., and Pita, S. S. R. (2016). Virtual Screening applied to search of inhibitors of trypanosoma cruzi trypanothione reductase employing the Natural Products Database from Bahia state (NatProDB). *Rev. Virtual Química* 8, 1289–1310. doi: 10.21577/1984-6835.20160093

Park, H., Eom, J. W., and Kim, Y. H. (2014). Consensus scoring approach to identify the inhibitors of AMP-activated protein kinase α2 with virtual screening. *J. Chem. Inf. Model.* 54, 2139–2146. doi: 10.1021/ci500214e

Paul, S. M., Mytelka, D. S., Dunwiddie, C. T., Persinger, C. C., Munos, B. H., Lindborg, S. R., et al. (2010). How to improve R&D productivity: the pharmaceutical industry's grand challenge. *Nat. Rev. Drug Discov.* 9, 203–214. doi: 10.1038/nrd3078

Pence, H. E., and Williams, A. (2010). ChemSpider: an online chemical information resource. *J. Chem. Educ.* 87, 1123–1124. doi: 10.1021/ed100697w

Pereira, J. C., Caffarena, E. R., and Dos Santos, C. N. (2016). Boosting docking-based virtual screening with deep learning. *J. Chem. Inf. Model.* 56, 2495–2506. doi: 10.1021/acs.jcim.6b00355

Peterson, Y. K., Wang, X. S., Casey, P. J., and Tropsha, A. (2009). The discovery of geranylgeranyltransferase-i inhibitors with novel scaffolds by the means of quantitative structure-activity relationship modeling, virtual screening, and experimental validation. *J. Med. Chem.* 52, 83–88. doi: 10.1021/jm8013772

Poli, G., Martinelli, A., and Tuccinardi, T. (2016). Reliability analysis and optimization of the consensus docking approach for the development of virtual screening studies. *J. Enzyme Inhib. Med. Chem.* 31, 167–173. doi: 10.1080/14756366.2016.1193736

Rarey, M., Kramer, B., Lengauer, T., and Klebe, G. (1996). A fast flexible docking method using an incremental construction algorithm. *J. Mol. Biol.* 261, 470–489. doi: 10.1006/jmbi.1996.0477

Ripphausen, P., Nisius, B., and Bajorath, J. J. (2011). State-of-the-art in ligand-based virtual screening. *Drug Discov. Today* 16, 372–376. doi: 10.1016/j.drudis.2011.02.011

Ruiz-Carmona, S., Alvarez-Garcia, D., Foloppe, N., Garmendia-Doval, A. B., Juhos, S., Schmidtke, P., et al. (2014). rDock: a fast, versatile and open source program for docking ligands to proteins and nucleic acids. *PLoS Comput. Biol.* 10:e1003571. doi: 10.1371/journal.pcbi.1003571

Ruiz-Tagle, B., Villalobos-Cid, M., Dorn, M., and Inostroza-Ponta, M. (2018). "Evaluating the use of local search strategies for a memetic algorithm for the protein-ligand docking problem," *2017 36th International Conference of the Chilean Computer Science Society* (SCCC) (Arica), 1–12. doi: 10.1109/SCCC.2017.8405141

Sargsyan, K., Grauffel, C., and Lim, C. (2017). How molecular size impacts RMSD applications in molecular dynamics simulations. *J. Chem. Theory Comput.* 13, 1518–1524. doi: 10.1021/acs.jctc.7b00028

Schnecke, V., and Kuhn, L. A. (2000). Virtual screening with solvation and ligand-induced complementarity. *Perspect. Drug Discov. Des.* 20, 171–190. doi: 10.1023/A:1008737207775

Schneider, P., Tanrikulu, Y., and Schneider, G. (2009). Self-organizing maps in drug discovery: compound library design, scaffold-hopping, repurposing. *Curr. Med. Chem.* 16, 258–266. doi: 10.2174/092986709787002655

Sci Tegic Accelrys Inc (2019). *The MDL Drug Data Report (MDDR) database.* Available online at: http://accelrys.com/products/collaborative-science/databases/bioactivity-databases/mddr.html (accessed March 22, 2019).

Sengupta, S., and Bandyopadhyay, S. (2014). Application of support vector machines in virtual screening. *Int. J. Comput. Biol.* 1, 56–62. doi: 10.34040/IJCB.1.1.2012.20

Shin, W. H., Heo, L., Lee, J., Ko, J., Seok, C., and Lee, J. (2011). LigDockCSA: protein-ligand docking using conformational space annealing. *J. Comput. Chem.* 32, 3226–3232. doi: 10.1002/jcc.21905

Shin, W. H., Kim, J. K., Kim, D. S., and Seok, C. (2013). GalaxyDock2: protein-ligand docking using beta-complex and global optimization. *J. Comput. Chem.* 34, 2647–2656. doi: 10.1002/jcc.23438

Sliwoski, G., Kothiwale, S., Meiler, J., and Edward, W., Lowe, J. (2013). Computational methods in drug discovery. *Pharmacol. Rev.* 66, 334–395. doi: 10.1124/pr.112.007336

Spitzer, R., and Jain, A. N. (2012). Surflex-Dock: docking benchmarks and real-world application. *J. Comput. Aided. Mol. Des.* 26, 687–699. doi: 10.1007/s10822-011-9533-y

Sridhar, D. (2008). Improving access to essential medicines: how health concerns can be prioritised in the global governance system. *Public Health Ethics* 1, 83–88. doi: 10.1093/phe/phn012

Sterling, T., and Irwin, J. J. (2015). ZINC15–ligand discovery for everyone. *J. Chem. Inf. Model.* 55, 2324–2337. doi: 10.1021/acs.jcim.5b00559

Stevens, H., and Huys, I. (2017). Innovative approaches to increase access to medicines in developing countries. *Front. Med.* 4:218. doi: 10.3389/fmed.2017.00218

Stokes, J. M., Yang, K., Swanson, K., Jin, W., Cubillos-Ruiz, A., Donghia, N. M., et al. (2020). A deep learning approach to antibiotic discovery. *Cell* 180, 688-702.e13. doi: 10.1016/j.cell.2020.01.021

Surabhi, S., and Singh, B. (2018). Computer aided drug design: an overview. *J. Drug Deliv. Ther.* 8, 504–509. doi: 10.22270/jddt.v8i5.1894

Talele, T. T., Khedkar, S. A., and Rigby, A. C. (2010). Successful applications of computer aided drug discovery: moving drugs from concept to the clinic. *Curr. Top. Med. Chem.* 10, 127–41. doi: 10.2174/156802610790232251

Tanchuk, V. Y., Tanin, V. O., Vovk, A. I., and Poda, G. (2016). A new, improved hybrid scoring function for molecular docking and scoring based on AutoDock and AutoDock vina. *Chem. Biol. Drug Des.* 87, 618–625. doi: 10.1111/cbdd.12697

Taranto, A. G., dos R., Santos, B., Costa, M. S., Campos, V. A., Lima, I. G., et al. (2015). "Octopus: a virtual high thoughput screening plataform for multi-compouds and targets," in: *XVIIISimpósio Brasileiro de Química Teórica* (Pirenópolis - GO -Brasil: Editora da UnB), 266.

ten Brink, T., and Exner, T. E. (2009). Influence of protonation, tautomeric, and stereoisomeric states on protein–ligand docking results. *J. Chem. Inf. Model.* 49, 1535–1546. doi: 10.1021/ci800420z

Tietze, S., and Apostolakis, J. (2007). GlamDock: development and validation of a new docking tool on several thousand protein-ligand complexes. *J. Chem. Inf. Model.* 47, 1657–1672. doi: 10.1021/ci7001236

Tresadern, G., Bemporad, D., and Howe, T. (2009). A comparison of ligand based virtual screening methods and application to corticotropin releasing factor 1 receptor. *J. Mol. Graph. Model.* 27, 860–870. doi: 10.1016/j.jmgm.2009.01.003

Triballeau, N., Acher, F., Brabet, I., Pin, J., and Bertrand, H. (2005). Virtual screening workflow development guided by the "receiver operating characteristic" curve approach. application to high-throughput docking on metabotropic glutamate receptor subtype 4. *J. Med. Chem.* 48, 2534–2547. doi: 10.1021/jm049092j

Trott, O., and Olson, A. J. (2009). AutoDock vina: improving the speed and accuracy of docking with a new scoring function, efficient optimization, and multithreading. *J. Comput. Chem.* 31, 455–461. doi: 10.1002/jcc.21334

Truchon, J. F., and Bayly, C. I. (2007). Evaluating virtual screening methods: good and bad metrics for the "early recognition" problem. *J. Chem. Inf. Model.* 47, 488–508. doi: 10.1021/ci600426e

Tuccinardi, T., Poli, G., Romboli, V., Giordano, A., and Martinelli, A. (2014). Extensive consensus docking evaluation for ligand pose prediction and virtual screening studies. *J. Chem. Inf. Model.* 54, 2980–2986. doi: 10.1021/ci500424n

Verdonk, M. L., Cole, J. C., Hartshorn, M. J., Murray, C. W., and Taylor, R. D. (2003). Improved protein-ligand docking using GOLD. *Proteins Struct. Funct. Genet.* 52, 609–623. doi: 10.1002/prot.10465

Verschueren, E., Vanhee, P., Rousseau, F., Schymkowitz, J., and Serrano, L. (2013). Protein-peptide complex prediction through fragment interaction patterns. *Structure* 21, 789–797. doi: 10.1016/j.str.2013.02.023

Vilar, S., Cozza, G., and Moro, S. (2008). Medicinal chemistry and the molecular operating environment (MOE): application of QSAR and molecular docking to drug discovery. *Curr. Top. Med. Chem.* 8, 1555–1572. doi: 10.2174/156802608786786624

von Korff, M., Freyss, J., and Sander, T. (2009). Comparison of ligand- and structure-based virtual screening on the DUD data set. *J. Chem. Inf. Model.* 49, 209–231. doi: 10.1021/ci800303k

von Wartburg, A., and Traber, R. (1988). 1 cyclosporins, fungal metabolites with immunosuppressive activities. *Prog. Med. Chem.* 25, 1–33. doi: 10.1016/S0079-6468(08)70276-5

Wang, T., Wu, M., Chen, Z., Chen, H., Lin, J., and Yang, L. (2015). Fragment-based drug discovery and molecular docking in drug design. *Curr. Pharm. Biotechnol.* 16, 11–25. doi: 10.2174/1389201015666141122204532

Ward, W. H. J., Cook, P. N., Slater, A. M., Davies, D. H., Holdgate, G. A., and Green, L. R. (1994). Epidermal growth factor receptor tyrosine kinase. Investigation of catalytic mechanism, structure-based searching and discovery of a potent inhibitor. *Biochem. Pharmacol.* 48, 659–666. doi: 10.1016/0006-2952(94)90042-6

Willett, P. (2006). Similarity-based virtual screening using 2D fingerprints. *Drug Discov. Today* 11, 1046–1053. doi: 10.1016/j.drudis.2006.10.005

Wishart, D. S., Feunang, Y. D., Guo, A. C., Lo, E. J., Marcu, A., Grant, R., et al. (2018). DrugBank 5.0: a major update to the DrugBank database for 2018. *Nucleic Acids Res.* 46, 1074–1082. doi: 10.1093/nar/gkx1037

Wójcikowski, M., Ballester, P. J., and Siedlecki, P. (2017). Performance of machine-learning scoring functions in structure-based virtual screening. *Sci. Rep.* 7:46710. doi: 10.1038/srep46710

Wood, A., and Armour, D. (2005). The discovery of the CCR5 receptor antagonist, UK-427,857, a new agent for the treatment of HIV infection and AIDS. *Progress Med Chem.* 43, 239–271. doi: 10.1016/S0079-6468(05)43007-6

Xia, J., Feng, B., Shao, Q., Yuan, Y., Wang, X. S., Chen, N., et al. (2017). Virtual screening against phosphoglycerate kinase 1 in quest of novel apoptosis inhibitors. *Molecules* 22:1029. doi: 10.3390/molecules22061029

Yuriev, E., and Ramsland, P. A. (2013). Latest developments in molecular docking: 2010-2011 in review. *J. Mol. Recognit.* 26, 215–239. doi: 10.1002/jmr.2266

Zhao, W., Hevener, K. E., White, S. W., Lee, R. E., and Boyett, J. M. (2009). A statistical framework to evaluate virtual screening. *BMC Bioinform.* 10:225. doi: 10.1186/1471-2105-10-225

Zhao, Y., and Sanner, M. F. (2007). FLIPDock: docking flexible ligands into flexible receptors. *Proteins Struct. Funct. Bioinforma* 68, 726–737. doi: 10.1002/prot.21423

Zilian, D., and Sotriffer, C. A. (2013). SFCscoreRF: a random forest-based scoring function for improved affinity prediction of protein-ligand complexes. *J. Chem. Inf. Model.* 53, 1923–1933. doi: 10.1021/ci400120b

Zsoldos, Z., Reid, D., Simon, A., Sadjad, S. B., and Johnson, A. P. (2007). eHiTS: a new fast, exhaustive flexible ligand docking system. *J. Mol. Graph. Model.* 26, 198–212. doi: 10.1016/j.jmgm.2006.06.002

9

Could Quantum Mechanical Properties be Reflected on Classical Molecular Dynamics? The Case of Halogenated Organic Compounds of Biological Interest

Lucas de Azevedo Santos[1], Ingrid G. Prandi[1] and Teodorico C. Ramalho[1,2]*

[1] Department of Chemistry, Federal University of Lavras, Lavras, Brazil, [2] Department of Chemistry, Faculty of Science, University of Hradec Kralove, Hradec Kralove, Czechia

***Correspondence:**
Teodorico C. Ramalho
teo@ufla.br*

Essential to understanding life, the biomolecular phenomena have been an important subject in science, therefore a necessary path to be covered to make progress in human knowledge. To fully comprehend these processes, the non-covalent interactions are the key. In this review, we discuss how specific protein-ligand interactions can be efficiently described by low computational cost methods, such as Molecular Mechanics (MM). We have taken as example the case of the halogen bonds (XB). Albeit generally weaker than the hydrogen bonds (HB), the XBs play a key role to drug design, enhancing the affinity and selectivity toward the biological target. Along with the attraction between two electronegative atoms in XBs explained by the σ-hole model, important orbital interactions, as well as relief of Pauli repulsion take place. Nonetheless, such electronic effects can be only well-described by accurate quantum chemical methods that have strong limitations dealing with supramolecular systems due to their high computational cost. To go beyond the poor description of XBs by MM methods, reparametrizing the force-fields equations can be a way to keep the balance between accuracy and computational cost. Thus, we have shown the steps to be considered when parametrizing force-fields to achieve reliable results of complex non-covalent interactions at MM level for *In Silico* drug design methods.

Keywords: halogen bonds, force-fields, molecular dynamics, non-covalent interactions, drug design

INTRODUCTION

Biological systems are huge, they change in time and they are very sensitive to *in vivo* conditions like temperature and environment (Ramalho et al., 2009; Freitas et al., 2014; Nair and Miners, 2014; Jurinovich et al., 2015). These facts are remembered every day by drug designers, structural biologists, biophysicists and many other professionals that need to study these systems (Nair and Miners, 2014). In order to overcome these barriers, many scientists opt to model their systems using the classical atomistic Molecular Dynamics (MD) simulation method.

The classical MD is a computational method based on Molecular Mechanics (MM) physics and its first simulation was performed by Alder and Wainright (Alder and Wainwright, 1959) in the late '50s. In this pioneering work, the authors discussed the difficulties to treat the many-body problem and proposed a numerical scheme to deal with multiple interactions of particles by solving Newton's motion equations. Although Alder and Wainright gave the first spark for the beginning of classical MD, the first realistic MD simulation was performed just in 1969 (Allen et al., 1969). In this work, by the implementation of Lennard-Jones potentials (essential to describe van der Waals interactions), Dr. Rahman and co-authors successfully modeled 864 atoms of liquid argon. Over the last decades, MD modeling was refined, and many different codes have been launched. Nowadays, drug design is one of the areas that most benefits from the enormous development that the atomistic MD has acquired over the years. However, the mindset that it is difficult, unnecessary or too time-consuming to parameterize new molecules may turn to final works that mislead the real interactions. Unphysical models or catastrophic geometries with very inaccurate interaction energies can be found along with an MD simulation, especially if the modeled molecule has too many chemical functions or π-conjugations (Davis and Patel, 2010; Prandi et al., 2016; Aytenfisu et al., 2017).

Despite the great effort being made by scientific programmers to enhance the quality of classical molecular simulation techniques, much more can be done by the user to improve inter- and intramolecular interactions outcomes. It should be kept in mind that intramolecular interactions are the driving force of most biomolecular phenomena (Martins et al., 2003; Adesokan et al., 2004; Ramalho et al., 2009; Poater et al., 2011; Ben-Naim, 2012; Hongo et al., 2013; Poznanski and Shugar, 2013). They are known to be quantum chemical phenomena that go beyond the classical description of matter and, in particular cases, they cannot be understood by simple electrostatic or dispersion schemes (Ramalho and da Cunha, 2011; Esrafili and Ahmadi, 2012; Wolters et al., 2014). This is one of the greatest challenges to force-field modeling since there is no classical analog to the quantum behavior of electrons.

That is the case of halogen bonds (XB), a real and relevant tool for rational drug design (Auffinger et al., 2004; Lu et al., 2009, 2010, 2012; Wilcken et al., 2013; Mendez et al., 2017). The XBs are non-covalent interactions between an acceptor (A), often Lewis base, and a halogenated molecule acting as a donor (D) (**Figure 1**). On one hand, some researchers address the origin of the XBs to the existence of a positive electrostatic potential region on the halogen atom (X) bond called σ-hole (Clark et al., 2007; Politzer et al., 2007, 2013; Kolár et al., 2014). On the other hand, the literature also highlights the importance of the orbital interactions, revealing the covalency part of XB (Wolters and Bickelhaupt, 2012; Wang et al., 2014; Novák et al., 2015; Wolters et al., 2015; Dominikowska et al., 2016; Bora et al., 2017; Santos et al., 2017). In contrast to molecular mechanics approaches, the XB are purely quantum chemical phenomena, whose strength grows with the size of the halogens, making chlorine, bromine, and iodine promising alternatives to promote secondary side-chain interactions inside protein cavities (Lu et al., 2010; Cavallo et al., 2016; Santos et al., 2017).

Once many compounds with biological activity have halogen atoms in their composition, the accurate description of XBs by molecular mechanics is crucial. Now, the main questions we pursue to answer are: what can we do to solve this problem?; what

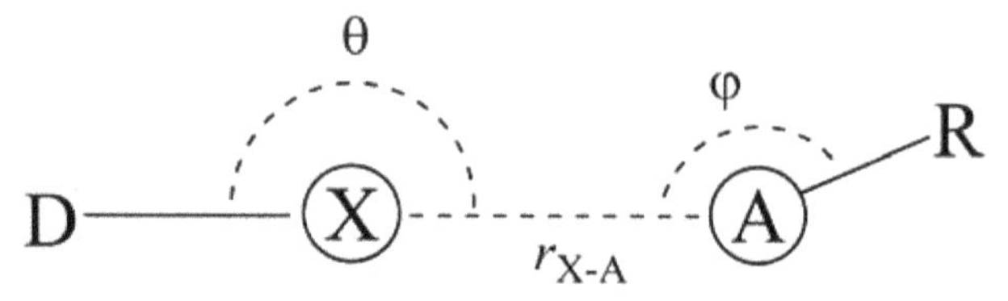

FIGURE 1 | General halogen-bond scheme. The donor (D) is bonded to a halogen atom (X) that interacts with the acceptor (A) in a distance *r*.

are the alternatives we have?; what is the best approach to build up accurate techniques to describe these interactions?

FORCE-FIELDS: AN OVERVIEW

Quantum Mechanics (QM) considers the electronic effects in molecules. On the other hand, Molecular Mechanics (MM) is based just on the interaction among classical charged particles, neglecting direct electronic effects.

Since the electronic environment around an atom changes accordingly to its neighborhood, we need an artifice to describe atoms with the same atomic numbers, but chemically different. For example, we need to distinguish the sp3 from sp2 carbons. To recover most of the electronic effects in MM based simulations different atom types should be employed. The atom types are atomic labels used to indicate chemically different atoms. In the example cited, different atom types should describe the carbons in ethanol.

After the atom types are set, the classical MD software associates each bonded or non-bonded molecular interaction to a set of parameters. In more detail, the MD software calculates the total potential (V_{TOT}) that acts in each particle.

$$V_{TOT} = V_S + V_A + V_D + V_{vdw} + V_C \tag{1}$$

The Equation (1) shows a generic form of a total potential: V_S, V_A, and V_D are the bonded terms, the stretching, angular, and dihedral potentials, respectively; and the last two terms are the non-bonded terms, in which accounts for the van der Waals interactions described by the Lennard-Jones potential (V_{vdw}) and Coulomb potential (V_C) that simulates the electrostatic interactions. It is important noticing that the terms in the total potential equation may vary depending on its implementation in the MD software. For instance, in Equation (1.1) we see the parameters k_μ^S, r_μ, and r_μ^0, that are the stretching force constant, the length of the bond and equilibrium distance, respectively; In Equation (1.2), k_μ^θ, θ_μ, and θ_μ^0 are the angular force constant, the angle, and equilibrium angle, respectively; The term $A_{j_\mu}^{SD}$ in Equation (1.3) is the dihedral torsional barrier, n_j^μ is the periodicity or the number of minima in the cosine function, δ_μ is the dihedral angle and γ_j^μ is a phase angle that represents the displacement of the dihedral angle (or torsional displacement); in Equation (1.4), ε_{ij}, σ_{ij}, and r_{ij} are the depth of the potential well, the distance at which V_{vdw} is a minimum and the distance between two particles, respectively; and finally

q and ϵ_0 in Equation (1.5) are the charge and the electrostatic constant, respectively. The description of each term in Equation (1) depends on these parameters and a complete set of equations together is named force-field (FF).

$$V_S = \sum_{\mu}^{N^{\underline{O}}_{bonds}} k^S_{\mu} (r_{\mu} - r^0_{\mu})^2 \quad (1.1)$$

$$V_A = \sum_{\mu}^{N^{\underline{O}}_{angles}} k^{\theta}_{\mu} (\theta_{\mu} - \theta^0_{\mu})^2 \quad (1.2)$$

$$V_D = \frac{1}{2} \sum_{\mu}^{N^{\underline{O}}_{Sdihedrals}} \sum_{j=1}^{N^{\underline{O}}_{\cos\mu}} A^{SD}_{j\mu} \left[1 + \cos\left(n^{\mu}_j \delta_{\mu} - \gamma^{\mu}_j\right)\right] \quad (1.3)$$

$$V_{vdw} = \sum_{i}^{N^{\underline{O}}_{vdw\ interactions}} \sum_{i<j}^{N^{\underline{O}}_{vdw\ interactions}} 4\varepsilon_{ij} \left[\left(\frac{\sigma_{ij}}{r_{ij}}\right)^{12} - \left(\frac{\sigma_{ij}}{r_{ij}}\right)^{6}\right] \quad (1.4)$$

$$V_C = \sum_{i}^{N^{\underline{O}}_{Coul.\ interac.}} \sum_{i<j}^{N^{\underline{O}}_{Coul.\ interac.}} \frac{q_i q_j}{4\pi \epsilon_0 r_{ij}} \quad (1.5)$$

In the last decades, the use of MD has been expanded to different areas, being necessary the creation of parameters to describe a huge set of molecular interactions at the same time or, at least, those more relevant to a certain purpose. Thus, large groups of transferable parameters have been created aiming to describe chemically similar molecules. Nowadays, there are many sets of specialized parameters for the description of many different molecular groups like polymers, proteins, solvents, small organic molecules, etc. (Jorgensen et al., 1996; Schuler et al., 2001; Wang et al., 2004; Vanommeslaeghe et al., 2010; Dickson et al., 2014).

Due to the wide use of classical MD for protein modeling, here we may highlight two of the most used sets of parameters for biomodelling: AMBER (Assisted Model Building with Energy Refinement) (Case et al., 2014), created by Peter Kollman and his group at the University of California, and CHARMM (Chemistry at Harvard using Molecular Mechanics) (Vanommeslaeghe et al., 2010), initially developed by Martin Karplus and co-workers at Harvard University. Over the years, CHARMM has expanded and gained new specific parameters for the modeling of smaller molecules.

Other diffused family of parameters for biomolecular systems are OPLS and GROMOS. The OPLS (Optimized Potentials for Liquid Simulations) (Jorgensen et al., 1996) force-field was developed by Jorgensen's group to simulate proteins in solution. In 1976, GROMOS (GROningen MOlecular Simulation) (Schuler et al., 2001) started to be developed at the University of Groningen. Originally created for biomolecules modeling, until today it is constantly updated for many different classes of molecules.

Another example of a set of parameters specially designed for small and medium-sized organic molecules is the MMn ($n = 1, 2, 3, 4$) family of parameters developed by Allinger and coauthors (Allinger et al., 1971, 1989, 1996; Allinger, 1977; Lii and Allinger, 1989a,b; Nevins et al., 1996; Langley et al., 2001; Langley and Allinger, 2002).

With the expansion of the use of MD simulations in the pharmaceutical field, the development of a set of parameters for drug design research was urgent. Thus, in 2004, the GAFF (General AMBER Force Field) (Wang et al., 2004) family of parameters was specifically created and tested for pharmaceutical purposes. In order to guarantee a great transferability, many GAFF equilibrium parameters were extracted from the average of X-ray and *ab initio* calculations of different molecules. Besides, pure GAFF is not yet able to model the major part of metallic interactions in complexes and can poorly describe halogen bonds (Rendine et al., 2011; Li and Merz, 2017).

PARAMETERIZATION: THE KEY TO REALISTIC RESULTS

In the last decade, the US Food and Drug Administration (FDA)[1] approved more than 230 New Molecular Entity (NME) drugs. Almost 42% of the new non-biological approved drugs contain halogen atoms, and more than 3% are metallic complexes (see data in **Figure 2**). These data show the importance of a specific parameterization for new drugs since most general FFs are not able to describe with high accuracy those bonds for molecular dynamics simulations (Santos et al., 2014, 2017).

Unfortunately, specificity and transferability usually have an inversely proportional relationship. Due to their good transferability, GAFF and other general force-fields are ideal to describe molecules that are indirectly involved in the studies that we would like to do. However, for very specific cases, sets of general parameters are not enough to model physical structures or interactions and we need to remodel them.

Then, theoretical scientists have realized that molecular models need to be accurate to perform a realistic simulation. For this reason, many tools were developed aiming more straightforward paths to parameterization. The greatest part of methodologies is based on the extraction of equilibrium distances, angles and dihedrals from a QM optimized structure and the force constants are derived from the diagonalization of the Hessian matrix (extracted from a QM calculation). Some examples of tools that help computational scientists to parameterize their molecules are the following: Automated Topology Builder (ATB) (Malde et al., 2011), Paratool (Mayne et al., 2013), and Joyce (Barone et al., 2013).

More specifically, ATB is much more than an on-line tool to build biomolecular force-fields for MD or Monte Carlo simulations, it can also calculate free energies and predict hydration free enthalpies. This website is very user-friendly, does not require any installation procedure and sends an e-mail to the user when the parameters are ready.

Paratool is a plugin of the software Visual Molecular Dynamics (VMD) (Humphrey et al., 1996). It was specifically developed to build parameters in CHARMM or AMBER format.

[1]US Food and Drug Administration (FDA). Available online at: https://www.fda.gov/ (accessed November 4, 2017).

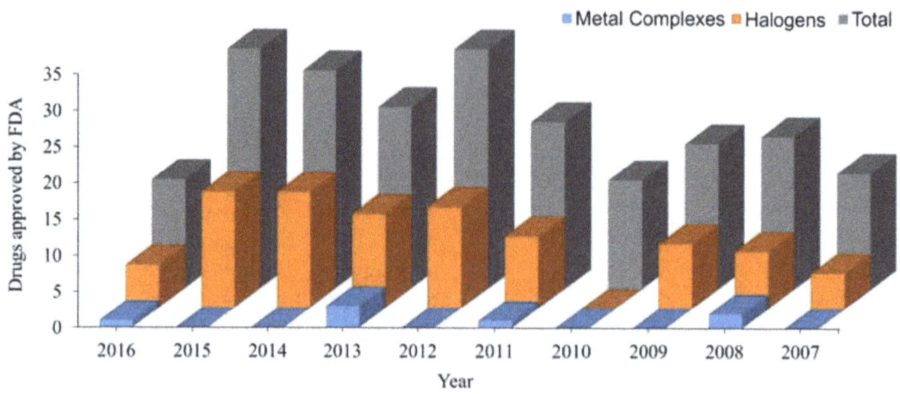

FIGURE 2 | New Molecular Entity (NME) approved by the US Food and Drug Administration (FDA) in the last 10 years. All data are taken from https://www.fda.gov.

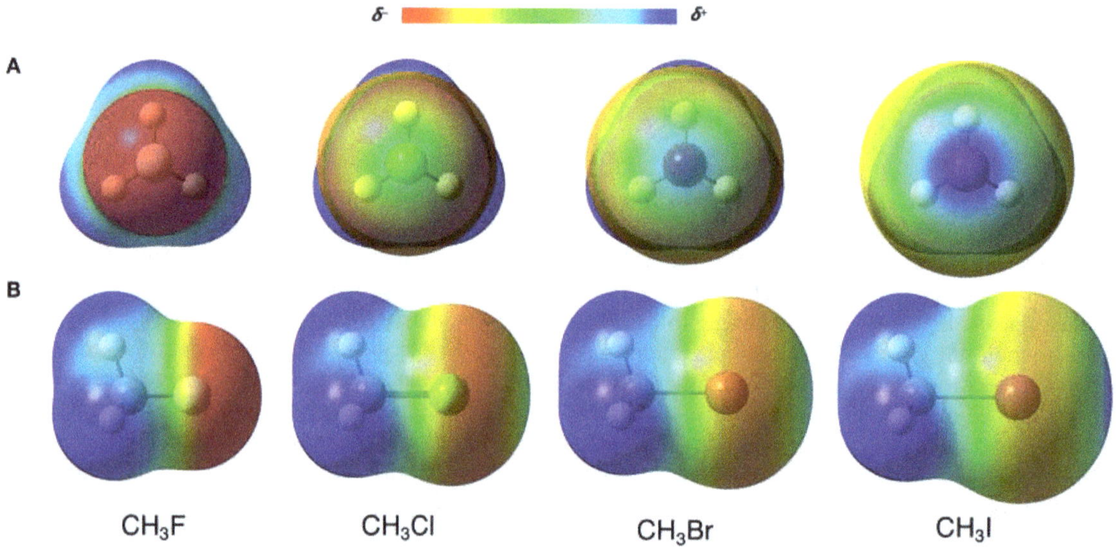

FIGURE 3 | (A) Front and **(B)** side view of the electrostatic potential surfaces (at 0.02 a.u.) from −0.3 (red) to 0.3 (blue) a.u. of CH_3X (X = F, Cl, Br, I) molecules. Computed at B3LYP-D3(BJ)/def2-TZVP, using Gaussian 09 (Frisch et al., 2009).

It is not as automated as ATB, but it is very user-friendly since it is linked to the VMD graphical interface.

Joyce is a software specially developed to assist the derivation of parameters in GROMACS (GROningen MAchine for Chemical Simulations) (van der Spoel et al., 2005) or Moscito (Paschek and Geiger, 2002) format for MD atomistic simulations. It is also a very versatile and flexible program, in which the user can symmetrize molecular groups, set dependencies between parameters and even impose specific values to the parameters.

The three aforementioned tools are just some examples of how a specific set of parameters can be derived. They were cited in ascendant order of time-consuming and effort to create a new specific FF. The choice of modeling a molecule with an FF created in a very automated way or a much more fitted one depends on the molecule, the required accuracy and how dependent the studied property is from the molecular geometry. However, another issue that cannot be neglected is the more complex intermolecular interactions, such as the halogen bonds. The difficulties of modeling intramolecular parameters are beyond the simple extraction and fitting of the parameters: they are also led by the MD software limitations.

Some MD software like AMBER do not distinguish intra from intermolecular parameters for van der Waals and Coulombic charges. Although MD simulations may give good results for many physical and macro properties of a large number of different systems, many times specific micro-interactions are not modeled in a refined way. This is the case of some vibrational modes: even if a very precise parameterization is done, coupled vibrational modes in very conjugated molecules are extremely hard to describe (Prandi et al., 2016; Andreussi et al., 2017). The difficulty of an accurate description is mirrored in the fact that most MD simulation programs do not couple molecular motions like a stretching mode with an angular bending or the stretching modes of two adjacent atom pairs (Andreussi et al., 2017; Cerezo et al., 2018). More precisely, all mentioned terms in Equation (1) are expressed as sums of contributions, each one depending on a single internal coordinate. In this way, the off-diagonal terms (or hybrid terms) of the Hessian are not explicitly taken into account. Here, it is important to emphasize that it is mathematically and physically possible to derive parameters considering the cited couplings (Cerezo et al., 2018), but the implementation of a force-field functional form that describes the coupled terms can still not be done in many MD software.

It is evident that neither the best set of parameters can completely recover the electronic effects of a given molecule along an MD trajectory. Although some MD simulation programs are starting to be more flexible in terms of a force-field functional implementation, like GROMACS and Moscito (Cerezo et al., 2018). There is a still long path to achieve the full force-field functional form flexibility. Indeed, the maximum refinement that a normal user of mostly MD programs can do is to construct his own set of parameters. However, diving into very specific cases simple parameterizations can still be not enough.

BEYOND THE LIMITS

As defined in the introduction, the halogen bonds (XB) are non-covalent interactions between the halogen bond donor (D) and the halogen-bond acceptor (A) (**Figure 1**). Thus, the force-fields will describe these phenomena through the van der Waals term (Equation 1.4) and by the Coulombic term (Equation 1.5).

Many researchers address the origin of the XBs to the σ-hole, classifying them as σ-hole interactions (Clark et al., 2007; Politzer et al., 2008). The σ-hole is a positive region on the electrostatic potential surface (ESP), that arises from a charge anisotropy effect along with the D–X bond (Clark et al., 2007; Politzer et al., 2013). In other words, the electron density polarizes toward the D–X, generating an electron depletion in the back of the halogen (X) toward the D–X bond axis (see the blue regions over the halogens in **Figure 3**, in which D = CH_3) (Politzer et al., 2012). For the σ-hole model, the strength of the XBs, which increases along X = F < Cl < Br < I, is directly correlated to the increase of the positive electrostatic potential on the halogen. In this sense, to perform a classical FF description of the XBs, the attraction between A and X should be rigorously described by the Coulomb potential. However, here we have at least two barriers to overcome: firstly, the XB cannot be seen as the attraction of two points charges as described by Equation (1.5), but the interaction of two densities; secondly, even using the point charge scheme, halogen atoms often have negative charges that would cause an electrostatic repulsion between X and A, not allowing the XB to happen. The fact is, something totally different from the usual parameterization must be done.

The first attempt to describe the XB through molecular mechanics was suggested by Ibrahim who introduced the Explicit σ-hole (ESH) theory (Ibrahim, 2011, 2012; Kolár et al., 2013). The ESH is a way to model the σ-hole as a massless positive point charge bonded to the halogen atom at a certain distance (r_{ESH})

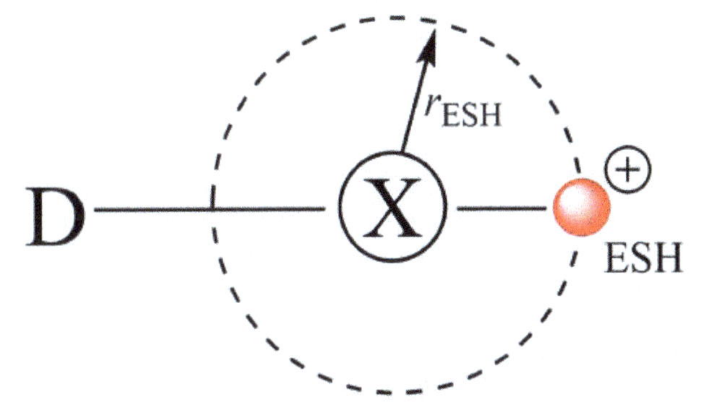

FIGURE 4 | The explicit σ-hole (ESH) scheme to model halogen bonds via the molecular mechanics approach.

(**Figure 4**). In general, there are two parameters to be fitted: the charge of the massless point and its distance to X (r_{ESH}).

The ESH strategy has promoted huge advances for the modeling of XB in a biological environment predicting energy minima points in halogen-bonded systems along the potential energy surfaces. However, it is totally based on the classical electrostatic point of view of chemical interactions, that is, the electrostatic attraction between two point charges.

In fact, the XBs are a mix of attractive dispersion, electrostatics and orbital interactions in balance with repulsive orbital interactions (Pauli repulsion) and should not be described neglecting either one of them (Huber et al., 2013; Wolters et al., 2014; Santos et al., 2017). **Figure 5** shows a simplified scheme of the halogen-bonding mechanism by Wolters and Bickelhaupt in the sight of Kohn-Sham density functional molecular orbital theory (Wolters and Bickelhaupt, 2012). An occupied molecular orbital of the acceptor, described by *np* orbitals of the halides, interacts with an unoccupied molecular orbital of the halogenated molecule (DX) to promote an attractive orbital interaction. Here, the doubly occupied orbital can be further extrapolated to any doubly occupied MO. See that the unoccupied molecular orbital of the DX molecule will have a strong sigma anti-bonding orbital (σ^*_{D-X}) character. The Pauli repulsion originates from the interaction between the doubly occupied orbitals.

In practice, the σ-hole model often seems to work, but just by coincidence. In previous work, we have shown that the maximum ESP values on σ-hole (V_{max}) and the unoccupied orbital which contains the contribution of σ^*_{D-X} may have a similar origin (Santos et al., 2017). In other words, by increasing the value of V_{max}, the σ^*_{D-X} will be stabilized and the interaction energy will become more stable.

Once the XBs have an important contribution of non-classical interactions, they cannot be described only by the Coulomb potential to get the ideal parameterization. In the traditional FF equation (Equation 1), the other alternative is to look at the van der Waals term. The Equation (2) is the Lennard-Jones 12-6 potential (Lennard-Jones, 1931) written in a different way than in Equation (1.4). Here, the positive part is the repulsion term and the negative part is the attractive term. The parameters are reduced to ε, the potential energy depth, and r_e, the equilibrium distance.

$$V_{vdw} = V_{LJ\ 12-6} = \varepsilon \left\{ \left(\frac{r_e}{r}\right)^{12} - 2\left(\frac{r_e}{r}\right)^{6} \right\} \tag{2}$$

In theory, the repulsive part of Equation (2) would account for the Pauli repulsion, which is decently described by the traditional FF being the result of the steric hindrance between two atoms. The attractive term would account for the dispersive and orbital interactions. The first is also quite well-parametrized but the same cannot be said for the orbital interactions (Wu et al., 2012; Santos et al., 2014). The main problem of neglecting the orbital interactions in molecular mechanics is to get overestimated destabilizing energies at low range distances (Santos et al., 2014, 2017). At this interaction bond length, the Pauli repulsion and charge transfer are exponentially intensified.

One way to minimize this problem is to use the LJ 10-6 potential (Equation 3). With a lower exponential factor in the repulsion term, the interaction energies at low range distances are less destabilized (Du et al., 2013; Santos et al., 2014, 2017). However, the LJ 10-6 does not bring geometric improvements in comparison with the LJ 12-6, mainly in the cases that the non-covalent interactions are extremely directional, as the halogen bonds. The Lennard-Jones potential can model if a Lewis base will approximate toward the σ_{D-X} bond axis or not and how it would affect the interaction energy (Soteras Gutiérrez et al., 2016; Bernardes and Canongia Lopes, 2017).

$$V_{vdw} = V_{LJ\ 10-6} = \varepsilon \left\{ \left(\frac{r_e}{r}\right)^{10} - 2\left(\frac{r_e}{r}\right)^{6} \right\} \tag{3}$$

CHANGING THE POTENTIAL EQUATIONS

If the actual model does not work for a specific system, we must reformulate it. So, why not do the same for FF equations? Nevertheless, it is not necessary to build an equation from scratch. Wiser is to modify a well-known model. In the case of reformulating new non-bonded force-field terms, subtly modifications into the V_C or V_{LJ} have been done to get more accurate functions.

The directional dependence of halogen bonds can be understood by looking at the σ-hole and MO theories together. The interaction angle θ must be close to 180° to lead the interaction toward the D–X bond axis (**Figure 1**). This is the geometry configuration that would maximize the electrostatic and orbital interactions for both σ-hole and MO theories (Riley et al., 2009, 2013; Esrafili and Ahmadi, 2012; Santos et al., 2017). The angle φ depends on the electronic structure of the acceptor (A) in order to maximize the attractive donor-acceptor orbital overlaps (see **Figure 5**). For instance, having an sp^2 oxygen as acceptor, φ would be around 120° to provide the frontal overlap between the lone pair of the oxygen (LP_O) and the σ^*_{D-X} orbital. By the same perspective, for an *sp* nitrogen as acceptor, φ would be around 180° and, for π acceptors, φ would be around 90° (Cavallo et al., 2016; Nziko and Scheiner, 2016; Santos et al., 2017).

In a very clever way, Carter and co-workers (Carter et al., 2012; Scholfield et al., 2015; Koebel et al., 2016) have introduced the angular dependence into the LJ 12-6 and Coulombic potentials to describe bromine bonds, which was later extended to chlorine and iodine. The Equations (4) and (5) are the *ff*BXB functions to describe the non-bonding terms of XBs. The effective halogen charge (Z_X) is defined by the amplitude (A) and the baseline (B) of the cosine function, which has the period ν and $\alpha = 180 - \theta$. In V_{LJ}, $\langle r_{vdw(X)} \rangle$ is now the average radius of the bromine at the energy minimum.

$$V_C = \frac{Z_X Z_A e^2}{D r^n} \quad ; \quad Z_X = A\cos(\nu\alpha) + B \tag{4}$$

$$V_{LJ} = \sqrt{\varepsilon_X \varepsilon_A} \left\{ \left(\frac{r_{vdw(A)} + \langle r_{vdw(X)} \rangle - \Delta r_X \cos(\nu\alpha)}{r} \right)^{12} - 2\left(\frac{r_{vdw(A)} + \langle r_{vdw(X)} \rangle}{r} \right)^{6} \right\} \tag{5}$$

Parameterized to predict the halogen bonds in DNA junctions, the variation in the interaction energies were ~0.06 to ~0.7 kcal.mol^{-1} in comparison to the experimental data. The *ff*BXB functions also give good values of θ, from ~146 to ~122°.

Du et al. have introduced new polarizable non-bonded functions to the force-field equations in order to reproduce the XBs, the PEff model (Du et al., 2013). The electrostatic potential is defined by (6), in which Q is a constant, α, β, and ς are parameters from *ab initio* electrostatic potential, r_1 is a coordinate in the equatorial area, R is the distance from the halogen atom toward the D–X axis and r is the halogen-bond length.

$$V_{elst}(r_1, R, r) = Q \cdot \left[\exp(-\alpha r_1 - \beta R) - exp(\varsigma r)\right] / r \tag{6}$$

The Lennard-Jones potential was used to simulate the repulsion and dispersion interactions (7), in which r_e is a function of θ, $r_{e,T}$ is the transverse distance, $r_{e,L}$ is the longitudinal distance and λ is a steepness parameter manually set to 1.26.

$$V_{rd} = 4\varepsilon \left\{ \left(\frac{r_e(\theta)}{r}\right)^{10} - \left(\frac{r_e(\theta)}{r}\right)^{6} \right\}; \quad r_e(\theta) = r_{e,T} sin^2(\lambda\theta) + r_{e,L} cos^2(\lambda\theta) \tag{7}$$

The third and last term is the polarization energy (8), in which E is the electronic field, E_{tot} incorporates the induce dipole effects and α is the isotropic polarizability of the halogen.

$$V_{pol} = -\frac{1}{2}\alpha E \cdot E_{tot} \exp\left(1.0 - \left(\frac{r}{r_{min}}\right)^2\right) \tag{8}$$

The PEff functions have demonstrated a good performance in comparison with MP2 methods to predict the binding energies for chlorine, bromine, and iodine. Applied to well-known crystal structures, the deviation of the halogen-bond lengths was <0.1 Å and giving bond angles close to 180°.

Both *ff*BXB and PEff are complete force-field and already functional, albeit some tests with molecular dynamics must be

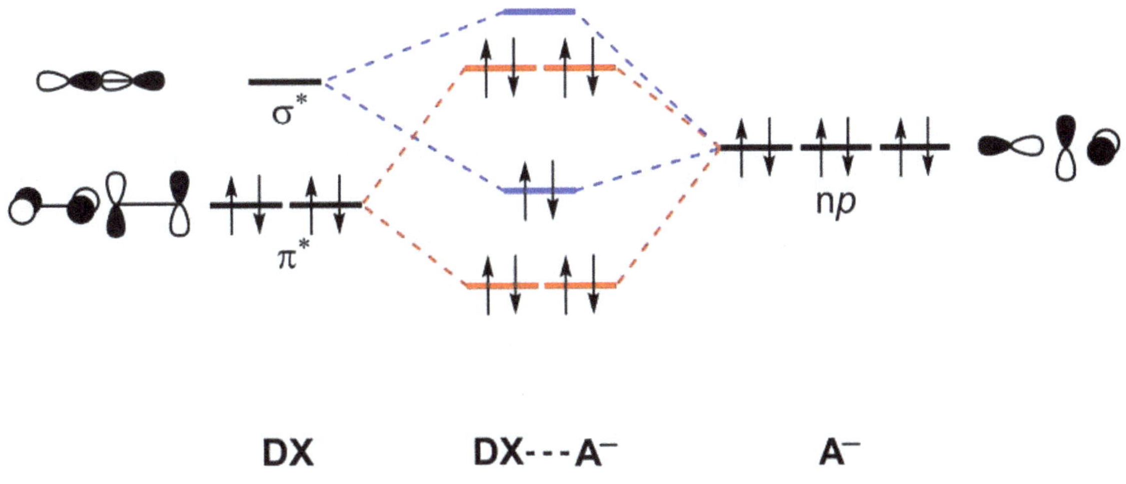

FIGURE 5 | Simplified molecular orbital perspective of halogen-halide bonds. Main attractive interactions (blue) and repulsive interactions (red) are highlighted. X, D, A = F, Cl, Br, I.

carried out. Moreover, they only consider Cl, Br, and I as donors and Lewis basis with available electron lone pairs (i.e., A = S, O, N) as acceptors. Nonetheless, molecules with π orbitals can also act as halogen bond acceptors and must be considered since there are several aromatic structures in the biological environment. In this sight, a new LJ 10-6 function has been proposed that takes into account the halogen-bond acceptor nature and also includes the fluorine in the XB donor, the E_{mod} (Equation 10) (Santos et al., 2017). Indeed, at certain conditions regarding the electronic structure of the whole donor molecule, the fluorine atom can form strong halogen-bonded complexes, sometimes as strong as the chlorine bonds (Wolters and Bickelhaupt, 2012; Santos et al., 2017).

$$V_{LJ} = E_{mod} = \varepsilon \left\{ \left(\frac{r_{e+\frac{\delta cos\Theta}{6}}}{r} \right)^{10} - 2\left(\frac{r_e}{r+\gamma} \right)^{6} \right\} \quad (9)$$

The E_{mod} empirical potential (10) has two new parameters: δ and γ (11). The parameter δ accounts for the attractive orbital interactions regarding the angular dependence to minimize the repulsion term, based on the synergy between V_{max} and the σ^*_{D-X} energies, as aforementioned. The V_{max} is calculated by QM methods, α is the van der Waals radius of the halogen atom and β is a constant, in which $\beta = 2.5$ for lone pair acceptors and $\beta = 0.432$ for aromatic acceptors. The parameter γ is a function of δ to rebalance the potential.

$$\delta = \frac{\beta V_{max}}{4\pi\alpha^3} \;;\; \gamma = \left[\frac{2^{2-\delta}(1-\delta)}{25r} \right] \quad (10)$$

The E_{mod} was designed to use the r_e already parameterized by any force-field without halogen-bond corrections. In practice, V_{max} should be obtained by a QM calculation and used to fully define the parameters in Equation (11). Also, the E_{mod} could be used the general V_{LJ} function of the FF, since when V_{max} is not given (i.e., equal to zero), the parameters δ and γ will tend to zero, and this function will behave like a traditional LJ 10-6 potential. However, E_{mod} has not been tested with a complete force-field equation and there are no parameters for iodine.

Performing subtle modifications in the traditional empirical potentials is a good strategy to improve force-field equations. There are many other examples of modified potentials fitted to obtain reliable results of complex properties at the molecular mechanics level (Bernardes and Canongia Lopes, 2017; Franchini et al., 2018; Lin and MacKerell, 2018; Nunes et al., 2018). This approach eases the implementation of these functions by not requiring a huge effort to build a code from the beginning but using an already existing open-access and well-working code.

The use parameters obtained from previous quantum mechanical calculations can surely improve the results of a molecular dynamics simulation, but the next step is to rework the potentials in Equation (1) to further decrease the level of empiricism. That is where we find the *ab initio* force-fields (McDaniel et al., 2016; Xu et al., 2018; Pérez-Conesa et al., 2019). In principle, it would be possible to properly describe any non-covalent interactions with *ab initio* derived potentials, considering their specific properties, with a manageable computational cost.

SUMMARY AND OUTLOOK

Through the last decades, computational methods have been employed in the investigations around chemical properties of the matter. The evolution of technology has allowed us to go deeper into the atomic level to retrieve information about chemical bonds and non-covalent interactions. However, the computational cost has been the border of how further our knowledge could go. To overcome these borders, cheap computational approaches based on classical mechanics have emerged.

In this review, we have discussed how cheap approaches, like molecular dynamics (MD) and molecular mechanics

(MM) calculations, can be improved. Toward this goal, the parameterization of their force field (FF) equations is the key. Most of the parameters can be obtained by quantum mechanical (QM) calculations together with specific tools to modify and generate more accurate FF. Nevertheless, we have further explored one case that only setting up better parameters is not enough to retrieve the real information from a non-covalent interaction.

Being purely quantum chemical phenomena, the halogen bonds (XBs) have required the replacement of some FF potentials, since simple classical equations could not describe the properties of systems they are involved in. This replacement has been wisely done by modifying and introducing new parameters to well-known potentials. The new potentials to describe XBs were fit to high-level QM calculations, showing good agreement with crystal structure data. Thus, we strongly believe that the classical mechanical approaches will evolve by introducing new potentials based on *ab initio* calculations. The scope of this review is to highlight the relevance of ab initio parameterizations if the recovering of quantum chemical effects, lost by MM simulations, is wanted.

AUTHOR CONTRIBUTIONS

LS and IP held the literature research and prepared the initial draft of this review. LS, IP, and TR were responsible for proofing and preparing the final copy of this review.

FUNDING

We thank the Brazilian agencies FAPEMIG, CNPq, and CAPES for the financial support. This work was also supported by University of Hradec Kralove (Faculty of Science, VT2019-2021).

REFERENCES

Adesokan, A. A., Roberts, V. A., Lee, K. W., Lins, R. D., and Briggs, J. M. (2004). Prediction of HIV-1 integrase/viral DNA interactions in the catalytic domain by fast molecular docking. *J. Med. Chem.* 47, 821–828. doi: 10.1021/jm0301890

Alder, B. J., and Wainwright, T. E. (1959). Studies in molecular dynamics. General method. *J. Chem. Phys.* 31:459. doi: 10.1063/1.1730376

Allen, R. E., de Wette, F. W., and Rahman, A. (1969). Calculation of dynamical surface properties of noble-gas crystals. II. *Phys. Rev.* 179:887. doi: 10.1103/PhysRev.179.887

Allinger, N. L. (1977). Conformational analysis. 130. MM2. a hydrocarbon force field utilizing V1 and V2 torsional terms. *J. Am. Chem. Soc.* 99, 8127–8134. doi: 10.1021/ja00467a001

Allinger, N. L., Chen, K., and Lii, J. H. (1996). An improved force field (MM4) for saturated hydrocarbons. *J. Comput. Chem.* 17, 642–668. doi: 10.1002/(SICI)1096-987X(199604)17:5/6<;642::AID-JCC6>;3.0.CO;2-U

Allinger, N. L., Thomas Tribble, M., Miller, M. A., and Wertz, D. H. (1971). Conformational analysis. LXIX. an improved force field for the calculation of the structures and energies of hydrocarbons. *J. Am. Chem. Soc.* 93, 1637–1648. doi: 10.1021/ja00736a012

Allinger, N. L., Yuh, Y. H., and Lii, J. H. (1989). Molecular mechanics. the MM3 force field for hydrocarbons. 1. *J. Am. Chem. Soc.* 111, 8551–8566. doi: 10.1021/ja00205a001

Andreussi, O., Prandi, I. G., Campetella, M., Prampolini, G., and Mennucci, B. (2017). Classical force fields tailored for QM applications: is it really a feasible strategy? *J. Chem. Theory Comput.* 13, 4636–4648. doi: 10.1021/acs.jctc.7b00777

Auffinger, P., Hays, F. A., Westhof, E., and Ho, P. S. (2004). Halogen bonds in biological molecules. *Proc. Natl. Acad. Sci. U.S.A.* 100, 8742–8747. doi: 10.1073/pnas.0407607101

Aytenfisu, A. H., Spasic, A., Grossfield, A., Stern, H. A., and Mathews, D. H. (2017). Revised RNA dihedral parameters for the Amber force field improve RNA molecular dynamics. *J. Chem. Theory Comput.* 13, 900–915. doi: 10.1021/acs.jctc.6b00870

Barone, V., Cacelli, I., De Mitri, N., Licari, D., Monti, S., and Prampolini, G. (2013). Joyce and Ulysses: integrated and user-friendly tools for the parameterization of intramolecular force fields from quantum mechanical data. *Phys. Chem. Chem. Phys.* 15, 3736–3751. doi: 10.1039/c3cp44179b

Ben-Naim, A. (2012). Levinthal's question revisited, and answered. *J. Biomol. Struct. Dyn.* 30, 113–124. doi: 10.1080/07391102.2012.674286

Bernardes, C. E. S., and Canongia Lopes, J. N. (2017). Modeling halogen bonds in ionic liquids: a force field for imidazolium and halo-imidazolium derivatives. *J. Chem. Theory Comput.* 13, 6167–6176. doi: 10.1021/acs.jctc.7b 00645

Bora, P. L., Novák, M., Novotný, J., Foroutan-Nejad, C., and Marek, R. (2017). Supramolecular covalence in bifurcated chalcogen bonding. *Chem. Eur. J.* 23, 7315–7323. doi: 10.1002/chem.201700179

Carter, M., Rappé, A. K., and Ho, P. S. (2012). Scalable anisotropic shape and electrostatic models for biological bromine halogen bonds. *J. Chem. Theory Comput.* 8, 2461–2473. doi: 10.1021/ct3001969

Case, D. A., Babin, V., Berryman, J. T., Betz, R. M., Cai, Q., Cerutti, D. S., et al. (2014), *AMBER 14*. San Francisco, CA: University of California.

Cavallo, G., Metrangolo, P., Milani, R., Pilati, T., Priimagi, A., Resnati, G., et al. (2016). The halogen bond. *Chem. Rev.* 116, 2478–2601. doi: 10.1021/acs.chemrev.5b00484

Cerezo, J., Prampolini, G., and Cacelli, I. (2018). Developing accurate intramolecular force fields for conjugated systems through explicit coupling terms. *Theor. Chem. Acc.* 137:80. doi: 10.1007/s00214-018-2254-8

Clark, T., Hennemann, M., Murray, J. S., and Politzer, P. (2007). Halogen bonding: the σ-Hole. *J. Mol. Model.* 13, 291–296. doi: 10.1007/s00894-006-0130-2

Davis, J. E., and Patel, S. (2010). Revised charge equilibration parameters for more accurate hydration free energies of alkanes. *Chem. Phys. Lett.* 484, 173–176. doi: 10.1016/j.cplett.2009.09.061

Dickson, C. J., Madej, B. D., Skjevik, A. A., Betz, R. M., Teigen, K., Gould, I. R., et al. (2014). Lipid14: the amber lipid force field. *J. Chem. Theory Comput.* 10, 865–879. doi: 10.1021/ct4010307

Dominikowska, J., Bickelhaupt, F. M., Palusiak, M., and Fonseca Guerra, C. (2016). Source of cooperativity in halogen-bonded haloamine tetramers. *Chem. Phys. Chem.* 17, 474–480. doi: 10.1002/cphc.201501130

Du, L., Gao, J., Bi, F., Wang, L., and Liu, C. (2013). A polarizable ellipsoidal force field for halogen bonds. *J. Comput. Chem.* 34, 2032–2040. doi: 10.1002/jcc.23362

Esrafili, M. D., and Ahmadi, B. (2012). A theoretical investigation on the nature of Cl. . . N and Br. . . N halogen bonds in FArX. . . NCY complexes (X=Cl, Br and Y=H, F, Cl, Br, OH, NH2, CH3 and CN). *Comput. Theor. Chem.* 997, 77–82. doi: 10.1016/j.comptc.2012.07.038

Franchini, D., Dapiaggi, F., Pieraccini, S., Forni, A., and Sironi, M. (2018). Halogen bonding in the framework of classical force fields: the case of chlorine. *Chem. Phys. Lett.* 712, 89–94. doi: 10.1016/j.cplett.2018.09.052

Freitas, L. B., Borgati, T. F., de Freitas, R. P., Ruiz, A. L., Marchetti, G. M., de Carvalho, J. E., et al. (2014). Synthesis and antiproliferative activity of 8-hydroxyquinoline derivatives containing a 1,2,3-triazole moiety. *Eur. J. Med. Chem.* 84, 595–604. doi: 10.1016/j.ejmech.2014.07.061

Frisch, M. J., Trucks, G. W., Schlegel, H. B., Scuseria, G. E., Robb, M. A., Cheeseman, J. R., et al. (2009). *Gaussian 09, Revision D.01*. Wallingford, CT: Gaussian Inc.

Hongo, K., Cuong, N. T., and Maezono, R. (2013). The importance of electron correlation on stacking interaction of adenine-thymine base-pair step in B-DNA: a quantum Monte Carlo study. *J. Chem. Theory Comput.* 9, 1081–1086. doi: 10.1021/ct301065f

Huber, S. M., Scanlon, J. D., Jimenez-Izal, E., Ugalde, J. M., and Infante, I. (2013). On the directionality of halogen bonding. *Phys. Chem. Chem. Phys.* 15:10350. doi: 10.1039/c3cp50892g

Humphrey, W., Dalke, A., and Schulten, K. (1996). VMD: visual molecular dynamics. *J. Mol. Graph.* 14, 33–38. doi: 10.1016/0263-7855(96)00018-5

Ibrahim, M. A. (2011). Molecular mechanical study of halogen bonding in drug discovery. *J. Comput. Chem.* 32, 2564–2574. doi: 10.1002/jcc.21836

Ibrahim, M. A. (2012). Molecular mechanical perspective on halogen bonding. *J. Mol. Model.* 18, 4625–4638. doi: 10.1007/s00894-012-1454-8

Jorgensen, W. L., Maxwell, D. S., and Tirado-Rives, J. (1996). Development and testing of the OLPS all-atom force field on conformational energetics and properties of organic liquids. *J. Am. Chem. Soc.* 118, 11225–11236. doi: 10.1021/ja9621760

Jurinovich, S., Viani, L., Prandi, I. G., and Mennucci, B. (2015). Towards an *ab initio* description of the optical spectra of light-harvesting antennae: application to the CP29 complex of photosystem II. *Phys. Chem. Chem. Phys.* 17, 14405–14416. doi: 10.1039/C4CP05647G

Koebel, M. R., Schmadeke, G., Posner, R. G., and Sirimulla, S. (2016). AutoDock VinaXB: implementation of XBSF, new empirical halogen bond scoring function, into AutoDock Vina. *J. Chem. Inform.* 8:27. doi: 10.1186/s13321-016-0139-1

Kolár, M., Hobza, P., and Bronowska, A. K. (2013). Plugging the explicit σ-holes in molecular docking. *Chem. Commun.* 49, 981–983. doi: 10.1039/C2CC37584B

Kolár, M., Hostaš, J., and Hobza, P. (2014). The strength and directionality of a halogen bond are co-determined by the magnitude and size of the σ-Hole. *Phys. Chem. Chem. Phys.* 16, 9987–9996. doi: 10.1039/C3CP55188A

Langley, C. H., and Allinger, N. L. (2002). Molecular mechanics (MM4) calculations on amides. *J. Phys. Chem. A* 106, 5638–5652. doi: 10.1021/jp014426r

Langley, C. H., Lii, J. H., and Allinger, N. L. (2001). Molecular mechanics (MM4) calculations on carbonyl compounds part I: aldehydes. *J. Comput. Chem.* 24, 1283–1286. doi: 10.1002/jcc.1177

Lennard-Jones, J. E. (1931). Cohesion. *Proc. Phys. Soc.* 43, 461–482. doi: 10.1088/0959-5309/43/5/301

Li, P., and Merz, K. M. Jr. (2017). Metal ion modeling using classical mechanics. *Chem. Rev.* 117, 1564–1686. doi: 10.1021/acs.chemrev.6b00440

Lii, J. H., and Allinger, N. L. (1989a). Molecular mechanics. the MM3 force field for hydrocarbons. 2. Vibrational frequencies and thermodynamics. *J. Am. Chem. Soc.* 111, 8566–8575. doi: 10.1021/ja00205a002

Lii, J. H., and Allinger, N. L. (1989b). Molecular mechanics. the MM3 force field for hydrocarbons. 3. The van Der Waals' potentials and crystal data for aliphatic and aromatic hydrocarbons. *J. Am. Chem. Soc.* 111, 8576–8582. doi: 10.1021/ja00205a003

Lin, F. Y., and MacKerell, A. D. (2018). Polarizable empirical force field for halogen-containing compounds based on the classical drude oscillator. *J. Chem. Theory Comput.* 14, 1083–1098. doi: 10.1021/acs.jctc.7b01086

Lu, Y., Liu, Y., Xu, Z., Li, H., Liu, H., and Zhu, W. (2012). Halogen bonding for rational drug design and new drug discovery. *Expert Opin. Drug Discov.* 7, 375–383. doi: 10.1517/17460441.2012.678829

Lu, Y., Shi, T., Wang, Y., Yang, H., Yan, X., Luo, X., et al. (2009). Halogen bonding-a novel interaction for rational drug design? *J. Med. Chem.* 52, 2854–2862. doi: 10.1021/jm9000133

Lu, Y., Wang, Y., and Zhu, W. (2010). Nonbonding interactions of organic halogens in biological systems: implications for drug discovery and biomolecular design. *Phys. Chem. Chem. Phys.* 12, 4543–4551. doi: 10.1039/b926326h

Malde, A. K., Zuo, L., Breeze, M., Stroet, M., Poger, D., Nair, P. C., et al. (2011). An automated force field topology builder (ATB) and repository: version 1.0. *J. Chem. Theory Comput.* 7, 4026–4037. doi: 10.1021/ct200196m

Martins, T. L. C., Ramalho, T. C., Figueroa-Villar, J. D., Flores, A. F. C., and Pereira, C. M. P. (2003). Theoretical and experimental ^{13}C and ^{15}N NMR investigation of guanylhydrazones in solution. *Magn. Reson. Chem.* 41, 983–988. doi: 10.1002/mrc.1299

Mayne, C. G., Saam, J., Schulten, K., Tajkhorshid, E., and Gumbart, J. C. (2013). Rapid parameterization of small molecules using the force field toolkit. *J. Comput. Chem.* 34, 2757–2770. doi: 10.1002/jcc.23422

McDaniel, J. G., Choi, E., Son, C. Y., Schmidt, J. R., and Yethiraj, A. (2016). *Ab Initio* force fields for imidazolium-based ionic liquids. *J. Phys. Chem. B* 120, 7024–7036. doi: 10.1021/acs.jpcb.6b05328

Mendez, L., Henriquez, G., Sirimulla, S., and Narayan, M. (2017). Looking back, looking forward at halogen bonding in drug discovery. *Molecules* 22, 22–25. doi: 10.3390/molecules22091397

Nair, P. C., and Miners, J. O. (2014). Molecular dynamics simulations: from structure function relationships to drug discovery. *In Silico Pharmacol.* 2:4. doi: 10.1186/s40203-014-0004-8

Nevins, N., Chen, K., and Allinger, N. L. (1996). Molecular mechanics (MM4) calculations on alkenes. *J. Comput. Chem.* 17, 669–694. doi: 10.1002/(SICI)1096-987X(199604)17:5/6<;669::AID-JCC7>;3.0.CO;2-S

Novák, M., Foroutan-Nejad, C., and Marek, R. (2015). Asymmetric bifurcated halogen bonds. *Phys. Chem. Chem. Phys.* 17, 6440–6450. doi: 10.1039/C4CP05532B

Nunes, R., Vila-Viçosa, D., Machuqueiro, M., and Costa, P. J. (2018). Biomolecular simulations of halogen bonds with a GROMOS force field. *J. Chem. Theory Comput.* 14, 5383–5392. doi: 10.1021/acs.jctc.8b00278

Nziko, V. P. N., and Scheiner, N. (2016). Comparison of π-hole tetrel bonding with σ-hole halogen bonds in complexes of XCN (X = F, Cl, Br, I) and NH_3. *Phys. Chem. Chem. Phys.* 18, 3581–3590. doi: 10.1039/C5CP07545A

Paschek, D., and Geiger, A. (2002). *MOSCITO 4.* Dortmund: Department of Physical Chemistry; University of Dortmund.

Pérez-Conesa, S., Torrico, F., Martínez, J. M., Pappalardo, R. R., and Marcos, E. S. (2019). A general study of actinyl hydration by molecular dynamics simulations using *ab initio* force fields. *J. Chem. Phys.* 150:104504. doi: 10.1063/1.5083216

Poater, J., Swart, M., Fonseca Guerra, C., and Bickelhaupt, F. M. (2011). Selectivity in DNA replication. interplay of steric shape, hydrogen bonds, π-stacking and solvent effects. *Chem. Commun.* 47, 7326–7328. doi: 10.1039/c0cc04707d

Politzer, P., Lane, P., Concha, M. C., Ma, Y., and Murray, J. S. (2007). An overview of halogen bonding. *J. Mol. Model.* 13, 305–311. doi: 10.1007/s00894-006-0154-7

Politzer, P., Murray, J. S., and Clark, T. (2013). Halogen bonding and other σ-hole interactions: a perspective. *Phys. Chem. Chem. Phys.* 15, 11178–11189. doi: 10.1039/c3cp00054k

Politzer, P., Murray, J. S., and Concha, M. C. (2008). σ-hole bonding between like atoms; a fallacy of atomic charges. *J. Mol. Model.* 14, 659–665. doi: 10.1007/s00894-008-0280-5

Politzer, P., Riley, K. E., Bulat, F. A., and Murray, J. S. (2012). Perspectives on halogen bonding and other σ-hole interactions: lex parsimoniae (Occam's Razor). *Comput. Theor. Chem.* 998, 2–8. doi: 10.1016/j.comptc.2012.06.007

Poznanski, J., and Shugar, D. (2013). Halogen bonding at the ATP binding site of protein kinases: preferred geometry and topology of ligand binding. *Biochim. Biophys. Acta* 1834, 1381–1396. doi: 10.1016/j.bbapap.2013.01.026

Prandi, I. G., Viani, L., Andreussi, O., and Mennucci, B. (2016). Combining classical molecular dynamics and quantum mechanical methods for the description of electronic excitations: the case of carotenoids. *J. Comput. Chem.* 37, 981–991. doi: 10.1002/jcc.24286

Ramalho, T. C., and da Cunha, E. F. F. (2011). Thermodynamic framework of the interaction between protein and solvent drives protein folding. *J. Biomol. Struct. Dyn.* 28, 645–646. doi: 10.1080/073911011010524975

Ramalho, T. C., Rocha, M. V. J., da Cunha, E. F. F., and Freitas, M. P. (2009). The search for new COX-2 inhibitors: a review of 2002-2008 patents. *Expert Opin. Ther. Pat.* 19, 1193–1228. doi: 10.1517/13543770903059125

Rendine, S., Pieraccini, S., Forni, A., and Sironi, M. (2011). Halogen bonding in ligand–receptor systems in the framework of classical force fields. *Phys. Chem. Chem. Phys.* 13, 19508–19516. doi: 10.1039/c1cp22436k

Riley, K. E., Murray, J. S., Politzer, P., Concha, M. C., and Hobza, P. (2009). Br... O complexes as probes of factors affecting halogen bonding: interactions of bromobenzenes and bromopyrimidines with acetone. *J. Chem. Theory Comput.* 5, 155–163. doi: 10.1021/ct8004134

Riley, K. E., Řezáč, J., and Hobza, P. (2013). Competition between halogen dihalogen and hydrogen bonds in bromo- and iodomethanol dimers. *J. Mol. Model.* 19, 2879–2883. doi: 10.1007/s00894-012-1727-2

Santos, L. A., da Cunha, E. F. F., Freitas, M. P., and Ramalho, T. C. (2014). Hydrophobic noncovalent interactions of inosine-phenylalanine: a theoretical model for investigating the molecular recognition of nucleobases. *J. Phys. Chem. A* 118, 5808–5817. doi: 10.1021/jp411230w

Santos, L. A., da Cunha, E. F. F., and Ramalho, T. C. (2017). Toward the classical description of halogen bonds: a quantum based generalized empirical potential for fluorine, chlorine, and bromine. *J. Phys. Chem. A* 121, 2442–2451. doi: 10.1021/acs.jpca.6b13112

Scholfield, M. R., Ford, M. C., Vander Zanden, C. M., Billman, M. M., Ho, P. S., and Rappé, A. K. (2015). Force field model of periodic trends in biomolecular halogen bonds. *J. Phys. Chem. B* 119, 9140–9149. doi: 10.1021/jp509003r

Schuler, L. D., Daura, X., and van Gunsteren, W. F. (2001). An improved GROMOS96 force field for aliphatic hydrocarbons in the condensed phase. *J. Comput. Chem.* 22, 1205–1218. doi: 10.1002/jcc.1078

Soteras Gutiérrez, I., Lin, F. Y., Vanommeslaeghe, K., Lemkul, J. A., Armacost, K. A., Brooks, C. L., et al. (2016). Parametrization of halogen bonds in the CHARMM general force field: improved treatment of ligand–protein interactions. *Bioorg. Med. Chem.* 24, 4812–4825. doi: 10.1016/j.bmc.2016.06.034

van der Spoel, D., Lindahl, E., Hess, B., Groenhof, G., Mark, A. E., and Berendsen, H. J. C. (2005). GROMACS: fast, flexible, and free. *J. Comput. Chem.* 26, 1701–1718. doi: 10.1002/jcc.20291

Vanommeslaeghe, K., Hatcher, E., Acharya, C., Kundu, S., Zhong, S., Shim, J., et al. (2010). CHARMM general force field: a force field for drug-like molecules compatible with the CHARMM all-atom additive biological force fields. *J. Comput. Chem.* 31, 671–690. doi: 10.1002/jcc.21367

Wang, C., Danovich, D., Mo, Y., and Shaik, S. (2014). On the nature of the halogen bond. *J. Chem. Theory Comput.* 10, 3726–3737. doi: 10.1021/ct500422t

Wang, J., Wolf, R. M., Caldwell, J. W., Kollman, P. A., and Case, D. A. (2004). Development and testing of a general amber force field. *J. Comput. Chem.* 25, 1157–1174. doi: 10.1002/jcc.20035

Wilcken, R., Zimmermann, M. O., Lange, A., Joerger, A. C., and Boeckler, F. M. (2013). Principles and applicationsof halogen bonding in medicinal chemistry and chemical biology. *J. Med. Chem.* 56, 1363–1388. doi: 10.1021/jm3012068

Wolters, L. P., and Bickelhaupt, F. M. (2012). Halogen bonding versus hydrogen bonding: a molecular orbital perspective. *Chem. Open* 1, 96–105. doi: 10.1002/open.201100015

Wolters, L. P., Schyman, P., Pavan, M. J., Jorgensen, W. L., Bickelhaupt, F. M., and Kozuch, S. (2014). The many faces of halogen bonding: a review of theoretical models and methods. *Wiley Interdiscip. Rev. Comput. Mol. Sci.* 4, 523–540. doi: 10.1002/wcms.1189

Wolters, L. P., Smits, N. W. G., and Fonseca Guerra, C. (2015). Covalency in resonance-assisted halogen bonds demonstrated with cooperativity in *n*-halo-guanine quartets. *Phys. Chem. Chem. Phys.* 17, 1585–1592. doi: 10.1039/C4CP03740E

Wu, X., Sun, Y., Li, C., and Yang, W. (2012). Parametric effects of the potential energy function on the geometrical features of ternary Lennard-Jones clusters. *J. Phys. Chem. A* 116, 8218–8225. doi: 10.1021/jp3037395

Xu, P., Guidez, E. B., Bertoni, C., and Gordon, M. S. (2018). Perspective: *ab initio* force field methods derived from quantum mechanics. *J. Chem. Phys.* 148:090901. doi: 10.1063/1.5009551

10

Docking, Interaction Fingerprint and Three-Dimensional Quantitative Structure–Activity Relationship (3D-QSAR) of Sigma1 Receptor Ligands, Analogs of the Neuroprotective Agent RC-33

José Luis Velázquez-Libera [1], Giacomo Rossino [2], Carlos Navarro-Retamal [1], Simona Collina [2] and Julio Caballero [1]*

[1] *Centro de Bioinformática y Simulación Molecular, Facultad de Ingeniería, Universidad de Talca, Talca, Chile,*
[2] *Pharmaceutical and Medicinal Chemistry Section, Drug Sciences Department, Università di Pavia, Pavia, Italy*

Correspondence:
Julio Caballero
jcaballero@utalca.cl

The human Sigma1 receptor (S1R), which has been identified as a target with an important role in neuropsychological disorders, was first crystallized 3 years ago. Since S1R structure has no relation with another previous crystallized structures, the presence of the new crystal is an important hallmark for the design of agonists and antagonists against this important target. Some years ago, our group identified RC-33, a potent and selective S1R agonist, endowed with neuroprotective properties. In this work, drawing on new structural information, we studied the interactions of RC-33 and its analogs with the S1R binding site by using computational methods such as docking, interaction fingerprints, and receptor-guided alignment three dimensional quantitative structure–activity relationship (3D-QSAR). We found that RC-33 and its analogs adopted similar orientations within S1R binding site, with high similitude with orientations of the crystallized ligands; such information was used for identifying the residues involved in chemical interactions with ligands. Furthermore, the structure-activity relationship of the studied ligands was adequately described considering classical QSAR tests. All relevant aspects of the interactions between the studied compounds and S1R were covered here, through descriptions of orientations, binding interactions, and features that influence differential affinities. In this sense, the present results could be useful in the future design of novel S1R modulators.

Keywords: sigma1 receptor ligands, RC-33, arylalkylamine derivates, docking, quantitative structure–activity relationships, interaction fingerprints

INTRODUCTION

The Sigma receptors (SR) have attracted the interest of the scientific community thoroughly in the last decades owing to their potential role in cell survival and function modulation (Walker et al., 1990; Chu and Ruoho, 2016). They were originally misclassified as a subtype of opioid receptors (Martin et al., 1976), but they were later classified as unique class of intracellular proteins, distinct from other receptors such as GPCRs (G protein-coupled receptors). Sigma receptors (SRs), comprise two subtypes σ_1 and σ_2 receptors (S1R and S2R, respectively) associated with aging- and mitochondria-associated disorders (Tesei et al., 2018). Both subtypes are highly expressed in the central nervous system, but they are derived from completely different genes. S1R was cloned in 1996 (Hanner et al., 1996) and was crystallized for the first time 3 years ago, in 2016 (Schmidt et al., 2016), whereas S2R was cloned only very recently, in 2017, by Alon et al. (2017).

S1R is an intracellular modulator between the endoplasmic reticulum and the mitochondria, the cell nuclei, the membrane, and it also modulates intracellular signaling. It plays a key role in neuropsychological disorders such as depression, enhances the glutamatergic neurotransmission (DeCoster et al., 1995; Meyer et al., 2002), and modulates second messenger systems, such as the phospholipase C/protein kinase C/inositol 1,4,5-trisphosphate system (Morin-Surun et al., 1999). Multiple biological roles of S1R have been identified, which made this protein a relevant target for the future treatment of epilepsy, schizophrenia, sclerosis, Alzheimer, and Parkinson's diseases, cancer, etc. (Mishina et al., 2005; Hashimoto, 2009; Furuse and Hashimoto, 2010; Mavlyutov et al., 2015; Vavers et al., 2017; Tesei et al., 2018). Moreover, S1R agonists enhanced neuroplasticity, and may be effective in amyotrophic lateral sclerosis (Peviani et al., 2014) and multiple sclerosis (Collina et al., 2017b).

Not less important, preclinical studies carried out on different models of memory impairment have revealed that S1R ligands could be promising drugs to treat cognitive dysfunctions (Hayashi and Su, 2004; Monnet and Maurice, 2006; Yagasaki et al., 2006; Collina et al., 2017a). Therefore, the identification of potent and selective S1R modulators is of great interest to develop novel therapeutic strategies focused mainly in the treatment of central nervous system disorders. The list of S1R ligands in the last years includes thioxanthene-derived compounds (Glennon et al., 2004), fenpropimorph-derived analogs (Hajipour et al., 2010), 2(3*H*)-benzothiazolones (Yous et al., 2005), cyclopropylmethylamines (Prezzavento et al., 2007), benzo[d]oxazol-2(3H)-one derivatives (Zampieri et al., 2009), etc. All these compounds were developed when the three-dimensional (3D) structure of S1R was unknown. Despite this, the pharmacophoric features of S1R were identified and these compounds comply with the general accepted pharmacophoric pattern. It was demonstrated that at least one N positively charged atom is important for binding at sigma receptors and this atom must be flanked by two hydrophobic regions of different sizes (Ablordeppey et al., 2000; Glennon, 2005; Caballero et al., 2012).

In the last years, we designed and synthesized compounds that comply with the proposed pharmacophore model and evaluated them as S1R ligands (Collina et al., 2007; Urbano et al., 2007; Rossi et al., 2010, 2011), leading to the finding of compound RC-33 as a potent and selective S1R agonist (Rossi et al., 2013a; Marra et al., 2016). The structure-activity relationship (SAR) of the majority of these compounds was previously described by us by using 2D-QSAR methodologies (Quesada-Romero et al., 2015). With the recent report of the S1R 3D structure (Schmidt et al., 2016), structure-based molecular modeling methods could be used to investigate S1R ligands with a new glance. With this in mind, we propose in this work the analysis of the SAR of RC-33 and its analogs (in total there were 80 compounds) by combining docking and a 3D-QSAR methodology. This is the first study focused on describing the SAR of S1R ligands by using structure-based molecular modeling methods, after the report of the crystallographic structure of this important biological target.

MATERIALS AND METHODS

Dataset Preparation

The studied compounds were extracted from references (Collina et al., 2007; Urbano et al., 2007; Rossi et al., 2010, 2011, 2015, 2017; Rui et al., 2016). This dataset yielded a total of 80 compounds with reported activities as Ki ranging from 0.00069 to 1 μM. Ki values were converted into logarithmic pKi values prior 3D-QSAR models' elaboration. The compound chemical structures and their pKi values are depicted in **Table 1**. The molecular structures were sketched using Maestro's molecular editor (Maestro 10.2.011, Schrödinger LLC). Thereafter, the 3D structures were obtained with the help of the LigPrep module (LigPrep, Maestro 10.2.011, Schrödinger LLC); ionization states were generated at pH 7.0 $\pm$ 2.0 using Epik (Shelley et al., 2007). For compounds containing two possible enantiomers which are reported in racemic form, the *R* enantiomer was chosen for QSAR experiments because it was determined that both RC-33 enantiomers showed similar affinities for the S1R and they are almost equally effective as S1R agonists (Rossi et al., 2013b). However, both enantiomers were chosen for docking experiments to explore the interactions in the S1R binding site.

Molecular Docking

The ligand-receptor molecular docking experiments of RC-33 analogs into the active site of S1R were performed by using the software Glide from the Schrödinger suite (Friesner et al., 2004). Glide is one of the most effective docking programs at this moment with many successful applications relating to rational design of novel drugs and investigation of protein-ligand interactions. Such applications encompass *in silico* search of novel drugs (Osguthorpe et al., 2012; Amaning et al., 2013), analysis of the SAR of congeneric series of compounds (Almerico et al., 2012; Quesada-Romero and Caballero, 2014; Quesada-Romero et al., 2014; Mena-Ulecia et al., 2015), evaluation of enzymatic reaction pathways (Wu et al., 2011; Batra et al., 2013), etc.

Protein coordinates were extracted from the crystal structure of S1R bound to the selective antagonist PD144418 (code 5HK1 in Protein Data Bank) (Schmidt et al., 2016). A grid box of 20 × 20 × 20Å was centered on the center of mass of the ligand in this crystal structure covering the binding site of S1R. Glide standard (SP) and extra-precision (XP) modes were employed with the same protocol and parameters that were used by us in previous works (Quesada-Romero and Caballero, 2014; Quesada-Romero et al., 2014; Mena-Ulecia et al., 2015). Glide SP was used to evaluate the capability of the Glide method to obtain poses that fit the known pharmacophore of S1R ligands,

TABLE 1 | Structures of RC-33 analogs as S1R ligands.

ID	Structure	Experimental pKi[b]	Predicted pKi[b]	References
1 (RC-33)	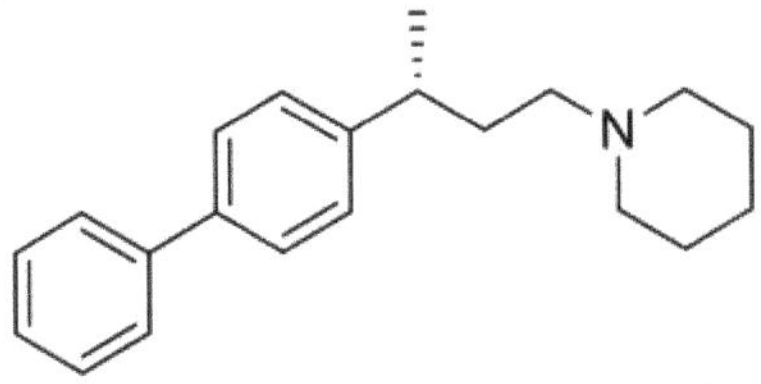	9.16	9.37	Rossi et al., 2011
2	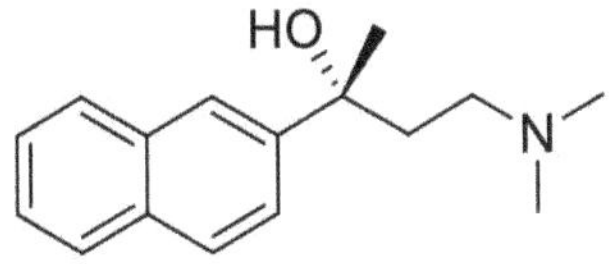	7.60	7.54	Collina et al., 2007
3	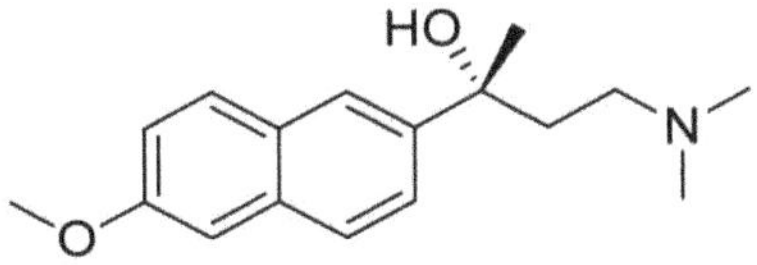	7.41	7.49	Rossi et al., 2010
4	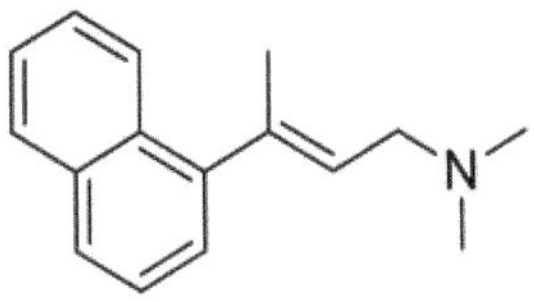	6.99	6.96	Collina et al., 2007
5	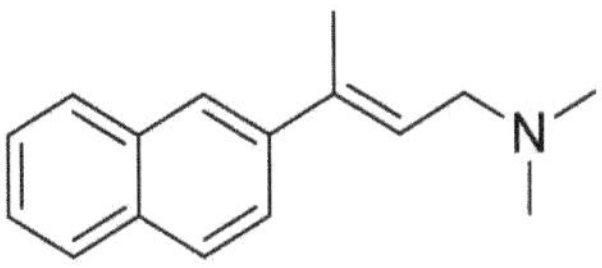	7.70	7.62	Collina et al., 2007
6	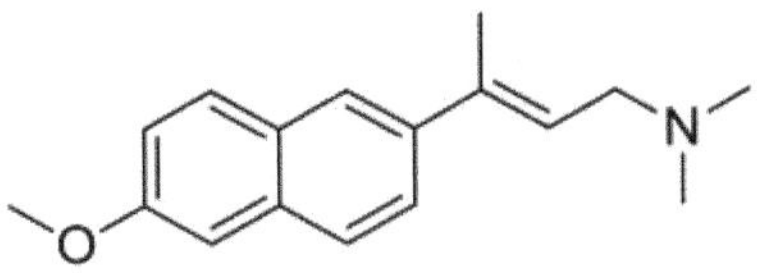	7.67	7.44	Collina et al., 2007
7	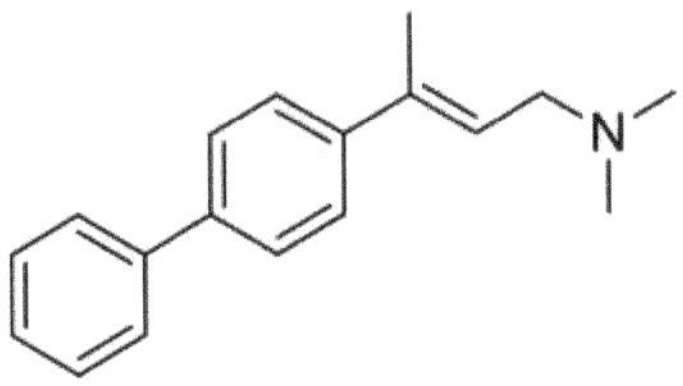	8.85	8.73	Rossi et al., 2011
8[a]	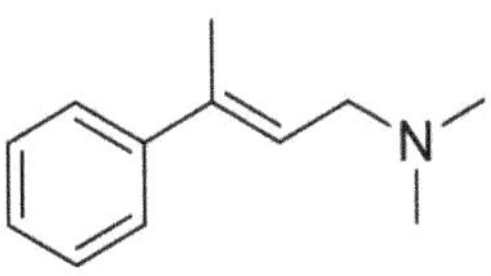	6.00	6.79	Rossi et al., 2011
9	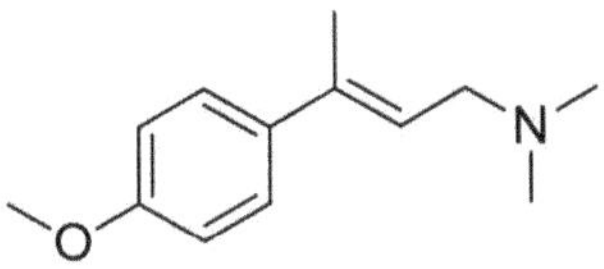	6.09	6.23	Rossi et al., 2011
10	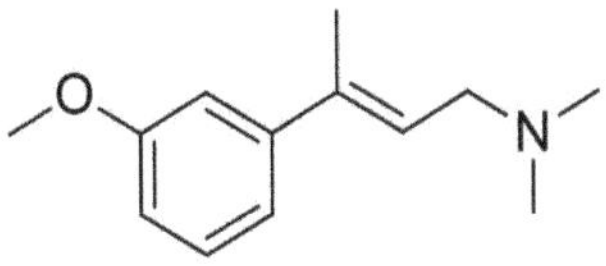	6.00	6.14	Rossi et al., 2011

(Continued)

TABLE 1 | Continued

ID	Structure	Experimental pKi[b]	Predicted pKi[b]	References
11	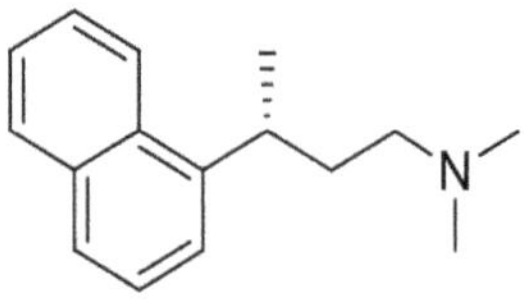	7.33	7.11	Collina et al., 2007
12[a]	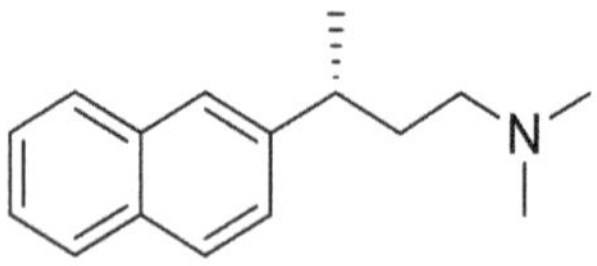	8.71	7.99	Collina et al., 2007
13	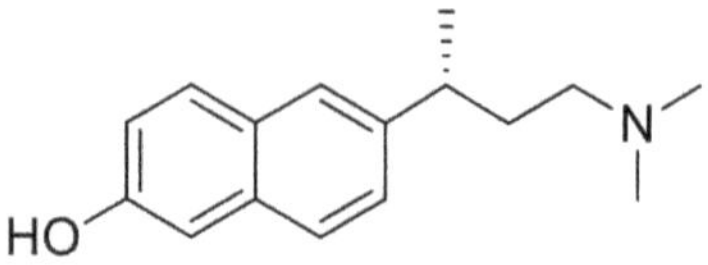	7.72	7.65	Collina et al., 2007
14	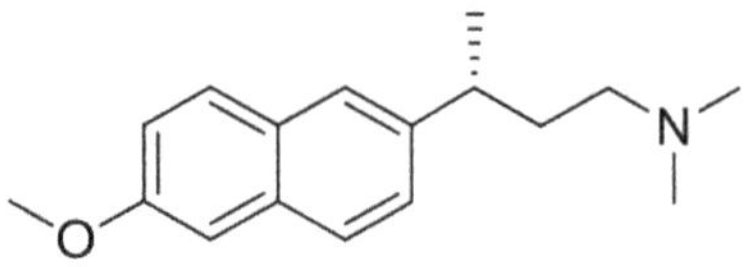	8.64	8.41	Collina et al., 2007
15	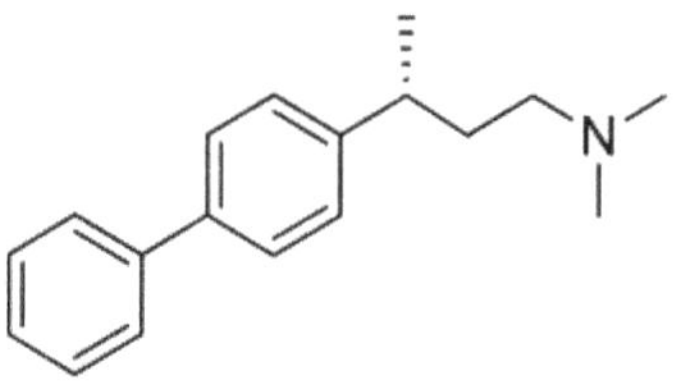	8.99	9.05	Collina et al., 2007
16	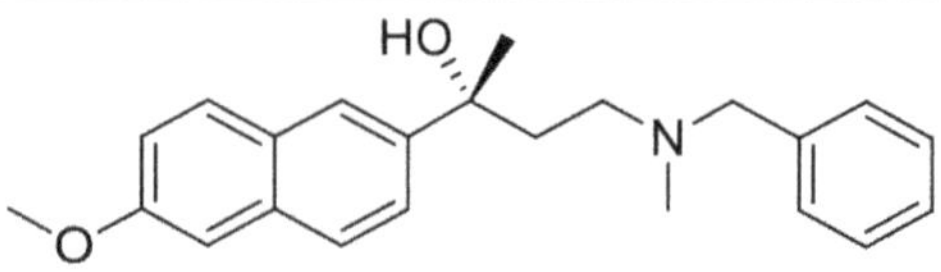	8.22	8.10	Rossi et al., 2010
17	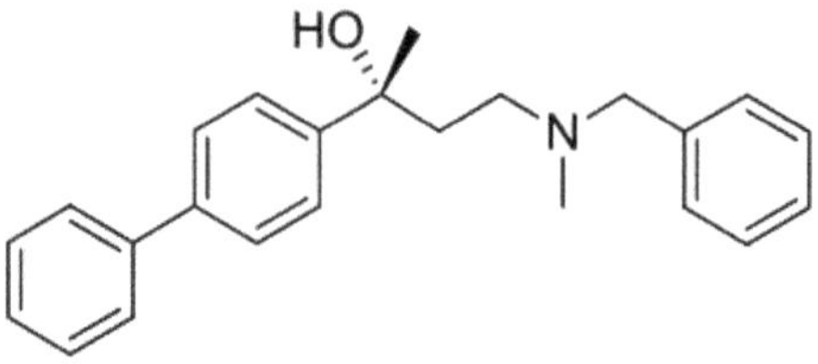	8.62	8.26	Rossi et al., 2010
18	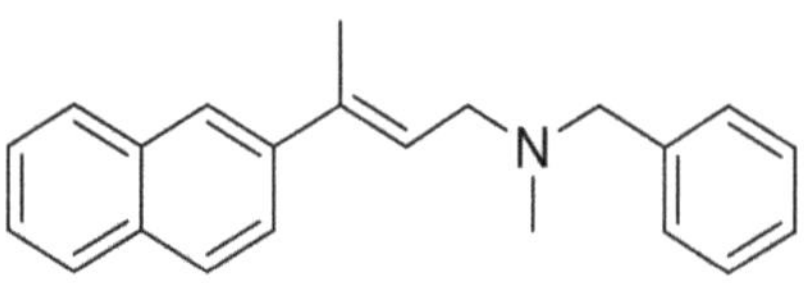	8.10	8.09	Collina et al., 2007
19	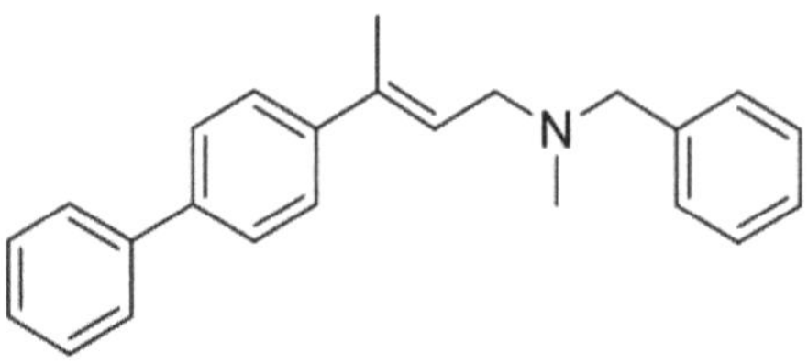	8.20	8.29	Collina et al., 2007

(Continued)

TABLE 1 | Continued

ID	Structure	Experimental pKi[b]	Predicted pKi[b]	References
20	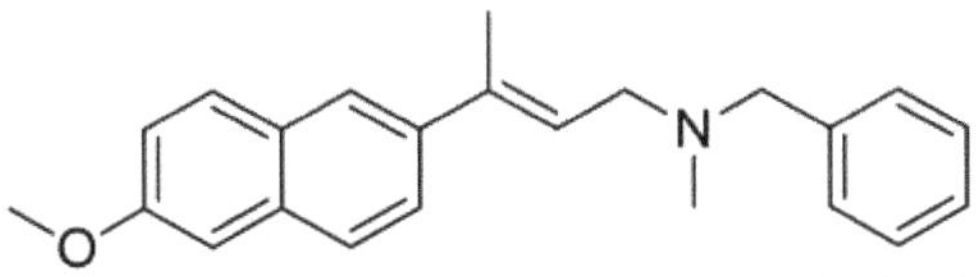	7.86	8.22	Rossi et al., 2010
21	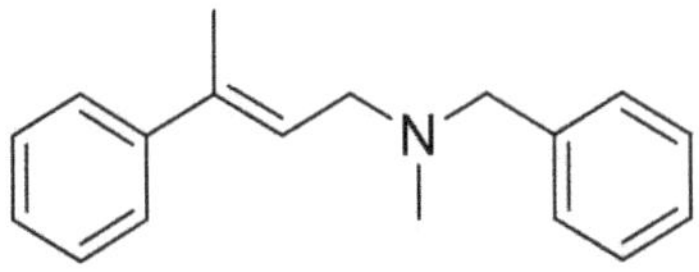	7.04	7.06	Collina et al., 2007
22	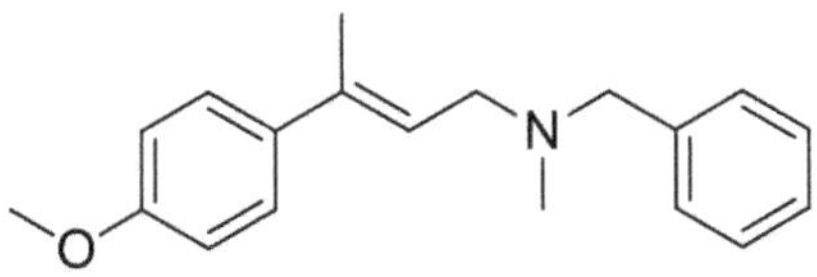	8.28	8.11	Collina et al., 2007
23[a]	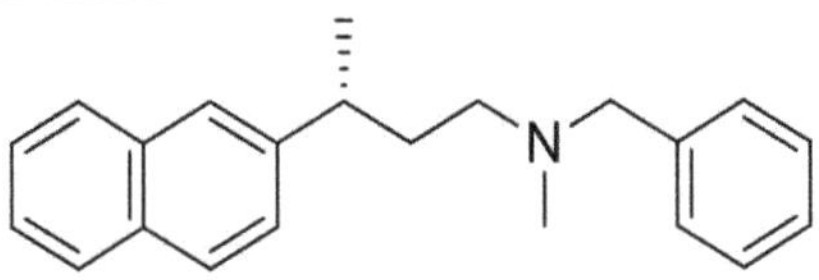	8.27	8.96	Collina et al., 2007
24	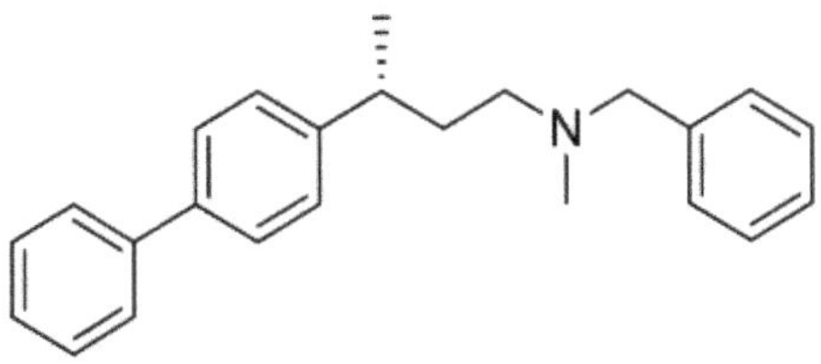	8.24	8.30	Collina et al., 2007
25	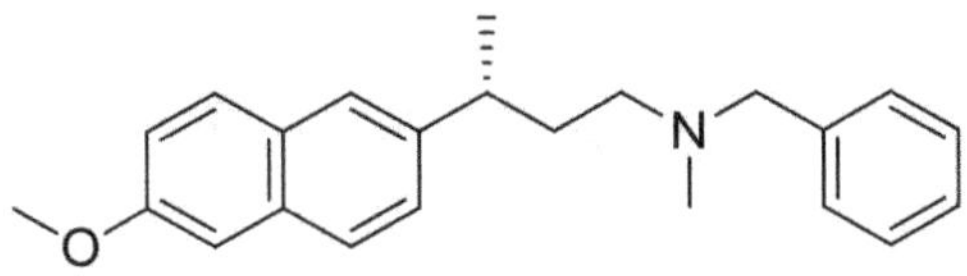	8.64	8.52	Rossi et al., 2010
26	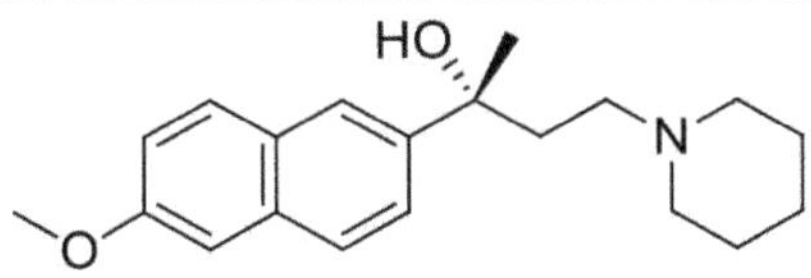	7.98	8.01	Rossi et al., 2010
27	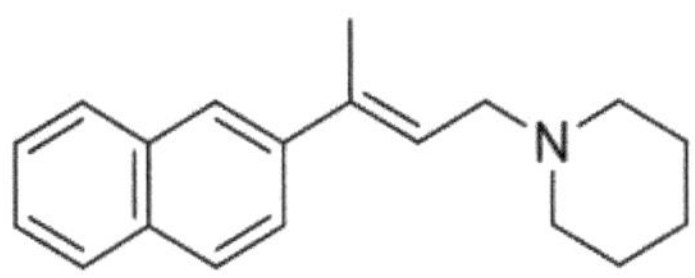	9.01	8.79	Rossi et al., 2011
28	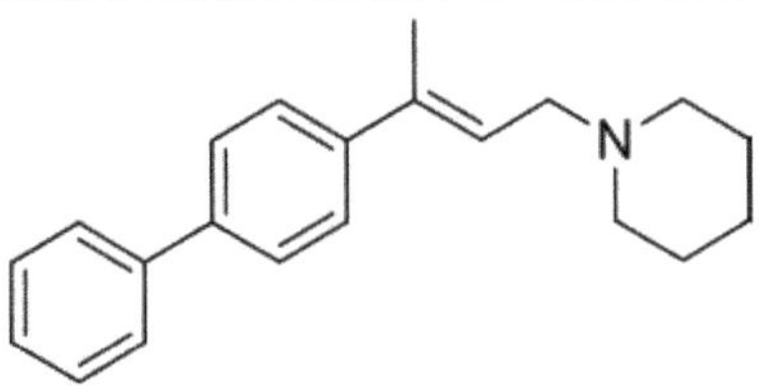	9.07	9.22	Rossi et al., 2011

(Continued)

TABLE 1 | Continued

ID	Structure	Experimental pKi[b]	Predicted pKi[b]	References
29[a]	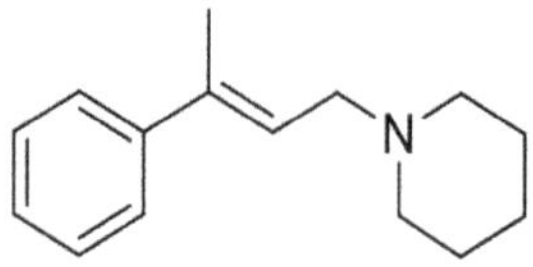	6.34	6.23	Rossi et al., 2011
30	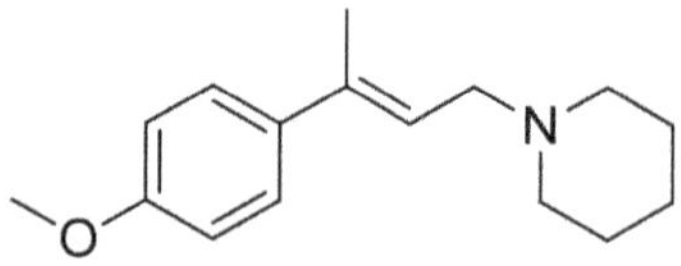	7.85	7.67	Rossi et al., 2011
31	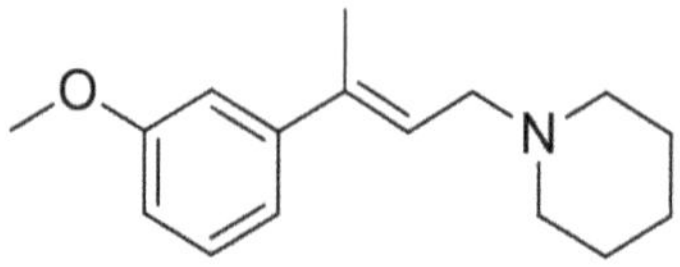	7.04	7.10	Rossi et al., 2011
32	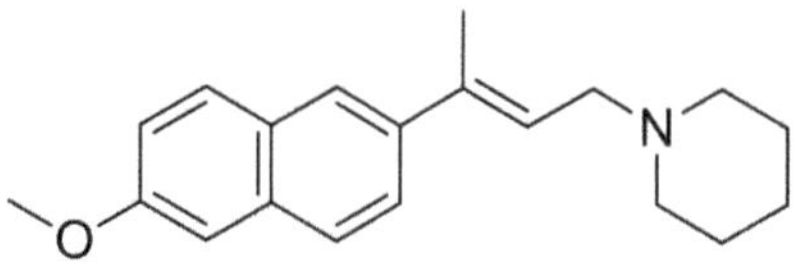	8.36	8.62	Rossi et al., 2010
33	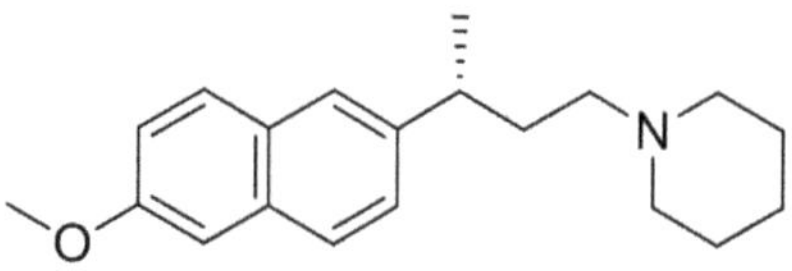	8.89	8.99	Rossi et al., 2010
34[a]	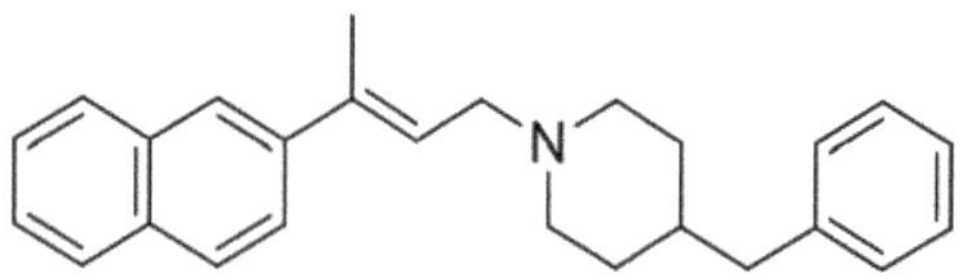	7.64	7.65	Rossi et al., 2011
35	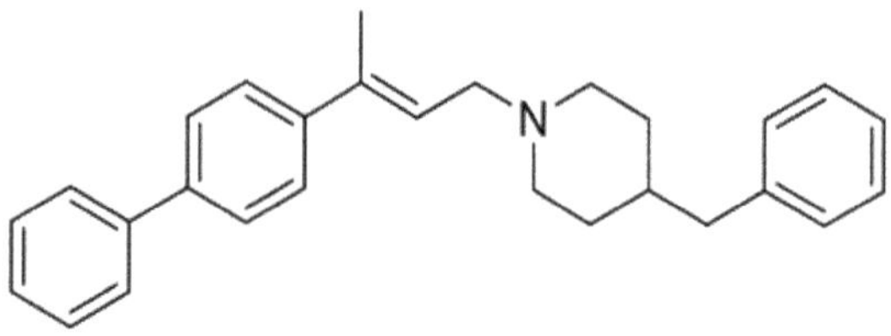	8.15	8.20	Rossi et al., 2011
36[a]	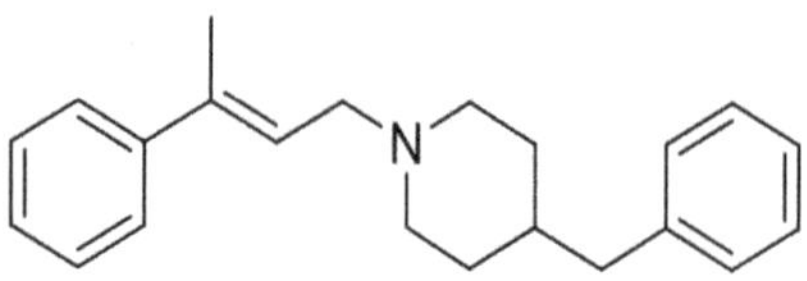	8.97	8.56	Rossi et al., 2011
37[a]	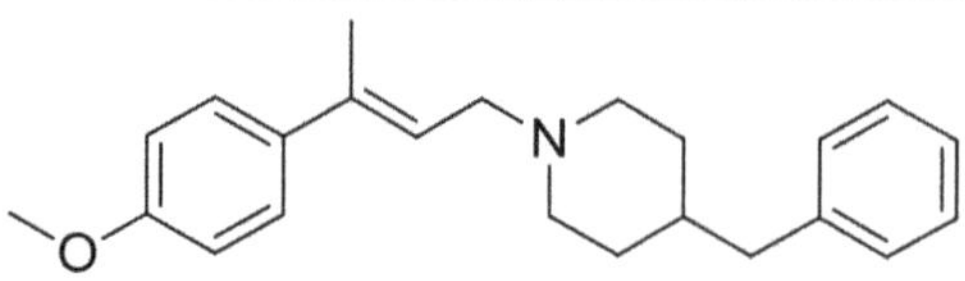	8.38	8.28	Rossi et al., 2011
38[a]	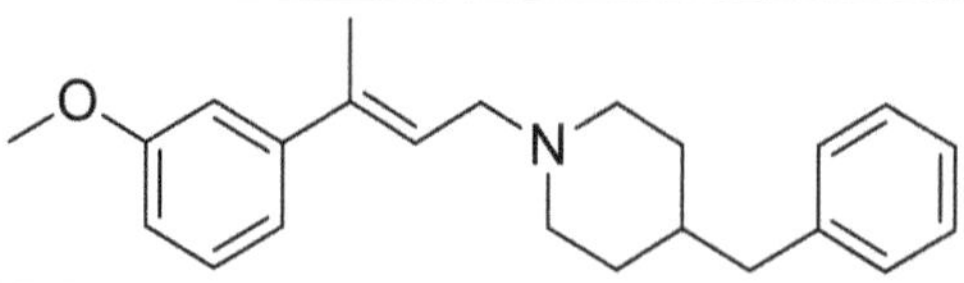	8.11	7.40	Rossi et al., 2011

(Continued)

TABLE 1 | Continued

ID	Structure	Experimental pKi[b]	Predicted pKi[b]	References
39	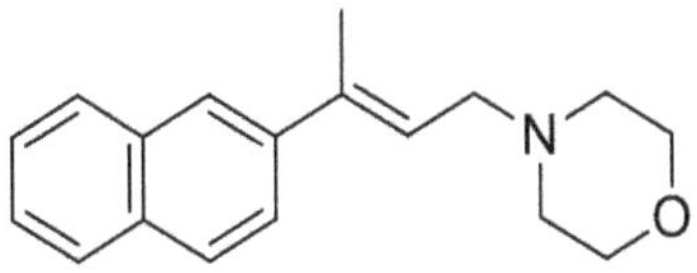	8.02	8.04	Rossi et al., 2011
40	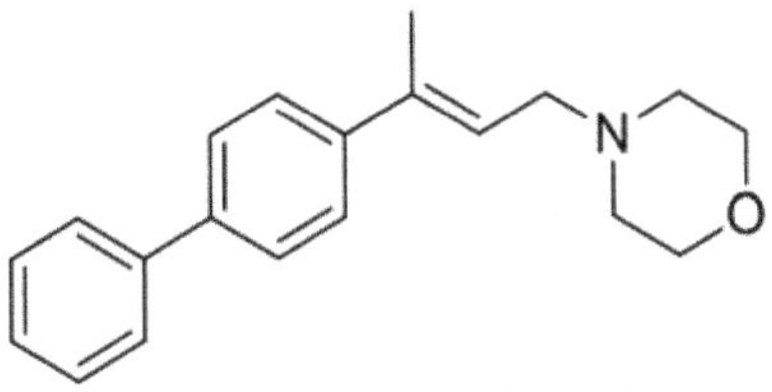	7.94	7.83	Rossi et al., 2011
41	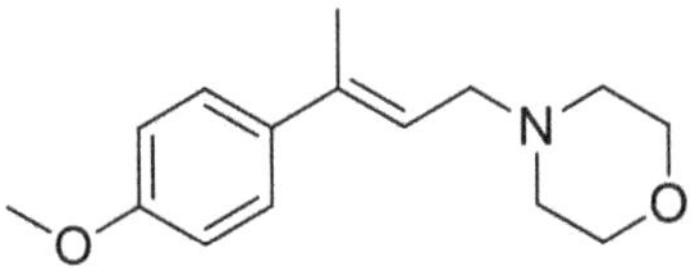	6.00	6.38	Rossi et al., 2011
42	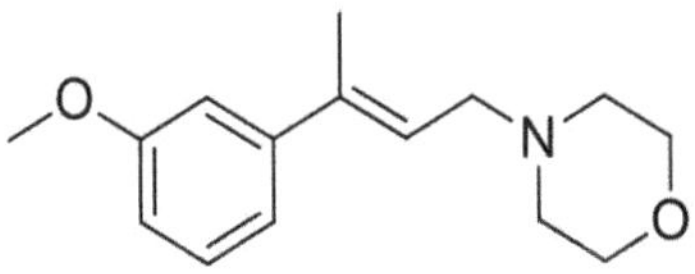	6.00	5.98	Rossi et al., 2011
43[a]	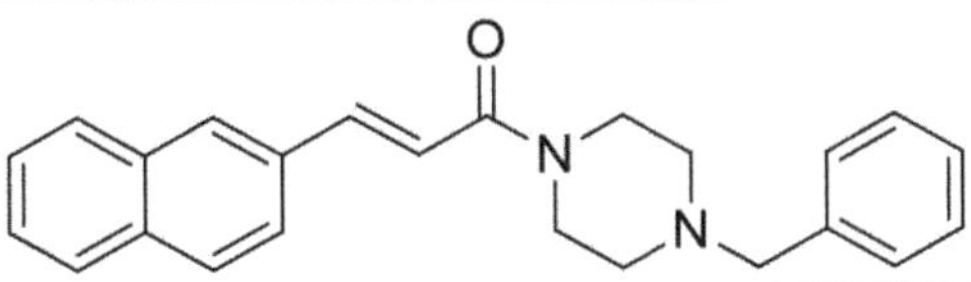	6.00	7.29	Urbano et al., 2007
44	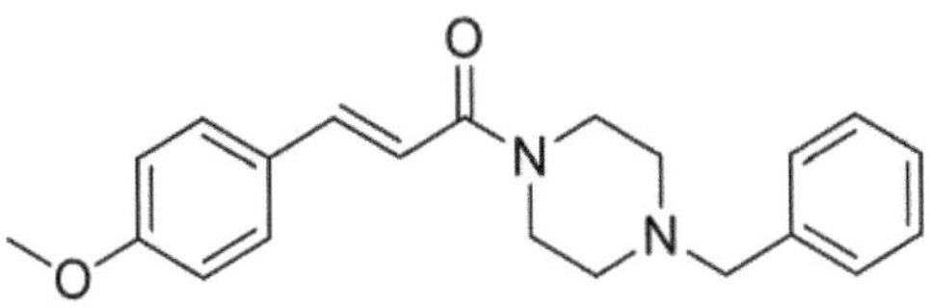	6.00	6.03	Urbano et al., 2007
45	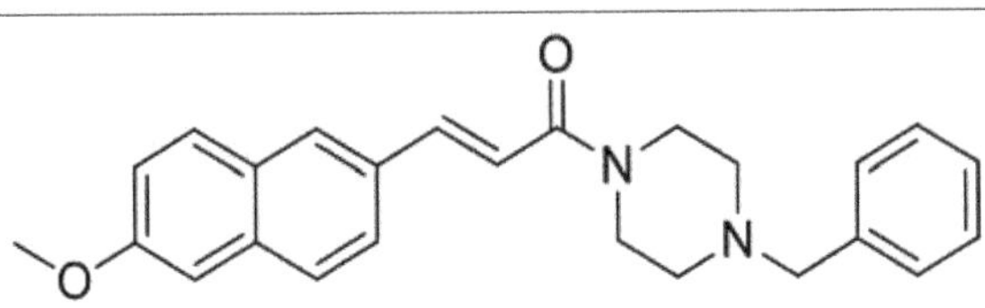	6.00	6.16	Urbano et al., 2007
46	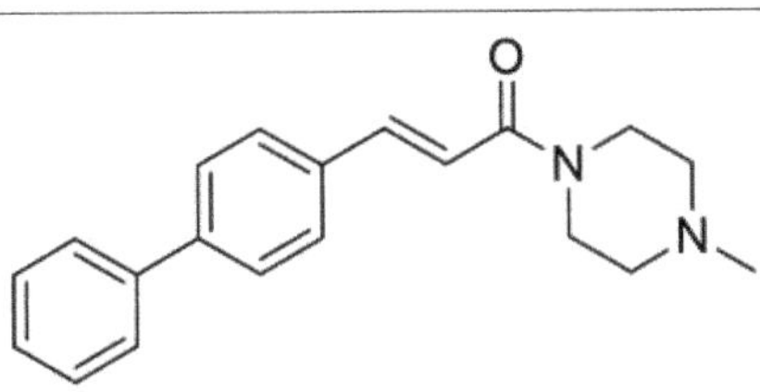	6.00	5.78	Urbano et al., 2007
47[a]	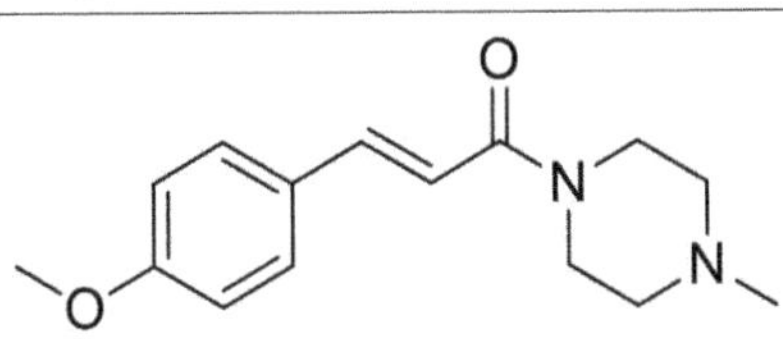	6.00	6.36	Urbano et al., 2007

(Continued)

TABLE 1 | Continued

ID	Structure	Experimental pKi[b]	Predicted pKi[b]	References
48	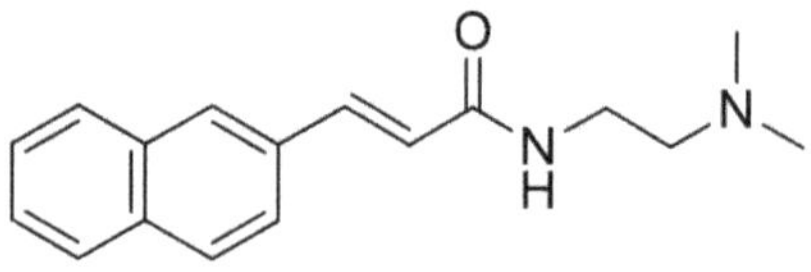	6.00	5.89	Urbano et al., 2007
49	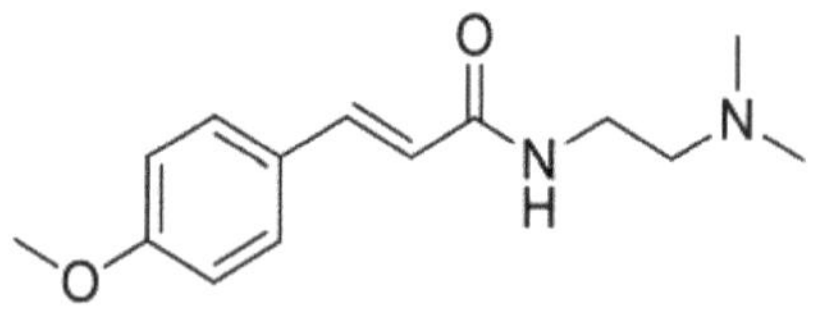	6.00	5.75	Urbano et al., 2007
50	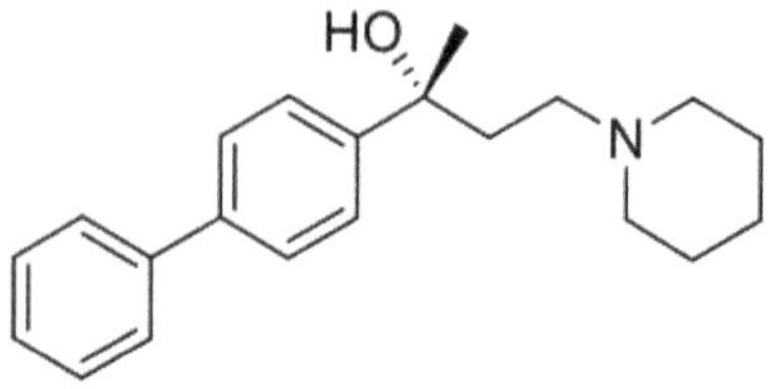	7.41	7.52	Rossi et al., 2015
51	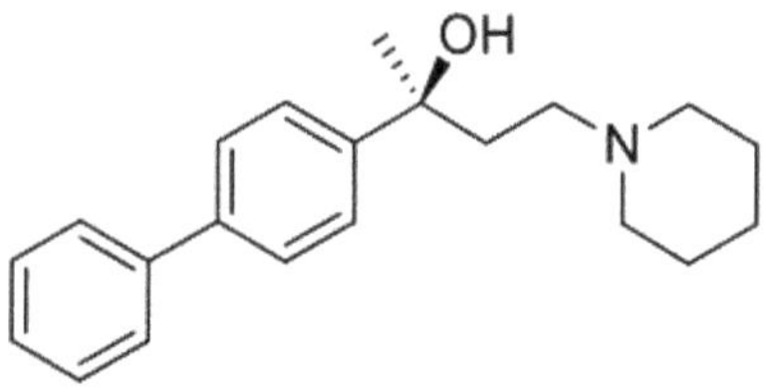	8.33	8.37	Rossi et al., 2015
52	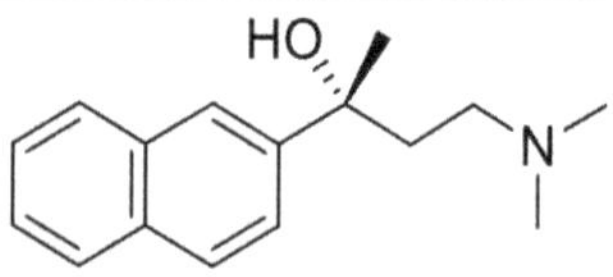	6.69	6.81	Rossi et al., 2015
53	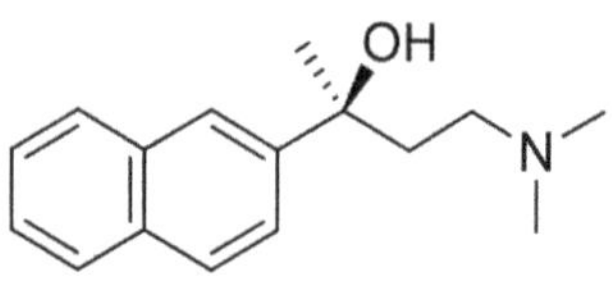	7.20	7.40	Rossi et al., 2015
54[a]	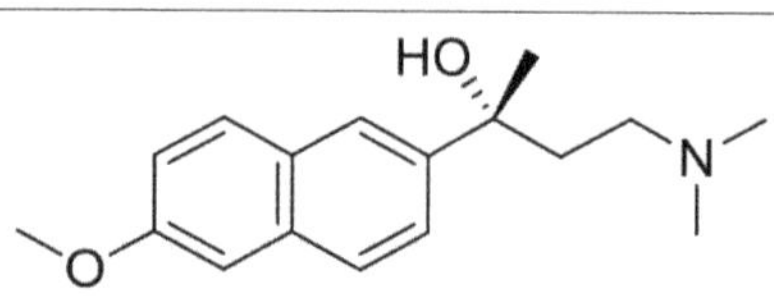	7.29	7.44	Rossi et al., 2015
55	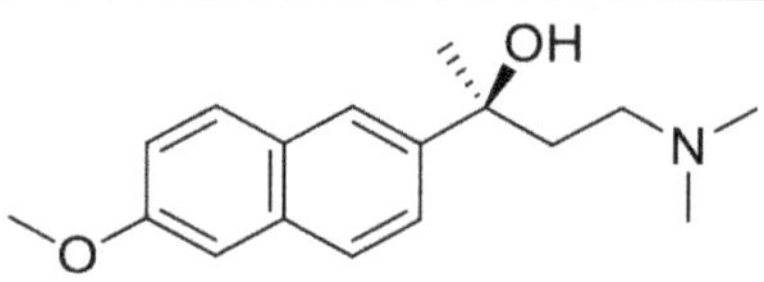	7.60	7.90	Rossi et al., 2015
56	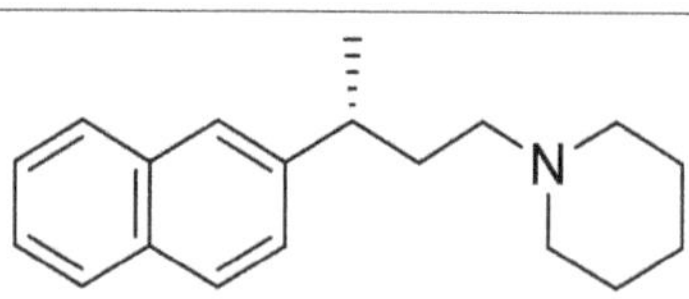	8.82	8.57	Rossi et al., 2017

(Continued)

TABLE 1 | Continued

ID	Structure	Experimental pKi[b]	Predicted pKi[b]	References
57	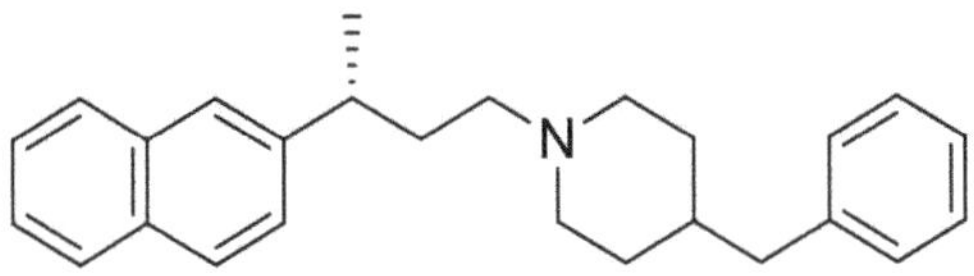	8.22	8.29	Rossi et al., 2017
58	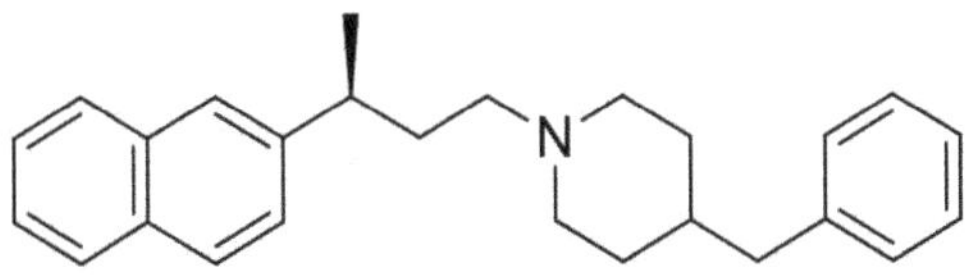	8.16	8.14	Rossi et al., 2017
59	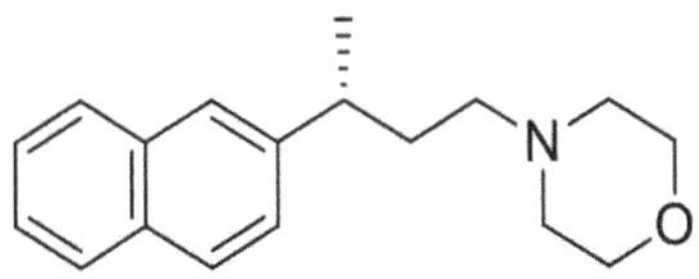	8.27	8.20	Rossi et al., 2017
60	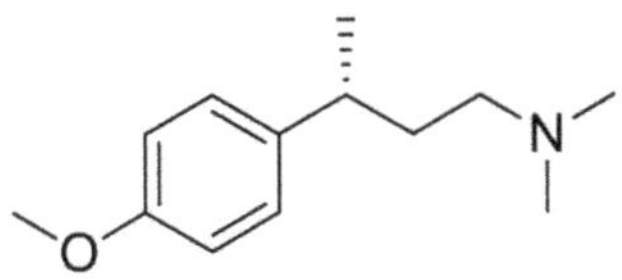	6.94	6.91	Rossi et al., 2017
61	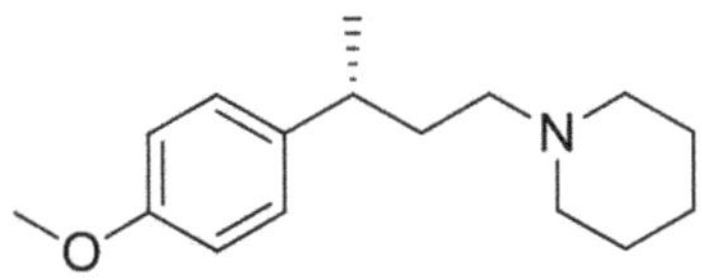	7.70	7.68	Rossi et al., 2017
62	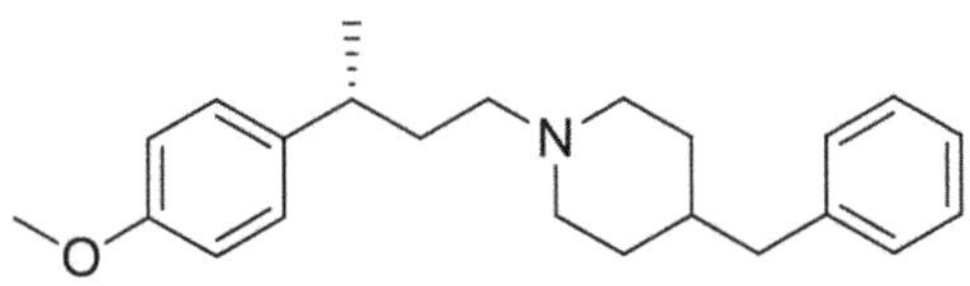	8.46	8.37	Rossi et al., 2017
63	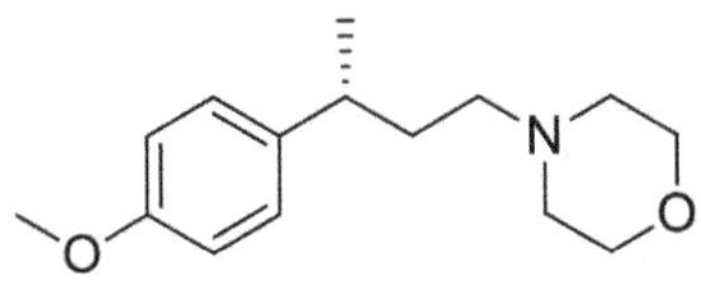	7.12	7.20	Rossi et al., 2017
64	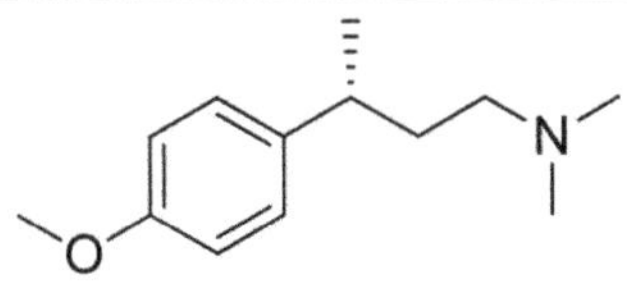	6.62	6.75	Rossi et al., 2017
65[a]	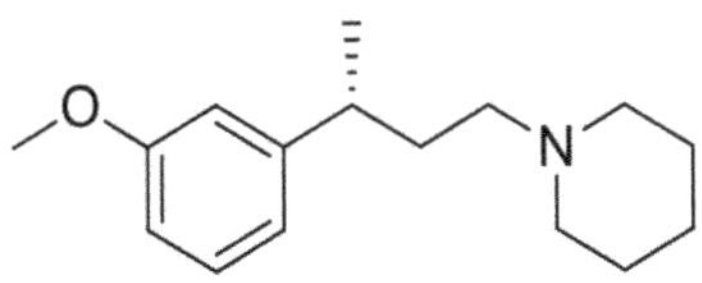	7.44	6.42	Rossi et al., 2017
66	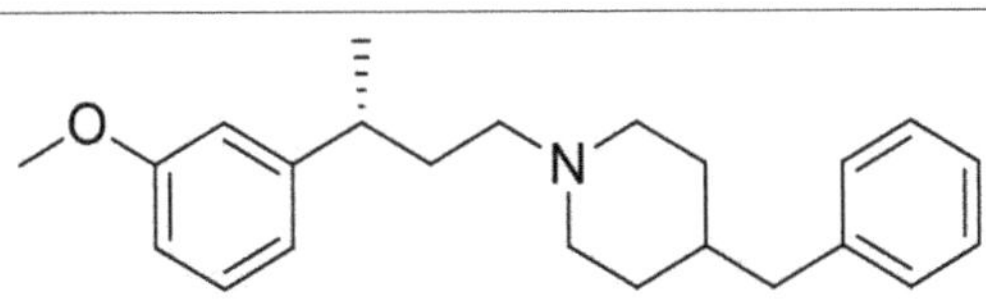	8.54	8.56	Rossi et al., 2017

(Continued)

TABLE 1 | Continued

ID	Structure	Experimental pKi[b]	Predicted pKi[b]	References
67[a]	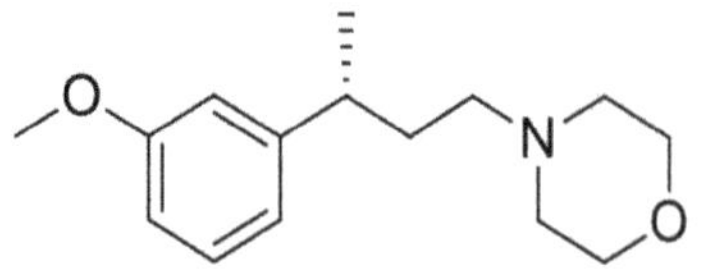	6.86	7.25	Rossi et al., 2017
68	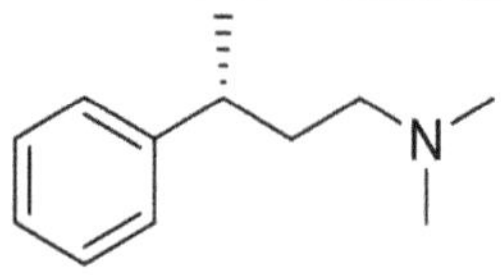	6.37	6.35	Rossi et al., 2017
69	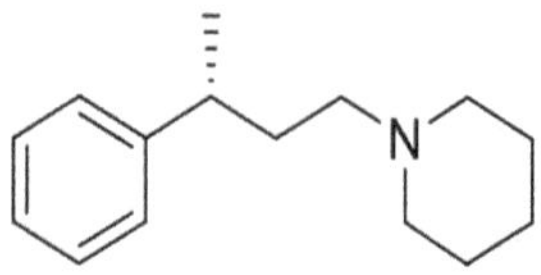	7.34	7.37	Rossi et al., 2017
70[a]	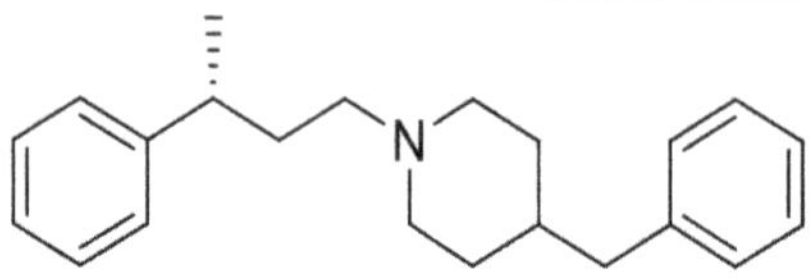	8.54	8.62	Rossi et al., 2017
71	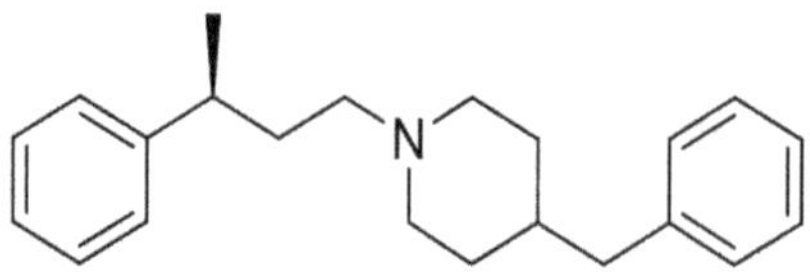	8.52	8.45	Rossi et al., 2017
72[a]	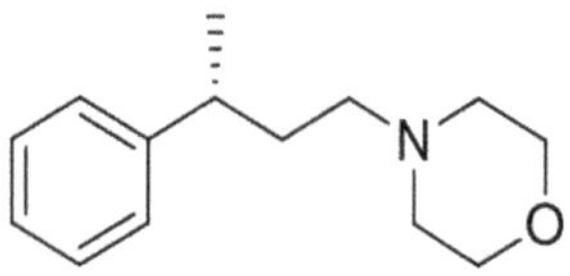	7.07	6.56	Rossi et al., 2017
73	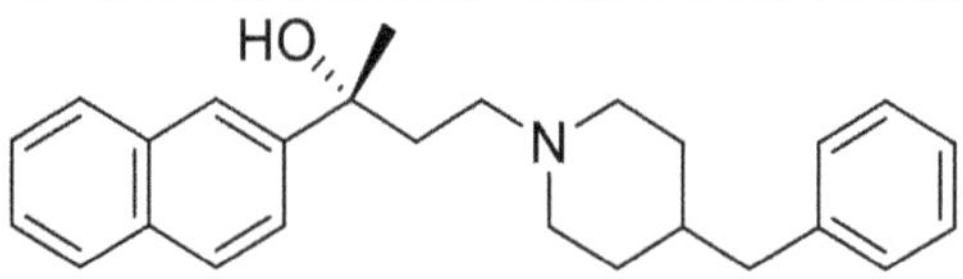	8.00	8.01	Rui et al., 2016
74	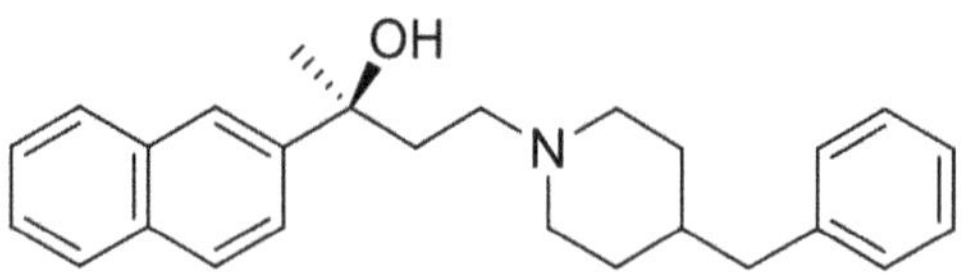	7.96	7.92	Rui et al., 2016
75	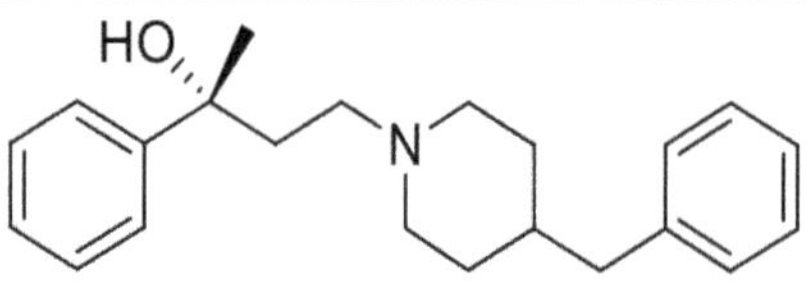	7.57	7.73	Rui et al., 2016
76	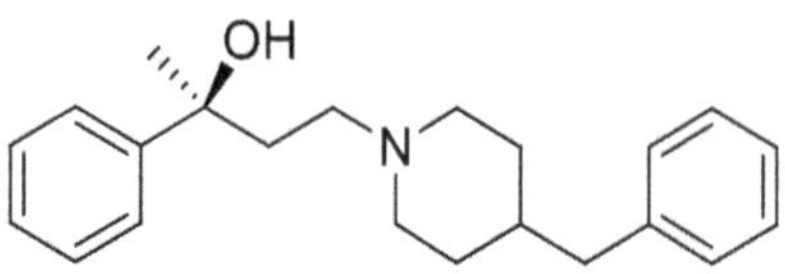	7.40	7.45	Rui et al., 2016

(Continued)

TABLE 1 | Continued

ID	Structure	Experimental pKi[b]	Predicted pKi[b]	References
77	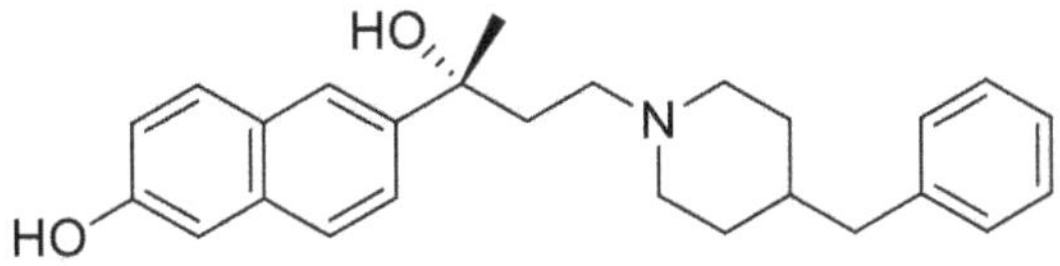	7.15	7.09	Rui et al., 2016
78	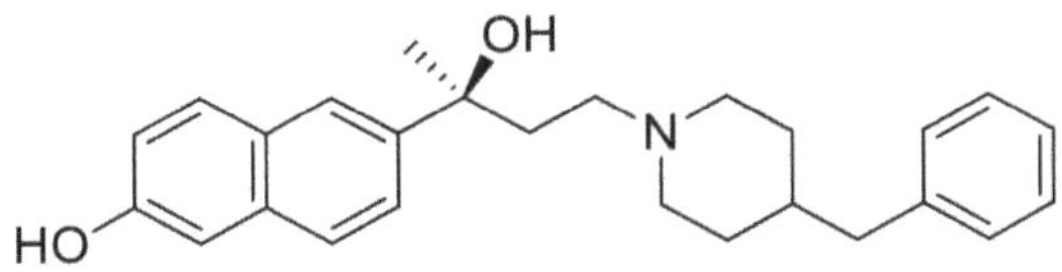	7.21	7.18	Rui et al., 2016
79	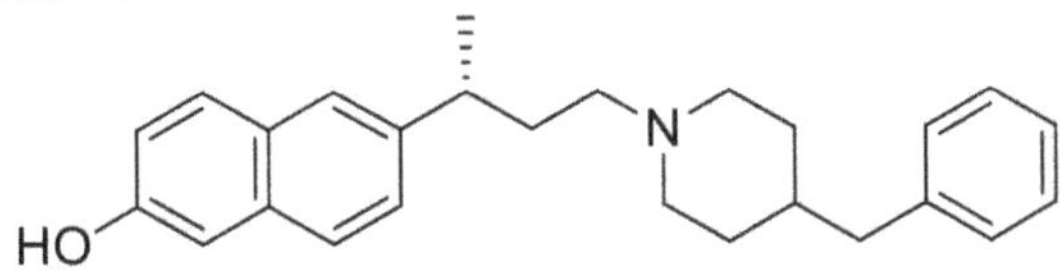	7.46	7.42	Rui et al., 2016
80[a]	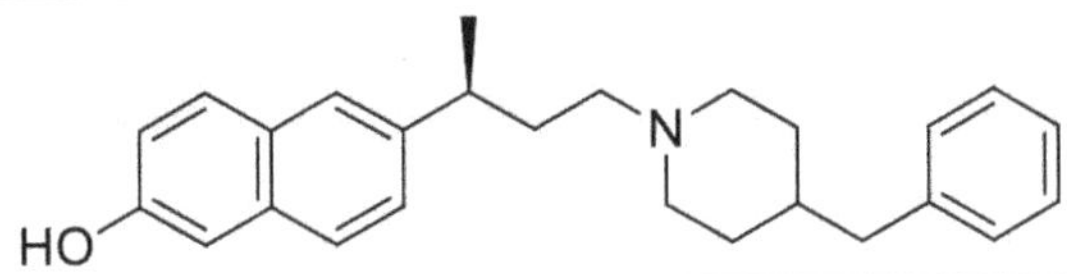	7.89	7.19	Rui et al., 2016

[a] *Test set compounds.*
[b] *Experimental and predicted pKi values using Model SE.*

and the more precise Glide XP was used for finding the final docking poses.

After several poses were found for each compound, the ones that showed the best scoring energies were considered. The information of PD144418, 4-IBP, haloperidol, NE-100, and (+)-pentazocine in the crystallographic structures recently reported (Schmidt et al., 2016, 2018) was considered for the selection of the best solutions; these compounds show how the previously reported pharmacophoric pattern (Glennon, 2005) is oriented inside the S1R binding site. The essential chemical interactions described for analog ligands (ECIDALs) (Muñoz-Gutierrez et al., 2016; Ramírez and Caballero, 2018) defined for S1R ligands were identified using this information. The most obvious essential chemical interaction is that charged amino group of the ligands must be close to the side chain carboxylate group of the residue Glu172, forming an electrostatic interaction. Therefore, the best docking solution for each compound was the pose that had the best scoring energy and complies with this essential chemical interaction.

The "Interaction Fingerprints Panel" of Maestro (Maestro 10.2.011, Schrödinger LLC) was used for deriving the Interaction fingerprints (IFPs) as described in Singh et al. reports (Deng et al., 2004; Singh et al., 2006). The method accounts for the presence of different types of chemical interactions between ligands and the binding site residues of the target receptor by using bits. For this purpose, distance cutoffs are defined for the binding site, and the interacting set encompasses the residues that contain atoms within the specified cutoff distance from ligand atoms. An interaction matrix is constructed including the bits with relevant information of the defined chemical interactions.

QSAR Modeling

After docking experiments, 3D-QSAR models were performed to explain the SAR of the RC-33 analogs. Their bioactive conformations predicted by using docking were used as the alignment rule for deriving the models. The structural features that affect their activities against the S1R were identified by describing steric and electrostatic fields.

The 80 compounds dataset was randomly partitioned into training (64 compounds) and external (16 compounds) sets. A homogenous distribution of the activities was granted in both training and test sets. 3D-QSAR models were generated using Open3DQSAR (Tosco and Balle, 2011), an open access tool with all the capacities to construct 3D-QSAR models. Steric and electrostatic fields were computed according to classical molecular mechanics equations using the Merck Molecular Force Field (Halgren, 1996).

The field variables were calculated by describing the interaction energies between probe atoms (sp^3 carbon atoms with a charge +1) and structures in a 1.0 Å step size grid box surrounding the whole set. Variables were processed as follows: (i) high energies adopted the top value of 30 kcal/mol, (ii) energy values very close to zero (below 0.05 kcal/mol) were set to zero in order to reduce noise, (iii) variables which only assumed a few different values (n-level variables) were removed. Thereafter, variables were scaled using the Block Unscaled Weighting procedure (Kastenholz et al., 2000; Boháč et al., 2002) and the predictive power of the models was improved by using the Smart Region Definition algorithm (Pastor et al., 1997).

Partial Least Square (PLS) regression was used to construct 3D-QSAR models, including from one to five Principal Components (PCs) and different combinations of fields. Models were derived by using one field and by combining them; the best model was selected by considering the higher value of the internal leave-one-out (LOO) cross-validation Q^2.

RESULTS AND DISCUSSION

Docking Predictions

We have a structural information of the binding poses of S1R ligands such as PD144418, 4-IBP, haloperidol, and NE-100 that similar in shape to RC-33. This information was used for evaluating the quality of the obtained docking results for RC-33 and its analogs. It is known that S1R ligands contain a charged nitrogen central atom flanked by two hydrophobic regions of different size (Glennon, 2005). The above mentioned S1R ligands form electrostatic interactions between the ligand charged nitrogen atoms and the side chain carboxylate of Glu172. In addition, their larger hydrophobic groups locate near the residues Val84, Met93, Leu95, Leu105, Tyr206, Ile178, Leu182, and Tyr103 (primary hydrophobic site), and their smaller hydrophobic groups locate near the residues Phe107, Trp164, His154, and Ile124 (secondary hydrophobic site). It is expected that the studied compounds establish such interactions.

Docking orientations of RC-33 and its analogs are represented in **Figure 1**. The best docking pose obtained for RC-33 was compared with the orientations of PD144418, 4-IBP, haloperidol, NE-100, and (+)-pentazocine in the reference crystallographic structures 5HK1, 5HK2, 6DJZ, 6DK0, and 6DK1, respectively. (+)-Pentazocine is an agonist as RC-33, but it is shorter than RC-33 and the other crystallized ligands; therefore, it is the least suitable ligand for the structural comparison between the crystallized ligands and the docked RC-33 analogs. **Figure 1A** shows that the docked structure of RC-33 was similarly oriented as the other crystallized ligands. On the other hand, **Figure 1B** shows that suitable binding modes of the ligands were found for all the RC-33 analogs. All of them form the conserved salt bridge between the charged N atom of the ligands and the residue Glu172 of the S1R. They also oriented their large hydrophobic groups to the primary hydrophobic site, and oriented their small hydrophobic groups to the secondary hydrophobic site. Representations in **Figure 1** show that our docking poses are similar to the S1R-ligand X-ray structures reported to date.

We calculated RMSD values for the studied compounds with respect to the docking result of RC-33 inside the S1R by using an *in-house* script (Velázquez-Libera et al., 2018). These calculations show the similarity in orientations between RC-33 and its analogs in an easy way. Since the RC-33 derivatives are different from the reference compound, RMSD values were calculated by considering only the common graphs between molecules. %RefMatch and %MolMatch values were defined, where %RefMatch refers to the percent of common graphs between the docked compound and RC-33 regarding the total number of atoms of RC-33; meanwhile, %MolMatch refers to the percent of common graphs between the docked compound, and RC-33 regarding the total number of atoms of the docked compound. These values allow identifying the maximal similitude between the docked compound and RC-33; therefore, an RMSD value with high %RefMatch and %MolMatch values reflects that the compound under analysis bears a strong resemblance with RC-33.

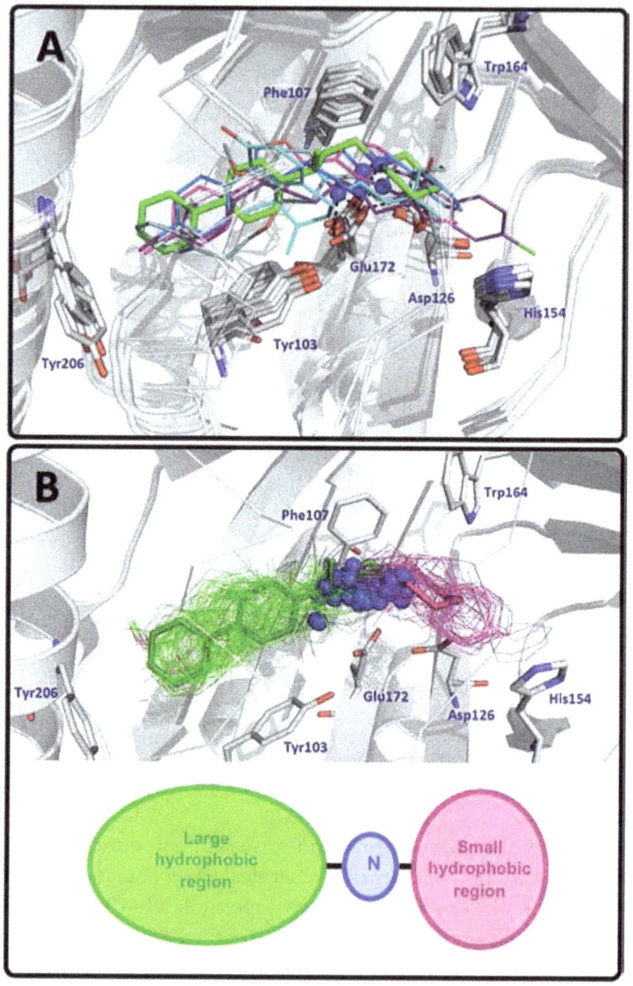

FIGURE 1 | Docking results for RC-33 and its analogs. **(A)** Docking pose obtained for RC-33 (stick representation in green) and comparison with X-ray crystallographic structures of the antagonist PD144418 (thin stick representation in purple, PDB code 5HK1), the ambiguous ligand 4-IBP (thin stick representation in light blue, PDB code 5HK2), the antagonist haloperidol (thin stick representation in lilac, PDB code 6DJZ), the antagonist NE-100 (thin stick representation in teal, PDB code 6DK0), and the agonist (+)-pentazocine (thin stick representation in cyan, PDB code 6DK1). N positively charged atom for each compound is represented by a blue sphere. **(B)** (top) Docking of RC-33 (in sticks representation) and comparison with its analogs (in lines representation); for each compound large hydrophobic group is in green at the left, small hydrophobic group is in purple at the right, and N positively charged atom is a sphere in blue. (bottom) Pharmacophoric model for S1R ligands: N positively charged atom (blue) flanked by large hydrophobic (green) and small hydrophobic (purple) regions.

The majority of the compounds under study have the 1-(3-phenylbutyl)piperidine or parts of this group in common with RC-33. Their RMSD values are reported in **Table 2**. In general, RMSD values reflect that the majority of compounds had the 1-(3-phenylbutyl)piperidine (or part of this group) similarly oriented with respect to RC-33 (RMSD < 2 Å). However,

TABLE 2 | RMSD values of the obtained docking pose common fragments for the studied compounds with respect to the docking result of RC-33 inside the S1R.

ID	RMSD (Å)[a]	%RefMatch[b]	%MolMatch[c]	RMSD (Å)[a,d]	%RefMatch[b,d]	%MolMatch[c,d]
1 (RC-33)				0.86	100	100
2	1.70	50	61	2.30	50	61
3	1.40	50	55	1.82	50	55
4	2.61	36	47			
5	2.20	36	47			
6	1.42	36	42			
7	0.46	64	74			
8	2.94	36	62			
9	1.67	36	53			
10	2.50	36	53			
11	2.80	50	65	2.89	50	65
12	2.05	50	65	2.16	50	65
13	2.21	50	61	1.50	50	61
14	1.43	50	58	1.46	50	58
15	0.43	77	89	0.86	77	89
16	1.45	50	42	1.07	50	42
17	0.97	77	65	0.69	77	65
18	1.58	36	35			
19	0.42	64	56			
20	1.29	36	32			
21	2.85	36	42			
22	0.38	36	38			
23	2.09	50	48	1.94	50	48
24	0.94	77	68	0.83	77	68
25	1.22	50	44	0.82	50	44
26	1.23	73	70	1.98	73	70
27	1.38	36	40			
28	0.59	64	64			
29	2.24	36	50			
30	0.85	36	44			
31	1.15	36	44			
32	1.11	36	36			
33	2.15	73	73	1.78	73	73
34	2.14	36	30			
35	0.45	64	48			
36	3.70	36	35			
37	4.17	36	32			
38	2.41	36	32			
39	1.16	36	40			
40	0.63	64	64			
41	0.77	36	44			
42	0.72	36	44			
43	2.10	32	26			
44	1.10	32	28			
45	1.66	32	24			
46	0.67	59	57			
47	1.05	32	37			
48	2.28	32	35			
49	2.23	32	39			
50	0.96	100	96			
51	0.64	100	96			

(Continued)

TABLE 2 | Continued

ID	RMSD (Å)[a]	%RefMatch[b]	%MolMatch[c]	RMSD (Å)[a,d]	%RefMatch[b,d]	%MolMatch[c,d]
52	1.50	50	61			
53	1.87	50	61			
54	1.48	50	55			
55	1.07	50	55			
56	2.19	73	80	1.96	73	80
57	2.63	73	59			
58	2.22	73	59			
59	1.95[e]	91	100	1.98[e]	91	100
60	1.80	50	73	2.54	50	73
61	2.63	73	89	1.52	73	89
62	3.02	73	64	6.97	73	64
63	2.38[e]	82	100	2.51[e]	82	100
64	2.11	50	73	2.58	50	73
65	2.45	73	89	1.01	73	89
66	2.68	73	64	4.26	73	64
67	2.19[e]	82	100	1.98[e]	82	100
68	0.63	50	85	2.96	50	85
69	2.65	73	100	2.73	73	100
70	3.87	73	70			
71	6.66	73	70			
72	2.58[e]	73	100	1.49[e]	73	100
73	2.29	73	57			
74	2.20	73	57			
75	4.65	73	67			
76	4.39	73	67			
77	2.72	73	55			
78	2.34	73	55			
79	1.74	73	57			
80	2.08	73	57			

[a]*RMSD values considering only the common chemical fragments between the docked compound and the reference compound RC-33.*
[b]*%RefMatch refers to the percent of common graphs between the docked and reference compound RC-33 concerning the total number of atoms of the reference compound RC-33.*
[c]*%MolMatch refers to the percent of common graphs between the docked and reference compound RC-33 regarding the total number of atoms of the docked compound.*
[d]*RMSD, %RefMatch, and %MolMatch values for the S enantiomer of the compounds reported as racemic pairs.*
[e]*In this case, difference in ring heavy atoms were not considered between the docked compound and the reference compound RC-33.*

Table 2 reports compounds with RMSD > 2.5 Å (for instance, compounds **11** (R and S), **57**, **60** (S), and **77**). The 1-(3-phenylbutyl)piperidine group of these compounds is displaced toward the helices α4 and α5; however, their amine groups keep the salt bridge interaction with the residue Glu172. In addition, we found in **Table 2** compounds with RMSD > 4 Å (for instance, compounds **37**, **62** (S), **66** (S), **75**, and **76**). The 1-(3-phenylbutyl)piperidine group of these compounds is oriented to the reverse with respect to this group in RC-33; their amine groups also keep the salt bridge interaction with the residue Glu172. These compounds have larger hydrophobic substituents at position 4 of the piperidine, increasing the size of this group. The changed groups fit better inside the bigger hydrophobic cavity close to the helices α4 and α5 when their orientations are opposed to the orientation of the 1-(3-phenylbutyl)piperidine group in RC-33. In this way, these compounds are also adapted to the previous described pharmacophore pattern for S1R ligands (Ablordeppey et al., 2000; Glennon, 2005; Caballero et al., 2012) (the N positively charged atom flanked by two hydrophobic groups of different sizes), where the charged atom is salt-bridged to Glu172, the bigger hydrophobic group is placed near the helices α4 and α5 at the membrane proximal, and the smaller hydrophobic group is placed near the narrow end of the cupin barrel that is further from the membrane.

The chemical interactions between the RC-33 analogs and the residues at the S1R binding site can be described in detail by using IFPs. This method has been commonly used for identifying the relevant residues involved in protein-ligand affinities (Caballero et al., 2018; Navarro-Retamal and Caballero, 2018; Velázquez-Libera et al., 2018). IFPs capture and label the chemical contacts between a target protein and a set of its ligands as a whole. The chemotypes are identified with the following labels: P (polar groups), H (hydrophobic groups), A (hydrogen bonds where the residue is the acceptor), D (hydrogen bonds where the residue is the donor), Ar (aromatic groups), and Ch (electrostatic interactions with charged groups). IFPs also differentiate between contacts with backbone and contacts with side-chain functional groups. We calculated IFPs by considering the S1R-ligand complexes formed by our docked structures.

The calculated IFPs are reported in **Figure 2**. The IFP analysis applied to the complexes between S1R and the RC-33 analogs obtained by docking revealed that 29 S1R residues had contacts with ligands. These residues and their positions in the S1R secondary structure are depicted in **Figure 2A**. The S1R binding site is mainly hydrophobic; in fact, the vast majority of the observed interactions are hydrophobic or aromatic when analyzing the occurrence of chemical contacts in the studied structures (**Figure 2C**).

The residues with polar interactions were identified in the plots of percent of occurrence obtained from IFP calculations (**Figure 2**). The residue E172 at the sheet β10 has polar contributions in 100% of the total structures, forming a salt-bridge and it also acts as HB acceptor in 80% of the studied structures. The residue D126 at the sheet β5 was identified with polar contributions in more than 50% of the studied structures. The residue T181 at the helix α4 has polar contributions in more than 80% of the studied structures. Finally, the residues S117 (backbone and side chain), H154 (side chain), and T202

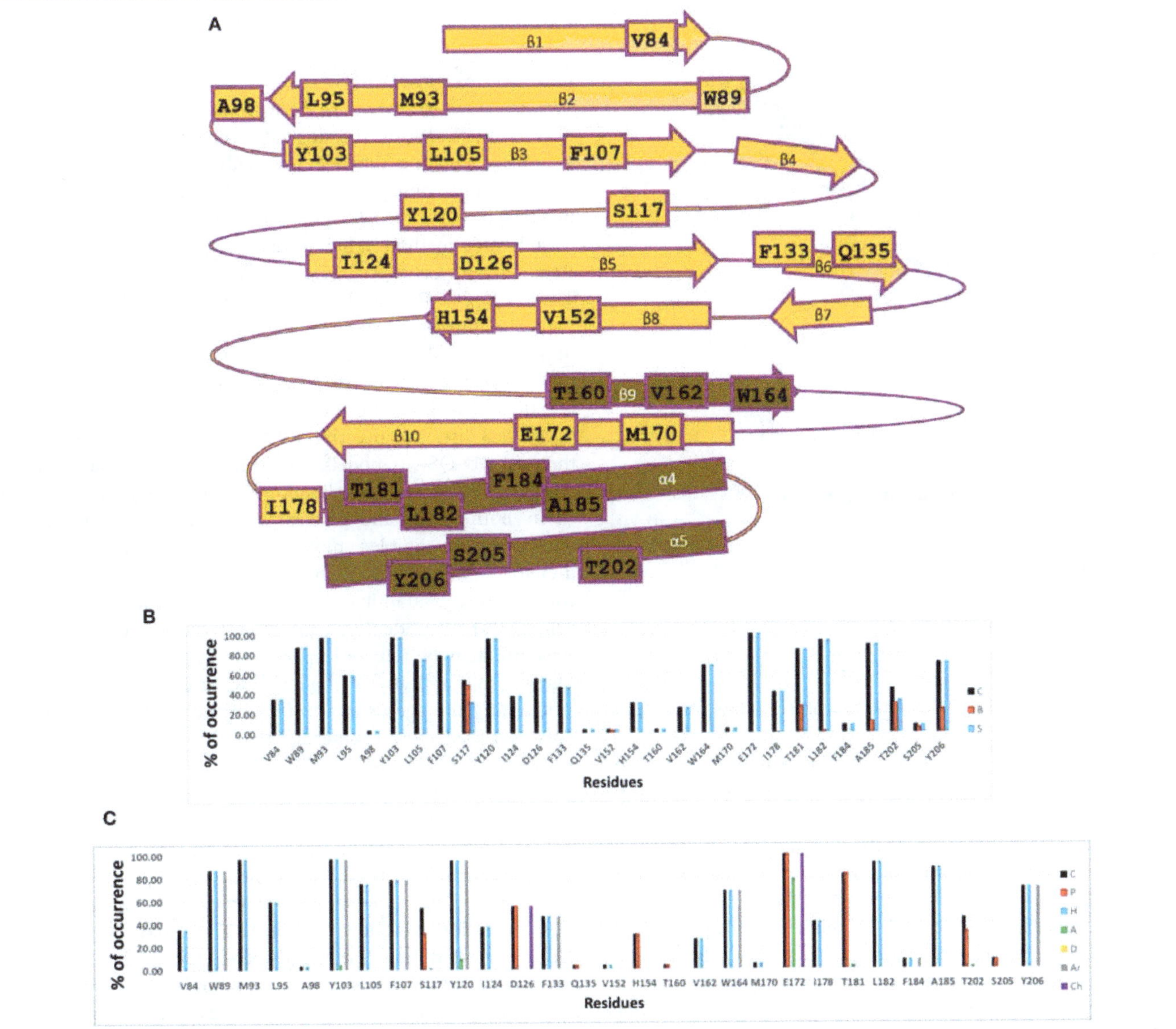

FIGURE 2 | Occurrence of interaction types at the S1R–ligand binding interface. **(A)** Residues with observed interactions, their position in the S1R sequence. **(B)** Percentages of occurrence of contacts C, interactions with the backbone of the residue B, and interactions with the side chain of the residue S. **(C)** Percentages of occurrence of chemical interactions: contacts C, polar P, hydrophobic H, HBs where the residue is acceptor A, HBs where the residue is donor D, aromatic Ar, and electrostatic with charged groups Ch. The S1R–ligand structures obtained by docking were used for calculations of the percentages of occurrence represented here.

TABLE 3 | Statistical information of the 3D-QSAR models.

Fields	NC	R^2	S	Q^2	S_{LOO}	R^2_{test}	S_{test}	%S	%E
S	8	0.98	0.13	0.64	0.54	0.34	0.81	1	
E	4	0.81	0.39	0.54	0.62	0.59	0.63	–	1
SE	7	0.97	0.15	0.70	0.50	0.61	0.62	0.88	0.12

NC is the number of components; S is the standard deviation of the fitted activity of the training set; R^2, Q^2, and R^2_{test} are the coefficients of correlation of the training set, LOO cross validation, and test set, respectively; S_{LOO} is the standard deviation of the LOO cross validation, and S_{test} is the standard deviation of the test predictions. %S and %E are the relative contributions of the steric (S) and the electrostatic (E) fields, respectively.

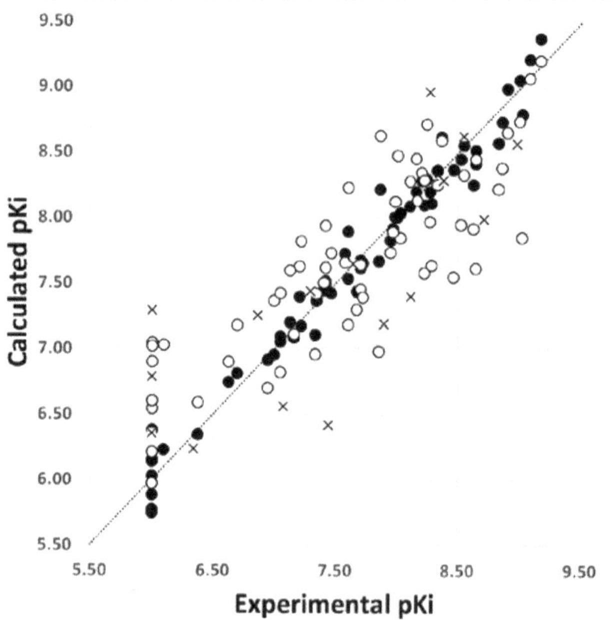

FIGURE 3 | Scatter plot of the experimental activities vs. predicted activities for the model SE: (•) training set predictions, (○) LOO cross-validation predictions, and (×) test set predictions.

(backbone and side chain) have polar contributions in around 30% of the studied structures.

Several residues with aromatic interactions were also identified in the plots of percent of occurrence obtained from IFP calculations (**Figure 2**). The residues with aromatic interactions were important for the shape of the S1R binding site because they restrict the space of the pockets. Four aromatic residues located at the center of the binding site (W89, Y103, F107, and Y120) were identified by the IFP calculations with percent of occurrence values above 80%. These residues cause a bottleneck just in front of the residue E172; therefore they could help to orient the positively charged N of the ligands to form the salt bridge. At the same time, they could stabilize the presence of the positive charge by means of π-cation interactions. The aromatic residues F133 at the sheet β6 and W164 the sheet β9, located close to the narrower end of the cupin β-barrel, have percent of occurrence values of 50 and 70%, respectively. On the other hand, the residue Y206, located at the helix α5, has a percent of occurrence value of 70%.

The remaining residues with hydrophobic interactions were also identified in the plots of percent of occurrence obtained from IFP calculations (**Figure 2**). The residues identified with percent of occurrence above 75% M93 (at β2), L105 (at β3), and L182/A185 (at α4) are located at the bigger hydrophobic pocket. The residues V84 (at β1), L95 (at β2), and I178 (at the loop between β10 and α4) are also located at the bigger hydrophobic pocket and were identified by IFP calculations with lower percent of occurrences, and the residue I124 at β5, located at the smaller hydrophobic pocket, had a percent of occurrence below 40%.

In general, the reported IFPs identify the most important S1R residues which establish chemical interactions with RC-33 analogs. Furthermore, it could be useful for the understanding of the interactions between S1R and its ligands.

3D-QSAR Results

We constructed the 3D-QSAR models based on docking alignment; therefore, the docked structures were included in a box for creating the relevant fields, since they are models of the ligand conformations inside the S1R binding site. The docking-based or receptor-guided alignment 3D-QSAR is a well-documented method in literature (Guasch et al., 2012; Navarro-Retamal and Caballero, 2016; Muñoz-Gutiérrez et al., 2017). Three 3D-QSAR models were trained using the steric field (Model S), the electrostatic field (Model E), and the combination of both fields (Model SE). The most reliable models were selected by measuring the LOO cross-validation performance (Q^2 > 0.5) and the test set predictions (R^2_{test} > 0.5).

Table 3 lists the description and statistical information of the best 3D-QSAR models. This report proved that model S has better (LOO) cross-validation Q^2 than model E. However, when both steric and electrostatic fields are tied together in the more complex model SE, the Q^2 value increases; therefore, this model, which had a $Q^2 = 0.70$ including seven components, containing a major contribution of the steric field (88%), was identified as the model best describing the structure-activity relationship of the studied RC-33 analogs. These results reflect that the steric features are mandatory for modulating the agonistic activities of the studied compounds. This is reasonable considering that the S1R binding site is mostly hydrophobic.

The model SE explains 97% of the variance and has a low standard deviation ($S = 0.15$). The predictions of pKi values for the 64 RC-33 analogs in the training set using the model SE are reported in **Table 1** and the correlations between the predicted and experimental pKi values (from training and LOO cross validation) are shown in **Figure 3**. It is possible to observe that the selected model fitted adequately the whole dataset; it is noteworthy that the more potent compounds had an outstanding performance. When the model SE was used to predict the pKi values of the test set compounds, well results were also found, reflected by the value of $R^2_{test} = 0.61$. The predicted pKi values for the test set are listed in **Table 1**, and the correlation between the calculated and experimental pKi values are plotted in **Figure 3**.

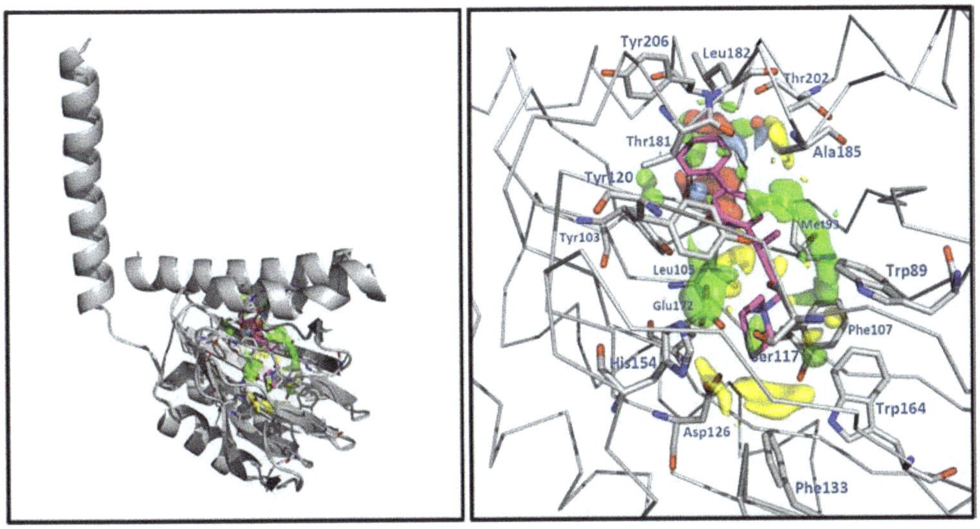

FIGURE 4 | 3D-QSAR contour maps for the RC-33 analogs (model SE). The steric field is represented by green and yellow isopleths: the green ones indicate regions where bulky groups enhance the activity, and the yellow ones indicate regions where bulky groups disfavor the activity. The electrostatic field is represented by blue and red isopleths: the blue ones indicate regions where an increase of positive charge enhances the activity and the red ones indicate regions where an increase of negative charge enhances the activity. RC-33 is shown inside the fields.

Figure 4 shows contour plots of the steric and electrostatic fields projected onto the docked structure of RC-33 for association between the fields, the compounds of the whole set, and the residues at the S1R binding site. In this figure, green and yellow contours represent regions with positive and negative steric components, respectively. It is noted that positive steric components have a major role. A great green contour in front of the 3-phenylbutylamine, and near the residues V84, W89, F107, and A185, indicates that bulk groups are desired in this region. It is noteworthy that the most active compounds such as RC-33, **7**, **15**, **27**, **28**, and **33** has the methyl group of the 3-phenylbutylamine in this region, but the majority of the less active compounds such as **8**, **29**, **41**, **64**, and **67** have this group deeper into the bigger hydrophobic pocket. Another three green contours are located near the piperidine of RC-33 and the residues Y120, S117, and W164 indicating that this group or another bulky group in this region is needed. In general, compounds with a dimethylamine in this region (compounds **2–15**) are less active than similar compounds that contain piperidine. Another green contour near the residues Y103 and E172 reflects that several active compounds contain the methyl group of the 3-phenylbutylamine in this region. Another green contours are located at the bigger hydrophobic pocket near the residues Y103, Y206, and T202, indicating the preference of a bulky group in this region. For instance, the biphenyl group in compound **7** is preferred instead the phenyl group in compound **8** because the former group fills the entire space of the bigger hydrophobic pocket. Several yellow contours were identified near the residues W164, L105, F107, and T202. All of them are close to the green contours both in the bigger and smaller pockets, and reflect the complexity of the steric field inside the S1R binding site.

In **Figure 4**, blue and red contours represent regions with positive and negative electrostatic components, respectively; all of them are small and are located inside the bigger hydrophobic pocket. The blue contours are near the residues T181, A185, L182, and the backbone of Y206, and the red contours are near the residues A92, L95, L105, L182, and T202. The blue contours are located in regions where ligands placed hydroxyl groups and their pKi values are between 7 and 7.8 (moderate activities). For instance, compounds **13** and **77** have hydroxyl close to the backbone of Y206, **75,** and **76** have hydroxyl close to A185, and **53**, 55, and **78** have hydroxyl close to T181. The red contours are located in regions where ligands placed OMe groups and the activity is increased. For instance, compounds **22** and **30** that contain OMe have better activities than compounds **21** and **29** without this group.

The docking-based 3D-QSAR methodology allows establishing a comparison between the chemical features that describe the structure-activity relationship of bioactive ligands and the protein binding site (Alzate-Morales and Caballero, 2010; Caballero et al., 2011; Quesada-Romero et al., 2014; Mena-Ulecia et al., 2015; Muñoz-Gutiérrez et al., 2017). The contour plots in receptor-based 3D-QSAR are not receptor maps, but they solve another key point of the description of the differential activities: different potency in activities is connected with different chemical environments and interactions. The docking and 3D-QSAR methods applied to the study of RC-33 analogs give more information about the structure of S1R-ligand complexes, and identify important chemical features to take into account in the future design of potent S1R ligands. We feel that another similar studies on other series of compounds will be reported during next years.

CONCLUSION

This is the first structure-based molecular modeling investigation a few years after the elucidation of the S1R crystallographic structure; therefore, details of the binding poses and the chemical interactions in the binding site are described. Binding orientations and structure-activity relationship of RC-33 analogs as S1R agonists were studied by using molecular docking and 3D-QSAR methods.

Docking poses obtained for the studied compounds inside the S1R binding site explain the interactions between the well-known theoretical pharmacophore model reported for these compounds (elucidated before the knowledge of the S1R 3D structure) and the residues located at the binding site. They also reproduced structural features reported for complexes between S1R and PD144418, 4-IBP, and other active ligands. The docking analysis, including the IFP calculations, confirmed the preponderant role of E172 forming a salt bridge with the positively charged N of the ligands. Furthermore, docking experiments also identified the importance role of the aromatic residues delimiting the shape of the S1R binding site: specifically, W89, Y103, F107, and Y120 which are at the center of the binding site, F133 and W164 which are close to the narrower end of the cupin β-barrel, and Y206 which is close to the helix α5.

A receptor-guided alignment 3D-QSAR model with adequate statistical significance and acceptable prediction power was obtained. Steric and electrostatic features had contributions to the differential potency of the agonists, with a major role of the steric ones. The 3D-QSAR model demonstrated that an implicit correlation is found in the data under analysis between the chemical features of the compounds in their active conformations and their interactions in the pockets of the S1R binding site.

Overall, the information reported here, derived from the recently reported S1R structure, will be useful for the future research in the design of novel S1R ligands.

AUTHOR CONTRIBUTIONS

The work was completed by cooperation of all authors. JC was responsible for the study of concept and design of the project. JV-L performed the docking RMSD analysis, IFPs, and 3D-QSAR calculations. GR and CN-R performed the docking calculations. SC and JC drafted and revised the manuscript.

FUNDING

This research was funded by FONDECYT Regular grant number 1170718 (JC) and FONDECYT Postdoc grant number 3170434 (CN-R). The authors gratefully acknowledge MIUR for the doctoral fellowship to GR and thankfully recognize Scuola di Alta Formazione Dottorale of University of Pavia for the mobility research scholarship provided to GR.

REFERENCES

Ablordeppey, S. Y., Fischer, J. B., and Glennon, R. A. (2000). Is a nitrogen atom an important pharmacophoric element in sigma ligand binding? *Bioorg. Med. Chem.* 8, 2105–2111. doi: 10.1016/S0968-0896(00)00148-6

Almerico, A. M., Tutone, M., and Lauria, A. (2012). Receptor-guided 3D-QSAR approach for the discovery of c-kit tyrosine kinase inhibitors. *J. Mol. Model.* 18, 2885–2895. doi: 10.1007/s00894-011-1304-0

Alon, A., Schmidt, H. R., Wood, M. D., Sahn, J. J., Martin, S. F., and Kruse, A. C. (2017). Identification of the gene that codes for the σ2 receptor. *Proc. Natl. Acad. Sci. U.S.A.* 114, 7160–7165. doi: 10.1073/pnas.1705154114

Alzate-Morales, J., and Caballero, J. (2010). Computational study of the interactions between guanine derivatives and cyclin-dependent kinase 2 (CDK2) by CoMFA and QM/MM. *J. Chem. Inf. Model.* 50, 110–122. doi: 10.1021/ci900302z

Amaning, K., Lowinski, M., Vallee, F., Steier, V., Marcireau, C., Ugolini, A., et al. (2013). The use of virtual screening and differential scanning fluorimetry for the rapid identification of fragments active against MEK1. *Bioorg. Med. Chem. Lett.* 23, 3620–3626. doi: 10.1016/j.bmcl.2013.04.003

Batra, J., Szabó, A., Caulfield, T. R., Soares, A. S., Sahin-Tóth, M., and Radisky, E. S. (2013). Long-range electrostatic complementarity governs substrate recognition by human chymotrypsin C, a key regulator of digestive enzyme activation. *J. Biol. Chem.* 288, 9848–9859. doi: 10.1074/jbc.M113.457382

Boháč, M., Loeprecht, B., Damborský, J., and Schüürmann, G. (2002). Impact of Orthogonal Signal Correction (OSC) on the predictive ability of CoMFA models for the ciliate toxicity of nitrobenzenes. *Q. Struct. Activit. Relationsh.* 21, 3–11. doi: 10.1002/1521-3838(200205)21:1<3::AID-QSAR3>3.0.CO;2-D

Caballero, J., Morales-Bayuelo, A., and Navarro-Retamal, C. (2018). *Mycobacterium tuberculosis* serine/threonine protein kinases: structural information for the design of their specific ATP-competitive inhibitors. *J. Comput. Aided Mol. Des.* 32, 1315–1336. doi: 10.1007/s10822-018-0173-3

Caballero, J., Quiliano, M., Alzate-Morales, J. H., Zimic, M., and Deharo, E. (2011). Docking and quantitative structure–activity relationship studies for 3-fluoro-4-(pyrrolo[2,1-f][1,2,4]triazin-4-yloxy)aniline, 3-fluoro-4-(1H-pyrrolo[2,3-b]pyridin-4-yloxy)aniline, and 4-(4-amino-2-fluorophenoxy)-2-pyridinylamine derivatives as c-Met kinase inhibitors. *J. Comput. Aided Mol. Des.* 25, 349–369. doi: 10.1007/s10822-011-9425-1

Caballero, J., Zilocchi, S., Tiznado, W., Rossi, D., and Collina, S. (2012). Models of the pharmacophoric pattern and affinity trend of methyl 2-(aminomethyl)-1-phenylcyclopropane-1-carboxylate derivatives as σ1 ligands. *Mol. Simul.* 38, 227–235. doi: 10.1080/08927022.2011.614243

Chu, U. B., and Ruoho, A. E. (2016). Biochemical pharmacology of the sigma-1 receptor. *Mol. Pharmacol.* 89, 142–153. doi: 10.1124/mol.115.101170

Collina, S., Bignardi, E., Rui, M., Rossi, D., Gaggeri, R., Zamagni, A., et al. (2017a). Are sigma modulators an effective opportunity for cancer treatment? A patent overview (1996–2016). *Expert Opin. Ther. Pat.* 27, 565–578. doi: 10.1080/13543776.2017.1276569

Collina, S., Loddo, G., Urbano, M., Linati, L., Callegari, A., Ortuso, F., et al. (2007). Design, synthesis, and SAR analysis of novel selective [sigma]1 ligands. *Bioorg. Med. Chem.* 15, 771–783. doi: 10.1016/j.bmc.2006.10.048

Collina, S., Rui, M., Stotani, S., Bignardi, E., Rossi, D., Curti, D., et al. (2017b). Are sigma receptor modulators a weapon against multiple sclerosis disease? *Future Med. Chem.* 9, 2029–2051. doi: 10.4155/fmc-2017-0122

DeCoster, M. A., Klette, K. L., Knight, E. S., and Tortella, F. C. (1995). σ receptor-mediated neuroprotection against glutamate toxicity in primary rat neuronal cultures. *Brain Res.* 671, 45–53. doi: 10.1016/0006-8993(94)01294-R

Deng, Z., Chuaqui, C., and Singh, J. (2004). Structural interaction fingerprint (SIFt): a novel method for analyzing three-dimensional protein-ligand binding interactions. *J. Med. Chem.* 47, 337–344. doi: 10.1021/jm030331x

Friesner, R. A., Banks, J. L., Murphy, R. B., Halgren, T. A., Klicic, J. J., Mainz, D. T., et al. (2004). Glide: a new approach for rapid, accurate docking and scoring. 1. Method and assessment of docking accuracy. *J. Med. Chem.* 47, 1739–1749. doi: 10.1021/jm0306430

Furuse, T., and Hashimoto, K. (2010). Sigma-1 receptor agonist fluvoxamine for delirium in patients with Alzheimer's disease. *Ann. Gen. Psychiatry* 9:6. doi: 10.1186/1744-859X-9-6

Glennon, R. A. (2005). Pharmacophore identification for sigma-1 (sigma1) receptor binding: application of the "deconstruction-reconstruction-elaboration" approach. *Mini Rev. Med. Chem.* 5, 927–940. doi: 10.2174/1389557057743295l9

Glennon, R. A., Ismaiel, A. M., Ablordeppey, S., El-Ashmawy, M., and Fisher, J. B. (2004). Thioxanthene-derived analogs as sigma(1) receptor ligands. *Bioorg. Med. Chem. Lett.* 14, 2217–2220. doi: 10.1016/j.bmcl.2004.02.018

Guasch, L., Sala, E., Valls, C., Mulero, M., Pujadas, G., and Garcia-Vallvé, S. (2012). Development of docking-based 3D-QSAR models for PPARgamma full agonists. *J. Mol. Graph. Model.* 36, 1–9. doi: 10.1016/j.jmgm.2012.03.001

Hajipour, A. R., Fontanilla, D., Chu, U. B., Arbabian, M., and Ruoho, A. E. (2010). Synthesis and characterization of N,N-dialkyl and N-alkyl-N-aralkyl fenpropimorph-derived compounds as high affinity ligands for sigma receptors. *Bioorg. Med. Chem.* 18, 4397–4404. doi: 10.1016/j.bmc.2010.04.078

Halgren, T. A. (1996). Merck molecular force field. II. MMFF94 van der Waals and electrostatic parameters for intermolecular interactions. *J. Comput. Chem.* 17, 520–552. doi: 10.1002/(SICI)1096-987X(199604)17:5/6<520::AID-JCC2>3.0.CO;2-W

Hanner, M., Moebius, F. F., Flandorfer, A., Knaus, H. G., Striessnig, J., Kempner, E., et al. (1996). Purification, molecular cloning, and expression of the mammalian sigma1-binding site. *Proc. Natl. Acad. Sci. U.S.A.* 93, 8072–8077. doi: 10.1073/pnas.93.15.8072

Hashimoto, K. (2009). Can the sigma-1 receptor agonist fluvoxamine prevent schizophrenia? *CNS Neurol. Disord. Drug Targets* 8, 470–474. doi: 10.2174/187152709789824633

Hayashi, T., and Su, T.-P. (2004). Sigma-1 receptor ligands: potential in the treatment of neuropsychiatric disorders. *CNS Drugs* 18, 269–284. doi: 10.2165/00023210-200418050-00001

Kastenholz, M. A., Pastor, M., Cruciani, G., Haaksma, E. E., and Fox, T. (2000). GRID/CPCA: a new computational tool to design selective ligands. *J. Med. Chem.* 43, 3033–3044. doi: 10.1021/jm000934y

Marra, A., Rossi, D., Pignataro, L., Bigogno, C., Canta, A., Oggioni, N., et al. (2016). Toward the identification of neuroprotective agents: g-scale synthesis, pharmacokinetic evaluation and CNS distribution of (R)-RC-33, a promising SIGMA1 receptor agonist. *Future Med. Chem.* 8, 287–295. doi: 10.4155/fmc.15.191

Martin, W. R., Eades, C. G., Thompson, J. A., Huppler, R. E., and Gilbert, P. E. (1976). The effects of morphine- and nalorphine- like drugs in the non-dependent and morphine-dependent chronic spinal dog. *J. Pharmacol. Exp. Ther.* 197, 517–532.

Mavlyutov, T. A., Guo, L.-W., Epstein, M. L., and Ruoho, A. E. (2015). Role of the sigma-1 receptor in Amyotrophic Lateral Sclerosis (ALS). *J. Pharmacol. Sci.* 127, 10–16. doi: 10.1016/j.jphs.2014.12.013

Mena-Ulecia, K., Tiznado, W., and Caballero, J. (2015). Study of the differential activity of thrombin inhibitors using docking, QSAR, molecular dynamics, and MM-GBSA. *PLoS ONE* 10:e0142774. doi: 10.1371/journal.pone.0142774

Meyer, D. A., Carta, M., Partridge, L. D., Covey, D. F., and Valenzuela, C. F. (2002). Neurosteroids enhance spontaneous glutamate release in hippocampal neurons possible role of metabotropic σ1-like receptors. *J. Biol. Chem.* 277, 28725–28732. doi: 10.1074/jbc.M202592200

Mishina, M., Ishiwata, K., Ishii, K., Kitamura, S., Kimura, Y., Kawamura, K., et al. (2005). Function of sigma1 receptors in Parkinson's disease. *Acta Neurol. Scand.* 112, 103–107. doi: 10.1111/j.1600-0404.2005.00432.x

Monnet, F. P., and Maurice, T. (2006). The sigma1 protein as a target for the non-genomic effects of neuro(active)steroids: molecular, physiological, and behavioral aspects. *J. Pharmacol. Sci.* 100, 93–118. doi: 10.1254/jphs.CR0050032

Morin-Surun, M. P., Collin, T., Denavit-Saubié, M., Baulieu, E. E., and Monnet, F. P. (1999). Intracellular sigma1 receptor modulates phospholipase C and protein kinase C activities in the brainstem. *Proc. Natl. Acad. Sci. U.S.A.* 96, 8196–8199. doi: 10.1073/pnas.96.14.8196

Muñoz-Gutierrez, C., Adasme-Carreño, F., Fuentes, E., Palomo, I., and Caballero, J. (2016). Computational study of the binding orientation and affinity of PPARγ agonists: inclusion of ligand-induced fit by cross-docking. *RSC Adv.* 6, 64756–64768. doi: 10.1039/C6RA12084A

Muñoz-Gutiérrez, C., Cáceres-Rojas, D., Adasme-Carreño, F., Palomo, I., Fuentes, E., and Caballero, J. (2017). Docking and quantitative structure-activity relationship of bi-cyclic heteroaromatic pyridazinone and pyrazolone derivatives as phosphodiesterase 3A (PDE3A) inhibitors. *PLoS ONE* 12:e0189213. doi: 10.1371/journal.pone.0189213

Navarro-Retamal, C., and Caballero, J. (2016). Flavonoids as CDK1 inhibitors: insights in their binding orientations and structure-activity relationship. *PLoS ONE* 11:e0161111. doi: 10.1371/journal.pone.0161111

Navarro-Retamal, C., and Caballero, J. (2018). "Molecular modeling of tau Proline-Directed Protein Kinase (PDPK) inhibitors," in *Computational Modeling of Drugs Against Alzheimer's Disease Neuromethods*, ed K. Roy (New York, NY: Humana Press), 305–345. doi: 10.1007/978-1-4939-7404-7_13

Osguthorpe, D. J., Sherman, W., and Hagler, A. T. (2012). Generation of receptor structural ensembles for virtual screening using binding site shape analysis and clustering. *Chem. Biol. Drug Des.* 80, 182–193. doi: 10.1111/j.1747-0285.2012.01396.x

Pastor, M., Cruciani, G., and Clementi, S. (1997). Smart region definition: a new way to improve the predictive ability and interpretability of three-dimensional quantitative structure-activity relationships. *J. Med. Chem.* 40, 1455–1464. doi: 10.1021/jm9608016

Peviani, M., Salvaneschi, E., Bontempi, L., Petese, A., Manzo, A., Rossi, D., et al. (2014). Neuroprotective effects of the Sigma-1 receptor (S1R) agonist PRE-084, in a mouse model of motor neuron disease not linked to SOD1 mutation. *Neurobiol. Dis.* 62, 218–232. doi: 10.1016/j.nbd.2013.10.010

Prezzavento, O., Campisi, A., Ronsisvalle, S., Li Volti, G., Marrazzo, A., Bramanti, V., et al. (2007). Novel sigma receptor ligands: synthesis and biological profile. *J. Med. Chem.* 50, 951–961. doi: 10.1021/jm0611197

Quesada-Romero, L., and Caballero, J. (2014). Docking and quantitative structure–activity relationship of oxadiazole derivates as inhibitors of GSK3beta. *Mol. Divers.* 18, 149–159. doi: 10.1007/s11030-013-9483-5

Quesada-Romero, L., Mena-Ulecia, K., Tiznado, W., and Caballero, J. (2014). Insights into the interactions between maleimide derivates and GSK3β combining molecular docking and QSAR. *PLoS ONE* 9:e102212. doi: 10.1371/journal.pone.0102212

Quesada-Romero, L., Mena-Ulecia, K., Zuñiga, M., De-la-Torre, P., Rossi, D., Tiznado, W., et al. (2015). Optimal graph-based and simplified molecular input line entry System-based descriptors for quantitative structure–activity relationship analysis of arylalkylaminoalcohols, arylalkenylamines, and arylalkylamines as σ1 receptor ligands. *J. Chemom.* 29, 13–20. doi: 10.1002/cem.2650

Ramírez, D., and Caballero, J. (2018). Is it reliable to take the molecular docking top scoring position as the best solution without considering available structural data? *Molecules* 23:1038. doi: 10.3390/molecules23051038

Rossi, D., Marra, A., Picconi, P., Serra, M., Catenacci, L., Sorrenti, M., et al. (2013a). Identification of RC-33 as a potent and selective σ1 receptor agonist potentiating NGF-induced neurite outgrowth in PC12 cells. Part 2: g-scale synthesis, physicochemical characterization and *in vitro* metabolic stability. *Bioorg. Med. Chem.* 21, 2577–2586. doi: 10.1016/j.bmc.2013.02.029

Rossi, D., Marra, A., Rui, M., Laurini, E., Fermeglia, M., Pricl, S., et al. (2015). A step forward in the sigma enigma: a role for chirality in the sigma1 receptor–ligand interaction? *Med. Chem. Commun.* 6, 138–146. doi: 10.1039/C4MD00349G

Rossi, D., Pedrali, A., Gaggeri, R., Marra, A., Pignataro, L., Laurini, E., et al. (2013b). Chemical, pharmacological, and *in vitro* metabolic stability studies on enantiomerically pure RC-33 compounds: promising neuroprotective agents acting as σ1 receptor agonists. *ChemMedChem* 8, 1514–1527. doi: 10.1002/cmdc.201300218

Rossi, D., Pedrali, A., Urbano, M., Gaggeri, R., Serra, M., Fernández, L., et al. (2011). Identification of a potent and selective σ1 receptor agonist potentiating NGF-induced neurite outgrowth in PC12 cells. *Bioorg. Med. Chem.* 19, 6210–6224. doi: 10.1016/j.bmc.2011.09.016

Rossi, D., Rui, M., Di Giacomo, M., Schepmann, D., Wünsch, B., Monteleone, S., et al. (2017). Gaining in pan-affinity towards sigma 1 and sigma 2 receptors. SAR studies on arylalkylamines. *Bioorg. Med. Chem.* 25, 11–19. doi: 10.1016/j.bmc.2016.10.005

Rossi, D., Urbano, M., Pedrali, A., Serra, M., Zampieri, D., Mamolo, M. G., et al. (2010). Design, synthesis and SAR analysis of novel selective sigma1 ligands (Part 2). *Bioorg. Med. Chem.* 18, 1204–1212. doi: 10.1016/j.bmc.2009.12.039

Rui, M., Rossi, D., Marra, A., Paolillo, M., Schinelli, S., Curti, D., et al. (2016). Synthesis and biological evaluation of new aryl-alkyl(alkenyl)-4-benzylpiperidines, novel Sigma Receptor (SR) modulators, as potential anticancer-agents. *Eur. J. Med. Chem.* 124, 649–665. doi: 10.1016/j.ejmech.2016.08.067

Schmidt, H. R., Betz, R. M., Dror, R. O., and Kruse, A. C. (2018). Structural basis for σ1 receptor ligand recognition. *Nat. Struct. Mol. Biol.* 25, 981–987. doi: 10.1038/s41594-018-0137-2

Schmidt, H. R., Zheng, S., Gurpinar, E., Koehl, A., Manglik, A., and Kruse, A. C. (2016). Crystal structure of the human σ1 receptor. *Nature* 532, 527–530. doi: 10.1038/nature17391

Shelley, J. C., Cholleti, A., Frye, L. L., Greenwood, J. R., Timlin, M. R., and Uchimaya, M. (2007). Epik: a software program for pK(a) prediction and protonation state generation for drug-like molecules. *J. Comput. Aided Mol. Des.* 21, 681–691. doi: 10.1007/s10822-007-9133-z

Singh, J., Deng, Z., Narale, G., and Chuaqui, C. (2006). Structural interaction fingerprints: a new approach to organizing, mining, analyzing, and designing protein-small molecule complexes. *Chem. Biol. Drug Des.* 67, 5–12. doi: 10.1111/j.1747-0285.2005.00323.x

Tesei, A., Cortesi, M., Zamagni, A., Arienti, C., Pignatta, S., Zanoni, M., et al. (2018). Sigma receptors as endoplasmic reticulum stress "Gatekeepers" and their modulators as emerging new weapons in the fight against cancer. *Front. Pharmacol.* 9:711. doi: 10.3389/fphar.2018.00711

Tosco, P., and Balle, T. (2011). Open3DQSAR: a new open-source software aimed at high-throughput chemometric analysis of molecular interaction fields. *J. Mol. Model.* 17, 201–208. doi: 10.1007/s00894-010-0684-x

Urbano, M., Collina, S., Rossi, D., Baraglia, A. C., Alcaro, S., Artese, A., et al. (2007). Design and synthesis of a (N-Alkylaminoalkyl-Substituted)arylalkenylamide drug discovery library. *Lett. Drug Des. Discov.* 4, 605–610. doi: 10.2174/157018007782794581

Vavers, E., Svalbe, B., Lauberte, L., Stonans, I., Misane, I., Dambrova, M., et al. (2017). The activity of selective sigma-1 receptor ligands in seizure models *in vivo*. *Behav. Brain Res.* 328, 13–18. doi: 10.1016/j.bbr.2017.04.008

Velázquez-Libera, J. L., Navarro-Retamal, C., and Caballero, J. (2018). Insights into the structural requirements of 2(S)-amino-6-boronohexanoic acid derivatives as arginase I inhibitors: 3D-QSAR, docking, and interaction fingerprint studies. *Int. J. Mol. Sci.* 19:2956. doi: 10.3390/ijms19102956

Walker, J. M., Bowen, W. D., Walker, F. O., Matsumoto, R. R., De Costa, B., and Rice, K. C. (1990). Sigma receptors: biology and function. *Pharmacol. Rev.* 42, 355–402.

Wu, D., Wang, Q., Assary, R. S., Broadbelt, L. J., and Krilov, G. (2011). A computational approach to design and evaluate enzymatic reaction pathways: application to 1-butanol production from pyruvate. *J. Chem. Inf. Model.* 51, 1634–1647. doi: 10.1021/ci2000659

Yagasaki, Y., Numakawa, T., Kumamaru, E., Hayashi, T., Su, T.-P., and Kunugi, H. (2006). Chronic antidepressants potentiate via sigma-1 receptors the brain-derived neurotrophic factor-induced signaling for glutamate release. *J. Biol. Chem.* 281, 12941–12949. doi: 10.1074/jbc.M508157200

Yous, S., Wallez, V., Belloir, M., Caignard, D. H., McCurdy, C. R., and Poupaert, J. H. (2005). Novel 2(3H)-benzothiazolones as highly potent and selective sigma-1 receptor ligands. *Med. Chem. Res.* 14, 158–168. doi: 10.1007/s00044-005-0131-1

Zampieri, D., Grazia Mamolo, M., Laurini, E., Zanette, C., Florio, C., Collina, S., et al. (2009). Substituted benzo[d]oxazol-2(3H)-one derivatives with preference for the sigma1 binding site. *Eur. J. Med. Chem.* 44, 124–130. doi: 10.1016/j.ejmech.2008.03.011

11

In silico Methods for Design of Kinase Inhibitors as Anticancer Drugs

Zarko Gagic[1], *Dusan Ruzic*[2], *Nemanja Djokovic*[2], *Teodora Djikic*[2] *and Katarina Nikolic*[2*]

[1] *Department of Pharmaceutical Chemistry, Faculty of Medicine, University of Banja Luka, Banja Luka, Bosnia and Herzegovina,* [2] *Department of Pharmaceutical Chemistry, Faculty of Pharmacy, University of Belgrade, Belgrade, Serbia*

Correspondence:
Katarina Nikolic
knikolic@pharmacy.bg.ac.rs

Rational drug design implies usage of molecular modeling techniques such as pharmacophore modeling, molecular dynamics, virtual screening, and molecular docking to explain the activity of biomolecules, define molecular determinants for interaction with the drug target, and design more efficient drug candidates. Kinases play an essential role in cell function and therefore are extensively studied targets in drug design and discovery. Kinase inhibitors are clinically very important and widely used antineoplastic drugs. In this review, computational methods used in rational drug design of kinase inhibitors are discussed and compared, considering some representative case studies.

Keywords: kinase inhibitors, rational drug design, molecular modeling, drug discovery, pharmacophore

KINASES AS TARGETS FOR DEVELOPING ANTICANCER DRUGS

Kinases belong to a large family of enzymes that catalyze transfer of high energy phosphate group from adenosine triphosphate (ATP) to substrates, such as proteins (the protein-tyrosine kinases, the serine-threonine specific kinases), lipids (phosphatidylinositol kinases, sphingosine kinases), carbohydrates, and nucleic acids (Duong-Ly and Peterson, 2013). Phosphorylation of the substrate modulates its activity and/or interaction with other molecules leading to different physiological responses. It is estimated that 50% of all proteins are constantly undergoing reversible phosphorylation and dephosphorylation, which emphasizes the role of protein kinases in almost all aspects of cell function, including proliferation, cell growth, apoptosis, and signal transduction (Graves and Krebs, 1999; Manning et al., 2002).

Dysregulated, overexpressed, or mutated protein kinases are found in many diseases, including cancer, and over the past two decades they became extensively examined targets for the development of new antineoplastic drugs (Blume-Jensen and Hunter, 2001; Cohen, 2002). There are 53 kinase inhibitors (KIs) currently approved by the FDA (FDA, 2019), while over 200 potential inhibitors are in different phases of clinical trials worldwide (Carles et al., 2018). Majority of the approved drugs are orally active and effective against various malignancies (**Table 1**; Roskoski, 2019a,b).

Structures of the selected KIs commonly used for treatment of cancer are shown in **Figure 1**. These drugs target different protein kinases that are frequently upregulated in cancer cells. The epidermal growth factor receptor (EGFR) is a member of the ErbB family of tyrosine kinase receptors that is overexpressed or mutated in non-small cell lung cancer and represents the primary target for drugs such erlotinib and gefitinib (Bethune et al., 2010). Lapatinib and neratinib bind to intracellular domain of the human epidermal growth factor receptor 2 (HER2/neu), another member of the ErbB tyrosine kinases, which elevated levels are found in approximately 20–30% of breast cancers (Collins et al., 2019). Imatinib possesses activity against non-receptor breakpoint cluster region (Bcr)-Abelson leukemia virus (Abl) tyrosine kinase that is formed as a result of a chromosome rearrangement and has been implicated in the pathogenesis of nearly all cases of chronic myeloid leukemia (CML) and acute lymphoblastic leukemia with the Philadelphia chromosome (Iqbal and Iqbal, 2014). Although imatinib is a relatively specific Bcr-Abl inhibitor, it also inhibits the CD117 tyrosine kinase associated with gastrointestinal stromal tumors and has consequently been approved for this indication (Buchdunger et al., 2000). The vascular endothelial growth factor family of receptors (VEGFR) contains a tyrosine kinase domain which activation can lead to induction of signaling pathways that regulate cell proliferation, survival, and promotion of tumor angiogenesis (Morabito et al., 2006). Agents that target VEGFR, including lenvatinib, sorafenib and vandetanib, are frequently used for treatment of thyroid cancers. Vemurafenib, dabrafenib, and encorafenib target BRAF, a serine/threonine protein kinase which mutation is expressed at about 50–60% of cutaneous melanomas where it leads to continuous activation of mitogen-activated protein kinase (MAPK) pathway and uncontrolled proliferation of cancer cells (Yu et al., 2019).

TABLE 1 | Therapeutic indications of selected FDA-approved protein kinase inhibitors.

Therapeutic indication	Drug
Breast cancer	Everolimus, lapatinib, neratinib, palbociclib, ribociclib
Non-small cell lung cancer	Afatinib, alectinib, brigatinib, ceritinib, crizotinib, dabrafenib, dacomitinib, erlotinib, gefitinib, lorlatinib, osimertinib
Leukemia	Bosutinib, dasatinib, gilteritinib, ibrutinib, imatinib, midostaurin, nilotinib, ponatinib
Melanoma	Binimetinib, cobimetinib, dabrafenib, encorafenib, trametinib, vemurafenib
Thyroid cancer	Cabozantinib, lenvatinib, vandetanib
Renal cancer	Axitinib, pazopanib, sorafenib, temsirolimus
Gastrointestinal cancer	Regorafenib, sunitinib

Structure of Protein Kinases

The human genome encodes at least 518 protein kinases (Manning et al., 2002). Out of them, 478 share highly conserved catalytic domains. The remaining 40 do not share the sequence similarity, but their folding is similar to the folding of "typical" PKs (Caballero and Alzate-Morales, 2012). In 1991, Knighton solved the X-ray structure of cyclic AMP-dependent PK and described its structure for the first time. This description can apply to all currently known protein kinases. The characteristic architecture of the catalytic domain of PK consists of a small, amino-terminal N-lobe and a large α-helical carboxy-terminal C-lobe which are connected with a small hinge region (**Figure 2**; Knighton et al., 1991). The N-terminal lobe is dominated by five β-strands (β1–β5) and one conserved α-helix (helix C) that occurs in active (αC-in) or inactive (αC-out) orientations. The C-lobe consists of eight α-helices and four short conserved β-strands (β6–β9) which include residues that participate in the phosphorylation of protein substrates. The small and large lobes form a catalytic cleft where ATP binds (Knighton et al., 1991; Roskoski, 2019a). The hydrophobic residues of the cleft form a binding pocket for ATP. The charged residues in the active site bind and position the γ-phosphate of ATP and divalent cation and take part in the catalysis (Knight et al., 2007).

Conserved residues play crucial roles in positioning ATP, stabilizing the active-conformation and in the catalytic mechanism, and they are mostly found in and around the active site but also in other parts of the protein kinase domain (Knight et al., 2007). Almost all protein kinases possess a conserved K/E/D/D (Lys/Glu/Asp/Asp) signature that is important for the

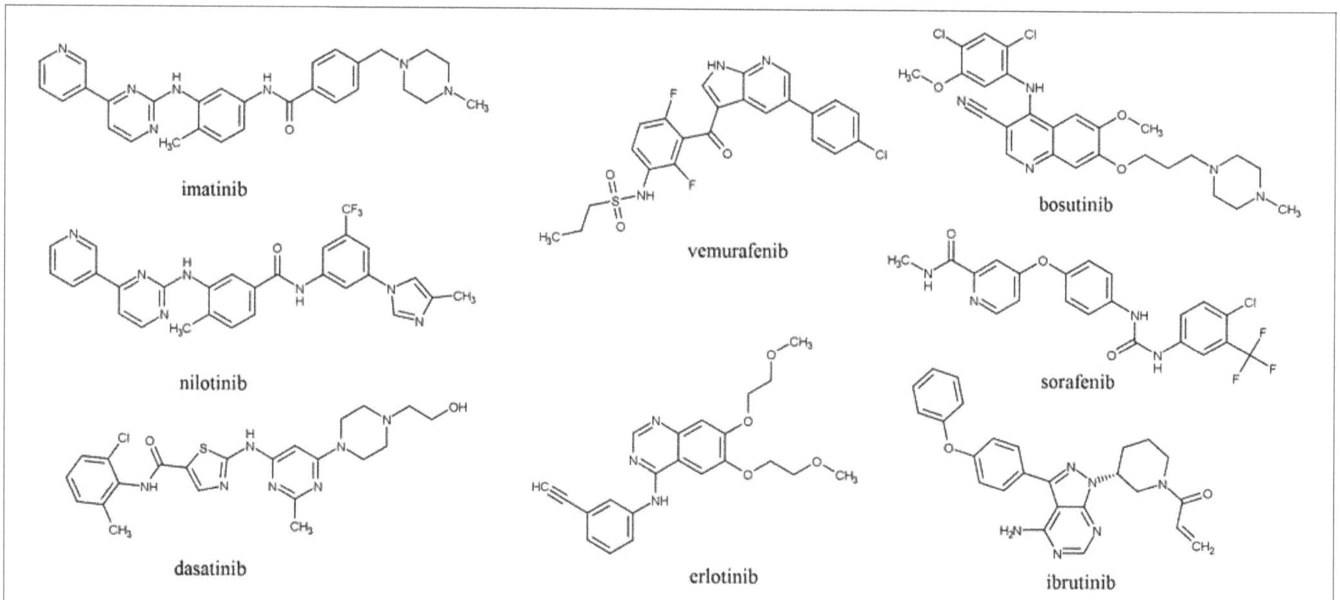

FIGURE 1 | Structures of selected protein kinase inhibitors that have been approved for clinical use.

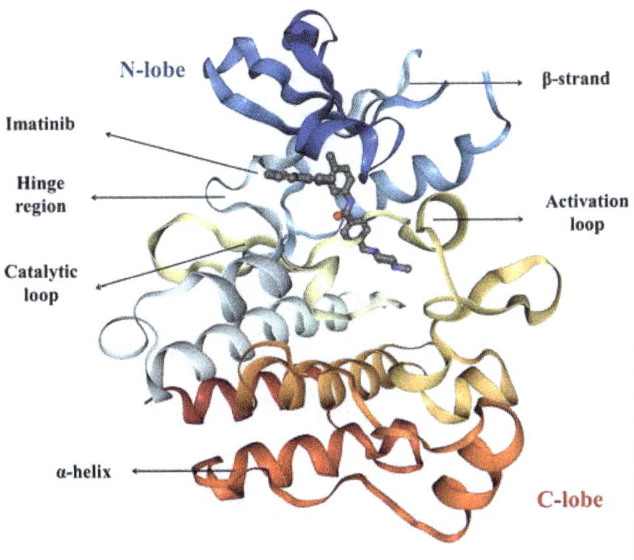

FIGURE 2 | The crystal structure of imatinib-bound form of the Abl kinase (PDB accession code: 2HYY), colored as rainbow from N-lobe (blue) to C-lobe (red). Imatinib is represented as ball and stick.

catalysis. Lysine and glutamic acid residues belong to the N-lobe, and the two aspartic acid residues are found in the C-lobe. Lysine residue binds to the α- and β-phosphates of ATP. Formation of the salt bridge between the carboxylate group of aspartic acid and the amino group of lysine stabilizes its interactions with the α- and β-phosphates, and it is required for kinase activation (Roskoski, 2015, 2019a,b).

The N-lobe contains a conserved flexible glycine-rich GxGxxG motif (also called P-loop) between $\beta 1$ and $\beta 2$ that folds over the nucleotide and places the γ-phosphate of ATP during the catalysis (Taylor and Kornev, 2011). As mentioned above, lysine from the $\beta 3$-strand forms a salt bridge with the conserved glutamate near the center of the protein-kinase αC-helix which is necessary for the formation of the active enzyme, and this structure corresponds to the "αC-in" conformation (Roskoski, 2015, 2019a,b).

The C-lobe is important for both the protein-substrate binding as well as nucleotide binding (Roskoski, 2015). The C-lobe contains a mobile activation loop of 20–30 residues which can take open or closed conformation. The activation loop begins with the DFG motif (Asp-Phe-Gly) and extends up to an APE motif (Ala-Pro-Glu) (Modi and Dunbrack, 2019). In the active conformation a divalent metal ion, Mg^{2+} (or sometimes Mn^{2+}), interacts with a highly conserved aspartic acid residue from the DFG motif. It coordinates with the α and γ phosphates of ATP and facilitates the phosphorylation and coordinates the ATP binding (Adams, 2001). At the other end, glutamic acid from APE motif is fixed by the formation of a salt bridge with arginine from the C-lobe (Roskoski, 2015, 2019b). In addition to these, another motif on the C-lobe is highly conserved suggesting it plays an important role in the catalysis—HRD (rarely YRD) motif. The aspartate residue of this motif is required for the orientation of the hydroxyl group of the substrate peptide at the P-site and the transfer of the phosphoryl group. Arginine residue interacts with the phosphorylated activation segment thereby contributing to its correct orientation. Histidine (or in rare cases tyrosine) is considered to be involved in the maintenance of the conserved rigid organization of the catalytic core (La Sala et al., 2016).

The main differences between tyrosine kinases and serine/threonine kinases are found in the protein-substrate binding site. In serine/threonine kinases, the phosphorylatable serine or threonine of the protein substrate interacts with backbone residues near the end of the activation segment. Basic residues of the protein-substrate N-terminal interact with surface acidic residues of the C-lobe. Additionally, peptide substrate is fixed by serine in the glycine rich loop and lysine in the catalytic loop and also to threonine in the P+1 loop. These three residues are highly conserved in the majority of protein-serine/threonine kinases, and they are positioning the target hydroxyl group of a substrate in the catalytic cleft (near the γ-phosphate of ATP) where the phosphotransfer reaction happens (P-site). Since both serine and threonine hydroxyls are linked to the β-carbon, they have similar mechanisms of the catalysis. On the other hand, in tyrosine kinases, after DFG motif, there is a very stable region that contains the three tyrosine phosphorylation sites. The protein substrate chain positions in a manner that one of the tyrosines is oriented with its hydroxyl group lying in phosphorylation site P-site. The following tyrosine residue lies in the P+1 site. Proline residue interacts with the tyrosyl residue of the protein-substrate and is responsible for positioning the P-site tyrosine in the phosphotransfer site. The tyrosine ring is also positioned by Arg (Hubbard et al., 1994; Taylor et al., 1995; Roskoski, 2015).

Moreover, many protein kinases are regulated by different mechanisms such as dimerization, binding of allosteric effectors, or other modifications important for subcellular localization that can modulate their activity. Binding of an allosteric modulator leads to conformational changes that mostly involve structural reorganization of the activation loop, making it a primary end point of allosteric regulation. Effectors or regulatory subunits bind outside the catalytic site, causing the changes in loop conformation through conformational changes of other substructural elements. In most of the cases, regulators bind the αC helix at different locations, allowing control of catalysis from distal regions (Shi et al., 2006). Nevertheless, the αC helix is not the only allosteric binding site, in fact, they are very diverse (**Figure 3**; Ohren et al., 2004; Vanderpool et al., 2009; Jahnke et al., 2010; Martin et al., 2012; Park et al., 2015; Rettenmaier et al., 2015; Ung et al., 2018). Therefore, understanding the diversity of allosteric regulatory sites among the kinase superfamily gives a unique opportunity for the creation of novel selective allosteric kinase antagonists (Lamba and Ghosh, 2012).

Active/Inactive States

Basically, protein kinases reside in one active state and multiple inactive states (**Figure 4**). In active kinase conformation, activation loop forms a cleft that binds the substrate. When the substrate peptide binds, it interacts with the HRD motif (His-Arg-Asp). Asp from the DFG motif binds a magnesium ion that interacts directly with an oxygen atom of the β phosphate of

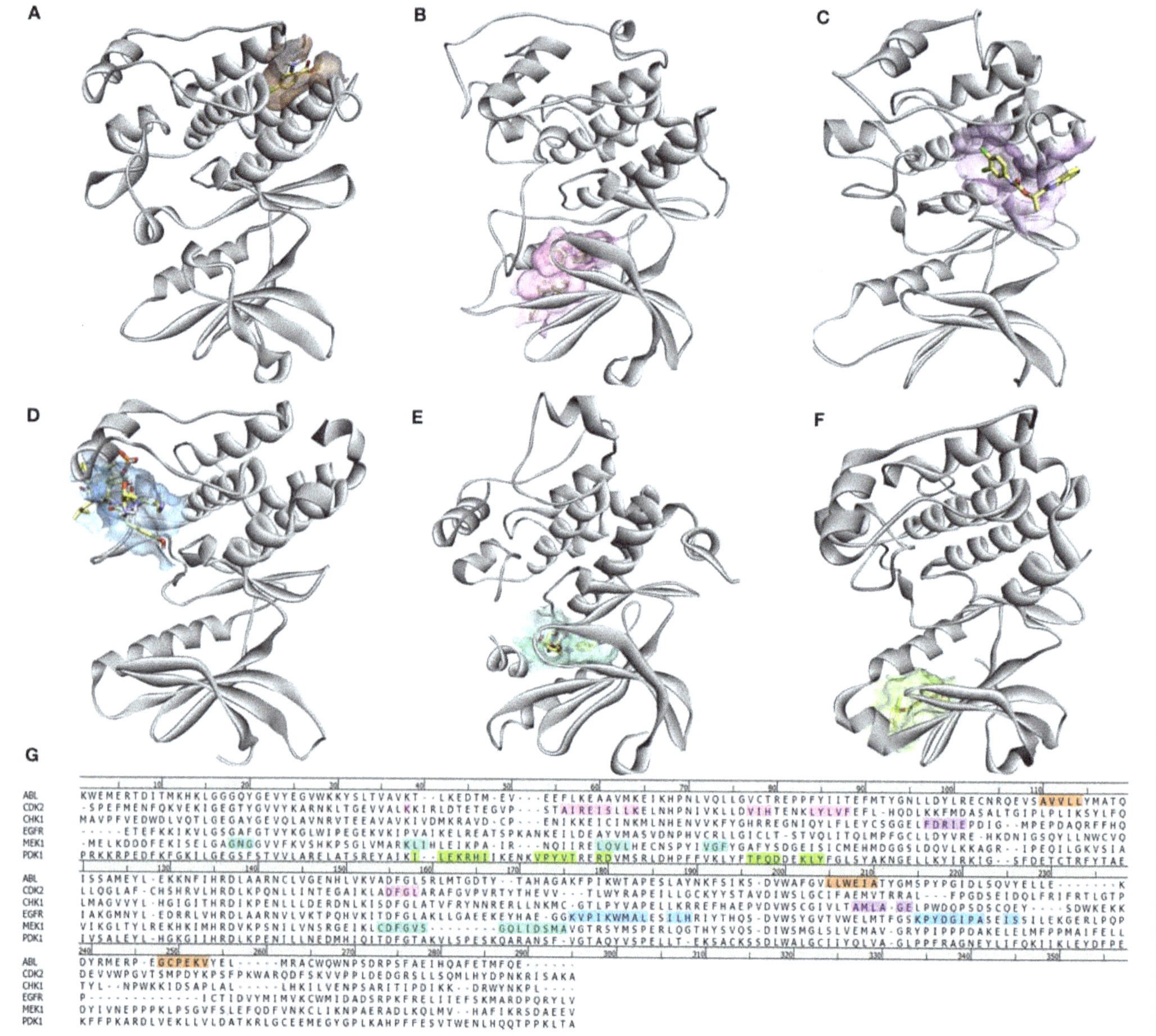

FIGURE 3 | Diversity of allosteric binding pockets in different protein kinases. **(A)** ABL kinase in complex with fragment FRAG1 (PDB: 3MS9) (Jahnke et al., 2010); **(B)** CDK2 in complex with 2 molecules of 8-anilino-1-naphthalene sulfonic acid (PBD: 4EZ7) (Martin et al., 2012); **(C)** CHK1 bound to allosteric inhibitor (1S)-1-(1H-benzimidazol-2-yl)ethyl (3,4-dichlorophenyl)carbamate (PDB: 3JVR) (Vanderpool et al., 2009); **(D)** EGFR in complex with Mig6 protein (PDB: 4R3P) (Park et al., 2015); **(E)** PDK1 with PIF pocket inhibitor RF4 (Rettenmaier et al., 2015); **(F)** MEK1 in complex with 5-bromo-N-(2,3-dihydroxyprpoxy)-3,4-difluoro-2-[(2fluoro-4-iodophenyl)amino]benzamide (PDB: 1S9J) (Ohren et al., 2004); **(G)** Sequence alignment of these kinases showing which amino acids are involved in the binding of allosteric modulators.

ATP. This is followed by formation of a salt bridge between the Glu from the C-helix with a Lys residue in the $\beta 3$ strand. When the salt bridge is formed, the lysine side chain forms hydrogen bonds with oxygen atoms of α and β phosphates of ATP. The Glycine-rich Loop of the N-lobe stabilizes the phosphates of the bound ATP molecule during catalysis (Taylor and Kornev, 2011; Modi and Dunbrack, 2019). In an inactive conformation, usually the activation loop is blocking the substrate binding, and DFG motif is incompatible with the binding ATP and magnesium ion required for catalysis. Many attempts have been made in order to achieve classification for these conformations and to study interaction of inhibitors in different states (Mobitz, 2015; Ung et al., 2018; Modi and Dunbrack, 2019), and they are all based on the position of highly conserved DFG motif.

The most recent classification was published by Modi and Dunbrack. They have divided kinase structures into three clusters based on the spatial position of the DFG-Phe side chain into DFG-in, DFG-out, and DFG-inter (intermediate) conformations.

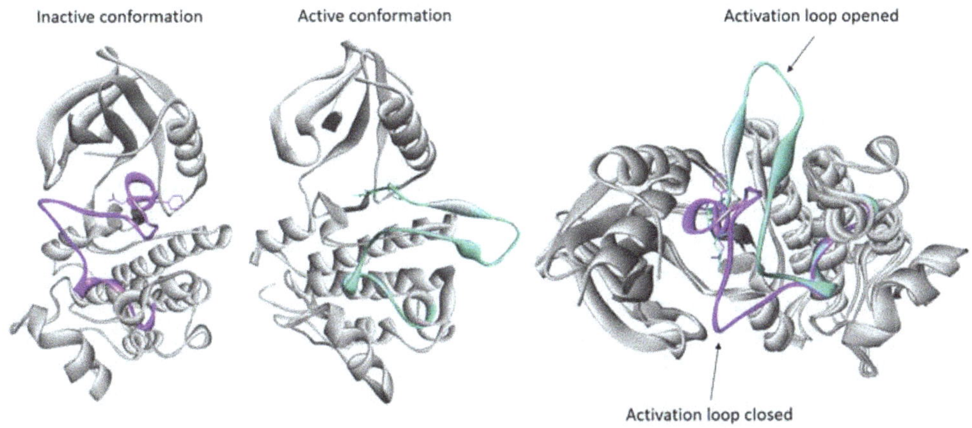

FIGURE 4 | Examples of inactive and active conformations of epidermal growth factor receptor (EGFR) kinase (PDB accession codes: 4HJO and 2GS6, respectively), and their superimposition. The activation loop of inactive conformation (purple) is closed therefore blocking the substrate to enter catalytic loop, while activation loop in active conformation (turquoise) is opened allowing the ATP to bind.

Each of these three clusters was further divided based on the dihedral angles required to place the Phe side chain, resulting in total of eight clusters: six for DFG-in and one cluster each for the DFG-out and DFG-inter groups. DFG-in represents the DFG motif orientations where DFG-Phe is packed against or under the C-helix. It contains many conformations, among all the typical DFG-in active conformation belongs to this group. DFG-out represents the structures where DFG-Phe is moved into the ATP binding pocket. DFG-inter represents the conformations in which the DFG-Phe side chain is out of the C-helix pocket but has not moved completely to a DFG-out conformation. Usually in this conformation DFG-Phe is pointing upward toward the β-sheets while dividing the active site into two halves (Modi and Dunbrack, 2019). This classification offers insight into active and inactive kinase conformations which are of great importance in structure-based design of kinase inhibitors.

Types of Kinase Inhibitors

Many reviewers have categorized KIs based on their binding modes into three classes, labeled as types I, II, and III kinase inhibitors (Roskoski, 2016; Bhullar et al., 2018). Type I inhibitors, such as gefitinib, bind to the active DFG-in conformation of a kinase in the phosphorylated ATP catalytic site, and they usually contain a heterocycle that mimic the purine ring of ATP. Considering that the ATP active site is highly conserved among different protein kinases, these ATP-competitive inhibitors display low selectivity profile which may lead to off-target side effects. While the physiological relevance of many off-target effects is still unclear, it was demonstrated that the lack of selectivity is connected with preclinical and clinical cardiotoxicity of kinase inhibitors (Force and Kolaja, 2011; Yang and Papoian, 2012). Possible mechanism behind the KI induced cardiotoxicity lies in binding of these drugs to colony-stimulating factor 1 receptor (CSF1R) (Hasinoff, 2010). Type II inhibitors, such as imatinib, bind to the inactive (DFG-out) conformation of a kinase in the unphosphorylated ATP catalytic site (Dar and Shokat, 2011). Zuccotto introduced type I½ inhibitors as compounds that bind to active ATP catalytic site as type I inhibitors but elongate into the back cavity of the ATP site giving rise to interactions specific for type II pharmacophore. These inhibitors represented by dasatinib, lapatinib, and vemurafenib, display higher selectivity profile as compared to Type I KIs (Zuccotto et al., 2010). Types III and IV are allosteric inhibitors that bind outside the ATP-binding site. Type III includes trametinib that binds to the allosteric site close to the ATP pocket, whereas Type IV inhibitors bind to a pocket distant from the ATP-binding site. Bivalent inhibitor spanning two regions of the protein kinase is termed as Type V (Wong et al., 2017), while KIs that form an irreversible covalent bond with the catalytic site represent Type VI inhibitors (afatinib and ibrutinib) (Roskoski, 2016).

Developing and Overcoming Resistance to Kinase Inhibitors

Despite the significant advances achieved by the use of protein kinase inhibitors, drug resistance remains one of the greatest challenges toward successful cancer treatment. Various mechanisms can underpin the development of resistance to KIs, including alterations in protein kinases, aberration of downstream pathways, or bypass mechanism that activates parallel signaling pathways (Holohan et al., 2013). Mutations of Bcr-Abl kinase domain were found in over 90% of patients with CML who relapsed after an initial response to imatinib. These mutations include different amino acid substitutions at the active site residues or changes in the kinase flexibility that impair its ability to adopt the inactive conformation required for optimal imatinib binding (Shah et al., 2002). Dasatinib is a novel Abl kinase inhibitor that can bind to both the active (mutated) and inactive (normal) conformations of Bcr-Abl, and its activity has been demonstrated in all imatinib-resistant CML patients, with the exception of those with the

T315I mutation that prevents formation of critical hydrogen bond (Shah et al., 2004; Burgess et al., 2005). Docking of dasatinib to three Bcr-Abl conformations (active, inactive, and intermediate inactive) showed that dasatinib binds preferentially to an active conformation, and that binding affinity significantly decreases when the kinase adopts inactive conformation (Laurini et al., 2013). Drug combinations targeting different upstream and downstream components within a single pathway, or targeting parallel kinase pathways, have been proved in clinical trials as an efficient method to overcame or delay therapeutic resistance. For instance, treatment with dabrafenib, a selective BRAF inhibitor, and trametinib, a selective MAPK kinase inhibitor, significantly improved progression-free survival of melanoma patients (Flaherty et al., 2012).

IN SILICO METHODS USED IN DRUG DESIGN

Since the approval of imatinib in 2001, protein kinases have received significant attention from academic and pharmaceutical companies, reflected in a large number of publications, solved crystal structures, and identified small molecule inhibitors for about one-fifth of the human kinome (Wu et al., 2015b). Considerable progress in this field is much owed to the use of computational methods that were able to provide valuable information on structural characteristic of both the kinase and the ligand that are important for favorable interaction and desired inhibitory activity (Agafonov et al., 2015). To design inhibitors for protein kinases it is necessary to understand the structure and dynamics of these enzymes, substrate recognition, and reaction of phosphorylation, product release as well as differences between active and inactive conformations.

There are two main approaches within the framework of computer-aided drug design (CADD): structure-based drug design (SBDD), and ligand-based drug design (LBDD). SBDD is based on structural information gathered from biological targets and includes *in silico* methods such as molecular docking, structure-based virtual screening (SBVS), and molecular dynamics (MD). In contrast, in the absence of information on targets, LBDD relies on the knowledge of ligands that interact with a specific target, and these methods include ligand-based virtual screening (LBVS), similarity searching, quantitative structure-activity relationship (QSAR) modeling, and pharmacophore generation (Ferreira et al., 2015). Over the last years, a large number of studies have reported successful use of CADD in design and discovery of new drugs (Lu et al., 2018b). In this study we provide the comprehensive review of computational tools that led to discovery, design and optimization of KIs as anticancer drugs.

Ligand-Based Methods in Drug Design

QSAR modeling involves the formation of a mathematical relationship between experimentally determined biological activity and quantitatively defined chemical characteristics that describe the analyzed molecule (descriptors) within a set of structurally similar compounds. The QSAR concept originated in the 1860s, when Crum-Brown and Fraser proposed the idea that the physiological action of a compound in a particular biological system is a function of its chemical constituent, while the modern era of QSAR modeling is associated with the work of Hansch et al. in the early 1960s (Hansch et al., 1962). The aim of the QSAR modeling is to utilize the information on structure and activity obtained from a relatively small series of data to ensure that the best lead compounds enter further studies, minimizing the time and the expense of drug development process (Cherkasov et al., 2014).

Classical 2D-QSAR models correlate physicochemical parameters, such as electronic, hydrophobic or steric characteristics of compounds, to biological activity, while the more advanced 3D-QSAR modeling adds quantum chemical parameters. One of the first approaches used in deriving 3D-QSAR models was CoMFA (comparative molecular field analysis). With this analysis, molecules were described with electrostatic and steric fields, which were correlated to biological activity by means of partial least squares regression (PLS) (Cramer et al., 1988). In addition to the steric and electrostatic descriptors, another approach used in deriving 3D-QSAR models was Comparative Molecular Similarity Index Analysis (CoMSIA). CoMSIA approach additionally uses three novel fields comparing to CoMFA, describing the ligand's hydrophobic properties, the presence of the hydrogen bond donors (HBD), and the presence of hydrogen bond acceptors (HBA) (Klebe et al., 1994). The main limitation of the CoMFA/CoMSIA methods is that they are largely dependent on the alignment of 3D-molecular structures which is often a slow process prone to subjectivity. Recently, modern QSAR programs that use new generation of 3D-descriptors, so-called grid-independent (GRIND) descriptors, have been developed and used for multivariate analyses and 3D-QSAR modeling (Pastor et al., 2000; Duran et al., 2009; Smajić et al., 2015; Gagic et al., 2016b).

Recent cases of reported QSAR studies aimed at providing useful information to guide the discovery of new potent KIs are listed in **Table 2**. Some of them will be discussed in this chapter.

Koneru et al. have used QSAR combined with molecular dynamics to redesign second-generation Src kinase inhibitor RL-45 in order to withstand the gatekeeper residue mutation

TABLE 2 | Selected studies that have used QSAR in the design of kinase inhibitors.

Target kinase	QSAR method	Software package	References
Mer	3D	Pentacle	Shiri et al., 2016
Lyn	2D	JMP	Naboulsi et al., 2018
HER2, EGFR	3D	SYBYL	de Angelo et al., 2018
EGFR	2D and 3D	SYBYL	Simeon et al., 2019
IKK-β	2D and 3D	Discovery studio; Schrödinger suite	Wang et al., 2019a
EGFR	3D	SYBYL	Zhao et al., 2019a
Src	3D	Vlife MDS	Koneru et al., 2019
VEGFR-2	3D	MOE	Mohamed et al., 2019
PKMYT1	2D	MOE	Najjar et al., 2019

and enhance binding affinity. They integrated fragment-based drug discovery (FBDD) technique with QSAR and molecular dynamics to assess novel Src kinase inhibitors. Newly designed compounds were assumed to be able to mitigate mutation-related Src kinase resistance and to bind more efficiently to the kinase active site and were proposed for further synthesis (Koneru et al., 2019). Wang et al. applied QSAR studies on a series of 2-acylamino-3-aminothienopyridine analogs in order to design new IKK-β inhibitors (Wang et al., 2019a). Obtained information on physicochemical, structural, electrostatic, and steric properties revealed that bulky aryl substituents at position C3 on the piperidine ring have favorable effect on activity, which led to the design of an in-house library. Compounds with best predicted activities were further subjected to docking studies. Based on these results two new compounds B01 and B02 were identified as potential IKK-β inhibitors, with predicted pIC_{50} activities of 7.18 and 7.17, and binding affinities of 41.6 and 40.1 kcal/mol, respectively.

Comparative 2D- and 3D-QSAR studies, followed by molecular docking were conducted on a series of quinazoline derivatives acting as EGFR inhibitors (Noolvi and Patel, 2013). According to the 2D-QSAR multiple linear regression (MLR) model, anticancer activity of quinazoline derivatives was influenced by lipophilicity and number of hydrogen bond donors. Presence of short chain ethers such as methoxy-, ethoxy- at C-6 and C-7 positions of quinazoline was found favorable for the activity, while N-containing groups should not be directly attached to the quinazoline ring. 3D-QSAR kNN-MFA (k-nearest neighbor molecular field analysis) revealed that the presence of electronegative groups on the anilino moiety site, electropositive groups at position C7, and a bulky aromatic substituent at C4 increases the EGFR kinase inhibitory activity.

Virtual screening (VS) refers to a group of *in silico* methods widely used in drug discovery to search large-scale compound databases in order to select a more manageable number of candidates with the highest probability of displaying the desired biological activity (Gagic et al., 2016a; Oluic et al., 2017; Vucicevic et al., 2017; Banegas-Luna et al., 2018). This method has been very popular among pharmaceutical companies since it enables developing drugs in time and cost-effective manner and increases the chance of selected candidates to reach clinical studies. Considering the constant improvement of computational power, it is expected that in the near future VS will be a reasonable alternative to high throughput screening (HTS) (Kumar et al., 2015). There are generally two approaches to screen molecular libraries: LBVS that will be discussed in this section and SBVS.

LBVS is often applied when there are known active compounds, but the target of action is not known, or the crystallographic structure of the protein is not available. These active compounds are then used as ligands to screen molecular libraries based on the similar property principle, which states that structurally similar compounds should possess similar biochemical properties (Nikolic et al., 2015; Bajorath, 2017). For each compound from the virtual library, the similarity with the known active is calculated. Many different strategies for measuring similarity have been developed, including Cosine coefficient, Euclidean distance, Soergel distance, and Tanimoto coefficient (Bajusz et al., 2015). Compounds are ranked based on the similarity score and those at the top are selected as virtual hit molecules for further optimization and synthesis. Modern VS protocols include additional filtering steps in order to exclude compounds that e.g., have low similarity score, do not fall within the Lipinski's rule of five, are not feasible for synthesis or are not available for purchase (Neves et al., 2018).

Besides similarity searches, pharmacophore search is one of the most commonly used LBVS techniques. Given a list of known actives, pharmacophore model can be derived to define the minimum structural requirements that molecule must possess in order to exhibit good activity profile (Vittorio et al., 2019). It is then possible to search large databases, such as PubChem (Kim et al., 2019), ChEMBL (Mendez et al., 2019), and DrugBank (Wishart et al., 2018), for identification of lead compounds that fit to the pharmacophore structure (Bacilieri and Moro, 2006). Several studies that describe the use of LBVS methodology in discovery of potential kinase inhibitors have been listed in **Table 3**. Pharmacophore-based VS model was employed to search for new tumor progression locus-2 (Tpl2) inhibitors (Teli and Rajanikant, 2012). Tpl2 is a serine/threonine kinase in the MAPK signaling pathway that regulates cell proliferation, survival, and death and participates in many processes of tumor development (Lee et al., 2015). For this purpose, Asinex database was screened using PHASE 3.0 module of the Schrodinger molecular modeling software which resulted in six potential Tpl2 kinase inhibitors. A 3D QSAR pharmacophore model was developed from the structures of known inhibitors of MAPK1 (ERK2) and used for virtual screening of ZINC database (Irwin et al., 2012) that contains over 750 million compounds, DrugBank with 13,443 drugs (Wishart et al., 2018), NCI (https://cactus.nci.nih.gov/ncidb2.2/) with 250,250 structures, Maybridge (https://www.maybridge.com) with over 53,000 compounds and Chembank database (Seiler et al., 2008). Top screened compounds were then subjected to molecular docking that identified new scaffolds with high potency and selectivity against ERK2 (Larif et al., 2014).

It can be concluded that VS strategies, especially Pharmacophore-based VS and combined use of VS and molecular docking, can be a reliable tool for future discovery of new KIs and have a potential to replace a HTS that is costly and time consuming process.

TABLE 3 | Selected studies that have used LBVS in the design of kinase inhibitors.

Target kinase	Software package	References
EGFR	PHASE	Sudha et al., 2015
CDK2	SYBYL	Zhang and Ren, 2018
ERK-1/2	QSAR-Co	Halder et al., 2019
VEGFR 2	Discovery studio	Sobhy et al., 2019
ALK	PHASE	James et al., 2019
CDK9/Cyclin T1	LigandScout	Hussain and Verma, 2019
FGFR1	Discovery studio	Liu et al., 2020

Case Studies

Application of quantitative structure-activity relationship in structure elucidation of Lyn kinase inhibitors

The generalized linear model (GLM) and the artificial neural network (ANN) QSAR models were combined with structural analysis in order to define pharmacophore of Lyn kinase inhibitors (Naboulsi et al., 2018). Lyn kinase is a member of the Src family of tyrosine kinases that was found to be correlated with chemotherapeutic resistance of cancer cells in patients with CML (Chakraborty et al., 2013; Aira et al., 2018). Derived pharmacophore for the inhibition of Lyn kinase suggested the presence of planar heterocyclic ring that contains HBD and HBA, a spacer that allows free bond rotation and central hydrophobic area that is linked to the aromatic ring substituted with lipophilic groups. These structural futures can be found in nilotinib and dasatinib that are approved for treatment of CML (**Figure 1**). Pyrimidine moiety of nilotinib has the role of the hydrogen bonding region; the attached amino group serves as a spacer that is linked to hydrophobic benzyl group connected with another aromatic ring that is substituted with lipophilic trifluoromethyl group and methylimidazole. Aminopyrimidine moiety is also present in dasatinib that is indicated in CML patients that developed resistance to nilotinib (Okabe et al., 2011). Dasatinib, instead of central hydrophobic benzene ring, contains thiazole connected to an aromatic ring with lipophilic substituents. Results of these QSAR studies can be of great help in future design and lead to optimization of new, more potent Lyn kinase inhibitors for treatment of patients with imatinib and nilotinib-resistant CML.

Quantum mechanical based quantitative structure-activity relationship of N-phenylquinazolin-4-amine derivatives as epidermal growth factor receptor inhibitors

Recently, Simeon at al. applied several 2D- and 3D-QSAR methodologies on a series of EGFR inhibitors, derivatives of N-phenylquinazolin-4-amine (Simeon et al., 2019). 2D QSAR models were created using physico-chemical descriptors, e-state indices and molecular fingerprints, while 3D-QSAR models were developed using CoMFA, CoMSIA, and quantum mechanical (QM) methods. Based on the calculated statistical parameters, the QM-QSAR model displayed better predictive power compared to the other models. Development of this model started with docking of N-phenylquinazolin-4-amine analogs to the EGFR active site and calculation of pairwise interaction energies between each inhibitor and amino acid residues using quantum mechanics. Distances that hold information about the position of the quinazoline ring and the aniline pharmacophores within the active site of the EGFR were extracted and used as descriptors for the QM-QSAR model. Combined 2D- physico-chemical and QM-QSAR model showed even better predictivity and provided more precise information about structural characteristics that are important for EGFR inhibitory activity. Based on the results of this study, it can be concluded that a combination of classical and more advanced quantum mechanical QSAR methodologies represents a good concept for future design of new EGFR inhibitors.

Discovery of potential FGFR1 inhibitors using pharmacophore-based virtual screening

Pharmacophore-based VS protocol was developed in Maestro 9.0 software package (https://www.schrodinger.com/) and used to screen SPECS database (http://www.specs.net) for potential FGFR1 inhibitors (Zhou et al., 2015). Database was previously filtered to extract only compounds with drug-like properties that comply with the Lipinski's rule of 5. Activities of top ranked compounds were predicted with constructed atom-based 3D-QSAR model, and those with highest activities were purchased for experimental enzyme assay. Nineteen hits exhibited moderate inhibitory activity with more than 50% FGFR1 inhibition at 50 μM concentration and IC_{50} values of most active compounds were 7.9 and 55.5 μM. It should be mentioned that the identified compounds had low structural similarity with previously reported FGFR1 inhibitors and offered novel chemical scaffolds for future optimization of FGFR1 inhibitors.

Structure based methods in drug design

Recent progresses in the field of X-ray crystallography, Nuclear Magnetic Resonance (NMR) techniques, and cryo-electron microscopy (CEM) caused a significant increase in the number of known 3D structures of proteins (Sun et al., 2011). With known 3D structures of proteins, docking became a method of choice in drug design.

Molecular docking predicts the most probable orientation of one molecule toward another (Lengauer and Rarey, 1996). It can be performed between a small molecule and a target protein (ligand-protein docking) or between two proteins (protein-protein docking). In ligand-protein docking, which will be discussed here, the samples of conformations of small molecules–ligands are placed into the binding sites of protein, where scoring functions are used to calculate which of these conformations best fits the target protein binding site (Sousa et al., 2006; Warren et al., 2006). Overall, docking protocols include search algorithm and a scoring function. Initially, the search algorithm is used to orient small molecules in the target binding site (Taylor et al., 2002). Sampling of conformational space has to be carried out with acceptable accuracy to determine the conformation that best fits the binding site, but fast enough to evaluate a large number of docked ligands. With today's computer power it would be impossible to explore all the degrees of freedom for ligand and protein complex. Therefore, there are different ways to overcome this problem. Search algorithms can be systematic and stochastic and deterministic (Novič et al., 2016). Systematic search algorithms sample the search space at predefined intervals while stochastic make random changes until a user-defined termination criterion is met, and because of that outcome can vary (Morris and Lim-Wilby, 2008). Search algorithm is then followed by scoring function that estimates the affinity of ligand through the assessment of interactions between ligands and potential targets (Kitchen et al., 2004). Scoring functions can be physics-based, empirical, knowledge-based, and machine learning-based (Liu and Wang, 2015; Li et al., 2019). The physic-based scoring function computes the free energy of binding by summing up the van der Waals and electrostatic interactions between the protein–ligand (enthalpy), and adding the torsion entropy of ligand as well as the solvation/desolvation effect described by explicit and implicit solvent models (Huang et al., 2006; Liu and Wang, 2015). Empirical scoring function estimates the binding affinity of a complex by accumulating significant energetic factors for protein–ligand binding (hydrogen bonds, hydrophobic effects, steric clashes, etc.). It uses a training set with known binding affinities of protein–ligand complex and optimizes the weights of the energetic factors by the means of regression analysis (Eldridge et al., 1997; Liu and Wang, 2015). The knowledge-based scoring functions also uses structural information of large set of known protein–ligand complexes and converts it into distance-dependent Helmholtz free interaction energies (Muegge and Martin, 1999; Li et al., 2019). Machine-learning based scoring functions for docking are getting more interests nowadays. These methods combine QSAR analysis and protein–ligand interaction evaluation. They combine QSAR analysis and protein–ligand interaction evaluation. The training set of protein–ligand complexes with known structures and binding affinities is required for a model calculation. Structural interaction fingerprints between a protein and a ligand are coded with certain descriptors (electrostatic interactions, hydrogen bonds, or aromatic stacking, surface or shape properties, molecular weight, number of rotatable single bonds, etc.). Then, different machine-learning algorithms are employed for variable selection (Deng et al., 2004; Zhang et al., 2006).

Molecular docking can be employed in many parts of drug discovery process, such as structure–activity studies, lead optimization, structure based virtual screening, binding modes defining, chemical mechanism studies, etc. (Nikolic et al., 2013; Bautista-Aguilera et al., 2014; Oluic et al., 2017; Albert et al., 2019). Most popular docking programs are DOCK (Kuntz et al., 1982), Autodock (Morris et al., 2009), AD Vina (Trott and Olson, 2010), GOLD (Verdonk et al., 2003), GLIDE from Schrödinger suite (Halgren et al., 2004), and they mostly differ in search algorithms and scoring functions they use. It is always recommendable to explore several different docking programs and then decide on the best one for the specific protein-ligand complexes.

For the last decade, molecular docking has been widely used in design of protein kinase inhibitors (**Table 4**). Tsou et al. designed 4-(phenylaminomethylene) isoquinoline-1, 3(2H, 4H)-dione derivatives, an original class of potent inhibitors that selectively inhibit CDK4 over CDK2 and CDK1 activities. They used SAR and docking to identify interactions between the ligands and residues of the protein's ATP binding pocket and to find interactions with amino acids unique to CDK4 (His82, Val83, and Asp84) and to optimize compounds with improved activity and selectivity toward CDK4 (Tsou et al., 2008). Gopalsamy et al. identified a compound as B-Raf inhibitor from high throughput screening (HTS) and used docking into the crystal structure of B-Raf-Sorafenib complex (1UWH) (Wan et al., 2004) to identify important protein–ligand interactions (two hydrogen bonds with Glu500 and Asp593, and hydrophobic interactions with Ile462, Trp530, Phe582, Ile 512, His 573, and Ile 571) and to optimize the scaffold to obtain compound with improved potency (Gopalsamy et al., 2009). In 2018, Amr et al. synthetized a series of macrocyclic pyrido-pentapeptide candidates, and identified their activity *in vitro* on several kinases. Following docking study of the best compound into VEGFR-2, EGFR, PDGFR, provided information of the binding mode and important protein-ligand interactions which can be further used as a guideline for future design (Amr et al., 2018). In their efforts to design 2-phenazinamine derivatives as Bcr-Abl tyrosine kinase inhibitors, Kale and Sonwane combined molecular docking studies with G-QSAR (Group-Based QSAR). Their *in silico* studies predicted better activity for the thiazolidones and benzenesulfonyl derivatives of phenazinamines than doxorubicin. However, *in vitro* cytotoxic activity was good, though still less than of doxorubicin (Kale and Sonwane, 2018).

TABLE 4 | Selected studies that have used docking in the design of kinase inhibitors.

Target kinase	Software package	References
EGFR	Maestro	Hu et al., 2017
VEGFR-2, CDK-2 and PDGFRβ	MOE	Amr et al., 2018
Bcr-Abl	Autodock	Kale and Sonwane, 2018
PKMYT1	GOLD	Platzer et al., 2018
EGFR, PDGFR-β	GOLD	Fischer et al., 2018
Pim-1	MOE	Mohareb et al., 2019
PAK4	Glide	Gao et al., 2019
Bcr-Abl	Discovery studio	Melge et al., 2019
EGFR	Glide	Debnath et al., 2019
PI3K	AutoDock	Wang et al., 2019b
Pim-1	AutoDock	Hazhazi et al., 2019
VEGFR-2	GOLD	Zhao et al., 2019b
PKC	Glide	Wang et al., 2019c
EGFR	MOE	Khodair et al., 2019

Molecular dynamics (MD) is a simulation technique for studying time dependent evolution of molecular system. Relying on principles of classical mechanics, in MD simulations, positions, and velocities of atoms are computed by classical (Newtonian) laws of motion (Klepeis et al., 2009). The forces acting on these atoms are computed using potential energy functions known as force fields. All common force fields express potential energy through bonded terms (covalent bond-stretching, angle-bending, torsion potential, improper torsions) and non-bonded terms (Lenard Jones repulsion and dispersion and Coulomb electrostatics) (Vanommeslaeghe et al., 2014). Several force fields were found to provide quite accurate representations of the structure and dynamics of a number of small globular proteins on the sub-microsecond timescale (Beauchamp et al., 2012). Most commonly used force fields today are CHARMM (Yin and MacKerell, 1998), AMBER (Weiner et al., 1984; Cornell et al., 1995), GROMOS (Oostenbrink et al., 2004), OPLS (Jorgensen et al., 1996), and COMPASS (Sun, 1998) force fields since they include various chemical groups present in macromolecules and drug-like entities.

Recent algorithmic advances and increase in computational power have enabled simulation studies of protein systems on biophysically-relevant timescales. Combined with modern improvements in the quality of force field parameters, protein structure prediction and modeling has advanced impressively (Beauchamp et al., 2012; Raval et al., 2012; Piana et al., 2014). Providing structural and dynamical insight into the studied molecular system difficult to obtain experimentally, as well as thermodynamics and kinetic understanding of the system, MD simulations are usually referred to as "computational microscopes" (Dror et al., 2012). In this review, we discuss the usefulness of MD and MD-based methods in the discovery of kinase inhibitors through different case studies presented below.

Structure-based virtual screening (SBVS) is based on the knowledge of the 3D structure of the target protein, obtained by X-ray crystallography, NMR, cryo-EM or homology modeling (Lionta et al., 2014). Nowadays, the SBVS methods are enabled thanks to a large number of 3D structural information deposited in the PDB. As described above, by using the 3D structural information of the protein target, we are now able to investigate the basic molecular interactions involved in ligand-protein binding and understand experimental results up to atomic levels. In SBVS, large libraries of commercially available drug-like compounds that are computationally screened against proteins of known structure and those that are predicted to bind well can be experimentally tested (Benod et al., 2013; Vucicevic et al., 2016; Oluic et al., 2017).

Case Studies

Structure-based design of imidazo [4,5-b]pyridin-2-one-based p38 mitogen-activated protein kinase inhibitors

Using structure-based drug design, Kaieda et al. have identified a series of potent p38 mitogen-activated protein kinase inhibitors. First they identified the lead compound with moderate inhibitory activity toward p38 MAP kinase by means of high-throughput screening. The lead compound was then crystalized with the MAP kinase. The X-ray crystallographic results showed that carbonyl group of the compound forms two hydrogen bonds with the backbone amide of Met109 and Gly110 of the enzyme (**Figure 5A**). The hinge backbone conformation of their crystal structure was different from that typically seen in protein kinases. Namely, usually the backbone amide and carbonyl group of Met109 are directed toward the ATP binding site and accessible for creation of hydrogen bonding with ligand. In the obtained crystal structure a flip of the peptide bond between Met109 and Gly110 was noticed which led to a switching of the hydrogen-bond acceptor and donor distribution around the peptide plane, instead. It was assumed that this flip could be responsible for the high kinase selectivity. After switching the scaffold of the carbonylpiperidine group while maintaining this binding mode, a series of synthetized imidazo[4,5-b]pyridin-2-one derivatives were identified as potent inhibitors of the p38 MAP kinase (**Figure 5B**; Kaieda et al., 2019).

Discovery of novel Pim-1 kinase inhibitors by support vector machine, pharmacophore modeling and molecular docking

In 2011 Ren et al. reported the discovery of novel potent Pim-1 inhibitors by combining ligand- and structure-based filtering methods. In order to find new molecules, a pipeline was created that consisted of support vector machine-based VS (SVM-based VS), pharmacophore-based VS (PB-VS), and docking-based VS (DB-VS) and screened approximately 20 million molecules. Protocol was evaluated by using the library which contained 203 known Pim-1 inhibitors and around 117,000 generated decoys. For validation of the performance of VS, the percentage of predicted compounds in known inhibitors, percentage of known inhibitors in predicted compounds, as well as enrichment factor were calculated. The combined protocol showed much better performance than solely SB-VS, PB-VS, and DB-VS. Finally, 47 compounds were selected for further *in vitro* Pim-1 kinase inhibitory assay for an inhibitor concentration of 10 μM, and 15 compounds showed nanomolar level or low micromolar inhibition potency against Pim-1. In conclusion, new scaffolds with the potential for the future chemical development were found (Ren et al., 2011).

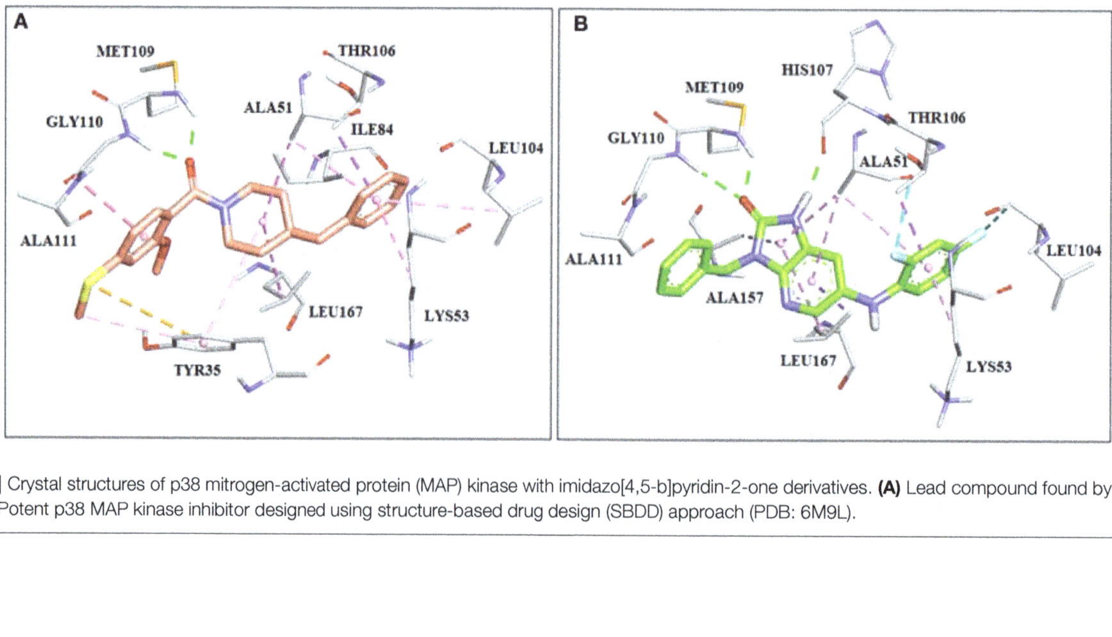

FIGURE 5 | Crystal structures of p38 mitrogen-activated protein (MAP) kinase with imidazo[4,5-b]pyridin-2-one derivatives. **(A)** Lead compound found by HTS (PDB: 6M95). **(B)** Potent p38 MAP kinase inhibitor designed using structure-based drug design (SBDD) approach (PDB: 6M9L).

Discovery of pazopanib, vascular endothelial growth factor family of receptor inhibitor

In 2008 Harris et al. published a paper explaining their discovery of pazopanib. That was a good example of usage of homology modeling and SBDD in the discovery of a drug that is today on the market. Since the crystal structure of VEGFR2 was not available at that time, a homology model of the VEGFR2 enzyme based on FGFR crystal structures was created to predict the binding mode of dimethoxyquinazoline analogs. It was noticed that the pyrimidine and the quinazoline bound similarly in the ATP binding site, making the hydrogen bonds with the Cys919 of the backbone (**Figure 6**). Crystallization of these compounds with VEGFR2 confirmed *in silico* results (PDB: 1Y6A, 1Y6B). Finally a series of new analogs was designed, synthetized, and tested *in vitro*, which led to the discovery of pazopanib (Harris et al., 2005, 2008).

Rational discovery of dual-indication multitarget phosphodiesterase/ kinase inhibitor

One of the latest studies published this year by Lim et al. combined molecular docking with other bioinformatics tools, with the goal of finding multi-target-multi-indication drugs (Lim et al., 2019). They have used structural and chemical genomics data and combined tools from bioinformatics, chemoinformatics, protein-ligand docking, and machine learning to create a novel structural systems pharmacology platform—3D-REMAP. It used four networks as input: 1. protein–ligand association, 2. off-target, 3. ligand–ligand similarity, and 4. protein–protein similarity. The protein–ligand associations were obtained from ChEMBL, DrugBank, and from other publications about kinome assays (Christmann-Franck et al., 2016; Drewry et al., 2017; Klaeger et al., 2017; Merget et al., 2017) and protein structure-based off-target prediction from binding pocket similarity search and protein–ligand docking. Ligand–ligand similarity was calculated in MadFast software from ChemAxon, and protein–protein similarity was run through BLAST. Moreover, to validate and show advantages of their platform, they searched for marketed drugs that could be dual-indication agents. In their study, they focused on drugs that could reduce the cardiotoxicity of anti-cancer therapy. They predicted that levosimendan, a phosphodiesterase (PDE) inhibitor which is used for heart failure, also inhibits serine/threonine-protein kinase RIO kinase 1 (RIOK1) and several other kinases [Ca2+/calmodulin-dependent protein kinase II (CAMK2), FMS-like tyrosine kinase 3 (FLT3), RIOK3, etc.]. To validate their results they tested anti-cancer activity of levosimendan for more than 200 cancer cell lines. Their experimental results showed that levosimendan is active against several cancers, particularly lymphoma, through the inhibition of RIOK1 and its RNA processing pathway (Lim et al., 2019). Since this study is brand new, the time will tell whether levosimendan will be a candidate for clinical research.

Fragment-based drug design of kinase inhibitors

Discovery of kinase inhibitors is a highly competitive process wherein teams of experienced researchers, both from academia and industry, use all the previous knowledge and new ideas to provide more effective therapies for patients. Depending on the available methodologies, one research group may start their drug discovery project with a high-throughput screening (HTS) campaign and search for the bioactive (HIT) compounds against the studied kinase. Selected HIT molecules usually possess drug-like properties and should be further optimized with the aid of lead optimization techniques. Contrary to drug-like molecules, fragments have a smaller number of heavy atoms (HA) and they should comply with Rule of Three (RO3), in which molecular weight is <300 Da, number of hydrogen bond donors and acceptors should be ≤ 3 and clogP is ≤ 3 (Congreve et al., 2003).

Fragment molecules tend to show high micromolar to millimolar affinities for a certain biological target. The advantages of using fragments in drug design studies of novel kinase inhibitors are numerous:

- Fragments displaying affinity to the examined biological target can overcome the entropy barrier and their binding is related to the favorable enthalpy contribution (Murray and Verdonk, 2002);

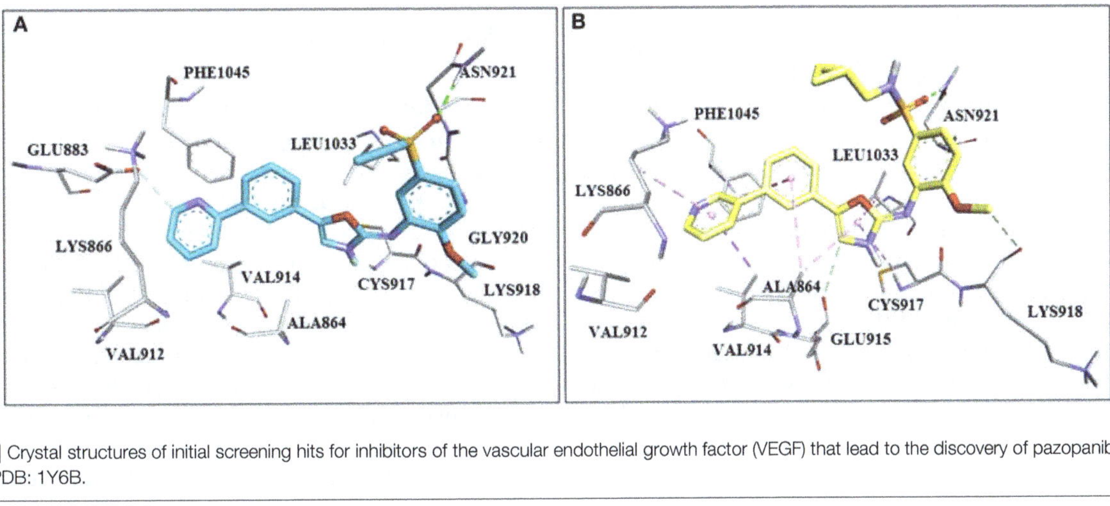

FIGURE 6 | Crystal structures of initial screening hits for inhibitors of the vascular endothelial growth factor (VEGF) that lead to the discovery of pazopanib. **(A)** PDB: 1Y6A, **(B)** PDB: 1Y6B.

- Comparing to drug-sized molecules, pharmacokinetic and physicochemical properties of fragments could be more efficiently optimized (Leach and Hann, 2011);
- Drug-sized molecules may suffer from a potential loss of complementarity with the studied targets, whereas the fragments seldom possess functional groups that establish ligand–protein intermolecular clashes (Hann et al., 2001);
- Given all the above, FBDD projects can lead to increased HIT rates and discovery of novel fragments interesting from different points of view (binding affinity, synthetic accessibility, intellectual property).

Historically, first FBDD projects were applied by a technique named "SAR by NMR" (structure-activity relationship by nuclear magnetic resonance) (Shuker et al., 1996). In this paper, authors successfully developed a potent compound with nanomolar affinity to FK506 binding protein (FKBP) by merging two building blocks. Except for NMR, protein-fragment interacting patterns are characterized by other biophysical methods such as X-ray crystallography, surface plasmon resonance (SRC), high concentration screening (HCS) assays, isothermal titration calorimetry (ITC), fluorescence correlation spectroscopy and many more (Sun et al., 2011). The choice of a particular method depends on the previous experience in FBDD projects and also the size of fragment libraries.

Until now, fragment-based drug discovery (FBDD) method resulted in FDA approval of three kinase inhibitors—vemurafenib (Bollag et al., 2012), venetoclax (Deeks, 2016), and erdafitinib (Markham, 2019). These excellent textbook examples of FBDD are developed by different biophysical methods; nevertheless, the present review focuses on various *in silico* techniques frequently used in fragment identification and optimization.

In recent years, experimental screening procedures may be replaced by computational methods to reduce the costs and time for early stages of FBDD project (Alves Avelar et al., 2019; Ruzic et al., 2019). It appears that *in silico* studies may support kinase drug discovery at almost every stage of fragment-based drug design projects. Various ligand-based virtual screening (Giordanetto et al., 2011), structure-based (Warner et al., 2006; Zhao et al., 2012), and quantum mechanical (Machrouhi et al., 2010) techniques have been proved as successful in novel fragment identification. Before running any virtual screening protocol, computational chemists must pay attention to the valid preparation of fragment library database. The fragment library databases should obey the aforementioned Rule of 3 (RO3); additionally, their chemical properties are filtered through certain software which removes possible toxicophores and pan-assay interference compounds (PAINS) (Baell and Walters, 2014). Nowadays, computational chemists may use kinase fragment libraries which may assist faster identification of novel hinge binding motifs. Moreover, fragments that target distal pockets from the ATP binding pocket could be scanned by allosteric kinase library, such as Enamine Allosteric Kinase Library (https://enamine.net).

Case Studies

Identification of PI3K p110β selective fragment

Intracellular lipid kinases that transfer a phosphate group from ATP to certain cell membrane's phospholipids (Phosphoinositide-4,5-biphosphate, PIP_2) belong to the family of phosphoinositide 3-kinases (PI3K). These enzymes regulate important cellular events and present interesting drug targets in anticancer drug discovery. Giordanetto et al. (2011) successfully identified fragments that showed selective p110β inhibition. At the time this study was performed, the crystal structure of p110β isoform was not available. Consequently, the homology model was built in MODELLER (Webb and Sali, 2016) by using the crystal structure of p110γ isoform. In this study, authors used AstraZeneca's virtual fragment database and subjected 183,330 fragments to a molecular docking study in GLIDE software (Schrödinger, New York). The poses and orientation of the fragments in the ATP binding pocket were inspected, as well as hydrogen bonding interactions with amino acid residues in the hinge region, affinity and selectivity pocket. The authors reported five chemical classes of fragments (**Figure 7A**) based on the different heterocyclic rings interacting with the hinge region in p110β and their *in vitro* enzymatic profiles against four human PI3K isoforms (p110α, p110β, p110γ, and p110δ). Overall, the hit rate achieved from this screening was 8.57%, indicating good performance of the molecular docking-based search for novel and chemically interesting fragments as PI3K hinge binders. The authors continued this study with the morpholine derivative, compound (**1**) (**Figure 7B**), which showed moderate potency against p110β (IC_{50} = 34 μM), but its inhibition of the other p110 isoforms was not determined at the tested concentrations.

In the following study, authors aimed to improve the affinity of the compound (**1**) by substituting the dimethylamino group with a more voluminous 2-(benzylamino) moiety (Giordanetto et al., 2012). The novel compound (**2**) showed improved potency (IC_{50} = 1.9 μM) and efficiency (LE = 0.37 and LLE = 4.52) toward p110β. The rationale for this chemical modification relies on the observation that the bulkier substituents might target amino acid residues M804 and W812 in the proximal selectivity pocket. Finally, compound (**3**) was synthesized by introducing the naphthyl group, which in turn attributed to the nanomolar potency (IC_{50} = 0.093 μM) and improved p110β selectivity profile of compound (**3**).

Identification of mitogen-activated protein kinase-interacting kinase 1 inhibitors

Mitogen-activated protein (MAP) kinase interacting kinases 1 and 2 (**MNK1** and **MNK2**) carry out phosphorylation reaction of eukaryotic translation initiation factor 4E (eIF4E) on serine 209 (Wendel et al., 2007). This translation factor is involved in different cellular pathways, such as Ras/Raf/MEK/ERK and PI3-kinase/protein kinase B (Akt) signaling pathways (Proud, 2015). The overexpression of phosphorylated eIF4E leads to several malignant diseases, such as lymphomas, breast cancer, and glioblastoma (Astanehe et al., 2012). The significance of MNK1/2 enzymes in malignant transformation of the cell has led to high demand for drug design of MNK1/2 inhibitors.

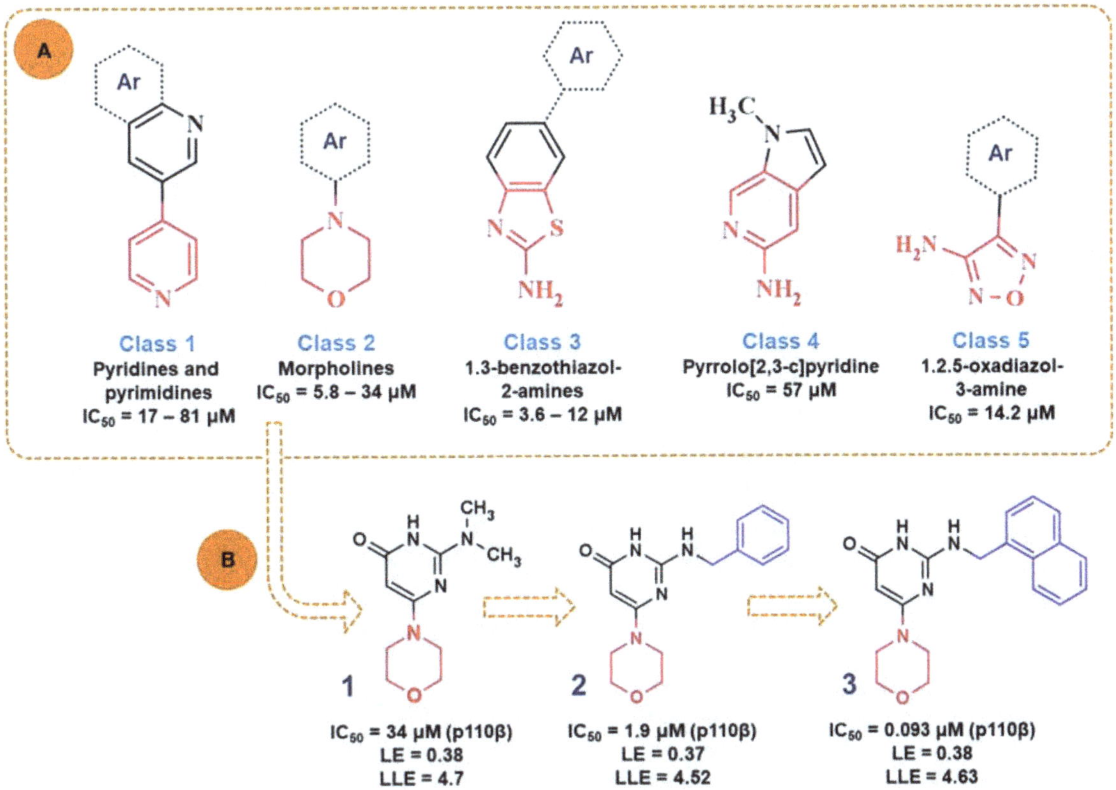

FIGURE 7 | (A) Presentation of the identified scaffolds by *in vitro* biochemical screening as PI3K inhibitors (hinge interacting moieties are labeled in red), *Ar*—presents carbocyclic or heterocyclic aromatic rings; **(B)** the scheme of lead optimization of the selected morpholine derivatives.

One remarkable study was performed in 2010, where Oyarzabal et al. identified a highly potent and efficient fragment entirely by *in silico* modeling. In this comprehensive study, authors combined different virtual screening techniques to identify pharmacological tools for MNK1 inhibition. Initially, the Centro Nacional de Investigaciones Oncológicas (CNIO) database was filtered according to the molecular weight (<300 Da) and calculated solubility values (threshold −4 mol/L). By performing this prefiltering procedure, the authors extracted 42,168 fragment-like compounds for virtual screenings (Oyarzabal et al., 2010).

Availability of the crystal structure of MNK2 complexed with staurosporine (PDB: 2HW7) enabled creating minimal substructure, required for crucial interactions with MNK2 (**Figure 8**). The GOLD software (Jones et al., 1997) used in this study was able to reproduce the binding mode of staurosporine in MNK2. The virtual substructure was docked in the crystal structure of MNK1 (PDB: 2HW6) to similarly elucidate crucial amino acid interactions in the ATP binding pocket. MNK1 pharmacophore prepared in this way was used for pharmacophore fitting study, as a molecular docking alternative and 92 compounds were extracted according to their goodness of fit with the pre-defined substructure.

Structure-based virtual screening protocols were combined with ligand-based virtual screenings of CNIO database and external virtual database of compounds collected by the authors who performed this study. These strategies involved 2D-substructural searches, 2D Tanimoto structural similarity, Feature Trees similarity, and three-dimensional shape and electrostatic similarities based on two reported MNK1 inhibitors. Finally, the authors selected 1,236 compounds for biochemical MNK1 assay and 26 of them were active. The hit ratio of this screening was 2.10% and 10 different scaffolds were represented. Interestingly, one compound (**Figure 8**, compound 29) demonstrated nanomolar MNK1 (IC_{50} = 646 nM) and MNK2 (IC_{50} = 575 nM) inhibition. Additionally, at the cellular level, compound 29 showed an antiproliferative effect against acute myeloid leukemia cell line (MV4:11, EC_{50} = 17 μM) with dose-dependent decrease in phosphorylation on serine 209 in eIF4E. In conclusion, this study identified 26 hit molecules as MNK1 inhibitors, with 19 of them as fragments with high ligand efficiency values. Among the 26 identified hits, there were 10 diverse chemotypes represented for further drug design studies.

Researchers from A-STAR were particularly interested in imidazopyridazine scaffold (chemotype III in the study of Oyarzabal et al.) as a starting fragment for lead optimization of MNK1/2 inhibitors (Yang et al., 2018). Extensive SAR study of imidazopyridazine derivatives was based on *in silico* conclusions defined in their previous computational study (Kannan et al., 2017). Concisely, researchers in this study aimed to modify the

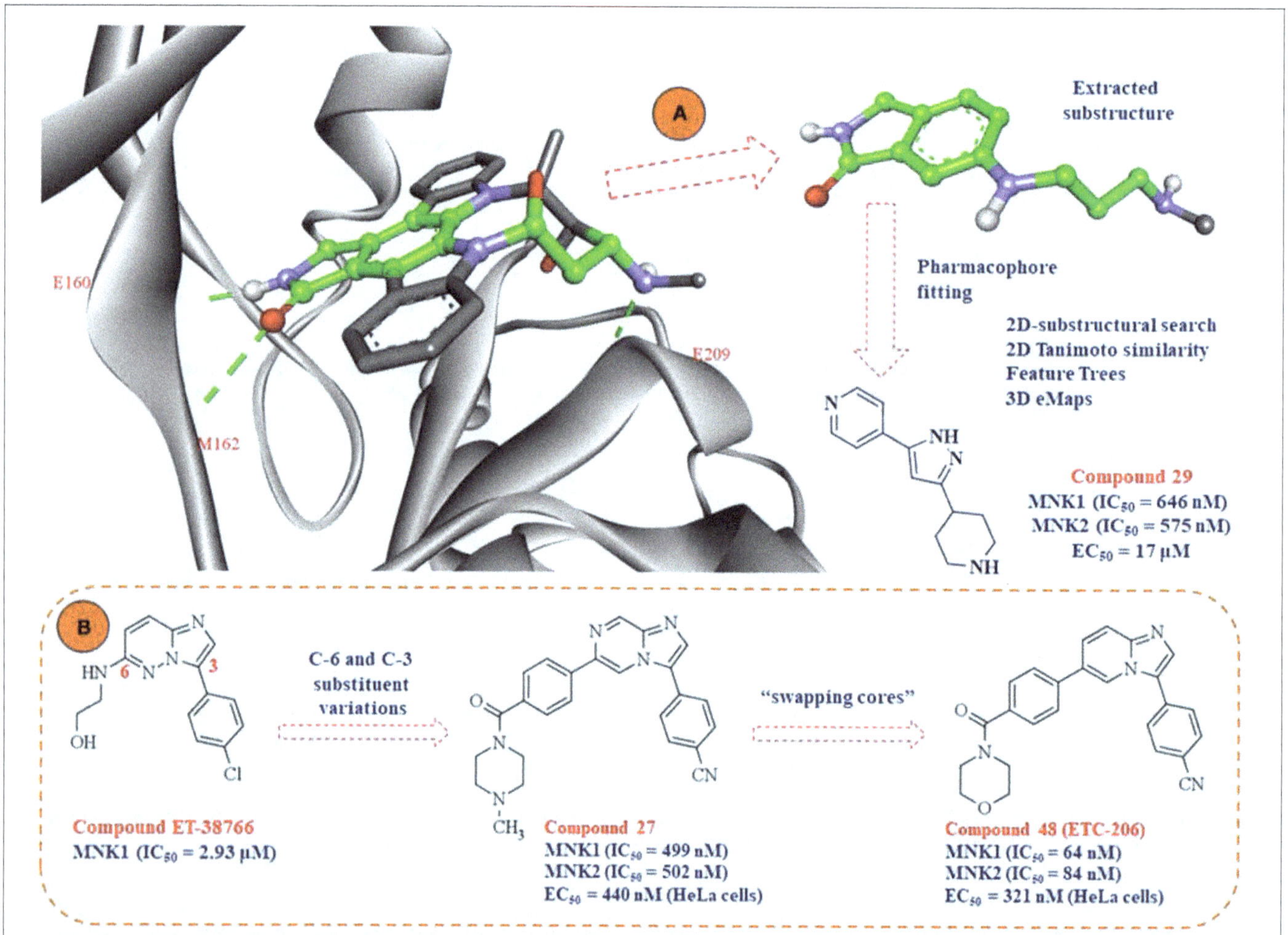

FIGURE 8 | (A) Crystal structure of MNK-2 complexed with staurosporine (PDB: 2HW7); the atoms of the substructure used in the study of pharmacophore fitting screening are labeled in green; **(B)** the lead optimization strategies starting from fragment ET-38766 to clinical candidate ETC-206.

heterocyclic core in positions 3 and 6, with later modification of the imidazopyridazine scaffold (swapping cores strategy). All the derivatives synthesized in this study were firstly examined by molecular docking studies in Glide 2017-3 software (www.schrodinger.com). By detailed computational analysis of the important amino acid residues in the ATP pocket of MNK1/2 kinases, researchers performed initial lead optimization of the fragment (compound ET-38766) to compound 27 (**Figure 8B**). Novel compound 27 bears imidazopyrazine scaffold, with improved potency against MNK-1 and MNK-2, cell permeability and improved pharmacokinetic properties. After finding optimal substituents in positions 3 and 6, the final step of lead optimization was focused on detailed DFT study to select the final heterocyclic core of MNK1/2 inhibitors. Initially, it was unclear from molecular dynamics (MD) simulations whether the imidazopyrazine N-7 contributes favorably to the binding affinity of MNK inhibitors. To examine this, the authors performed DFT study and demonstrated that N-7 is mostly solvent exposed, thus the final selected heterocyclic core was imidazopyridine. The most promising compound 48 (**Figure 8B**) later designated as ETC-206, was presented as superior compared to other derivatives in the study. This compound was investigated for the synergism with dasatinib *in vivo* and currently is in phase I clinical trial for the blast crisis chronic myeloid leukemia (BC-CML).

Computational approaches in rational discovery of allosteric kinase inhibitors

Although targeting of highly conserved ATP-binding site by Type I and Type II inhibitors provides limited selectivity, inhibiting multiple kinases with a single small-molecule inhibitor was proven to be a useful strategy for therapeutic intervention. However, development of highly selective small-molecule kinase inhibitors remains a pressing concern where targeting of allosteric sites emerged as a promising approach (Wu et al., 2015a). Some of the advantages of targeting allosteric sites include increased selectivity and low toxicity of such inhibitors due to low evolutional conservation of allosteric sites compared to orthosteric (ATP-binding) sites (Fang et al., 2013). Additionally, overcoming of point mutation-associated drug resistance, especially for mutations in the ATP-binding site reported for almost all of ATP-competitive inhibitors, could be another advantage of developing allosteric kinase inhibitors (Gibbons et al., 2012).

While exploitation of allosteric sites represents a very promising strategy, it remains challenging from the aspect of rational drug discovery. Some of the major obstacles include identification of allosteric binding sites, which are usually hidden in less populated higher energy conformations of the proteins. Those conformations are poorly accessible to current experimental methods of structural biology (Lu et al., 2018a). Additionally, allosteric effectors are susceptible to "mode switching," where minor chemical modification of ligand induces critical change in activity (Wenthur et al., 2014). Although known CADD workflows for discovery of drugs directed to orthosteric binding sites are being used in allosteric inhibitors discovery (Rastelli et al., 2014; Schoepfer et al., 2018), they provide limited utility rising the need for development of more spatialized tools and workflows (Greener and Sternberg, 2018).

Identification of allosteric pockets is a crucial first step in rational discovery of allosteric inhibitors. As will discussed below, a plethora of computationally inexpensive methodologies have been developed for this purpose and many of them are even implemented as web servers. While these methodologies provide fast and inexpensive highway in the discovery of druggable allosteric pockets, proper understanding of the allosteric mechanism is impossible without considering underlying conformational landscape and free-energy profiles where more computationally demanding molecular dynamics based approaches have a predominant role. In this review, we discuss few examples of computational methodologies used for direct discovery of novel allosteric sites and/or allosteric kinase inhibitors. For detailed description of recent breakthroughs in computational methodologies used for allosteric inhibitors discovery in general, the interested reader is referred to the recent reviews (Wagner et al., 2016; Lu et al., 2019).

Automatic Computational Tools/Web Servers to Investigate Allostery

Structure-based computational tools AlloSite and recently advanced descendant AllositePro (http://mdl.shsmu.edu.cn/AST/) are intended for fast detection of allosteric site in input PDB structures. Initial detection of allosteric sites is based on Fpocket, a fast open source protein pocket detection software package based on Voronoi tessellation (Le Guilloux et al., 2009). While Allosite uses a machine-learning model to re-rank detected pockets in terms of their allosteric character, AllositePro additionally implements normal-mode analysis (NMA) perturbation with elastic network models to account for protein flexibility. NMA is a technique developed for investigation of the vibrational motion of a harmonic oscillating system in the immediate vicinity of its equilibrium. Under assumption that the potential energy landscape in the vicinity of a minimized atomic structure is approximately harmonic, NMA eliminates the need to integrate the equations of motion and makes NMA much less computationally demanding compared to MD (Bahar and Rader, 2005). Zhang et al. demonstrated utility of AllositePro in identification of novel allosteric site on CDK2 kinase. Existence of novel site was validated in mutagenic analysis (Song et al., 2017). Recently, the same group developed AlloFinder, integrated allosterome mapping, and virtual screening workflow implemented as web server (http://mdl.shsmu.edu.cn/ALF/). AlloFinder relies on AllositePro algorithm for detection of allosteric sites, Allolike filter for pre-filtering of ligand library to enrich allosteric-like compounds (Wang et al., 2012), AutoDock Vina algorithm for docking (Trott and Olson, 2010), and Alloscore empirical scoring function for scoring allosteric modulator-protein complexes (Li et al., 2016). In the final step, alosterome mapping is used to detect highly similar allosteric sites among known human allosteric sites and to rule out selective ligands. This approach was retrospectively validated on several kinase targets (Huang et al., 2018).

CavityPlus (http://www.pkumdl.cn:8000/cavityplus/index.php) is another web server for detection of potential allosteric sites that works on similar principle (Xu et al., 2018). CavityPlus is aimed to detect potential binding sites on the surface of a given protein and rank them based on ligandability and druggability scores. This server integrates several functionalities: CAVITY for detection and scoring of potential binding sites (Yuan et al., 2013); CavPharmer for generation of receptor-based pharmacophores (Chen et al., 2014); CorrSite for prediction of allostery based on NMA motion correlation analysis between allosteric and orthosteric sites (Ma et al., 2016); CivCys for detection of binding sites for covalent inhibitors (Zhang et al., 2017). Functionalities of CavityPlus were successfully used for identification of allosteric binding site on Polo-like kinase 1 (Plk1). Subsequent molecular-docking-based virtual screening on allosteric site resulted in identification of few potent Plk1 inhibitors (Yun et al., 2016).

Another successful implementation of web server based tools for allosteric drug discovery is Kinase Atlas (https://kinase-atlas.bu.edu/) (Yueh et al., 2019). Kinase Atlas is systematic collection of mostly unexplored allosteric sites (binding hot spots) calculated for 4,910 PDB structures of 376 distinct kinases. The hot spots are identified by FTMap. This method places molecular probes (small organic molecules) on a dense grid around the protein and finds favorable positions using an empirical energy function and CHARMM potential. After clustering of obtained positions for each probe, regions that bind several probe clusters are marked as hot spots (Kozakov et al., 2015). Authors of the study identified novel allosteric site on CDK2 and screened library of 1,280 molecules using disulphide-based fragment screening. Two potent and novel allosteric inhibitors were described.

Molecular Dynamics-Based Approaches to Investigate Allostery

Molecular dynamics-based approaches in rational discovery of allosteric kinase inhibitors have potential to provide exclusive insight in atomic-level dynamical mechanism of allostery, to explore conformational landscape and capture kinase conformational states inaccessible to current experimental methodologies. Therefore, molecular-dynamics-based approaches, even though being computationally intensive, could detect previously unknown conformations and hidden allosteric binding pockets (Guo and Zhou, 2016; Lu et al., 2018a).

Combination of conventional MD simulations with other standard SBDD approaches resulted in identification of novel allosteric sites and discovery of novel allosteric ligands in several cases. For example, Perez et al. identified novel inhibitory allosteric site and inhibitors of p38α by using MD simulations starting from the X-ray structure of binary complex of p38α and its interacting partner MAPK-activated protein kinase 2 (MK2). MD simulations permitted definition of pharmacophoric features of small peptide inhibitors derived from sequence of MK2. Subsequent virtual screening study resulted in first small molecule allosteric inhibitor for identified binding site (Gomez-Gutierrez et al., 2016). Cournia et al. verified existence of allosteric site on human PI3Kα previously described in murine PI3Kα using combination of FTMap, MD, and *in vitro* assays. Intriguingly, MD simulations revealed different binding mode of studied allosteric inhibitor in murine, WT, and mutant forms of PI3Kα and consequent differences in propagation of allosteric signal to orthosteric ATP-binding site (Gkeka et al., 2015).

Computational costs of insufficient conformational sampling often limit application of conventional MD simulations in investigating allostery phenomena. Currently, there is a large gap between the time scale which can be reached in MD simulations and that observed in experiments. Several strategies for enhancing the sampling of MD simulations have been proposed (Aci-Seche et al., 2016; Yang et al., 2019). Two recently reported studies demonstrating full power of enhanced sampling methods (Markov-state modeling based adaptive sampling and parallel tempering in the well-tempered ensemble) are discussed below with special reference to atomic-level description of allosteric communication and discovery of cryptic allosteric pockets.

Pande et al. investigated activation pathway of c-Src kinase using massively distributed MD simulations (550 μs) on Folding@HOME (Shirts and Pande, 2000) Markov-state modeling (MSM) and adaptive sampling algorithms in order to provide description of factors underlying thermodynamics and kinetics of c-Src activation and to identify key structural intermediates (Shukla et al., 2014). Briefly, MSM models represent kinetical description of a system's underlying free-energy landscape, useful for characterization of probability of dynamical transitions between conformational states identified in many independent MD simulations and for extrapolation of long time system's behavior (Sengupta and Strodel, 2018). In this study intermediate conformational state which could be stabilized to block the c-Src activation pathway, was described through MSM analysis for the first time. Further analysis on identified c-Src conformational state revealed the existence of allosteric pocket and surprisingly high structural similarity to known complex of CDK2 bound to allosteric inhibitor—ANS (Betzi et al., 2011). Further simulations confirmed binding of ANS to the novel allosteric site of c-Src and blockage of activation process by stabilization of intermediate states. Additionally, the long-range residues coupling analysis identified myristate-binding pocket as another potential target for development of allosteric modulators of c-Src. Taken together, results of this study highlighted large-scale MD coupled with MSM modeling as an indispensable tool for identification of novel conformational states, potential allosteric pockets, and study of mechanisms of allostery in kinases.

In another example, authors explored the possibility of bidirectional communication between allosteric so-called PIF-pocket and ATP-binding site in PDK1 protein kinase using a combination of experimental techniques and enhanced-sampling simulations [parallel tempering simulations in the well-tempered ensemble (PT-WTE)] (Schulze et al., 2016). Results of PT-WTE MD revealed bidirectional mechanisms of communication between the ATP-binding site and allosteric site. Interestingly, this study for the first time demonstrated how different ligands which bind to the ATP-binding site differently modulate responses of allosteric site in interaction with a partner protein (e.g., enhance or inhibit interaction). Providing computer platform for rational design of allosteric modulators, the authors of this study opened an exciting avenue for future discovery of novel class of kinase inhibitors with less on-target side effects and more specific modulation of signaling pathways.

Case Study

Rational design of clinical candidate Asciminib—allosteric Bcr-Abl1 inhibitor

Asciminib belongs to a class of drugs designed to inhibit Bcr-Abl by binding to an allosteric pocket known as myristate-binding pocket. Rational development of Asciminib started with fragment-based screening using NMR assay (Schoepfer et al., 2018). Although determined NMR-based dissociation constants (Kd) for fragment hits were satisfactory, none of the fragments were active in biochemical and cellular assays. Subsequent X-ray studies revealed inability of fragment hits to induce assembled inactive state by bending of helix I, previously reported as conformational change important or autoinhibition of Abl by myristoilation (Nagar et al., 2003). Following this finding, the authors established another screening assay, the NMR-based conformational assay, which monitors the conformational state of C-terminal helix I (Jahnke et al., 2010). NMR-based conformational assay was used to investigate identified fragments and series of known allosteric modulators—derivatives of GNF-2 (Adrian et al., 2006; **Figure 9**). Results of the study revealed that compounds which bind to myristoyl pocket and do not induce helix I bending were actually functional activators of Abl1 (by interfering with autoinhibition mechanism of Abl1). Critical bending of helix I was found to be induced by the presence of CF_3O– group from GNF-2. Based on these findings, CADD techniques (molecular docking, similarity and pharmacophore searches) were used to design compound **X** in respect to X-ray structure with bent helix I conformation. Subsequent introduction of CF_3O– group finally led to the first active allosteric inhibitor. Molecular modeling techniques were used in combination with X-ray crystallography in order to optimize potency and drug-like properties of the compound. Although only standard CADD techniques were reported in the discovery of Asciminib, recent application of molecular dynamics-based approaches demonstrated utility of such techniques in examination of mechanisms of resistance

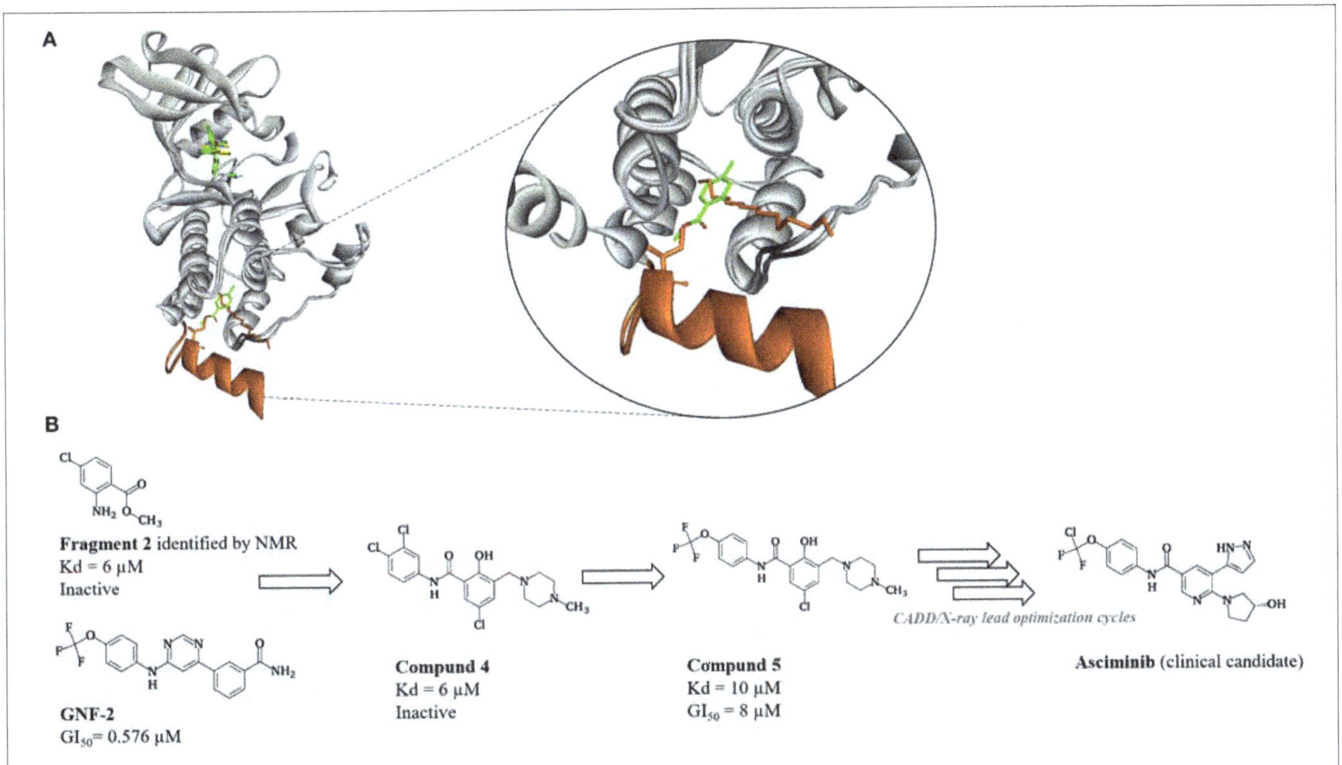

FIGURE 9 | Discovery of Asciminib (Schoepfer et al., 2018). **(A)** Representation of initial hypothesis regarding bending of helix I (orange). Assembled inactive state of ABL1 kinase in complex with myristic acid (orange sticks) (PDB: 1OPL, SH3, and SH2 domains omitted for clarity) is superimposed on ABL1 in complex with fragment 2 (green sticks) (PDB: 3MS9). Steric clash between isoleucin I521 (orange sticks) on helix I and fragment 2 prevents full bending of helix I and formation of assembled inactive state of ABL1. Helix I is not visible in the PDB: 3MS9. **(B)** Medicinal chemistry progression from fragment 2 to fragment derived hit 4, first active hit-compound 5 and finally clinical candidate—Asciminib.

and effects of dual targeting of ATP-binding and allosteric site providing rationale for development of novel drugs (El Rashedy et al., 2018; Meng et al., 2018; Zhan et al., 2019).

Machine learning methods to predict kinase-compound interactions

Nowadays, we are seeing the widespread use of machine learning in many areas, including pharmaceutical industry, especially in drug design. Popular computational methods initially used in pharmaceutical research were quantitative structure activity relationships (QSAR) and quantitative structure property relationship (QSPR), which were adequate for small datasets. However, with the rapid growth of databases (thanks to methods such as high-throughput *in vitro* screening and X-ray crystallography), it became inevitable to develop different *in silico* tools that can manage bigger data (Ekins, 2016). Today, many different machine learning methods such as support vector machines (SVM), k-Nearest Neighbors, Artificial Neural Networks (ANN), Deep Learning (DL), *etc.* are used in pharmaceutical research and they can be applied in various processes of drug design from virtual screening to *de novo* drug design (Buchwald et al., 2011; Drewry et al., 2017; Konze et al., 2019; Kuthuru et al., 2019; Lee et al., 2019; Zhavoronkov et al., 2019).

Many different machine learning models were created for the prediction of drug-target interactions (DTI), and many DTI methods have been applied to the protein kinases family (Kuthuru et al., 2019). Unlike LB and SB methods, DTI prediction uses the information from both protein and ligand and these methods can be similarity based or descriptor-based. One of the first similarity-based methods for identification of drug-target interactions was introduced by Yamanishi et al. in 2008. It used the known drug structure, protein sequence and drug-target interaction network to determine unknown ligand-target interactions. The main hypothesis is that two compounds that have high structure similarity might probably interact with similar target proteins, and *vice versa* two proteins with high sequence similarity might probably interact with similar drugs (Yamanishi et al., 2008). On the other hand, descriptor-based models use feature vectors from known drug structures and protein sequences, as inputs for machine learning methods, such SVM, AAN, DL, etc. In 2011, Buchwald et al. used SVM to prepare the model for prediction of protein kinases-ligand interactions. They used a set of binding data obtained from 113 different protein kinases and 20 inhibitors obtained through ATP site-dependent binding competition assays. They focused on vector features that describe the structure of molecules that are connected with certain chemical environment-protein active site sequence and created a SVM model with good predictivity (Buchwald et al., 2011).

Recently, the use of ANN, especially deep learning methods saw a significant increase in the process of drug design (Ekins, 2016; Merk et al., 2018; Putin et al., 2018; Konze et al., 2019). Deep generative models are utilizing neural networks to generate new objects (drugs) with desired properties (for example activity, Ki, IC_{50}). These methods should be able to produce chemically correct structures without the need for including fragment libraries and/or rules for their combination (Merk et al., 2018). The ability to produce novel chemical structures with certain properties makes deep generative models suitable for the discovery of novel possible therapeutics (Zhavoronkov et al., 2019). In 2018, Merk et al. applied generative models to come up with novel bioactive, synthesizable drugs. They trained the model with more than 500,000 SMILES of bioactive compounds with their activity properties extracted from the ChEMBL (K_D, K_i, IC/EC_{50} values $<1\,\mu M$). Additionally, the model was fine-tuned to enable the *de novo* generation of target-specific ligands on retinoid X receptors (RXR) and/or peroxisome proliferator-activated receptors (PPAR). Finally, none of the generated compounds was identical to compounds from the training sets, and they were residing within the RXR/PPAR region of the fine-tuning set (Merk et al., 2018).

Case Studies

Predictive proteochemometric models for kinases derived from 3D protein field-based descriptors

Subramanian et al. described the development of proteochemometric models for 1,572 inhibitors and 95 kinases obtained from Kinase SARfari (https://chembl.gitbook.io/chembl-interface-documentation/legacy-resources#kinase-sarfari) and CHEMBL database, using 3D structure of proteins and active and inactive ligands. Proteins were described with molecular interaction fields derived from Schrödinger's WaterMaps, while different 1D, 2D, and 3D descriptors were used to describe the ligands. Separate training sets were created for the ligands and targets. Different methods were used for preparation of the proteochemometric models: support vector machines (SVM) and random forests (RF). The ligand prediction model was trained on the ligand training set and was used for ligand prediction model and target training set for target predicting model. In the end, they validated all the models using internal and external validation. This approach allows creation of not only predictive proteochemometrics model for protein kinases, but also preparation of visually interpretable models. This allows interpretation of kinase–ligand interactions, which can be used, for example, for optimization of ligand in order to achieve optimal activity and/or selectivity. Having visually interpretable models is the advantage compared to classical DTI methods that use only 2D information (Subramanian et al., 2013, 2016).

Deep learning model for identification of potent discoidin domain receptor 1 kinase inhibitors

Recently, Zhavoronkov et al. created a deep generative model for *de novo* small-molecule design—GENTRL (GENerative Tensorial Reinforcement Learning). Besides the effectiveness of a compound against a given biological target, GENTRL also takes into account its dissimilarity from other molecules in the literature and patent space, as well as its synthetic feasibility. For the proof-of-concept GENTRL was used to design potential Discoidin domain receptor 1 (DDR1) kinase inhibitors. Data was collected from different data sets: ZINC data set, known DDR1 kinase inhibitors data set, common kinase inhibitors, molecules with activity on non-kinase targets, patent data, and used to train the model. The model was generated by combining reinforcement learning with a reward, variational inference, and tensor decompositions. Finally the randomly elected six compounds that have not been previously published or patented were designed, synthesized, and experimentally tested. The whole process lasted only 46 days, which suggests that the application of drug design methods such as this will reduce the time and cost of drug discovery process (Zhavoronkov et al., 2019).

CONCLUDING REMARKS

In silico approaches are viable, usually cheaper and faster alternative to experimental drug discovery techniques. This review summarizes the most important computational tools that have led to the discovery of kinase inhibitors, many of which are in clinical use today as promising anticancer drugs. Computational approaches, such as QSAR modeling, ligand-based and structure-based virtual screening, molecular docking, molecular dynamics, quantum mechanics, fragment-based drug design, and machine learning methods, provide unique insight in the conformational landscape of kinases, structural requirements for inhibitory activity, binding modes and atomistic mechanisms of allostery, which represent indispensable information for rational *de novo* design. One of the main advantages of computational approaches is the possibility of introduction of new groups on the known scaffolds and *in silico* prediction of activities and binding affinities. Known scaffolds of the approved KIs include pyrimidine (imatinib, dasatinib, nilotinib), quinazoline (erlotinib, gefitinib, afatinib, vandetanib), pyridine (sorafenib), pirrolopyridine (vemurafenib), pyrazolopyridine (ibrutinib) etc. *In silico* modification of these scaffolds resulted in the design of many kinase inhibitors with enhanced predicted activities and binding affinities which can serve as lead compounds for further synthesis and preclinical testing. New chemical scaffolds that possess kinase inhibitory activity (imidazopyridazine, imidazopyridine, isoquinoline, phenazinamine, etc.) have also been proposed by computational approach and represent a good starting point for discovery of new kinase inhibitors. Due to increases in computational power, algorithmic improvements and increased accuracy, *in silico* approaches are yet expected to radically shape the era of kinase inhibitor discovery. Of note is to emphasize that not all drug discovery projects could be initiated and guided only with computational studies. The computational chemist must be aware of the structural biology of the studied targets, their dynamical changes influenced upon fragment/ligand binding. Whenever possible, it is advised to start CADD studies with experimental data and continue *in silico* optimization with combined modeling approaches, as much as possible. This review highlights the recent advances in discovery of kinase inhibitors by *in silico* approaches and can be useful for future design and synthesis of new kinase inhibitors as anticancer drugs.

AUTHOR CONTRIBUTIONS

ZG wrote the introduction and LB methods. TD wrote the structure of protein kinases, machine learning methods, and SB methods. DR wrote FB methods. ND wrote modeling of allosteric kinase inhibitors. KN contributed to the conception of the manuscript, collection of the data, drafting and revising. All authors have contributed to the bibliographical research and interpretation of the work, to its critical revision, and approved the final version of the manuscript.

ACKNOWLEDGMENTS

The authors kindly acknowledge national project number 172033 supported by the Ministry of Education, Science and Technological development of the Republic of Serbia.

REFERENCES

Aci-Seche, S., Ziada, S., Braka, A., Arora, R., and Bonnet, P. (2016). Advanced molecular dynamics simulation methods for kinase drug discovery. *Future Med. Chem.* 8, 545–566. doi: 10.4155/fmc.16.9

Adams, J. A. (2001). Kinetic and catalytic mechanisms of protein kinases. *Chem. Rev.* 101, 2271–2290. doi: 10.1021/cr000230w

Adrian, F. J., Ding, Q., Sim, T., Velentza, A., Sloan, C., Liu, Y., et al. (2006). Allosteric inhibitors of Bcr-abl-dependent cell proliferation. *Nat. Chem. Biol.* 2, 95–102. doi: 10.1038/nchembio760

Agafonov, R. V., Wilson, C., and Kern, D. (2015). Evolution and intelligent design in drug development. *Front. Mol. Biosci.* 2:27. doi: 10.3389/fmolb.2015.00027

Aira, L. E., Villa, E., Colosetti, P., Gamas, P., Signetti, L., Obba, S., et al. (2018). The oncogenic tyrosine kinase Lyn impairs the pro-apoptotic function of Bim. *Oncogene* 37, 2122–2136. doi: 10.1038/s41388-017-0112-0

Albert, L., Penalver, A., Djokovic, N., Werel, L., Hoffarth, M., Ruzic, D., et al. (2019). Modulating protein-protein interactions with visible-light-responsive peptide backbone photoswitches. *Chembiochem* 20, 1417–1429. doi: 10.1002/cbic.201800737

Alves Avelar, L. A., Ruzic, D., Djokovic, N., Kurz, T., and Nikolic, K. (2019). Structure-based design of selective histone deacetylase 6 zinc binding groups. *J. Biomol. Struct. Dyn.* 1–12. doi: 10.1080/07391102.2019.1652687. [Epub ahead of print].

Amr, A. E. E., Abo-Ghalia, M. H., Moustafa, G. O., Al-Omar, M. A., Nossier, E. S., and Elsayed, E. A. (2018). Design, synthesis and docking studies of novel macrocyclic pentapeptides as anticancer multi-targeted kinase inhibitors. *Molecules* 23:2416. doi: 10.3390/molecules23102416

Astanehe, A., Finkbeiner, M. R., Krzywinski, M., Fotovati, A., Dhillon, J., Berquin, I. M., et al. (2012). MKNK1 is a YB-1 target gene responsible for imparting trastuzumab resistance and can be blocked by RSK inhibition. *Oncogene* 31, 4434–4446. doi: 10.1038/onc.2011.617

Bacilieri, M., and Moro, S. (2006). Ligand-based drug design methodologies in drug discovery process: an overview. *Curr. Drug Discov. Technol.* 3, 155–165. doi: 10.2174/157016306780136781

Baell, J., and Walters, M. A. (2014). Chemistry: chemical con artists foil drug discovery. *Nature* 513, 481–483. doi: 10.1038/513481a

Bahar, I., and Rader, A. J. (2005). Coarse-grained normal mode analysis in structural biology. *Curr. Opin. Struct. Biol.* 15, 586–592. doi: 10.1016/j.sbi.2005.08.007

Bajorath, J. (2017). Molecular similarity concepts for informatics applications. *Methods Mol. Biol.* 1526, 231–245. doi: 10.1007/978-1-4939-6613-4_13

Bajusz, D., Racz, A., and Heberger, K. (2015). Why is Tanimoto index an appropriate choice for fingerprint-based similarity calculations? *J. Cheminform.* 7:20. doi: 10.1186/s13321-015-0069-3

Banegas-Luna, A. J., Ceron-Carrasco, J. P., and Perez-Sanchez, H. (2018). A review of ligand-based virtual screening web tools and screening algorithms in large molecular databases in the age of big data. *Future Med. Chem.* 10, 2641–2658. doi: 10.4155/fmc-2018-0076

Bautista-Aguilera, O. M., Esteban, G., Bolea, I., Nikolic, K., Agbaba, D., Moraleda, I., et al. (2014). Design, synthesis, pharmacological evaluation, QSAR analysis, molecular modeling and ADMET of novel donepezil-indolyl hybrids as multipotent cholinesterase/monoamine oxidase inhibitors for the potential treatment of Alzheimer's disease. *Eur. J. Med. Chem.* 75, 82–95. doi: 10.1016/j.ejmech.2013.12.028

Beauchamp, K. A., Lin, Y. S., Das, R., and Pande, V. S. (2012). Are protein force fields getting better? A systematic benchmark on 524 diverse NMR measurements. *J. Chem. Theory Comput.* 8, 1409–1414. doi: 10.1021/ct2007814

Benod, C., Carlsson, J., Uthayaruban, R., Hwang, P., Irwin, J. J., Doak, A. K., et al. (2013). Structure-based discovery of antagonists of nuclear receptor LRH-1. *J. Biol. Chem.* 288, 19830–19844. doi: 10.1074/jbc.M112.411686

Bethune, G., Bethune, D., Ridgway, N., and Xu, Z. (2010). Epidermal growth factor receptor (EGFR) in lung cancer: an overview and update. *J. Thorac. Dis.* 2, 48–51.

Betzi, S., Alam, R., Martin, M., Lubbers, D. J., Han, H., Jakkaraj, S. R., et al. (2011). Discovery of a potential allosteric ligand binding site in CDK2. *ACS Chem. Biol.* 6, 492–501. doi: 10.1021/cb100410m

Bhullar, K. S., Lagaron, N. O., McGowan, E. M., Parmar, I., Jha, A., Hubbard, B. P., et al. (2018). Kinase-targeted cancer therapies: progress, challenges and future directions. *Mol. Cancer* 17:48. doi: 10.1186/s12943-018-0804-2

Blume-Jensen, P., and Hunter, T. (2001). Oncogenic kinase signalling. *Nature* 411, 355–365. doi: 10.1038/35077225

Bollag, G., Tsai, J., Zhang, J., Zhang, C., Ibrahim, P., Nolop, K., et al. (2012). Vemurafenib: the first drug approved for BRAF-mutant cancer. *Nat. Rev. Drug Discov.* 11, 873–886. doi: 10.1038/nrd3847

Buchdunger, E., Cioffi, C. L., Law, N., Stover, D., Ohno-Jones, S., Druker, B. J., et al. (2000). Abl protein-tyrosine kinase inhibitor STI571 inhibits *in vitro* signal transduction mediated by c-kit and platelet-derived growth factor receptors. *J. Pharmacol. Exp. Ther.* 295, 139–145.

Buchwald, F., Richter, L., and Kramer, S. (2011). Predicting a small molecule-kinase interaction map: a machine learning approach. *J. Cheminform.* 3:22. doi: 10.1186/1758-2946-3-22

Burgess, M. R., Skaggs, B. J., Shah, N. P., Lee, F. Y., and Sawyers, C. L. (2005). Comparative analysis of two clinically active BCR-ABL kinase inhibitors reveals the role of conformation-specific binding in resistance. *Proc. Natl. Acad. Sci. U.S.A.* 102, 3395–3400. doi: 10.1073/pnas.0409770102

Caballero, J., and Alzate-Morales, J. H. (2012). Molecular dynamics of protein kinase-inhibitor complexes: a valid structural information. *Curr. Pharm. Des.* 18, 2946–2963. doi: 10.2174/138161212800672705

Carles, F., Bourg, S., Meyer, C., and Bonnet, P. (2018). PKIDB: a curated, annotated and updated database of protein kinase inhibitors in clinical trials. *Molecules* 23:908. doi: 10.3390/molecules23040908

Chakraborty, S., Lin, Y. H., Leng, X., Miranda, R. N., Medeiros, L. J., Shpall, E., et al. (2013). Activation of Jak2 in patients with blast crisis chronic myelogenous leukemia: inhibition of Jak2 inactivates Lyn kinase. *Blood Cancer J.* 3:e142. doi: 10.1038/bcj.2013.41

Chen, J., Ma, X., Yuan, Y., Pei, J., and Lai, L. (2014). Protein-protein interface analysis and hot spots identification for chemical ligand design. *Curr. Pharm. Des.* 20, 1192–1200. doi: 10.2174/13816128113199990065

Cherkasov, A., Muratov, E. N., Fourches, D., Varnek, A., Baskin, I. I., Cronin, M., et al. (2014). QSAR modeling: where have you been? Where are you going to? *J. Med. Chem.* 57, 4977–5010. doi: 10.1021/jm4004285

Christmann-Franck, S., van Westen, G. J., Papadatos, G., Beltran Escudie, F., Roberts, A., Overington, J. P., et al. (2016). Unprecedently large-scale kinase inhibitor set enabling the accurate prediction of compound-kinase activities: a way toward selective promiscuity by design? *J. Chem. Inf. Model.* 56, 1654–1675. doi: 10.1021/acs.jcim.6b00122

Cohen, P. (2002). Protein kinases — the major drug targets of the twenty-first century? *Nat. Rev. Drug Discov.* 1, 309–315. doi: 10.1038/nrd773

Collins, D. M., Conlon, N. T., Kannan, S., Verma, C. S., Eli, L. D., Lalani, A. S., et al. (2019). Preclinical characteristics of the irreversible pan-HER kinase inhibitor neratinib compared with lapatinib: implications for the treatment of HER2-positive and HER2-mutated breast cancer. *Cancers* 11:737. doi: 10.3390/cancers11060737

Congreve, M., Carr, R., Murray, C., and Jhoti, H. (2003). A 'Rule of Three' for fragment-based lead discovery? *Drug Discov. Today* 8, 876–877. doi: 10.1016/S1359-6446(03)02831-9

Cornell, W. D., Cieplak, P., Bayly, C. I., Gould, I. R., Merz, K. M., Ferguson, D. M., et al. (1995). A second generation force field for the simulation of proteins, nucleic acids, and organic molecules. *J. Am. Chem. Soc.* 117, 5179–5197. doi: 10.1021/ja00124a002

Cramer, R. D., Patterson, D. E., and Bunce, J. D. (1988). Comparative molecular field analysis (CoMFA). 1. Effect of shape on binding of steroids to carrier proteins. *J. Am. Chem. Soc.* 110, 5959–5967. doi: 10.1021/ja00226a005

Dar, A. C., and Shokat, K. M. (2011). The evolution of protein kinase inhibitors from antagonists to agonists of cellular signaling. *Annu. Rev. Biochem.* 80, 769–795. doi: 10.1146/annurev-biochem-090308-173656

de Angelo, R. M., Almeida, M. O., de Paula, H., and Honorio, K. M. (2018). Studies on the dual activity of EGFR and HER-2 inhibitors using structure-based drug design techniques. *Int. J. Mol. Sci.* 19:3728. doi: 10.3390/ijms19123728

Debnath, S., Kanakaraju, M., Islam, M., Yeeravalli, R., Sen, D., and Das, A. (2019). *In silico* design, synthesis and activity of potential drug-like chrysin scaffold-derived selective EGFR inhibitors as anticancer agents. *Comput. Biol. Chem.* 83:107156. doi: 10.1016/j.compbiolchem.2019.107156

Deeks, E. D. (2016). Venetoclax: first global approval. *Drugs* 76, 979–987. doi: 10.1007/s40265-016-0596-x

Deng, W., Breneman, C., and Embrechts, M. J. (2004). Predicting protein-ligand binding affinities using novel geometrical descriptors and machine-learning methods. *J. Chem. Inf. Comput. Sci.* 44, 699–703. doi: 10.1021/ci034246+

Drewry, D. H., Wells, C. I., Andrews, D. M., Angell, R., Al-Ali, H., Axtman, A. D., et al. (2017). Progress towards a public chemogenomic set for protein kinases and a call for contributions. *PLoS ONE* 12:e0181585. doi: 10.1371/journal.pone.0181585

Dror, R. O., Dirks, R. M., Grossman, J. P., Xu, H., and Shaw, D. E. (2012). Biomolecular simulation: a computational microscope for molecular biology. *Annu. Rev. Biophys.* 41, 429–452. doi: 10.1146/annurev-biophys-042910-155245

Duong-Ly, K. C., and Peterson, J. R. (2013). The human kinome and kinase inhibition. *Curr. Protoc. Pharmacol.*60, 2.9.1–2.9.14. doi: 10.1002/0471141755.ph0209s60

Duran, A., Zamora, I., and Pastor, M. (2009). Suitability of GRIND-based principal properties for the description of molecular similarity and ligand-based virtual screening. *J. Chem. Inf. Model.* 49, 2129–2138. doi: 10.1021/ci900228x

Ekins, S. (2016). The next era: deep learning in pharmaceutical research. *Pharm. Res.* 33, 2594–2603. doi: 10.1007/s11095-016-2029-7

El Rashedy, A. A., Olotu, F. A., and Soliman, M. E. S. (2018). Dual drug targeting of mutant Bcr-Abl induces inactive conformation: new strategy for the treatment of chronic myeloid leukemia and overcoming monotherapy resistance. *Chem. Biodivers.* 15:e1700533. doi: 10.1002/cbdv.201700533

Eldridge, M. D., Murray, C. W., Auton, T. R., Paolini, G. V., and Mee, R. P. (1997). Empirical scoring functions: I. The development of a fast empirical scoring function to estimate the binding affinity of ligands in receptor complexes. *J. Comput. Aided Mol. Des.* 11, 425–445. doi: 10.1023/A:1007996124545

Fang, Z., Grutter, C., and Rauh, D. (2013). Strategies for the selective regulation of kinases with allosteric modulators: exploiting exclusive structural features. *ACS Chem. Biol.* 8, 58–70. doi: 10.1021/cb300663j

FDA (2019). *Novel Drug Approvals for 2019*. Available online at: https://www.fda.gov/drugs/new-drugs-fda-cders-new-molecular-entities-and-new-therapeutic-biological-products/novel-drug-approvals-2019

Ferreira, L. G., Dos Santos, R. N., Oliva, G., and Andricopulo, A. D. (2015). Molecular docking and structure-based drug design strategies. *Molecules* 20, 13384–13421. doi: 10.3390/molecules200713384

Fischer, T., Najjar, A., Totzke, F., Schachtele, C., Sippl, W., Ritter, C., et al. (2018). Discovery of novel dual inhibitors of receptor tyrosine kinases EGFR and PDGFR-beta related to anticancer drug resistance. *J. Enzyme Inhib. Med. Chem.* 33, 1–8. doi: 10.1080/14756366.2017.1370583

Flaherty, K. T., Infante, J. R., Daud, A., Gonzalez, R., Kefford, R. F., Sosman, J., et al. (2012). Combined BRAF and MEK inhibition in melanoma with BRAF V600 mutations. *N. Engl. J. Med.* 367, 1694–1703. doi: 10.1056/NEJMoa1210093

Force, T., and Kolaja, K. L. (2011). Cardiotoxicity of kinase inhibitors: the prediction and translation of preclinical models to clinical outcomes. *Nat. Rev. Drug Discov.* 10, 111–126. doi: 10.1038/nrd3252

Gagic, Z., Ivkovic, B., Srdic-Rajic, T., Vucicevic, J., Nikolic, K., and Agbaba, D. (2016a). Synthesis of the vitamin E amino acid esters with an enhanced anticancer activity and *in silico* screening for new antineoplastic drugs. *Eur. J. Pharm. Sci.* 88, 59–69. doi: 10.1016/j.ejps.2016.04.008

Gagic, Z., Nikolic, K., Ivkovic, B., Filipic, S., and Agbaba, D. (2016b). QSAR studies and design of new analogs of vitamin E with enhanced antiproliferative activity on MCF-7 breast cancer cells. *J. Taiwan Inst. Chem. Eng.* 59, 33–44. doi: 10.1016/j.jtice.2015.07.019

Gao, Y., Wang, H., Wang, J., and Cheng, M. (2019). *In silico* studies on p21-activated kinase 4 inhibitors: comprehensive application of 3D-QSAR analysis, molecular docking, molecular dynamics simulations, and MM-GBSA calculation. *J. Biomol. Struct. Dyn.* 1–15. doi: 10.1080/07391102.2019.1673823. [Epub ahead of print].

Gibbons, D. L., Pricl, S., Kantarjian, H., Cortes, J., and Quintas-Cardama, A. (2012). The rise and fall of gatekeeper mutations? The BCR-ABL1 T315I paradigm. *Cancer* 118, 293–299. doi: 10.1002/cncr.26225

Giordanetto, F., Kull, B., and Dellsén, A. (2011). Discovery of novel class 1 phosphatidylinositide 3-kinases (PI3K) fragment inhibitors through structure-based virtual screening. *Bioorg. Med. Chem. Lett.* 21, 829–835. doi: 10.1016/j.bmcl.2010.11.087

Giordanetto, F., Wallberg, A., Cassel, J., Ghosal, S., Kossenjans, M., Yuan, Z. Q., et al. (2012). Discovery of 4-morpholino-pyrimidin-6-one and 4-morpholino-pyrimidin-2-one-containing Phosphoinositide 3-kinase (PI3K) p110beta isoform inhibitors through structure-based fragment optimisation. *Bioorg. Med. Chem. Lett.* 22, 6665–6670. doi: 10.1016/j.bmcl.2012.08.101

Gkeka, P., Papafotika, A., Christoforidis, S., and Cournia, Z. (2015). Exploring a non-ATP pocket for potential allosteric modulation of PI3Kalpha. *J. Phys. Chem. B* 119, 1002–1016. doi: 10.1021/jp506423e

Gomez-Gutierrez, P., Campos, P. M., Vega, M., and Perez, J. J. (2016). Identification of a Novel Inhibitory Allosteric Site in p38alpha. *PLoS ONE* 11:e0167379. doi: 10.1371/journal.pone.0167379

Gopalsamy, A., Ciszewski, G., Hu, Y., Lee, F., Feldberg, L., Frommer, E., et al. (2009). Identification of pyrazolo[1,5-a]pyrimidine-3-carboxylates as B-Raf kinase inhibitors. *Bioorg. Med. Chem. Lett.* 19, 2735–2738. doi: 10.1016/j.bmcl.2009.03.129

Graves, J. D., and Krebs, E. G. (1999). Protein phosphorylation and signal transduction. *Pharmacol. Ther.* 82, 111–121. doi: 10.1016/S0163-7258(98)00056-4

Greener, J. G., and Sternberg, M. J. (2018). Structure-based prediction of protein allostery. *Curr. Opin. Struct. Biol.* 50, 1–8. doi: 10.1016/j.sbi.2017.10.002

Guo, J., and Zhou, H. X. (2016). Protein allostery and conformational dynamics. *Chem. Rev.* 116, 6503–6515. doi: 10.1021/acs.chemrev.5b00590

Halder, A. K., Giri, A. K., and Cordeiro, M. (2019). Multi-target chemometric modelling, fragment analysis and virtual screening with ERK inhibitors as potential anticancer agents. *Molecules* 24:E3909. doi: 10.3390/molecules24213909

Halgren, T. A., Murphy, R. B., Friesner, R. A., Beard, H. S., Frye, L. L., Pollard, W. T., et al. (2004). Glide: a new approach for rapid, accurate docking and scoring. 2. Enrichment factors in database screening. *J. Med. Chem.* 47, 1750–1759. doi: 10.1021/jm030644s

Hann, M. M., Leach, A. R., and Harper, G. (2001). Molecular complexity and its impact on the probability of finding leads for drug discovery. *J. Chem. Inf. Comput. Sci.* 41, 856–864. doi: 10.1021/ci000403i

Hansch, C., Maloney, P. P., Fujita, T., and Muir, R. M. (1962). Correlation of biological activity of phenoxyacetic acids with Hammett substituent constants and partition coefficients. *Nature* 194, 178–180. doi: 10.1038/194178b0

Harris, P. A., Boloor, A., Cheung, M., Kumar, R., Crosby, R. M., Davis-Ward, R. G., et al. (2008). Discovery of 5-[[4-[(2,3-dimethyl-2H-indazol-6-yl)methylamino]-2-pyrimidinyl]amino]-2-methyl-b enzenesulfonamide (Pazopanib), a novel and potent vascular endothelial growth factor receptor inhibitor. *J. Med. Chem.* 51, 4632–4640. doi: 10.1021/jm800566m

Harris, P. A., Cheung, M., Hunter, R. N. III, Brown, M. L., Veal, J. M., Nolte, R. T., et al. (2005). Discovery and evaluation of 2-anilino-5-aryloxazoles as a novel class of VEGFR2 kinase inhibitors. *J. Med. Chem.* 48, 1610–1619. doi: 10.1021/jm049538w

Hasinoff, B. B. (2010). The cardiotoxicity and myocyte damage caused by small molecule anticancer tyrosine kinase inhibitors is correlated with lack of target specificity. *Toxicol. Appl. Pharmacol.* 244, 190–195. doi: 10.1016/j.taap.2009.12.032

Hazhazi, H., Melkemi, N., Salah, T., and Bouachrine, M. (2019). DFT-based reactivity and combined QSAR, molecular docking of 1,2,4,5-Tetrazine derivatives as inhibitors of Pim-1 kinase. *Heliyon* 5:e02451. doi: 10.1016/j.heliyon.2019.e02451

Holohan, C., Van Schaeybroeck, S., Longley, D. B., and Johnston, P. G. (2013). Cancer drug resistance: an evolving paradigm. *Nat. Rev. Cancer* 13, 714–726. doi: 10.1038/nrc3599

Hu, X., Wang, D., Tong, Y., Tong, L., Wang, X., Zhu, L., et al. (2017). Design, synthesis, and evaluation of ribose-modified anilinopyrimidine derivatives as EGFR tyrosine kinase inhibitors. *Front. Chem.* 5:101. doi: 10.3389/fchem.2017.00101

Huang, M., Song, K., Liu, X., Lu, S., Shen, Q., Wang, R., et al. (2018). AlloFinder: a strategy for allosteric modulator discovery and allosterome analyses. *Nucleic Acids Res.* 46, W451–W458. doi: 10.1093/nar/gky374

Huang, N., Kalyanaraman, C., Irwin, J. J., and Jacobson, M. P. (2006). Physics-based scoring of protein-ligand complexes: enrichment of known inhibitors in large-scale virtual screening. *J. Chem. Inf. Model.* 46, 243–253. doi: 10.1021/ci0502855

Hubbard, S. R., Wei, L., Ellis, L., and Hendrickson, W. A. (1994). Crystal structure of the tyrosine kinase domain of the human insulin receptor. *Nature* 372, 746–754. doi: 10.1038/372746a0

Hussain, A., and Verma, C. K. (2019). Ligand- and structure-based pharmacophore modeling, docking study reveals 2-[[4-[6-(isopropylamino) pyrimidin-4-yl]-1H-pyrrolo[2,3-b] pyridin-6-yl] amino] ethanol as a potential anticancer agent of CDK9/cyclin T1 kinase. *J. Cancer Res. Ther.* 15, 1131–1140. doi: 10.4103/jcrt.JCRT_47_18

Iqbal, N., and Iqbal, N. (2014). Imatinib: a breakthrough of targeted therapy in cancer. *Chemother. Res. Pract.* 2014:357027. doi: 10.1155/2014/357027

Irwin, J. J., Sterling, T., Mysinger, M. M., Bolstad, E. S., and Coleman, R. G. (2012). ZINC: a free tool to discover chemistry for biology. *J. Chem. Inf. Model.* 52, 1757–1768. doi: 10.1021/ci3001277

Jahnke, W., Grotzfeld, R. M., Pelle, X., Strauss, A., Fendrich, G., Cowan-Jacob, S. W., et al. (2010). Binding or bending: distinction of allosteric Abl kinase agonists from antagonists by an NMR-based conformational assay. *J. Am. Chem. Soc.* 132, 7043–7048. doi: 10.1021/ja101837n

James, N., Shanthi, V., and Ramanathan, K. (2019). Density functional theory and molecular simulation studies for prioritizing anaplastic lymphoma kinase inhibitors. *Appl. Biochem. Biotechnol.* doi: 10.1007/s12010-019-03156-1. [Epub ahead of print].

Jones, G., Willett, P., Glen, R. C., Leach, A. R., and Taylor, R. (1997). Development and validation of a genetic algorithm for flexible docking. *J. Mol. Biol.* 267, 727–748. doi: 10.1006/jmbi.1996.0897

Jorgensen, W. L., Maxwell, D. S., and Tirado-Rives, J. (1996). Development and testing of the OPLS all-atom force field on conformational energetics and properties of organic liquids. *J. Am. Chem. Soc.* 118, 11225–11236. doi: 10.1021/ja9621760

Kaieda, A., Takahashi, M., Fukuda, H., Okamoto, R., Morimoto, S., Gotoh, M., et al. (2019). Structure-based design, synthesis, and biological evaluation of imidazo[4,5-b]pyridin-2-one-based p38 MAP kinase inhibitors: part 1. *ChemMedChem* 14, 1022–1030. doi: 10.1002/cmdc.201900129

Kale, M. A., and Sonwane, G. M. (2018). Molecular docking, G-QSAR studies, synthesis and anticancer screening of some new 2-phenazinamines as Bcr-Abl tyrosine kinase inhibitors. *Curr. Drug Discov. Technol.* doi: 10.2174/1570163815666180913122542. [Epub ahead of print].

Kannan, S., Poulsen, A., Yang, H. Y., Ho, M., Ang, S. H., Eldwin, T. S. W., et al. (2017). Correction to probing the binding mechanism of Mnk inhibitors by docking and molecular dynamics simulations. *Biochemistry* 56, 5964–5965. doi: 10.1021/acs.biochem.7b00996

Khodair, A. I., Alsafi, M. A., and Nafie, M. S. (2019). Synthesis, molecular modeling and anti-cancer evaluation of a series of quinazoline derivatives. *Carbohydr. Res.* 486:107832. doi: 10.1016/j.carres.2019.107832

Kim, S., Chen, J., Cheng, T., Gindulyte, A., He, J., He, S., et al. (2019). PubChem 2019 update: improved access to chemical data. *Nucleic Acids Res.* 47, D1102–D1109. doi: 10.1093/nar/gky1033

Kitchen, D. B., Decornez, H., Furr, J. R., and Bajorath, J. (2004). Docking and scoring in virtual screening for drug discovery: methods and applications. *Nat. Rev. Drug Discov.* 3, 935–949. doi: 10.1038/nrd1549

Klaeger, S., Heinzlmeir, S., Wilhelm, M., Polzer, H., Vick, B., Koenig, P. A., et al. (2017). The target landscape of clinical kinase drugs. *Science* 358:eaan4368. doi: 10.1126/science.aan4368

Klebe, G., Abraham, U., and Mietzner, T. (1994). Molecular similarity indices in a comparative analysis (CoMSIA) of drug molecules to correlate and predict their biological activity. *J. Med. Chem.* 37, 4130–4146. doi: 10.1021/jm00050a010

Klepeis, J. L., Lindorff-Larsen, K., Dror, R. O., and Shaw, D. E. (2009). Long-timescale molecular dynamics simulations of protein structure and function. *Curr. Opin. Struct. Biol.* 19, 120–127. doi: 10.1016/j.sbi.2009.03.004

Knight, J. D., Qian, B., Baker, D., and Kothary, R. (2007). Conservation, variability and the modeling of active protein kinases. *PLoS ONE* 2:e982. doi: 10.1371/journal.pone.0000982

Knighton, D. R., Zheng, J. H., Ten Eyck, L. F., Ashford, V. A., Xuong, N. H., Taylor, S. S., et al. (1991). Crystal structure of the catalytic subunit of cyclic adenosine monophosphate-dependent protein kinase. *Science* 253, 407–414. doi: 10.1126/science.1862342

Koneru, J. K., Sinha, S., and Mondal, J. (2019). *In Silico* reoptimization of binding affinity and drug-resistance circumvention ability in kinase inhibitors: a case study with RL-45 and Src kinase. *J. Phys. Chem. B* 123, 6664–6672. doi: 10.1021/acs.jpcb.9b02883

Konze, K. D., Bos, P. H., Dahlgren, M. K., Leswing, K., Tubert-Brohman, I., Bortolato, A., et al. (2019). Reaction-based enumeration, active learning, and free energy calculations to rapidly explore synthetically tractable chemical space and optimize potency of cyclin-dependent kinase 2 inhibitors. *J. Chem. Inf. Model.* 59, 3782–3793. doi: 10.1021/acs.jcim.9b00367

Kozakov, D., Grove, L. E., Hall, D. R., Bohnuud, T., Mottarella, S. E., Luo, L., et al. (2015). The FTMap family of web servers for determining and characterizing ligand-binding hot spots of proteins. *Nat. Protoc.* 10, 733–755. doi: 10.1038/nprot.2015.043

Kumar, V., Krishna, S., and Siddiqi, M. I. (2015). Virtual screening strategies: recent advances in the identification and design of anti-cancer agents. *Methods* 71, 64–70. doi: 10.1016/j.ymeth.2014.08.010

Kuntz, I. D., Blaney, J. M., Oatley, S. J., Langridge, R., and Ferrin, T. E. (1982). A geometric approach to macromolecule-ligand interactions. *J. Mol. Biol.* 161, 269–288. doi: 10.1016/0022-2836(82)90153-X

Kuthuru, S., Szafran, A. T., Stossi, F., Mancini, M. A., and Rao, A. (2019). Leveraging image-derived phenotypic measurements for drug-target interaction predictions. *Cancer Inform.* 18:1176935119856595. doi: 10.1177/1176935119856595

La Sala, G., Riccardi, L., Gaspari, R., Cavalli, A., Hantschel, O., and De Vivo, M. (2016). HRD motif as the central hub of the signaling network for activation loop autophosphorylation in Abl kinase. *J. Chem. Theory Comput.* 12, 5563–5574. doi: 10.1021/acs.jctc.6b00600

Lamba, V., and Ghosh, I. (2012). New directions in targeting protein kinases: focusing upon true allosteric and bivalent inhibitors. *Curr. Pharm. Des.* 18, 2936–2945. doi: 10.2174/138161212800672813

Larif, S., Salem, C. B., Hmouda, H., and Bouraoui, K. (2014). *In silico* screening and study of novel ERK2 inhibitors using 3D QSAR, docking and molecular dynamics. *J. Mol. Graph. Model.* 53, 1–12. doi: 10.1016/j.jmgm.2014.07.001

Laurini, E., Posocco, P., Fermeglia, M., Gibbons, D. L., Quintas-Cardama, A., and Pricl, S. (2013). Through the open door: preferential binding of dasatinib to the active form of BCR-ABL unveiled by *in silico* experiments. *Mol. Oncol.* 7, 968–975. doi: 10.1016/j.molonc.2013.06.001

Le Guilloux, V., Schmidtke, P., and Tuffery, P. (2009). Fpocket: an open source platform for ligand pocket detection. *BMC Bioinformatics* 10:168. doi: 10.1186/1471-2105-10-168

Leach, A. R., and Hann, M. M. (2011). Molecular complexity and fragment-based drug discovery: ten years on. *Curr. Opin. Chem. Biol.* 15, 489–496. doi: 10.1016/j.cbpa.2011.05.008

Lee, H. W., Choi, H. Y., Joo, K. M., and Nam, D. H. (2015). Tumor progression locus 2 (Tpl2) kinase as a novel therapeutic target for cancer: double-sided effects of Tpl2 on cancer. *Int. J. Mol. Sci.* 16, 4471–4491. doi: 10.3390/ijms16034471

Lee, I., Keum, J., and Nam, H. (2019). DeepConv-DTI: prediction of drug-target interactions via deep learning with convolution on protein sequences. *PLoS Comput. Biol.* 15:e1007129. doi: 10.1371/journal.pcbi.1007129

Lengauer, T., and Rarey, M. (1996). Computational methods for biomolecular docking. *Curr. Opin. Struct. Biol.* 6, 402–406. doi: 10.1016/S0959-440X(96)80061-3

Li, J., Fu, A., and Zhang, L. (2019). An overview of scoring functions used for protein-ligand interactions in molecular docking. *Interdiscip. Sci.* 11, 320–328. doi: 10.1007/s12539-019-00327-w

Li, S., Shen, Q., Su, M., Liu, X., Lu, S., Chen, Z., et al. (2016). Alloscore: a method for predicting allosteric ligand-protein interactions. *Bioinformatics* 32, 1574–1576. doi: 10.1093/bioinformatics/btw036

Lim, H., He, D., Qiu, Y., Krawczuk, P., Sun, X., and Xie, L. (2019). Rational discovery of dual-indication multi-target PDE/Kinase inhibitor for precision anti-cancer therapy using structural systems pharmacology. *PLoS Comput. Biol.* 15:e1006619. doi: 10.1371/journal.pcbi.1006619

Lionta, E., Spyrou, G., Vassilatis, D. K., and Cournia, Z. (2014). Structure-based virtual screening for drug discovery: principles, applications and recent advances. *Curr. Top. Med. Chem.* 14, 1923–1938. doi: 10.2174/1568026614666140929124445

Liu, J., and Wang, R. (2015). Classification of current scoring functions. *J. Chem. Inf. Model.* 55, 475–482. doi: 10.1021/ci500731a

Liu, J., Wen, Y., Gao, L., Gao, L., He, F., Zhou, J., et al. (2020). Design, synthesis and biological evaluation of novel 1H-1,2,4-triazole, benzothiazole and indazole-based derivatives as potent FGFR1 inhibitors viafragment-based virtual screening. *J. Enzyme Inhib. Med. Chem.* 35, 72–84. doi: 10.1080/14756366.2019.1673745

Lu, S., He, X., Ni, D., and Zhang, J. (2019). Allosteric modulator discovery: from serendipity to structure-based design. *J. Med. Chem.* 62, 6405–6421. doi: 10.1021/acs.jmedchem.8b01749

Lu, S., Ji, M., Ni, D., and Zhang, J. (2018a). Discovery of hidden allosteric sites as novel targets for allosteric drug design. *Drug Discov. Today* 23, 359–365. doi: 10.1016/j.drudis.2017.10.001

Lu, W., Zhang, R., Jiang, H., Zhang, H., and Luo, C. (2018b). Computer-aided drug design in epigenetics. *Front. Chem.* 6:57. doi: 10.3389/fchem.2018.00057

Ma, X., Meng, H., and Lai, L. (2016). Motions of allosteric and orthosteric ligand-binding sites in proteins are highly correlated. *J. Chem. Inf. Model.* 56, 1725–1733. doi: 10.1021/acs.jcim.6b00039

Machrouhi, F., Ouhamou, N., Laderoute, K., Calaoagan, J., Bukhtiyarova, M., Ehrlich, P. J., et al. (2010). The rational design of a novel potent analogue of the 5'-AMP-activated protein kinase inhibitor compound C with improved selectivity and cellular activity. *Bioorg. Med. Chem. Lett.* 20, 6394–6399. doi: 10.1016/j.bmcl.2010.09.088

Manning, G., Whyte, D. B., Martinez, R., Hunter, T., and Sudarsanam, S. (2002). The protein kinase complement of the human genome. *Science* 298, 1912–1934. doi: 10.1126/science.1075762

Markham, A. (2019). Erdafitinib: first global approval. *Drugs* 79, 1017–1021. doi: 10.1007/s40265-019-01142-9

Martin, M. P., Alam, R., Betzi, S., Ingles, D. J., Zhu, J. Y., and Schonbrunn, E. (2012). A novel approach to the discovery of small-molecule ligands of CDK2. *Chembiochem* 13, 2128–2136. doi: 10.1002/cbic.201200316

Melge, A. R., Kumar, L. G., Pavithran, K., Nair, S. V., Manzoor, K., Gopi Mohan, C. (2019). Predictive models for designing potent tyrosine kinase inhibitors in chronic myeloid leukemia for understanding its molecular mechanism of resistance by molecular docking and dynamics simulations. *J. Biomol. Struct. Dyn.* 37, 4747–4766. doi: 10.1080/07391102.2018.1559765

Mendez, D., Gaulton, A., Bento, A. P., Chambers, J., De Veij, M., Felix, E., et al. (2019). ChEMBL: towards direct deposition of bioassay data. *Nucleic Acids Res.* 47, D930–D940. doi: 10.1093/nar/gky1075

Meng, Y., Gao, C., Clawson, D. K., Atwell, S., Russell, M., Vieth, M., et al. (2018). Predicting the conformational variability of Abl tyrosine kinase using molecular dynamics simulations and markov state models. *J. Chem. Theory Comput.* 14, 2721–2732. doi: 10.1021/acs.jctc.7b01170

Merget, B., Turk, S., Eid, S., Rippmann, F., and Fulle, S. (2017). Profiling prediction of kinase inhibitors: toward the virtual assay. *J. Med. Chem.* 60, 474–485. doi: 10.1021/acs.jmedchem.6b01611

Merk, D., Friedrich, L., Grisoni, F., and Schneider, G. (2018). *De novo* design of bioactive small molecules by artificial intelligence. *Mol. Inform.* 37. doi: 10.1002/minf.201700153

Mobitz, H. (2015). The ABC of protein kinase conformations. *Biochim. Biophys. Acta* 1854(10 Pt B), 1555–1566. doi: 10.1016/j.bbapap.2015.03.009

Modi, V., and Dunbrack, R. L. Jr. (2019). Defining a new nomenclature for the structures of active and inactive kinases. *Proc. Natl. Acad. Sci. U.S.A.* 116, 6818–6827. doi: 10.1073/pnas.1814279116

Mohamed, T. K., Batran, R. Z., Elseginy, S. A., Ali, M. M., and Mahmoud, A. E. (2019). Synthesis, anticancer effect and molecular modeling of new thiazolylpyrazolyl coumarin derivatives targeting VEGFR-2 kinase and inducing cell cycle arrest and apoptosis. *Bioorg. Chem.* 85, 253–273. doi: 10.1016/j.bioorg.2018.12.040

Mohareb, R. M., Samir, E. M., and Halim, P. A. (2019). Synthesis, and anti-proliferative, Pim-1 kinase inhibitors and molecular docking of thiophenes derived from estrone. *Bioorg. Chem.* 83, 402–413. doi: 10.1016/j.bioorg.2018.10.067

Morabito, A., De Maio, E., Di Maio, M., Normanno, N., and Perrone, F. (2006). Tyrosine kinase inhibitors of vascular endothelial growth factor receptors in clinical trials: current status and future directions. *Oncologist* 11, 753–764. doi: 10.1634/theoncologist.11-7-753

Morris, G. M., Huey, R., Lindstrom, W., Sanner, M. F., Belew, R. K., Goodsell, D. S., et al. (2009). AutoDock4 and AutoDockTools4: automated docking with selective receptor flexibility. *J. Comput. Chem.* 30, 2785–2791. doi: 10.1002/jcc.21256

Morris, G. M., and Lim-Wilby, M. (2008). Molecular docking. *Methods Mol. Biol.* 443, 365–382. doi: 10.1007/978-1-59745-177-2_19

Muegge, I., and Martin, Y. C. (1999). A general and fast scoring function for protein-ligand interactions: a simplified potential approach. *J. Med. Chem.* 42, 791–804. doi: 10.1021/jm980536j

Murray, C. W., and Verdonk, M. L. (2002). The consequences of translational and rotational entropy lost by small molecules on binding to proteins. *J. Comput. Aided Mol. Des.* 16, 741–753. doi: 10.1023/A:1022446720849

Naboulsi, I., Aboulmouhajir, A., Kouisni, L., Bekkaoui, F., and Yasri, A. (2018). Combining a QSAR approach and structural analysis to derive an SAR map of Lyn kinase inhibition. *Molecules* 23:3271. doi: 10.3390/molecules23123271

Nagar, B., Hantschel, O., Young, M. A., Scheffzek, K., Veach, D., Bornmann, W., et al. (2003). Structural basis for the autoinhibition of c-Abl tyrosine kinase. *Cell* 112, 859–871. doi: 10.1016/S0092-8674(03)00194-6

Najjar, A., Platzer, C., Luft, A., Assmann, C. A., Elghazawy, N. H., Erdmann, F., et al. (2019). Computer-aided design, synthesis and biological characterization of novel inhibitors for PKMYT1. *Eur. J. Med. Chem.* 161, 479–492. doi: 10.1016/j.ejmech.2018.10.050

Neves, B. J., Braga, R. C., Melo-Filho, C. C., Moreira-Filho, J. T., Muratov, E. N., and Andrade, C. H. (2018). QSAR-based virtual screening: advances and applications in drug discovery. *Front. Pharmacol.* 9:1275. doi: 10.3389/fphar.2018.01275

Nikolic, K., Agbaba, D., and Stark, H. (2015). Pharmacophore modeling, drug design and virtual screening on multi-targeting procognitive agents approaching histaminergic pathways. *J. Taiwan Inst. Chem. Eng.* 46, 15–29. doi: 10.1016/j.jtice.2014.09.017

Nikolic, K., Veljkovic, N., Gemovic, B., Srdic-Rajic, T., and Agbaba, D. (2013). Imidazoline-1 receptor ligands as apoptotic agents: pharmacophore modeling and virtual docking study. *Comb. Chem. High Throughput Screen* 16, 298–319. doi: 10.2174/1386207311316040004

Noolvi, M. N., and Patel, H. M. (2013). A comparative QSAR analysis and molecular docking studies of quinazoline derivatives as tyrosine kinase (EGFR)

inhibitors: a rational approach to anticancer drug design. *J. Saudi Chem. Soc.* 17, 361–379. doi: 10.1016/j.jscs.2011.04.017

Novič, M., Tibaut, T., Anderluh, M., Borišek, J., and Tomašič, T. (2016). "The comparison of docking search algorithms and scoring functions," in *Methods and Algorithms for Molecular Docking-Based Drug Design and Discovery*, ed S. Dastmalchi, M. Hamzeh-Mivehroud, B. Sokouti. (Hershey, PA: IGI Global), 99–127.

Ohren, J. F., Chen, H., Pavlovsky, A., Whitehead, C., Zhang, E., Kuffa, P., et al. (2004). Structures of human MAP kinase kinase 1 (MEK1) and MEK2 describe novel noncompetitive kinase inhibition. *Nat. Struct. Mol. Biol.* 11, 1192–1197. doi: 10.1038/nsmb859

Okabe, S., Tauchi, T., Tanaka, Y., and Ohyashiki, K. (2011). Dasatinib preferentially induces apoptosis by inhibiting Lyn kinase in nilotinib-resistant chronic myeloid leukemia cell line. *J. Hematol. Oncol.* 4:32. doi: 10.1186/1756-8722-4-32

Oluic, J., Nikolic, K., Vucicevic, J., Gagic, Z., Filipic, S., and Agbaba, D. (2017). 3D-QSAR, virtual screening, docking and design of dual PI3K/mTOR inhibitors with enhanced antiproliferative activity. *Comb. Chem. High Throughput Screen* 20, 292–303. doi: 10.2174/1386207320666170427143858

Oostenbrink, C., Villa, A., Mark, A. E., and van Gunsteren, W. F. (2004). A biomolecular force field based on the free enthalpy of hydration and solvation: the GROMOS force-field parameter sets 53A5 and 53A6. *J. Comput. Chem.* 25, 1656–1676. doi: 10.1002/jcc.20090

Oyarzabal, J., Zarich, N., Albarran, M. I., Palacios, I., Urbano-Cuadrado, M., Mateos, G., et al. (2010). Discovery of mitogen-activated protein kinase-interacting kinase 1 inhibitors by a comprehensive fragment-oriented virtual screening approach. *J. Med. Chem.* 53, 6618–6628. doi: 10.1021/jm1005513

Park, E., Kim, N., Ficarro, S. B., Zhang, Y., Lee, B. I., Cho, A., et al. (2015). Structure and mechanism of activity-based inhibition of the EGF receptor by Mig6. *Nat. Struct. Mol. Biol.* 22, 703–711. doi: 10.1038/nsmb.3074

Pastor, M., Cruciani, G., McLay, I., Pickett, S., and Clementi, S. (2000). GRid-INdependent descriptors (GRIND): a novel class of alignment-independent three-dimensional molecular descriptors. *J. Med. Chem.* 43, 3233–3243. doi: 10.1021/jm000941m

Piana, S., Klepeis, J. L., and Shaw, D. E. (2014). Assessing the accuracy of physical models used in protein-folding simulations: quantitative evidence from long molecular dynamics simulations. *Curr. Opin. Struct. Biol.* 24, 98–105. doi: 10.1016/j.sbi.2013.12.006

Platzer, C., Najjar, A., Rohe, A., Erdmann, F., Sippl, W., and Schmidt, M. (2018). Identification of PKMYT1 inhibitors by screening the GSK published protein kinase inhibitor set I and II. *Bioorg. Med. Chem.* 26, 4014–4024. doi: 10.1016/j.bmc.2018.06.027

Proud, C. G. (2015). Mnks, eIF4E phosphorylation and cancer. *Biochim. Biophys. Acta* 1849, 766–773. doi: 10.1016/j.bbagrm.2014.10.003

Putin, E., Asadulaev, A., Ivanenkov, Y., Aladinskiy, V., Sanchez-Lengeling, B., Aspuru-Guzik, A., et al. (2018). Reinforced adversarial neural computer for *de novo* molecular design. *J. Chem. Inf. Model.* 58, 1194–1204. doi: 10.1021/acs.jcim.7b00690

Rastelli, G., Anighoro, A., Chripkova, M., Carrassa, L., and Broggini, M. (2014). Structure-based discovery of the first allosteric inhibitors of cyclin-dependent kinase 2. *Cell Cycle* 13, 2296–2305. doi: 10.4161/cc.29295

Raval, A., Piana, S., Eastwood, M. P., Dror, R. O., and Shaw, D. E. (2012). Refinement of protein structure homology models via long, all-atom molecular dynamics simulations. *Proteins* 80, 2071–2079. doi: 10.1002/prot.24098

Ren, J. X., Li, L. L., Zheng, R. L., Xie, H. Z., Cao, Z. X., Feng, S., et al. (2011). Discovery of novel Pim-1 kinase inhibitors by a hierarchical multistage virtual screening approach based on SVM model, pharmacophore, and molecular docking. *J. Chem. Inf. Model.* 51, 1364–1375. doi: 10.1021/ci100464b

Rettenmaier, T. J., Fan, H., Karpiak, J., Doak, A., Sali, A., Shoichet, B. K., et al. (2015). Small-molecule allosteric modulators of the protein kinase PDK1 from structure-based docking. *J. Med. Chem.* 58, 8285–8291. doi: 10.1021/acs.jmedchem.5b01216

Roskoski, R. Jr. (2015). A historical overview of protein kinases and their targeted small molecule inhibitors. *Pharmacol. Res.* 100, 1–23. doi: 10.1016/j.phrs.2015.07.010

Roskoski, R. Jr. (2016). Classification of small molecule protein kinase inhibitors based upon the structures of their drug-enzyme complexes. *Pharmacol. Res.* 103, 26–48. doi: 10.1016/j.phrs.2015.10.021

Roskoski, R. Jr. (2019a). Cyclin-dependent protein serine/threonine kinase inhibitors as anticancer drugs. *Pharmacol. Res.* 139, 471–488. doi: 10.1016/j.phrs.2018.11.035

Roskoski, R. Jr. (2019b). Properties of FDA-approved small molecule protein kinase inhibitors. *Pharmacol. Res.* 144, 19–50. doi: 10.1016/j.phrs.2019.03.006

Ruzic, D., Petkovic, M., Agbaba, D., Ganesan, A., and Nikolic, K. (2019). Combined ligand and fragment-based drug design of selective histone deacetylase - 6 inhibitors. *Mol. Inform.* 38:e1800083. doi: 10.1002/minf.201800083

Schoepfer, J., Jahnke, W., Berellini, G., Buonamici, S., Cotesta, S., Cowan-Jacob, S. W., et al. (2018). Discovery of Asciminib (ABL001), an allosteric inhibitor of the tyrosine kinase activity of BCR-ABL1. *J. Med. Chem.* 61, 8120–8135. doi: 10.1021/acs.jmedchem.8b01040

Schulze, J. O., Saladino, G., Busschots, K., Neimanis, S., Suss, E., Odadzic, D., et al. (2016). Bidirectional allosteric communication between the ATP-binding site and the regulatory PIF pocket in PDK1 protein kinase. *Cell Chem. Biol.* 23, 1193–1205. doi: 10.1016/j.chembiol.2016.06.017

Seiler, K. P., George, G. A., Happ, M. P., Bodycombe, N. E., Carrinski, H. A., Norton, S., et al. (2008). ChemBank: a small-molecule screening and cheminformatics resource database. *Nucleic Acids Res.* 36, D351–D359. doi: 10.1093/nar/gkm843

Sengupta, U., and Strodel, B. (2018). Markov models for the elucidation of allosteric regulation. *Philos. Trans. R. Soc. Lond. B. Biol. Sci.* 373:20170178. doi: 10.1098/rstb.2017.0178

Shah, N. P., Nicoll, J. M., Nagar, B., Gorre, M. E., Paquette, R. L., Kuriyan, J., et al. (2002). Multiple BCR-ABL kinase domain mutations confer polyclonal resistance to the tyrosine kinase inhibitor imatinib (STI571) in chronic phase and blast crisis chronic myeloid leukemia. *Cancer Cell* 2, 117–125. doi: 10.1016/S1535-6108(02)00096-X

Shah, N. P., Tran, C., Lee, F. Y., Chen, P., Norris, D., and Sawyers, C. L. (2004). Overriding imatinib resistance with a novel ABL kinase inhibitor. *Science* 305, 399–401. doi: 10.1126/science.1099480

Shi, Z., Resing, K. A., and Ahn, N. G. (2006). Networks for the allosteric control of protein kinases. *Curr. Opin. Struct. Biol.* 16, 686–692. doi: 10.1016/j.sbi.2006.10.011

Shiri, F., Pirhadi, S., and Ghasemi, J. B. (2016). Alignment independent 3D-QSAR, quantum calculations and molecular docking of Mer specific tyrosine kinase inhibitors as anticancer drugs. *Saudi Pharm. J.* 24, 197–212. doi: 10.1016/j.jsps.2015.03.012

Shirts, M., and Pande, V. S. (2000). COMPUTING: screen savers of the world unite! *Science* 290, 1903–1904. doi: 10.1126/science.290.5498.1903

Shuker, S. B., Hajduk, P. J., Meadows, R. P., and Fesik, S. W. (1996). Discovering high-affinity ligands for proteins: SAR by NMR. *Science* 274, 1531–1534. doi: 10.1126/science.274.5292.1531

Shukla, D., Meng, Y., Roux, B., and Pande, V. S. (2014). Activation pathway of Src kinase reveals intermediate states as targets for drug design. *Nat. Commun.* 5:3397. doi: 10.1038/ncomms4397

Simeon, S., Jongkon, N., Chotpatiwetchkul, W., and Gleeson, M. P. (2019). Insights into the EGFR SAR of N-phenylquinazolin-4-amine-derivatives using quantum mechanical pairwise-interaction energies. *J. Comput. Aided Mol. Des.* 33, 745–757. doi: 10.1007/s10822-019-00221-z

Smajić, M., Nikoli,ć, K., Vujić, Z., Ahmetović, L., and Kuntić, V. (2015). 3D-QSAR studies and pharmacophore identification of AT1 receptor antagonists. *Med. Chem. Res.* 25, 51–61. doi: 10.1007/s00044-015-1470-1

Sobhy, M. K., Mowafy, S., Lasheen, D. S., Farag, N. A., and Abouzid, K. A. M. (2019). 3D-QSAR pharmacophore modelling, virtual screening and docking studies for lead discovery of a novel scaffold for VEGFR 2 inhibitors: design, synthesis and biological evaluation. *Bioorg. Chem.* 89:102988. doi: 10.1016/j.bioorg.2019.102988

Song, K., Liu, X., Huang, W., Lu, S., Shen, Q., Zhang, L., et al. (2017). Improved method for the identification and validation of allosteric sites. *J. Chem. Inf. Model.* 57, 2358–2363. doi: 10.1021/acs.jcim.7b00014

Sousa, S. F., Fernandes, P. A., and Ramos, M. J. (2006). Protein-ligand docking: current status and future challenges. *Proteins* 65, 15–26. doi: 10.1002/prot.21082

Subramanian, V., Prusis, P., Pietila, L. O., Xhaard, H., and Wohlfahrt, G. (2013). Visually interpretable models of kinase selectivity related features derived from field-based proteochemometrics. *J. Chem. Inf. Model.* 53, 3021–3030. doi: 10.1021/ci400369z

Subramanian, V., Prusis, P., Xhaard, H., and Wohlfahrt, G. (2016). Predictive proteochemometric models for kinases derived from 3D protein field-based descriptors. *Medchemcomm* 7, 1007–1015. doi: 10.1039/C5MD 00556F

Sudha, A., Srinivasan, P., and Rameshthangam, P. (2015). Exploration of potential EGFR inhibitors: a combination of pharmacophore-based virtual screening, atom-based 3D-QSAR and molecular docking analysis. *J. Recept. Signal Transduct. Res.* 35, 137–148. doi: 10.3109/10799893.2014.942461

Sun, C., Petros, A. M., and Hajduk, P. J. (2011). Fragment-based lead discovery: challenges and opportunities. *J. Comput. Aided Mol. Des.* 25, 607–610. doi: 10.1007/s10822-011-9451-z

Sun, H. (1998). COMPASS: An *ab initio* force-field optimized for condensed-phase applicationsoverview with details on alkane and benzene compounds. *J. Phys. Chem. B* 102, 7338–7364. doi: 10.1021/jp980939v

Taylor, R. D., Jewsbury, P. J., and Essex, J. W. (2002). A review of protein-small molecule docking methods. *J. Comput. Aided Mol. Des.* 16, 151–166. doi: 10.1023/A:1020155510718

Taylor, S. S., and Kornev, A. P. (2011). Protein kinases: evolution of dynamic regulatory proteins. *Trends Biochem. Sci.* 36, 65–77. doi: 10.1016/j.tibs.2010.09.006

Taylor, S. S., Radzio-Andzelm, E., and Hunter, T. (1995). How do protein kinases discriminate between serine/threonine and tyrosine? Structural insights from the insulin receptor protein-tyrosine kinase. *FASEB J.* 9, 1255–1266. doi: 10.1096/fasebj.9.13.7557015

Teli, M. K., and Rajanikant, G. K. (2012). Pharmacophore generation and atom-based 3D-QSAR of novel quinoline-3-carbonitrile derivatives as Tpl2 kinase inhibitors. *J. Enzyme Inhib. Med. Chem.* 27, 558–570. doi: 10.3109/14756366.2011.603128

Trott, O., and Olson, A. J. (2010). AutoDock Vina: improving the speed and accuracy of docking with a new scoring function, efficient optimization, and multithreading. *J. Comput. Chem.* 31, 455–461. doi: 10.1002/jcc.21334

Tsou, H. R., Otteng, M., Tran, T., Floyd, M. B. Jr., Reich, M., Birnberg, G., et al. (2008). 4-(Phenylaminomethylene)isoquinoline-1,3(2H,4H)-diones as potent and selective inhibitors of the cyclin-dependent kinase 4 (CDK4). *J. Med. Chem.* 51, 3507–3525. doi: 10.1021/jm800072z

Ung, P. M., Rahman, R., and Schlessinger, A. (2018). Redefining the protein kinase conformational space with machine learning. *Cell Chem. Biol.* 25, 916–924.e912. doi: 10.1016/j.chembiol.2018.05.002

Vanderpool, D., Johnson, T. O., Ping, C., Bergqvist, S., Alton, G., Phonephaly, S., et al. (2009). Characterization of the CHK1 allosteric inhibitor binding site. *Biochemistry* 48, 9823–9830. doi: 10.1021/bi900258v

Vanommeslaeghe, K., Guvench, O., and MacKerell, A. D. Jr. (2014). Molecular mechanics. *Curr. Pharm. Des.* 20, 3281–3292. doi: 10.2174/13816128113199990600

Verdonk, M. L., Cole, J. C., Hartshorn, M. J., Murray, C. W., and Taylor, R. D. (2003). Improved protein-ligand docking using GOLD. *Proteins* 52, 609–623. doi: 10.1002/prot.10465

Vittorio, S., Seidel, T., Germano, M. P., Gitto, R., Ielo, L., Garon, A., et al. (2019). A combination of pharmacophore and docking-based virtual screening to discover new tyrosinase inhibitors. *Mol. Inform.* doi: 10.1002/minf.201900054. [Epub ahead of print].

Vucicevic, J., Nikolic, K., and Mitchell, J. B. O. (2017). Rational drug design of antineoplastic agents using 3D-QSAR, cheminformatic, and virtual screening approaches. *Curr. Med. Chem.* 26, 3874–3889. doi: 10.2174/0929867324666170712115411

Vucicevic, J., Srdic-Rajic, T., Pieroni, M., Laurila, J. M., Perovic, V., Tassini, S., et al. (2016). A combined ligand- and structure-based approach for the identification of rilmenidine-derived compounds which synergize the antitumor effects of doxorubicin. *Bioorg. Med. Chem.* 24, 3174–3183. doi: 10.1016/j.bmc.2016.05.043

Wagner, J. R., Lee, C. T., Durrant, J. D., Malmstrom, R. D., Feher, V. A., and Amaro, R. E. (2016). Emerging computational methods for the rational discovery of allosteric drugs. *Chem. Rev.* 116, 6370–6390. doi: 10.1021/acs.chemrev.5b00631

Wan, P. T. C., Garnett, M. J., Roe, S. M., Lee, S., Niculescu-Duvaz, D., Good, V. M., et al. (2004). Mechanism of activation of the RAF-ERK signaling pathway by oncogenic mutations of B-RAF. *Cell* 116, 855–867. doi: 10.1016/S0092-8674(04)00215-6

Wang, J. L., Li, L., Hu, M. B., Wu, B., Fan, W. X., Peng, W., et al. (2019a). *In silico* drug design of inhibitor of nuclear factor kappa B kinase subunit beta inhibitors from 2-acylamino-3-aminothienopyridines based on quantitative structure-activity relationships and molecular docking. *Comput. Biol. Chem.* 78, 297–305. doi: 10.1016/j.compbiolchem.2018.12.021

Wang, Q., Zheng, M., Huang, Z., Liu, X., Zhou, H., Chen, Y., et al. (2012). Toward understanding the molecular basis for chemical allosteric modulator design. *J. Mol. Graph. Model.* 38, 324–333. doi: 10.1016/j.jmgm.2012.07.006

Wang, T., Peng, T., Wen, X., Wang, G., Sun, Y., Liu, S., et al. (2019b). Design, synthesis and preliminary biological evaluation of benzylsulfone coumarin derivatives as anti-cancer agents. *Molecules* 24:4034. doi: 10.3390/molecules24224034

Wang, Y., Tang, C., Yao, S., Lai, H., Li, R., Xu, J., et al. (2019c). Discovery of a novel protein kinase C activator from Croton tiglium for inhibition of non-small cell lung cancer. *Phytomedicine* 65:153100. doi: 10.1016/j.phymed.2019.153100

Warner, S. L., Bashyam, S., Vankayalapati, H., Bearss, D. J., Han, H., Mahadevan, D., et al. (2006). Identification of a lead small-molecule inhibitor of the Aurora kinases using a structure-assisted, fragment-based approach. *Mol. Cancer Ther.* 5, 1764–1773. doi: 10.1158/1535-7163.MCT-05-0524

Warren, G. L., Andrews, C. W., Capelli, A. M., Clarke, B., LaLonde, J., Lambert, M. H., et al. (2006). A critical assessment of docking programs and scoring functions. *J. Med. Chem.* 49, 5912–5931. doi: 10.1021/jm050362n

Webb, B., and Sali, A. (2016). Comparative Protein Structure Modeling Using MODELLER. *Curr. Protoc. Bioinformatics* 54, 5.6.1–5.6.37. doi: 10.1002/cpbi.3

Weiner, S. J., Kollman, P. A., Case, D. A., Singh, U. C., Ghio, C., Alagona, G., et al. (1984). A new force field for molecular mechanical simulation of nucleic acids and proteins. *J. Am. Chem. Soc.* 106, 765–784. doi: 10.1021/ja00315a051

Wendel, H. G., Silva, R. L., Malina, A., Mills, J. R., Zhu, H., Ueda, T., et al. (2007). Dissecting eIF4E action in tumorigenesis. *Genes Dev.* 21, 3232–3237. doi: 10.1101/gad.1604407

Wenthur, C. J., Gentry, P. R., Mathews, T. P., and Lindsley, C. W. (2014). Drugs for allosteric sites on receptors. *Annu. Rev. Pharmacol. Toxicol.* 54, 165–184. doi: 10.1146/annurev-pharmtox-010611-134525

Wishart, D. S., Feunang, Y. D., Guo, A. C., Lo, E. J., Marcu, A., Grant, J. R., et al. (2018). DrugBank 5.0: a major update to the DrugBank database for 2018. *Nucleic Acids Res.* 46, D1074–D1082. doi: 10.1093/nar/gkx1037

Wong, M. L., Murphy, J., Harrington, E., Gower, C. M., Jain, R. K., Schirle, M., et al. (2017). Examining the influence of specificity ligands and ATP-competitive ligands on the overall effectiveness of bivalent kinase inhibitors. *Proteome Sci.* 15:17. doi: 10.1186/s12953-017-0125-1

Wu, P., Clausen, M. H., and Nielsen, T. E. (2015a). Allosteric small-molecule kinase inhibitors. *Pharmacol. Ther.* 156, 59–68. doi: 10.1016/j.pharmthera.2015.10.002

Wu, P., Nielsen, T. E., and Clausen, M. H. (2015b). FDA-approved small-molecule kinase inhibitors. *Trends Pharmacol. Sci.* 36, 422–439. doi: 10.1016/j.tips.2015.04.005

Xu, Y., Wang, S., Hu, Q., Gao, S., Ma, X., Zhang, W., et al. (2018). CavityPlus: a web server for protein cavity detection with pharmacophore modelling, allosteric site identification and covalent ligand binding ability prediction. *Nucleic Acids Res.* 46, W374–W379. doi: 10.1093/nar/gky380

Yamanishi, Y., Araki, M., Gutteridge, A., Honda, W., and Kanehisa, M. (2008). Prediction of drug-target interaction networks from the integration of chemical and genomic spaces. *Bioinformatics* 24, i232–i240. doi: 10.1093/bioinformatics/btn162

Yang, B., and Papoian, T. (2012). Tyrosine kinase inhibitor (TKI)-induced cardiotoxicity: approaches to narrow the gaps between preclinical safety evaluation and clinical outcome. *J. Appl. Toxicol.* 32, 945–951. doi: 10.1002/jat.2813

Yang, H., Chennamaneni, L. R., Ho, M. W. T., Ang, S. H., Tan, E. S. W., Jeyaraj, D. A., et al. (2018). Optimization of selective mitogen-activated protein kinase interacting kinases 1 and 2 inhibitors for the treatment of blast crisis leukemia. *J. Med. Chem.* 61, 4348–4369. doi: 10.1021/acs.jmedchem.7b01714

Yang, Y. I., Shao, Q., Zhang, J., Yang, L., and Gao, Y. Q. (2019). Enhanced sampling in molecular dynamics. *J. Chem. Phys.* 151:070902. doi: 10.1063/1.5109531

Yin, D., and MacKerell, A. D. (1998). Combinedab initio/empirical approach for optimization of Lennard-Jones parameters. *J. Comp. Chem.* 19, 334–348. doi: 10.1002/(SICI)1096-987X(199802)19:3<334::AID-JCC7>3.0.CO;2-U

Yu, C., Liu, X., Yang, J., Zhang, M., Jin, H., Ma, X., et al. (2019). Combination of immunotherapy with targeted therapy: theory and practice in metastatic melanoma. *Front. Immunol.* 10:990. doi: 10.3389/fimmu.2019.00990

Yuan, Y., Pei, J., and Lai, L. (2013). Binding site detection and druggability prediction of protein targets for structure-based drug design. *Curr. Pharm. Des.* 19, 2326–2333. doi: 10.2174/1381612811319120019

Yueh, C., Rettenmaier, J., Xia, B., Hall, D. R., Alekseenko, A., Porter, K. A., et al. (2019). Kinase Atlas: druggability analysis of potential allosteric sites in kinases. *J. Med. Chem.* 62, 6512–6524. doi: 10.1021/acs.jmedchem.9b00089

Yun, T., Qin, T., Liu, Y., and Lai, L. (2016). Discovery of non-ATP-competitive inhibitors of polo-like kinase 1. *ChemMedChem* 11, 713–717. doi: 10.1002/cmdc.201600051

Zhan, J. Y., Ma, J., and Zheng, Q. C. (2019). Molecular dynamics investigation on the Asciminib resistance mechanism of I502L and V468F mutations in BCR-ABL. *J. Mol. Graph. Model.* 89, 242–249. doi: 10.1016/j.jmgm.2019.03.018

Zhang, G., and Ren, Y. (2018). Molecular modeling and design studies of purine derivatives as novel CDK2 inhibitors. *Molecules* 23:2924. doi: 10.3390/molecules23112924

Zhang, S., Golbraikh, A., and Tropsha, A. (2006). Development of quantitative structure-binding affinity relationship models based on novel geometrical chemical descriptors of the protein-ligand interfaces. *J. Med. Chem.* 49, 2713–2724. doi: 10.1021/jm050260x

Zhang, W., Pei, J., and Lai, L. (2017). Statistical analysis and prediction of covalent ligand targeted cysteine residues. *J. Chem. Inf. Model.* 57, 1453–1460. doi: 10.1021/acs.jcim.7b00163

Zhao, B., Zhao, C., Hu, X., Xu, S., Lan, Z., Guo, Y., et al. (2019a). Design, synthesis and 3D-QSAR analysis of novel thiopyranopyrimidine derivatives as potential antitumor agents inhibiting A549 and Hela cancer cells. *Eur. J. Med. Chem.* 185:111809. doi: 10.1016/j.ejmech.2019.111809

Zhao, H., Dong, J., Lafleur, K., Nevado, C., and Caflisch, A. (2012). Discovery of a novel chemotype of tyrosine kinase inhibitors by fragment-based docking and molecular dynamics. *ACS Med. Chem. Lett.* 3, 834–838. doi: 10.1021/ml3001984

Zhao, Y., Liu, F., He, G., Li, K., Zhu, C., Yu, W., et al. (2019b). Discovery of arylamide-5-anilinoquinazoline-8-nitro derivatives as VEGFR-2 kinase inhibitors: synthesis, *in vitro* biological evaluation and molecular docking. *Bioorg. Med. Chem. Lett.* 29:126711. doi: 10.1016/j.bmcl.2019.126711

Zhavoronkov, A., Ivanenkov, Y. A., Aliper, A., Veselov, M. S., Aladinskiy, V. A., Aladinskaya, A. V., et al. (2019). Deep learning enables rapid identification of potent DDR1 kinase inhibitors. *Nat. Biotechnol.* 37, 1038–1040. doi: 10.1038/s41587-019-0224-x

Zhou, N., Xu, Y., Liu, X., Wang, Y., Peng, J., Luo, X., et al. (2015). Combinatorial pharmacophore-based 3D-QSAR analysis and virtual screening of FGFR1 inhibitors. *Int. J. Mol. Sci.* 16, 13407–13426. doi: 10.3390/ijms160613407

Zuccotto, F., Ardini, E., Casale, E., and Angiolini, M. (2010). Through the "gatekeeper door": exploiting the active kinase conformation. *J. Med. Chem.* 53, 2681–2694. doi: 10.1021/jm901443h

12

In silico Strategies to Support Fragment-to-Lead Optimization in Drug Discovery

Lauro Ribeiro de Souza Neto [1†], *José Teófilo Moreira-Filho* [2†], *Bruno Junior Neves* [2,3†], *Rocío Lucía Beatriz Riveros Maidana* [1,4], *Ana Carolina Ramos Guimarães* [4], *Nicholas Furnham* [5*], *Carolina Horta Andrade* [2*] *and Floriano Paes Silva Jr.* [1*]

[1] *LaBECFar – Laboratório de Bioquímica Experimental e Computacional de Fármacos, Instituto Oswaldo Cruz, Fundação Oswaldo Cruz, Rio de Janeiro, Brazil,* [2] *LabMol – Laboratory for Molecular Modeling and Drug Design, Faculdade de Farmácia, Universidade Federal de Goiás, Goiânia, Brazil,* [3] *Laboratory of Cheminformatics, Centro Universitário de Anápolis – UniEVANGÉLICA, Anápolis, Brazil,* [4] *Laboratório de Genômica Funcional e Bioinformática, Instituto Oswaldo Cruz, Fundação Oswaldo Cruz, Rio de Janeiro, Brazil,* [5] *Department of Infection Biology, London School of Hygiene and Tropical Medicine, London, United Kingdom*

***Correspondence:**
Nicholas Furnham
nick.furnham@lshtm.ac.uk
Carolina Horta Andrade
carolina@ufg.br
Floriano Paes Silva Jr.
floriano@ioc.fiocruz.br

† *These authors have contributed*

Fragment-based drug (or lead) discovery (FBDD or FBLD) has developed in the last two decades to become a successful key technology in the pharmaceutical industry for early stage drug discovery and development. The FBDD strategy consists of screening low molecular weight compounds against macromolecular targets (usually proteins) of clinical relevance. These small molecular fragments can bind at one or more sites on the target and act as starting points for the development of lead compounds. In developing the fragments attractive features that can translate into compounds with favorable physical, pharmacokinetics and toxicity (ADMET—absorption, distribution, metabolism, excretion, and toxicity) properties can be integrated. Structure-enabled fragment screening campaigns use a combination of screening by a range of biophysical techniques, such as differential scanning fluorimetry, surface plasmon resonance, and thermophoresis, followed by structural characterization of fragment binding using NMR or X-ray crystallography. Structural characterization is also used in subsequent analysis for growing fragments of selected screening hits. The latest iteration of the FBDD workflow employs a high-throughput methodology of massively parallel screening by X-ray crystallography of individually soaked fragments. In this review we will outline the FBDD strategies and explore a variety of *in silico* approaches to support the follow-up fragment-to-lead optimization of either: growing, linking, and merging. These fragment expansion strategies include hot spot analysis, druggability prediction, SAR (structure-activity relationships) by catalog methods, application of machine learning/deep learning models for virtual screening and several *de novo* design methods for proposing synthesizable new compounds. Finally, we will highlight recent case studies in fragment-based drug discovery where *in silico* methods have successfully contributed to the development of lead compounds.

Keywords: fragment-based, drug discovery, lead discovery, *in silico* methods, machine learning, *de novo* design, optimization, hot spot analysis

INTRODUCTION

Fragment-Based Drug Discovery

Since the inception of fragment-based drug discovery (FBDD) over 20 years ago it has become an established technology used in both industry and academia (Hubbard, 2015). FBDD offers an attractive approach for effectively exploring the chemical space for binding a target protein. In conventional high-throughput screening (HTS) campaigns, large libraries of often complex compounds are screened for activity against a target (Hall et al., 2014). In contrast, FBDD use relatively small libraries of low complexity compounds representing fragments of larger more drug-like compounds. By reducing the complexity of the chemicals screened more of the potential binding sites of a target protein can be explored through the binding promiscuity of the fragments (Thomas et al., 2017). Where fragments do bind, albeit with lower potency than the drug-like molecules of HTS, they offer good starting points to design larger higher affinity binders using knowledge of the protein structure as a template to generate compounds with greater ligand efficiency (improved per atom binding energy to the target). This bottom-up approach means that a greater range of chemical space can be explored, leading quickly to higher affinity lead compounds with greater specificity (Patel et al., 2014).

FBDD projects require relatively lower investments in research and development (R&D) than HTS (Davis and Roughley, 2017). An example is the discovery of vemurafenib (Zelboraf^{TM}), the first fragment-derived drug, which moved relatively very quickly (6 years) between the phases of R&D pipeline before reaching Food and Drug Association (FDA) approval (Erlanson et al., 2016). Thus, FBDD provides attractive opportunities for the drug discovery field.

Output of Structure-Enabled Fragment Screening Campaigns

FBDD workflows are multi-step starting with target selection and protein isolation and followed by an initial screen of the fragment library using biophysical techniques such as nuclear magnetic resonance (NMR), surface plasmon resonance (SPR), thermal-shift assay, microscale thermophoresis (MST), mass spectrometry, and others. For fragments which show evidence of binding, a further step of hit validation and characterization occurs principally using X-ray crystallography (Verdonk and Hartshorn, 2004). Using hit characterization, an iterative cycle of fragment development can occur employing a range of *in silico* and experimental techniques. Advances in this protocol try to compress the process by combining the initial fragment screen with the hit characterization. This has been implemented in a high throughput FBDD platform called XChem located at the United Kingdom's national synchrotron the Diamond Light Source (Cox et al., 2016). It uses the ability to produce and handle a large number of crystals of the target protein to screen the fragment library by soaking each individual crystal with a fragment and then using X-ray crystallography to determine which fragments have bound and where. Though this high throughput technique often provides multiple hits, care needs to be taken in interpreting the significance of the hit. Promiscuous fragments may bind parts of the protein which are not involved in the protein function and therefore are unlikely to yield a successful inhibitor. Additionally, as the fragments are by their very nature weak binders and X-ray crystallography being a sensitive technique, observed binding events might be transient and not easily reproducible. It is therefore important to confirm hits with orthogonal structural (e.g., NMR), biophysical techniques (SPR, MST, etc.) or *in vitro* biological assays.

Fragment Libraries

A crucial step in FBDD process is in the development and choice of the fragment library used in the screening campaign. Several fragment libraries have been developed that exploit certain properties or chemistries. An example of a fragment library is the Diamond-SGC Poised Library (DSPL) (Cox et al., 2016). This has been developed for use with high-throughput XChem platform and consists of around 760 fragments that have been selected to contain at least one functional group that is open to rapid, cheap follow-up synthesis using robust well-characterized reactions (poised) and maximizing chemical diversity. Other fragment libraries optimize other properties such as solubility, 3D traits or based on subsets of existing drugs and related molecules such as natural products (Schuffenhauer et al., 2005). The fragment libraries generally share similar properties of "Rule of 3" compliant i.e., less than 300 Da molecular weight, 3 or less hydrogen bond donors, 3 or less hydrogen bond acceptors and CLogP no more than 3. In addition, they are soluble in dimethyl sulfoxide (DMSO) or phosphate buffered saline. Fragment libraries generally tend to be <1,000 fragments, which is significantly less than the many millions of compounds screened in high-throughput and high content screening campaigns (Trevizani et al., 2017).

Fragment Expansion Strategies

Once the fragment screen has been completed and hits characterized, the next step is the challenge of expanding these fragments to generate larger molecular entities with high binding affinity and demonstrating inhibition activity. There are several strategies that can be followed (Lamoree and Hubbard, 2017) (**Figure 1**). One option is to use expert medicinal chemistry advice to design and synthesize larger molecules based on the protein and the fragment pose. Another approach is to define vectors along the fragment molecule based on the steric hindrance of the protein target in which the fragment can be expanded. The fragment is then searched for within a large library of synthesizable (or purchasable) molecules which are bigger by between one and three heavy atoms along the identified vectors. These expanded fragments can be synthesized and soaked/co-crystallized and re-screened by X-ray crystallography. Expanded fragments that show improved binding can be further extended or structurally modified using the same process, with this cycle continuing until a larger high-affinity binding entity is reached.

An alternative to this "small steps" approach is to try to get a larger higher affinity binding molecule in a single step. This can be achieved by having an *in silico* method using the fragment in a substructure search of a large purchasable compound library (e.g., Zinc15), and to virtually screen the results using the pose

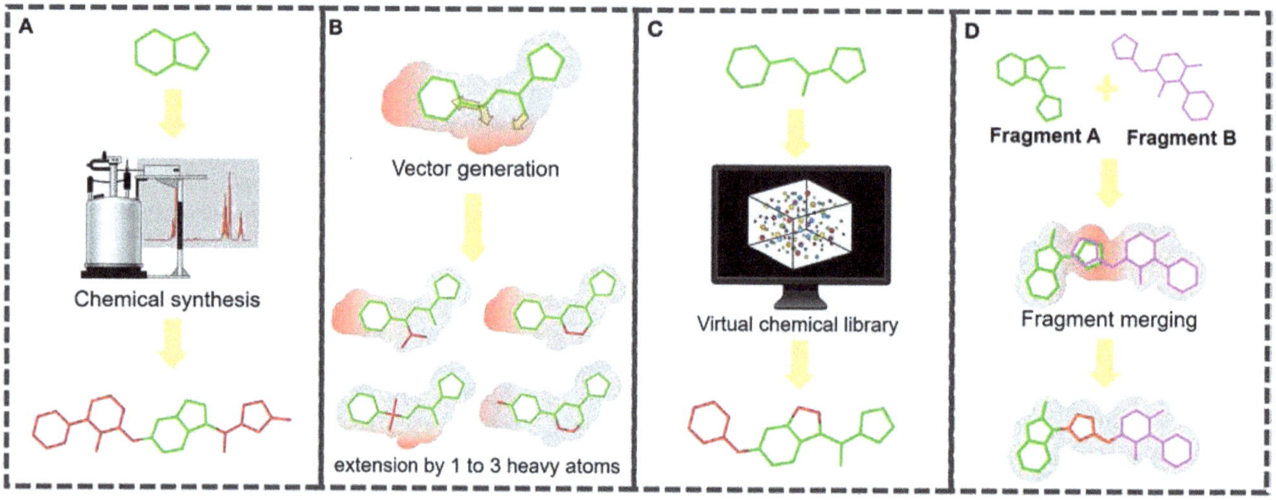

FIGURE 1 | Multiple routes to expanding fragment to more drug-like molecule with improved binding affinity. **(A)** Traditional medicinal chemistry route: knowledge-based design and synthesis. **(B)** "Small steps" route: successive cycles of extension of the fragment hit by 1–3 heavy atoms through vectors defined by high-resolution structural characterization methods, such as X-ray crystallography. **(C)** "Large leaps" or "SAR by catalog" route: from fragment to rule of 5 compliant molecules using virtual screening of commercial compound libraries. **(D)** Fragment merging route: bridging two overlapping fragments bound at neighbor sites. Regardless of the route, expanded fragments should be checked for biological activity using *in vitro*, *ex vivo*, or *in vivo* assays.

of the fragment to dock the molecules and rank them based on docking parameters (Trevizani et al., 2017). The top-ranking virtual screening hits can then be co-crystallized and well as evaluated *in vitro* and *in vivo*. A final expansion option is to link or merge fragments that hit near to each other or within the same site (Davis and Roughley, 2017). The combined fragments can then be further expanded using the approaches described previously. It is vital that as expansion progresses *in vitro* and *in vivo* assays are conducted to asses activity of the new molecules.

In the next section, we will discuss in depth the main optimization approaches used for a fragment structurally characterized in a binding site of its target. Further sections will describe existing software tools or modeling techniques (e.g., machine learning) employed for taking a fragment hit thorough the path for becoming a lead compound—a process known as fragment-to-lead (F2L)—for drug development and conclude by presenting case studies where *in silico* strategies have been successfully utilized to support the F2L optimization process.

FRAGMENT OPTIMIZATION APPROACHES

After the hit identification in a FBDD campaign, the fragment moves forward to the optimization phase. This optimization takes into account the structural characteristics of the ligand as well as its binding site. The principle in using fragments relies on the premise that these molecular entities are more efficient ligands compared to drug-like molecules, and their structures can be further optimized more efficiently. In fact, this constitutes one of its many advantages. As small entities, molecular fragments can be iteratively optimized to show a better pharmacokinetic profile in the later development stages. Drug-like molecules may contain functional groups that contribute poorly to protein binding or, in some cases, can even disrupt the protein-ligand interaction. On the other hand, fragments often form high-quality interactions able to more easily bind to the protein target, translating to a greater number of hits. **Figure 2** depicts schematically this concept.

Another advantage of FBDD is the potential for faster hit progression through the campaign, since the fragments are usually structurally simple and many follow-up compounds can be easily purchased from commercial databases (e.g., MolPort, ZINC15, and ChemBridge) instead of being synthesized. Another important characteristic often used to defend this approach is the high hit rates. In this sense, high hit rates means that the FBDD yields relatively more hits in comparison to the traditional methods such as HTS (Coutard et al., 2014; Mondal et al., 2015). This is due the inversely related nature between molecular complexity and the binding probability (Hann et al., 2001). Other advantages includes the more efficient chemical space sampling (Coutard et al., 2014; Mondal et al., 2015) and the relative low cost to implement the FBDD, as it can be seen from comparing the usual size of the HTS library (thousands of compounds) with fragment libraries (hundreds of compounds) (Macarron et al., 2011).

Assessment of the interactions between the fragment and its binding site should be carefully performed for further identification of synthetically accessible vectors on the ligand. Although x-ray crystallography data is a valuable technique in fragment optimization, is important to keep in mind that the observed structural data only represents a snapshot of the system under investigation. It's been known that the ligand affinity can be affected by the structural protein dynamics without changing the ligand-binding interface (Matias et al., 2000; Seo et al., 2014). This complex dynamic environment (Henzler-Wildman and Kern, 2007; Boehr et al., 2009) can affect small and weak ligands as

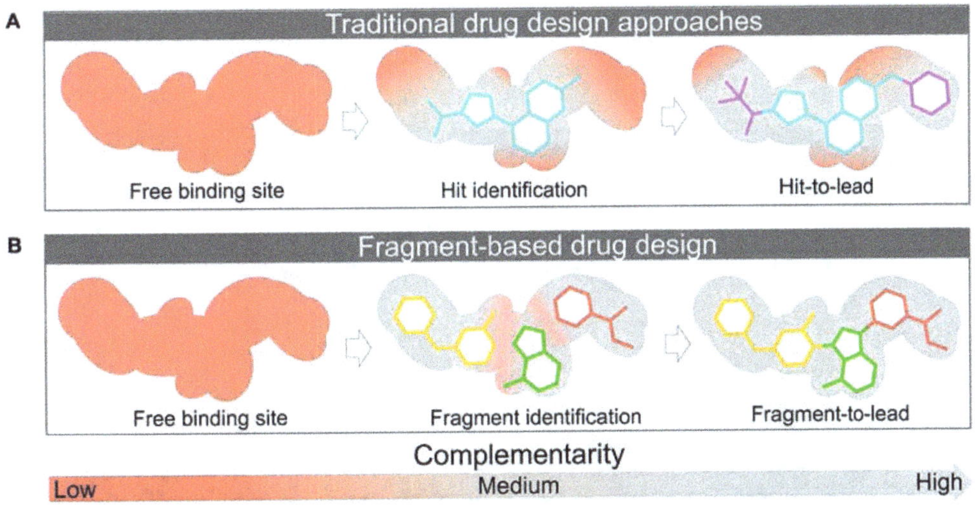

FIGURE 2 | Discovery and structural-optimization of drug-like molecules **(A)** and fragments **(B)** using protein target information. The surface represents the binding site. The red and gray colors represent the level of complementarity of ligand with the active site. Pockets with low complementarity with ligand are colored in red; pockets with high complementarity with ligand are highlighted in gray.

fragments. With this in mind, many methods can additionally be used to guide the fragment identification/optimization either providing complementary data (e.g., thermodynamic data) or acting as orthogonal approaches (Ciulli, 2013a). These methods are mostly biophysical (Shuker et al., 1996; Lo et al., 2004; Navratilova and Hopkins, 2010; Pedro and Quinn, 2016) and their use has some advantages such as, direct measurement of the binding, detection of small ligands with low affinity, and not needing any prior information about the protein function (Ciulli, 2013b). Despite the supremacy of biophysical methods, biochemical approaches are increasingly being used (Godemann et al., 2009; Boettcher et al., 2010; Mondal et al., 2015) in FBLD.

In addition to orthogonal and complementary methods, the ligand efficiency (LE) or one of its related metrics should ideally be used to keep track of the quality of follow-up ligands as they progress through the iterative optimization cycle. Some of these parameters are described below.

- **Ligand Efficiency (LE)** (Hopkins et al., 2004; Nissink, 2009; Davis and Roughley, 2017) = $\Delta G/HAC^{A}$;
- **Binding Efficiency Index (BEI)** (Abad-Zapatero, 2013) = pKi/MW^{B};
- **Percentage Efficiency Index (PEI)** (Abad-Zapatero, 2017; Davis and Roughley, 2017) = % inhibition/MW [B];
- **Surface-binding Efficiency Index (SEI)** (Abad-Zapatero, 2013) = $pIC_{50}/(TPSA^{C})$;
- **Lipophilic Efficiency (LipE/LLE)** (Shultz, 2013) = pIC_{50}-cLogP;
- **Size-Independent Ligand Efficiency (SILE)** (Nissink, 2009) = $\Delta G/HAC^{1-x}$;
- **Ligand Efficiency-Dependent Lipophlicity (LELP)** (Davis and Roughley, 2017) = logP/LE.

[A]Heavy Atom Count; [B]Molecular Weight; [C]Topological Polar Surface Area;

For the sake of brevity these metrics will not be further discussed and we recommend the references above for a deeper understanding. The structural complexity of the protein makes larger, more complex and less efficient molecules less likely to bind. This is one of the main reasons why fragment libraries often yield more hits when compared to a drug-like molecule commonly used in HTS (Hann et al., 2001). The use of fragments is a bottom-up approach, starting from less complex molecules with greater binding efficiency and ending up with a larger optimized molecule. As already highlighted, there are three main strategies that can be employed to optimize a ligand found bound in its target surface: linking, merging and growing (**Figure 3**). The next sections are dedicated to discussing in more depth each of them.

Growing

Fragment growing (**Figure 3A**) is the strategy most commonly employed during FBLD campaigns. As the name suggests, it consists of modifying the fragments to increase their size. Conceptually this approach is identical to the traditional compound modification methods employed in the optimization of hits from HTS campaigns. This modification occurs through the addition of groups.

A recent paper published by Strecker et al. (2019) is an example of how the growing strategy can be used to improve bind affinity. Using computer-aided drug design (CADD) and synthesis, the authors explored small structural modifications in a previously (PDB: 3U0X) identified compound (**1**) ($K_i = 800\ \mu M$).

These studies showed that a modification of a fragment phenyl moiety to a naphthyl allowed two new simultaneous π-π interactions, a parallel-displaced with Trp300 and an edge-to-face with His233. This minor modification led to a compound (**2**) with a 3-fold improved binding affinity ($K_i = 271\ \mu M$) (**Figure 4**).

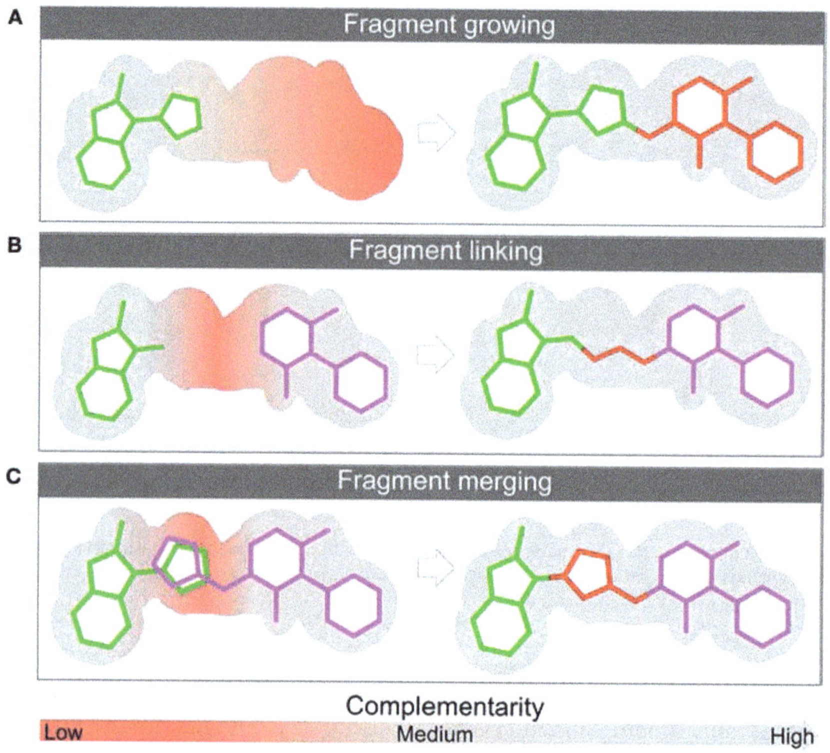

FIGURE 3 | Fragment optimization approaches: fragment growing **(A)**, fragment linking **(B)**, and fragment merging **(C)**. The surface of the binding site is depicted in gray. The red and gray colors represent the level of complementarity of ligand with the active site. Pockets with low complementarity with ligand are colored in red; pockets with high complementarity with ligand are highlighted in gray.

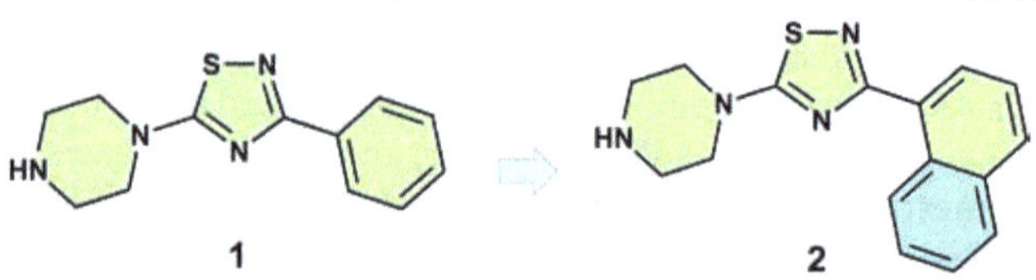

FIGURE 4 | Hit to lead progression of an initial fragment **(1)** to a compound **(2)** with improved affinity.

This example highlights the use of optimal growth vectors to introduce a rigid group, which led to an increased binding affinity. Alternatively, introduction of a moiety with increased number of rotatable bonds could impact negatively—due to the entropic penalty—in the affinity. Although this optimization approach can be computationally aided without further structural data, small modifications—as in the case of the hypothetical flexible moiety addition—can led to great changes in binding mode. When growing fragments is the chosen approach, structural data can be decisive to avoid misinterpretation.

Linking

Fragment linking (**Figure 3B**) describes the process of joining two non-competitive fragments (i.e., fragments that bind in two different sub-pockets of the binding site) with a chemical linker or spacer. Although conceptually simple, linking fragments is perhaps the most challenging strategy to implement. Although fragment linking is the most attractive approach in terms of rapid improvement of potency, the design of a linker with suitable flexibility while not disturbing the original binding modes of the fragments, makes it one of the most challenging optimization approaches.

As previously discussed, the introduction of flexible moieties affects these compounds properties and an optimal orientation should always be pursued. In fact, varying the degree of rigidity of a linker for the purpose of conformational restriction of the linked product can be used as a strategy for linker optimization, as it can be seen in Chung and colleagues work (Chung et al., 2009). This work shows how a conversion of oxime linkers into monoamine and diamines interferes with the rigidity and its impact on binding.

Although often neglected, the impact on the ADMET properties should also be taken in consideration. In the case of the linker, that usually adds rotatable bonds to the system (Ichihara et al., 2011; De Fusco et al., 2017), this modification can lead to poor PK features, like low permeability (Veber et al., 2002).

Merging

This strategy (**Figure 3C**) can be used in cases where two distinct fragments partially occupy the same region, or when two binding sites have regions in common and therefore their ligands are partially competitive with respect to the site. In such cases the overlapping parts form a nucleus where dissimilar parts come together. In a recent example, a gain of 2 orders of magnitude in potency was achieved for an inhibitor of flavin-dependent monooxygenase (EthA) transcriptional repressor (EthR) (Nikiforov et al., 2016) where the existence of overlapping groups within fragments bound to EthR allowed the use of merging as an optimization strategy.

Although not always possible, merging is a simpler strategy than linking, as there is no need to design a spacer that joins fragments together (Xu et al., 2017; Miyake et al., 2019). As also seen in this example, like linking (Davis and Roughley, 2017), this approach has the drawback of relying on high-quality structural data to go further in the optimization process.

Therefore, merging is an approach related to the "molecular hybridization" strategy, a long-consolidated approach in medicinal chemistry for designing new compounds with improved potency through the fusion of other active compound structures.

IN SILICO STRATEGIES FOR F2L OPTIMIZATION

Hot Spots Analysis and Pocket Druggability Prediction

Hot spots analysis is an important tool for structure-based F2L that allows the prediction of the small regions of the binding sites containing residues mostly contributing to the binding free energy (Cukuroglu et al., 2014). Once a fragment hit is experimentally identified, the hot spots analysis can be used to map the subsites around the fragment hit using small organic probes, driving the optimization into higher-affinity ligands (Hall et al., 2012).

One of the most used methods of hot spot analysis is the FTMap web server (Kozakov et al., 2015). This algorithm places 16 small organic probe molecules of different shape, size, and polarity on the protein surface to find favorable positions for each probe. Then, each probe type is clustered and overlapping clusters of different probes, called consensus sites (CSs), represent the hot spots. The consensus sites are ranked by the number of probe clusters, and the main hot spot is, generally, where the fragment hit binds and secondary hot spots are used to extend the fragment in the best direction (Hall et al., 2012; Ngan et al., 2012; Kozakov et al., 2015).

As an example, we used the FTMap server for predicting the hot spots for the oncogenic B-RAF kinase, the target of the first marketed drug from fragment-based drug design, vemurafenib (Bollag et al., 2012). **Figure 5A** shows the fragment hit experimentally bound to B-RAF kinase (PDB ID: 2UVX) (Donald et al., 2007), and the predicted hot spots around this fragment (shown in yellow dots) using the FTMap server. In **Figures 5B–D**, the iterative process of growing the fragment hit led to the discovery of the drug vemurafenib (PDB ID: 3OG7) (Bollag et al., 2010) with the hot spots shown in yellow dots. Although hot spot analysis was not used in the F2L process of vemurafenib, the results here showed that the predicted hot spots overlap the grown portions of vemurafenib.

During fragment screening, the fragment hits can bind in different sites of the protein (Giordanetto et al., 2019). If the binding site is not well-defined, the researchers can use the pocket druggability prediction to move forward in F2L with the most druggable site, capable to accommodate ligands orally bioavailable (Schmidtke and Barril, 2010; Hussein et al., 2015). There are many available methods for predicting pocket druggability and these are well-described and reviewed elsewhere (Barril, 2013; Abi Hussein et al., 2017).

SAR by Catalog

One fast and cheap way in F2L optimization is the SAR by catalog approach (Hall et al., 2017). This approach relies on the search of analogs of *in-house* or commercial databases that can be purchased or rapidly accessed for testing (Schulz et al., 2011). This process can use the fragment hit features for similarity, ligand-based pharmacophores, shape-based, fingerprints (Rogers and Hahn, 2010; Riniker and Landrum, 2013; Alvarsson et al., 2014), and substructure searches to find suitable compounds (Hubbard and Murray, 2011; Andrade et al., 2018). Some databases often used for SAR by catalog are ZINC (Sterling and Irwin, 2015), MolPort (https://www.molport.com), Mcule (https://mcule.com/), and eMolecules (https://www.emolecules.com) that contains collections of commercially available compounds. The databases Enamine (https://enaminestore.com), ChemDiv (http://www.chemdiv.com/) and ChemBridge (https://www.chembridge.com) are direct suppliers.

SAR by catalog approach only retrieves similar compounds or superstructures of the fragment hit. Thus, other filters should be applied to filter compounds with more optimized properties. These filters are molecular docking, ADMET, machine learning models, aqueous solubility, among others, and will be discussed later in this review.

Molecular Docking

Molecular docking is a computational approach used to predict the position, orientation, and the binding scores of small molecules to proteins (Torres et al., 2019). Hence, as the F2L process is commonly addressed as a combinatorial problem, molecular docking is a method that can be used in combination with other approaches to enhance the F2L process, and to increase the chances to convert a fragment hit into higher affinity ligands. The SAR by catalog approach in combination with molecular docking, for example, can be used to select compounds that maintain the fragment hit binding mode while the binding energy is optimized. Moreover, the number of generated optimized fragments can exceed the number that can be tested experimentally. Thus, applying molecular docking, large compound datasets are efficiently assessed using SAR by catalog, and a small subset of most promising compounds can be selected by binding modes and scores for experimental testing (Grove et al., 2016).

To overcome the problem that SAR by catalog has the limitation to cover only the finite chemical space of commercially available compounds (Hoffer et al., 2018), it is possible to

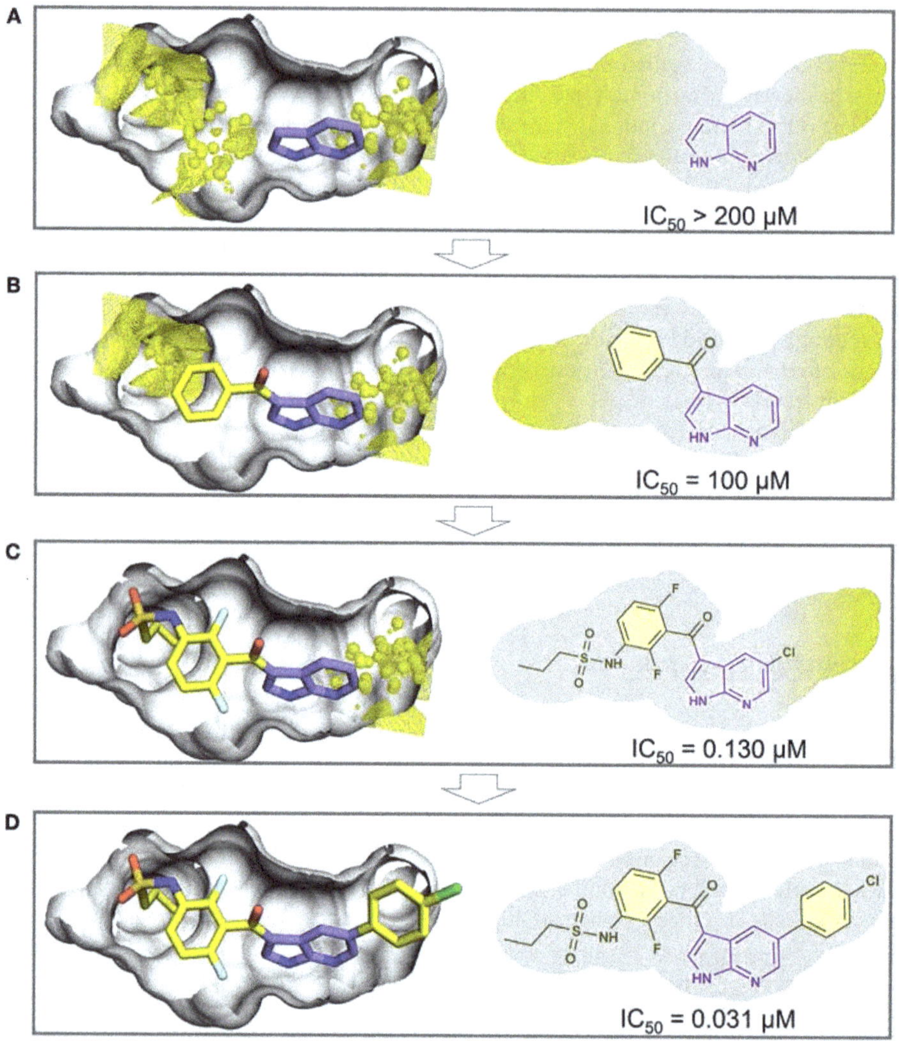

FIGURE 5 | Example of a hot spot analysis using FTMap web server of the oncogenic B-RAF kinase, the target of the first marketed drug from fragment-based drug design, vemurafenib. The surface of the binding site is depicted in gray. **(A)** (PDB ID: 2UVX) the fragment hit (carbon atoms in purple sticks) and the predicted hot spots (yellow dots and surface). **(B–D)** The iterative growing process of vemurafenib (PDB ID: 3OG7) overlapping the predicted hot spots (the carbon atoms of the fragment hit portion is shown in purple sticks and carbon atoms of the grown portions in yellow sticks).

generate virtual catalogs with analogs to hit fragments that can be easily synthesized, astronomically increasing the number of possible compounds. Then, a docking-based virtual screening can be applied to prioritize compounds for experimental evaluation (Rodríguez et al., 2016; Männel et al., 2017).

Another scenario in F2L is when the co-crystallization of a fragment hit commonly fails and no structural information about the binding mode is available. In these cases, alternative strategies for F2L process are required where the binding mode of a fragment can be predicted using molecular docking calculations (Kumar et al., 2012; Chevillard et al., 2018; Erlanson et al., 2019) on high-quality three-dimensional structures of the target in apo form or bound to other ligands. When neither of the latter are available, a theoretical model of the target protein can be obtained by homology modeling methods.

However, there are concerns about fragment docking in the scientific community. The assumption is that fragments, as low molecular weight compounds, are weak binders and promiscuous in binding modes, and consequently, the fragment docking implies in incorrect predictions of the binding modes. Also, there is a concern that scoring functions of the docking programs are parameterized to drug-like ligands, being inaccurate to differentiate native and other low-energy poses (Chen and Shoichet, 2009; Wang et al., 2015; Grove et al., 2016). To overcome these concerns, there are studies demonstrating no significant difference in docking performance between fragments and drug-like ligands (Verdonk et al., 2011; Joseph-mccarthy et al., 2013). They showed that molecular weight is not the principal parameter for docking performance, instead, for high LE compounds the docking performance fared better for both fragments and drug-like ligands (Verdonk et al., 2011; Kumar et al., 2012).

When available, the use of experimental structural information data can be used to support and improve docking performance. These data are used in docking programs including distance constraints, pharmacophore constraints, shape-based constraints, similarity or substructure overlap, interaction fingerprints, hydrogen-bond constraints, and others (Verdonk et al., 2011; Erlanson et al., 2019; Jacquemard et al., 2019).

Similarly to hot spot analysis, molecular docking can also be used to discover secondary binding pockets and guide the F2L process (Männel et al., 2017).

Machine Learning (ML) and Deep Learning (DL) Models

A large variety of F2L approaches use structure-based methods to optimize fragments into high-affinity ligands taking into consideration the steric and electronic constraints within binding pockets of the target of interest (Schneider and Fechner, 2005). However, the optimized compounds generated constantly present drawbacks of poor synthetic feasibility and/or undesirable biological properties, including absorption, distribution, metabolism, excretion, and toxicity (ADMET) properties (Yang et al., 2019b). In the last years, novel ligand-based methods, including machine learning (ML) models, have been used for F2L campaigns. ML models are statistical methods that present the capacity to learn from data without the explicit programming for this task, and then, make a prediction for new compounds (Mak and Pichika, 2019). The increase of storage capacity and the size of the datasets available, coupled to advances in computer hardware such as graphical processing units (GPUs) (Gawehn et al., 2018), provided means to move theoretical studies in ML to practical applications in drug discovery (Vamathevan et al., 2019).

The ML algorithms are widely used to construct quantitative structure-activity relationship (QSAR) models, able to find mathematical correlations between molecular features and compound activity/property, and this correlation can be categorical (active, inactive, toxic, nontoxic, etc.) or continuous (pIC_{50}, pEC_{50}, Ki, and others) by means of classification or regression techniques (Tropsha, 2010; Cherkasov et al., 2014). Thus, machine learning-based QSAR models can be constructed for biological activity, ADMET properties, solubility and synthetic feasibility, among other endpoints, and applied after fragment optimization, with aforementioned methods, in a cascade virtual screening for filtering compounds with the desired activities and properties (**Figure 6**) (Braga et al., 2014; Neves et al., 2018; Pérez-Sianes et al., 2018).

More recently, a subfield of ML called deep learning (DL) which utilizes artificial neural networks to learn from a large amount of data have been used to resolve complex problems (Mak and Pichika, 2019). DL models are not only able to learn from a dataset and to make predictions for new data but are also able to generate new data instances through a constructive process (Schneider, 2018). In this context, there has been a rising interest in using DL generative and predictive models for F2L optimization (Olivecrona et al., 2017; Gupta et al., 2018).

For this task, a combination of DL architectures is used and in many cases, generative DL models based on recurrent neural networks (RNNs) are trained on the simplified molecular input line entry system (SMILES) representation of compounds from large databases (DrugBank, ChEMBL, etc.) to learn the syntax of SMILES language and the chemical space distribution (Olivecrona et al., 2017). After training, the models are able to generate new strings that are new SMILES, corresponding to new compounds (Segler et al., 2018). Then, the transfer learning (TL) can be used to fine-tuning the model and generate compounds related to a fragment hit. As the name suggests, TL learns and transfers the information from an old source to a new application (Yang et al., 2019b). The aim of this integrative approach is to learn general features from a big dataset and, then, retrain the model focusing on a smaller dataset such as fragment hits, for F2L purposes (**Figure 7**) (Gupta et al., 2018; Segler et al., 2018). Gómez–Bombarelli et al. used variational autoencoder (VAE) to encode SMILES into a continuous latent-space, then a separate multilayer perceptron trained to predict several properties on the latent space was applied to generate new molecules with the desired properties. After this, a decoder was used to retrieve the molecules on the latent space into SMILES (Gómez-Bombarelli et al., 2018). Handling these DL methods in a multidimensional way, fragment hits can be optimized automatically taking into consideration several parameters such as bioactivity, solubility, synthetic feasibility, and ADMET properties, generating new compounds with optimized values for these parameters (**Figure 7**) (Olivecrona et al., 2017; Ramsundar et al., 2017; Gómez-Bombarelli et al., 2018; Harel and Radinsky, 2018; Li et al., 2018; Merk et al., 2018; Polykovskiy et al., 2018; Popova et al., 2018; Putin et al., 2018; Awale et al., 2019; Vamathevan et al., 2019).

De novo Design

The *de novo* approach looks for new chemical entities from scratch within a structurally defined binding site (Schneider and Clark, 2019). These entities are generated out of building blocks, either by growing from an initial fragment or by linking two or more non-overlapping fragments (Dey and Caflisch, 2008; Kumar et al., 2012). Since their arise, *in silico* methods have played an important role in FBDD (Kumar et al., 2012).

Software for Building New Compounds Within a Structurally-Defined Binding Site

De novo design software takes advantage of a known binding mode of a fragment, described experimentally or computationally, to propose modified analogs with improved binding affinities. The LUDI (Bohm, 1992) program was one of the first programs developed for *de novo* design. It calculates the interaction sites, maps the molecular fragments, and connects them using bridges, using an empirical scoring. Considering the vast chemical space, evolutionary algorithms are widely used (Srinivas Reddy et al., 2013). In this context, the program GANDI (Dey and Caflisch, 2008) connects pre-docked fragments with linker fragments using a genetic algorithm and a tabu search.

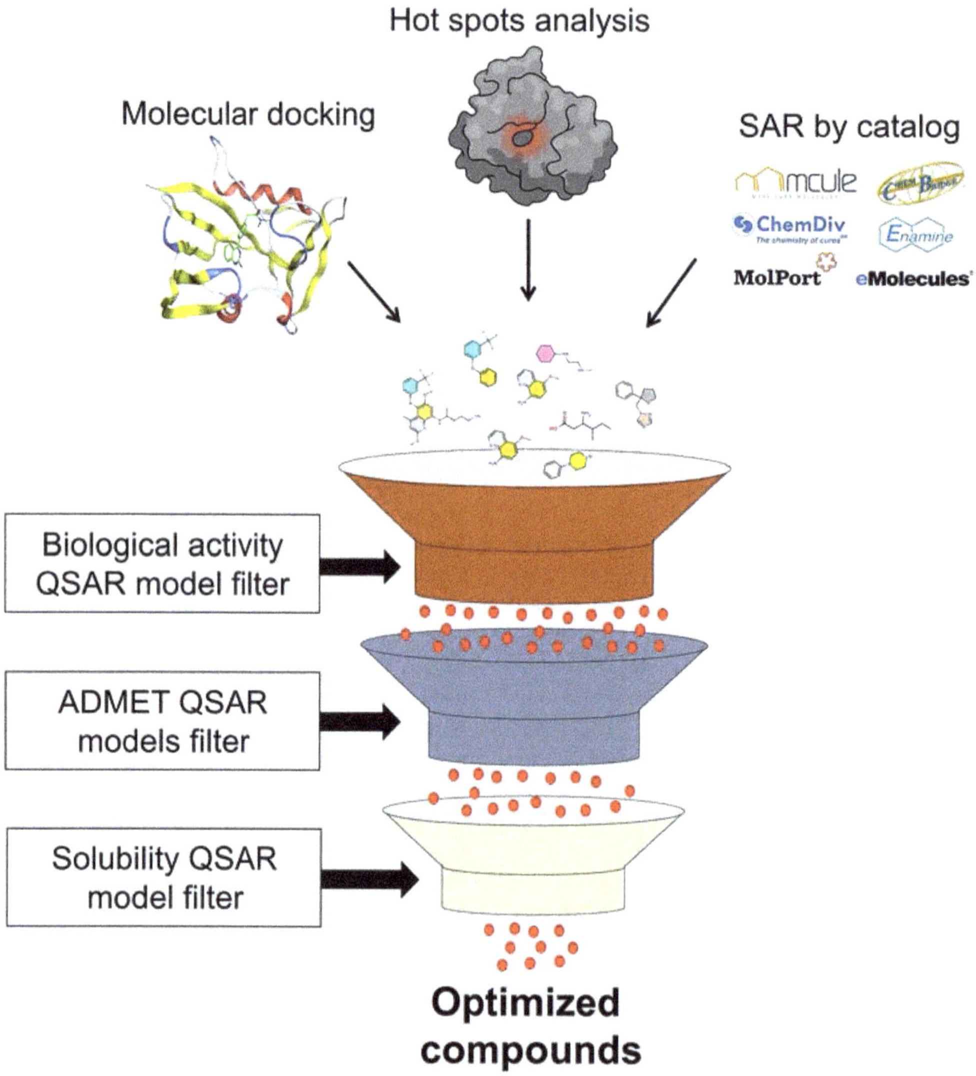

FIGURE 6 | Cascade virtual screening filtering optimized compounds with the desired activities and properties.

The scoring function is a linear combination of force-field binding energy and similarity measures. BREED (Pierce et al., 2004) is a computational method for merging fragments that is widely used. It aligns the 3D coordinates of two ligands and recombines the fragments or substructures into the overlapping bonds to generate new hybrid molecules in a strategy called fragment shuffling. LigBuilder (Wang et al., 2000; Yuan et al., 2011) is a program that uses a genetic algorithm to build up the ligands using a library of organic fragments. It contemplates the growing and linking approach. The 2.0 version includes the synthesis accessibility analysis through a chemical reaction database and retro-synthetic analysis. Autogrow (Durrant et al., 2009, 2013) is another growing approach algorithm that builds a fragment upon a "core" scaffold. The fragment is docked to the receptor. A genetic algorithm evaluates the docking score to select the best population which forms the subsequent generation. The last version considers the synthetic accessibility and the druggability. The program ADAPT (Pegg et al., 2001; Srinivas Reddy et al., 2013) applies a genetic algorithm which uses molecular interactions and docking calculations as a fitness function to reduce the search space. The initial sets of compounds are iteratively built until it reaches the predefined target value.

Prediction of ADMET Properties of New Compounds

The ADMET properties and synthetic accessibility (SA) constitutes the secondary constraints whereas primary constraints are geometric and chemical constraints derived from the receptor or target ligand(s) and internal constraints to the geometry and chemistry of the lead compound being constructed. Issues with these points result in the majority of clinical trial failures (Dong et al., 2018). Numerous software and web platforms were developed to predicted ADMET parameters but presented limitations due to narrow chemical

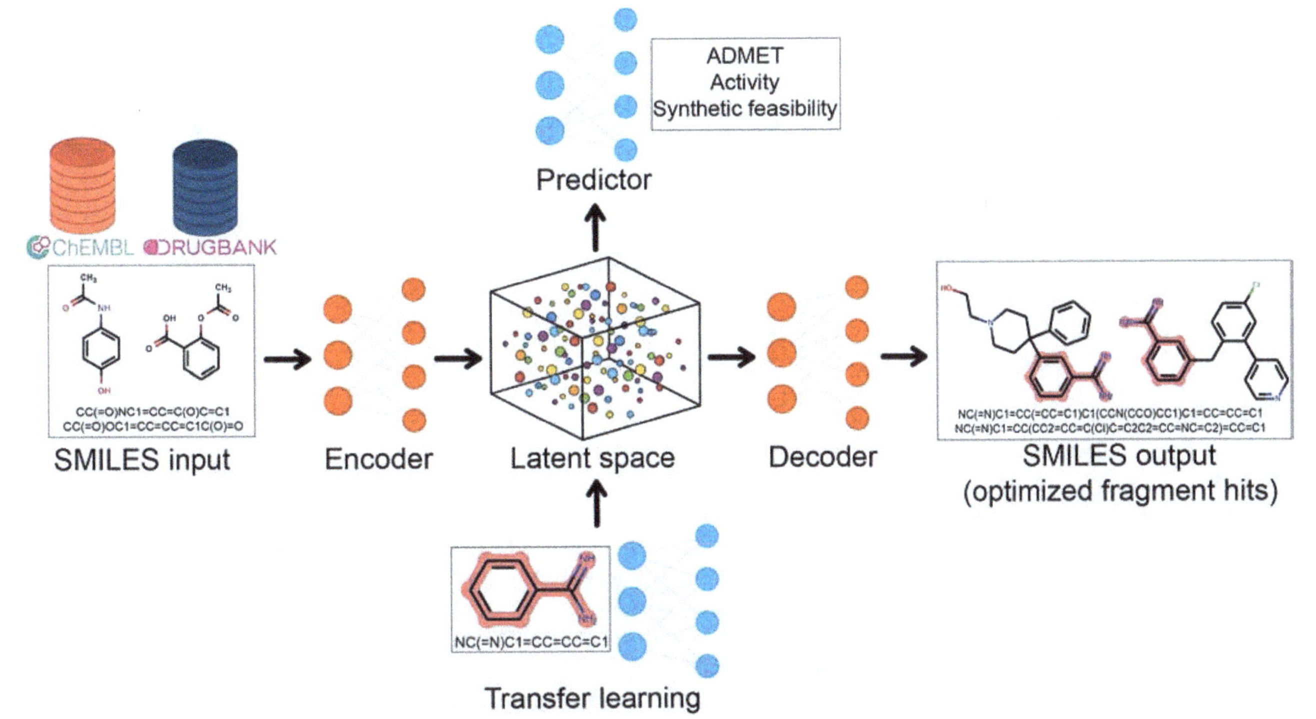

FIGURE 7 | Representation of the integrative approach of generative and predictive deep learning models and transfer learning for fragment-to-lead optimization.

space coverage or expensive prices (Cheng et al., 2012). Recent works predominantly rely on ML methods, like random forest (RF), support vector machine (SVM), and tree-based methods (Ferreira and Andricopulo, 2019). The vNN Web Server for ADMET predictions (Schyman et al., 2017) is a publicly available online platform to predict ADMET properties and to build new models based on the k-nearest neighbor (k-NN), which rest on the premise that compounds with similar structures have similar activities. vNN uses all nearest neighbors that are structurally similar to define the model's applicability domain. The similarity distance employed is Tanimoto's coefficient. The platform allows running pre-build ADMET models, and to build and run customized models. Those models assess cytotoxicity, mutagenicity, cardiotoxicity, drug-drug interactions, microsomal stability, and likelihood of causing drug-induced liver injury. Like all machine learning methods, the lack of training data is a limitation.

Pred-hERG (Braga et al., 2015; Alves et al., 2018) is a web app that allows users to predict blockers and non-blockers of the hERG channels, and important drug anti-target associated with lethal cardiac arrhythmia (Mitcheson et al., 2000). The current version of the app (v. 4.2) was developed using ChEMBL (Willighagen et al., 2013) version 23, containing 8,134 compounds with hERG blockage data after curation, using robust and predictive machine learning models based on RF. This app is publicly available at http://labmol.com.br/predherg/.

In admetSAR 2.0 (Cheng et al., 2012; Yang et al., 2019a) tool, the predictive models are built using RF, SVM and kNN algorithms. It presents 27 endpoints and also includes eco-toxicity models and an optimization module called ADMETopt that optimize the query molecule by scaffold hopping based on ADMET properties. The ADMETlab platform (Dong et al., 2018) performs its evaluations based on a database of collected entries and assess drug-likeness evaluation, ADMET prediction, systematic evaluation and database/similarity searching. It uses 31 endpoints applying RF, SVM, recursive partitioning regression (RP), naive Bayes (NB), and decision tree (DT).

SwissADME tool (Daina et al., 2017) uses predictive models for physicochemical properties, lipophilicity and water solubility. It also analyses pharmacokinetics models as BBB permeability, gastrointestinal absorption, P-gp binding, skin permeation (logKp), and CYP450 inhibition. Additionally, the tool presents five drug-likeness models (Lipinsky, Ghose, Veber, Egan, and Muegge) and medicinal chemistry alerts. It is integrated with the SwissDrugDesign workspace. The QikProp (Schrödinger, LLC, NY, 2019) provides rapid predictions of ADME properties for molecules with novel scaffolds as for analogs of well-known drugs and display information about octanol/water and water/gas logPs, logS, logBBB, overall CNS activity, Caco-2 and MDCK cell permeabilities, log Kd for human serum albumin binding, and log IC_{50} for HERG K+-channel blockage.

Prediction of Synthetic Tractability (Synthesizability) of New Compounds

Even though large numbers of molecules are generated by *de novo* design, many of them are synthetically infeasible

(Dey and Caflisch, 2008). To address this problem, methods to calculate the synthetic accessibility (SA) are being developed. SA can be addressed by estimating the complexity of the molecule or making a retrosynthetic approach, where the complete synthetic tree leading to the molecules needs to be processed (Ertl and Schuffenhauer, 2009). SYLVIA (Boda et al., 2007) is one of the programs that estimate the synthetic accessibility of an organic compound. It obtains the SA score by the addition of five variables as the molecular graph complexity, ring complexity, stereochemical complexity, starting material similarity and reaction center substructure, where the first three are structure-based and the other two utilize information from starting material catalogs and reaction databases. Ertl and Schuffenhauer (2009) developed another method that uses historical synthetic knowledge obtained by analyzing information from millions of already synthesized chemicals and also considers molecule complexity. The method is based on a combination of fragment contributions and a complexity penalty. Podolyan et al. (2010) presented two approaches to quickly predict the synthetic accessibility of chemical compounds by utilizing SVMs operating on molecular descriptors. The first approach (RSsvm) identifies compounds that can be synthesized using a specific set of reactions and starting materials and builds the model by training the compounds identified as synthetically or otherwise accessible by retrosynthetic analysis while the second approach (DRSVM) is constructed to generate a more general assessment. More recently, Fukunishi et al. (2014) designed a new method of predicting SA based on commercially available compound databases and molecular descriptors where the SA is estimated from the probability of the existence of substructures of the compound, the number of symmetry atoms, the graph complexity, and the number of the chiral center of the compound.

Synthesizability-Aware Methods

Given the difficulty of synthesis of most of the leads produced by *de novo* approaches, some programs added methods to score the SA. Lead+Op (Lin et al., 2018) is an example of these programs that takes an initial fragment, looks for associated reaction rules, virtually generate the reaction products and select the best binding conformation. Them it generates conformers and select one that becomes a reactant for another round. Also, programs mentioned above as LigBuilder and Autogrow include SA analysis on their current versions. In the medicinal chemistry component of **SwissADME,** a SA score is also included.

Different programs use distinct algorithms for *de novo* design compounds in CADD. **Table 1** summarizes some programs cited in this section.

TABLE 1 | FBDD programs with respective approaches.

Program	Algorithm	FBDD Approach	SA
AUTOGROW	Docking + Genetic Algorithm	Growing	YES (Latest version)
LUDI	Empirical scoring	Linking	NO
AUTO T and T	Transplants fragments into the lead	Merging	NO
LeadOp+R	Looks for associated reaction rules	Growing	YES
GANDI	Genetic Algorithm	Linking	NO
LigBuilder 2	Genetic Algorithm	Linking and Growing	YES
ADAPT	Genetic Algorithm	Growing	NO

CASE STUDIES IN THE LAST FIVE YEARS

Case 1: FBDD in the Development of New Anti-mycobacterium Drugs

A successful application of the FBDD techniques have been applied to early stage drug discovery of new therapeutics against *Mycobacterium sp.* and in particular *M. tuberculosis* (*Mtb*) and *M. abscessus (Mab)* (Thomas et al., 2017). *Mtb*, the causative agent of tuberculosis, has several therapeutic interventions developed to treat the disease. However, through their long-term use and misuse, the efficacy of these drugs is becoming reduced with strains currently circulating that are mono-resistant, multidrug-resistant, extensively drug-resistant and totally drug-resistant. Despite this little drug development activity has been undertaken since the 1960's. However, relatively in response to the growing drug-resistant threat many different approaches are being deployed to developing novel therapeutics, including FBDD. An example of such an effort is against the meta cleavage product hydrolase (HsaD) that is involved in cholesterol catabolism in *Mtb*. Initial screening was conducted on a library of 1,258 fragments using differential scanning fluorimetry, with hits confirmed by ligand-observed NMR spectroscopy and inhibition by enzymatic assay. The three confirmed fragment initial hits were structurally characterized by X-ray crystallography and fragment soaking. A small series of compounds based on these hits were further tested for activity both *in vitro* and *ex vivo* with promising results (Ryan et al., 2017).

Another target of *Mtb* where FBDD has been applied is the pantothenate synthetase (Pts) where a similar sized fragment library of 1,250 rule-of-three compliant fragments was investigated. An initial screen was performed using a thermal shift assay, followed by a secondary screen using 1-D NMR spectroscopy with ultimate hit validation by isothermal titration calorimetry and characterization by X-ray crystallography. Three distinct fragment binding sites were identified (Silvestre et al., 2013). Follow-up expansion of one of the fragment sites using a combination of fragment linking and fragment growing generated a new series of inhibitors. Though fragment linking seemed to be an attractive approach, the limitation in the repertoire of linkers compromised the binding mode. Greater success came from fragment growth using expert knowledge and the protein target as a template (Hung et al., 2009).

Targets in other pathogenic *Mycobacterium* sp. have also been subject to successful FBDD campaigns. Most notably the recent development of inhibitors against tRNA methyltransferase (TrmD) of *M. abscessus* (Mab). This multi-drug resistant pathogen is increasingly problematic in individuals with cystic fibrosis and other chronic lung conditions. A library of 960 fragments was screened biophysically using differential scanning fluorimetry in a similar fashion used for HsaD, with 53 hits taken to validation and structural characterization using X-ray crystallography (no NMR based validation was undertaken). Only 27 fragments could be validated all of which bound within the substrate binding pocket. A strategy of fragment-merging centered around the overlap of a 4-methoxyphenyl ring system with the indole ring system of two fragments that spanned the adenine and ribose binding pockets. This was explored successfully with a new combined compound providing a new aminopyrazole-indole scaffold with both improved affinity (K_d = 110 μM, LE of 0.36) and prospects for further elaboration relative to the parent fragments. It also exhibited inhibition activity *in vitro* and *ex vivo* with promising *in vivo* activity also against *M. leprae*, the causative agent of leprosy (Whitehouse et al., 2019).

These successful FBDD campaigns against a range of targets in pathogenic *Mycobacterium* have yielded promising leads with indications of efficacy in *ex vivo* and *in vivo* demonstrating both the power and efficacy of the approach. The ability of these leads to work across a range of pathogens is also highly encouraging. However, work still needs to be done to improve these leads to progress them into early clinical evaluations and into clinical use.

Case 2: Inhibitors of Dengue Virus Enzymes

A 2014 paper (Coutard et al., 2014) describes the use of FBLD in the discovery of inhibitors for an important subunit of dengue virus (DENV) viral replication complex. In this work, 500 fragments were screened against two subunits of the viral replication complex: NS3 helicase (Hel) and the NS5 mRNA methyltransferase (MTase) subunits. DENV Hel, located in the *C*-terminal region of the NS3 subunit of the replication complex, is involved in viral genome replication and RNA capping. The role of DENV NS5 MTase is related with a double methylation (N-7 and 2'-O) during the cap formation process in flavivirus (Dong et al., 2008).

The authors used a combination of Thermal Shift Assay (TSA), X-ray diffraction crystallography (XRD) and enzymatic assays in order to screen compounds against NS3 DENV Hel and NS5 DENV MTase subunits. The TSA was used as the primary screening technique. During the TSA screening, not surprisingly part of the fragments—used at high concentrations and with poorly optimized physicochemical properties—presented solubility problems. This was the reason for the exclusion of ~4.8% of the screened compounds during this phase. This initial screening yielded 68 hits, from those, 7 were found bound to the DENV MTase subunit by XRD.

Using a direct colorimetric ATPase-based assay to identify inhibitors, from those previous 7 crystallographic hits, 5 fragments (**Table 2**) were classified as hits with their potency varying between 180 μM and 9 mM.

In the most recent work, the fragments **3** and **4** (**Figure 8**) were found bound at the DENV MTase S-Adenosyl-L-methionine (AdoMet) binding site using XRD. A computer-aided fragment optimization gave rise to a new series of compounds using these

TABLE 2 | Inhibition and potency data from the final hits (Coutard et al., 2014).

	DENV 2'O-Mtase activity inhibition (%)	DENV 2'O-MTase activity IC_{50} (mM)
81	4	3.90 ± 0.16
91	11	2.83 ± 0.18
95	85	0.18 ± 0.01
157	9	9.39 ± 0.90
217	11	3.12 ± 0.27

two fragments. The urea was used as a linker to connect the fragments. Further modifications yielded compounds **5** and **6** (**Figure 8**).

During the optimization process, the authors had good insights about the important features to the molecule binding on this target. One of these features is the presence of phenyl rings substituted in meta position and is crucial for favoring binding.

This work yielded two inhibitors (**5** and **6**) with potency around 100 μM, even though no effect was observed on a cell assay. Despite this negative result, this work showed the feasibility of the FBDD approach in getting micromolar inhibitors from structurally simple fragments.

Case 3: MTH1 Inhibitors for Anticancer Drug Discovery

The mutT homolog 1 (MTH1) is an enzyme involved in the prevention of incorporation of deoxynucleoside triphosphates (dNTPs) oxidized by reactive oxygen species (ROS), e.g., 8-oxodGTP or 2-OH-dATP, into DNA, which prevents the killing of the cell. MTH1 is frequently overexpressed in cancer cells and is non-essential in normal cells, proving to be a druggable target for cancer treatment (Smits and Gillespie, 2014; Berglund et al., 2016).

Rudling et al. applied a combination of molecular docking, SAR by catalog, and experimental testing for discovering and optimizing MTH1 inhibitors (Rudling et al., 2017). Initially, a molecular docking-based virtual screening using a crystal structure of MTH1 was performed using 0.3 million fragments from the ZINC fragment-like database, all commercially available. Subsequently, for the 5,000 top-ranked fragments, allowed the search of analogs representing superstructures of the fragment or containing similar substructures in the ZINC database using the chemical structures encoded as circular fingerprints and the Tversky similarity index (Tversky, 1977). The criteria used to select analogs from 4.4 million commercially available compounds in the ZINC database was the following: (i) Tversky similarity >0.8; (ii) up to six additional heavy atoms (HAs) compared to the parent fragment; (iii) improved docking score 80% lower compared to the parent fragment; (iv) visual inspection of the binding modes. After these analyses, a set of 22 commercially available fragments with at least five analogs comprising the above-mentioned criteria were selected for experimental evaluation. Five of these 22 fragments showing IC_{50} values ranging from 5.6 to 79 μM were considered hits and were used for F2L (**Table 3**). The fragment **7** presented an

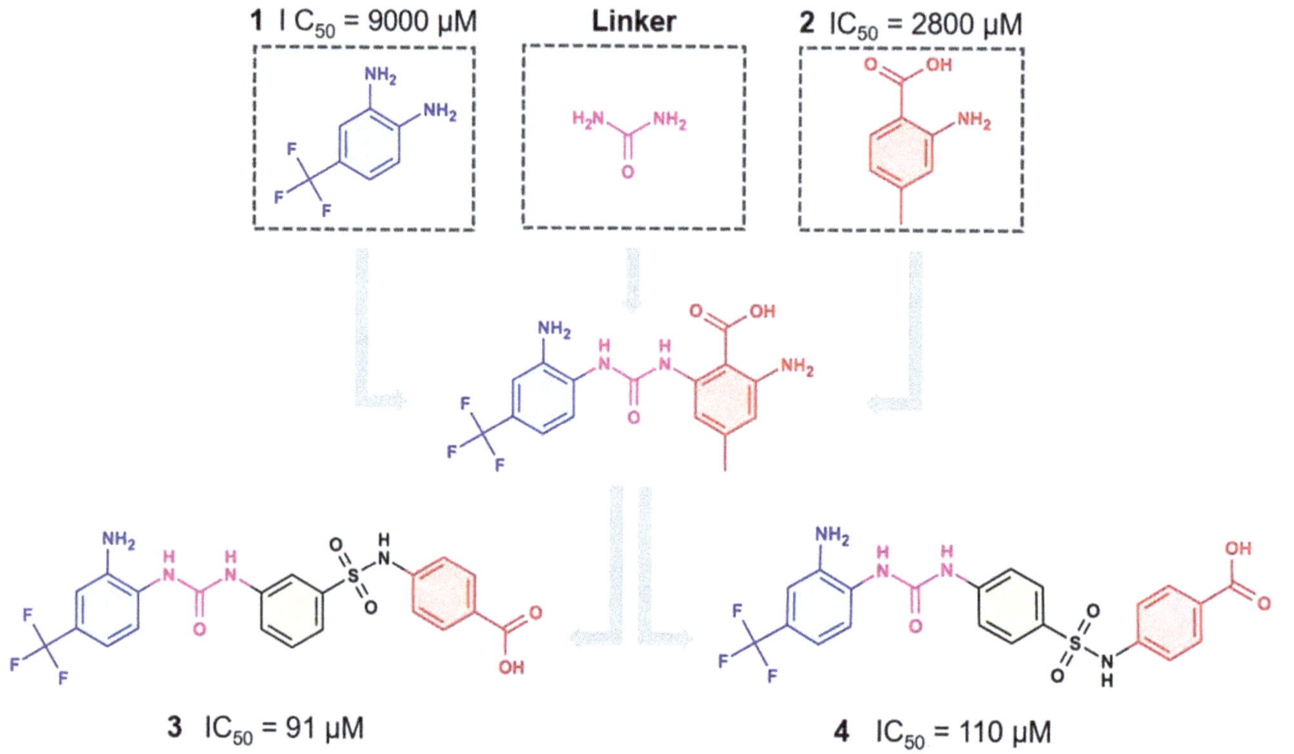

FIGURE 8 | Fragment optimization predecessors and products (Coutard et al., 2014; Benmansour et al., 2017).

IC_{50} value of 79 μM and its most potent analog presented an IC_{50} of 170 nM, representing a 470-fold improvement (**Table 3**). Although the crystal structure of the fragment **7** in complex with MTH1 was not obtained, the crystallization of its most potent analog and MTH1 was solved at 1.85 Å resolution, demonstrating an RMSD of 0.6 Å between the common atoms of the fragment **7** (binding mode predicted by molecular docking) and the analog (crystal structure). Because of the closely related structures and binding modes of fragments **8** and **9**, its analogs were analyzed together, but the most potent analog presented an IC_{50} of only 3.5 μM. The most potent analog of fragment **10** presented a 190-fold increase of the activity, with an IC_{50} of 120 nM (**Table 3**). The crystallization of fragment **10** with MTH1 was also unsuccessful, but the molecular docking was able to predict the binding mode, showing an RMSD of 0.9 comparing the overlapping atoms with the crystal of the most potent analog obtained at 1.50 Å resolution. The analogs of the fragment **11** were not available during the study. This work demonstrated that virtual screening and SAR by catalog can be used to rapidly identify and optimize fragments into nanomolar inhibitors (Rudling et al., 2017).

Case 4: New Acetylcholinesterase Inhibitors Against Alzheimer's Disease

Alzheimer's disease is a neurodegenerative disorder and has no cure. The actual treatments are based on drugs that leverage the transmission of electrical impulses. Pascoini et al. (2019), computationally developed new acetylcholinesterase (AChE) inhibitors. AChE is responsible for decreasing levels of acetylcholine in the synaptic cleft. Their inhibition enhances the transmission of the electric impulse (Polinsky, 1998; Talesa, 2001).

For the *in silico* inhibitor development, they divided the process into four steps. First, a *de novo* design was applied to generate an initial library of compounds. The first library was then filtered according to ADME properties at the second step. In the third step, the filtered library was filtered again using a similarity criterion. Finally, the resulting library was used in docking studies. The best three complexes were used for molecular dynamic studies. In this work, they used three reference drugs for AD treatment: donepezil, galantamine, and rivastigmine.

For the *de novo* design, the LigBuilder software was used. The CAVITY procedure was employed to detect and analyze ligand-binding sites of the target. It classified the cavities' druggability, who would be used for docking studies. The BUILD procedure was used in the exploring and growing/linking modes. In the explore mode, fragments from the program's database were added in the protein site and their interaction was scored. Then, the fragments with the best scores were linked. In the growing mode, seeds molecules were put at the binding site and fragments were added to the seeds. At the linking mode, the seed was divided into fragments and other fragments were added to them. After the BUILD procedure, they got a library of 2.5 million compounds. The resulting library was filtered according to ADME properties with the software QUIKPROP where molecules that infringed more than five properties (physicochemical properties, lipophilicity, water solubility, pharmacokinetics models) were discarded. A library

TABLE 3 | Experimental data for the five most potent MTH1 inhibitors (data taken from Rudling et al., 2017).

Fragment ID	Fragment 2D structure	Fragment IC_{50}	Most potent analog 2D structure	Analog IC_{50}
7	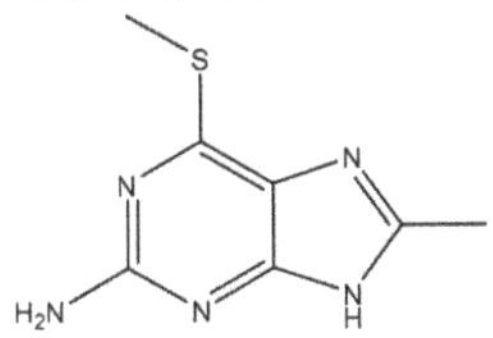	79 μM	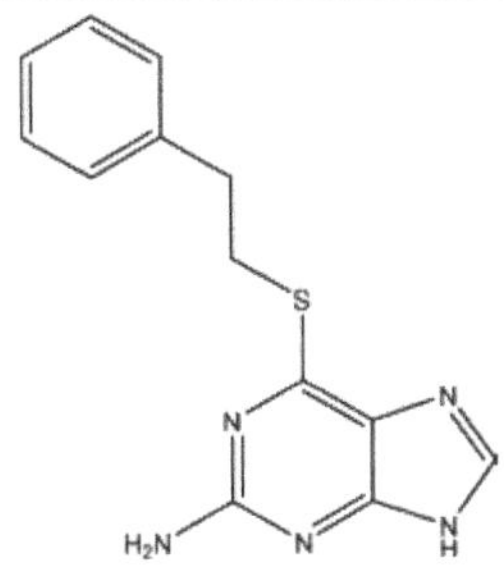	0.17 μM
8	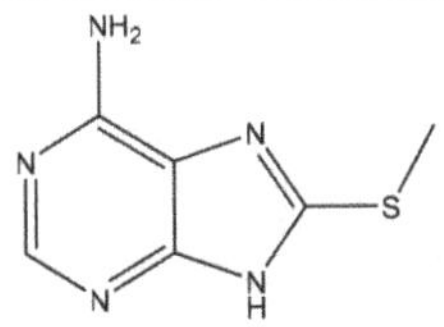	24 μM	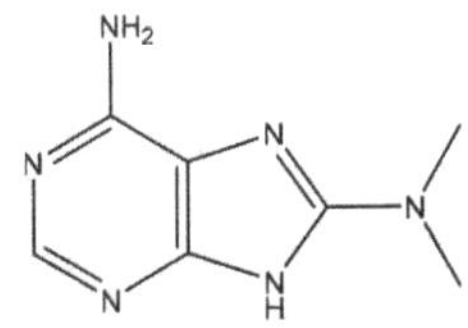	3.5 μM
9	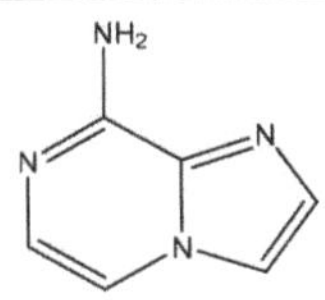	26 μM	n/a	n/a
10	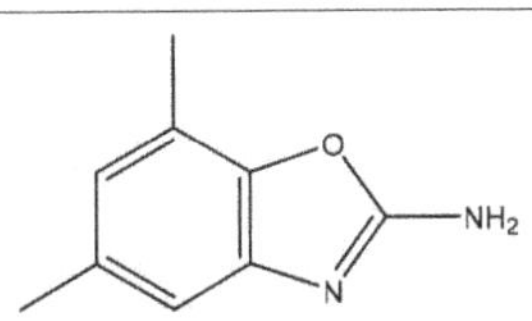	23 μM	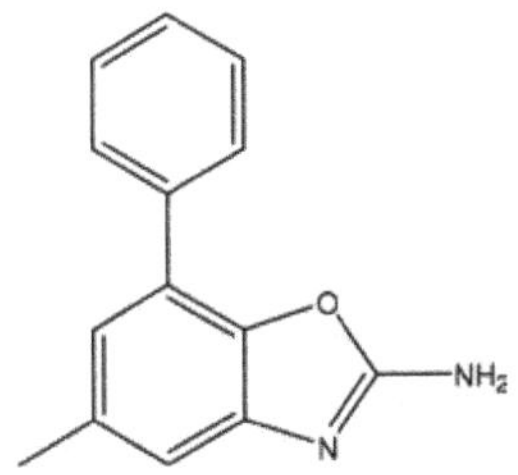	0.12 μM
11	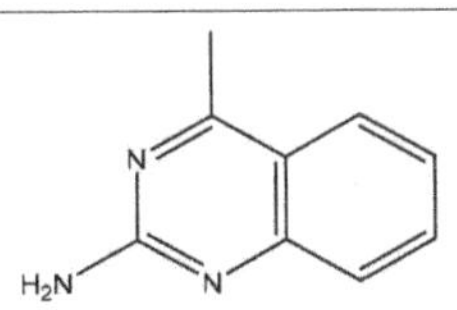	5.6 μM	n/a	n/a

n/a, not available.

of 6,000 compounds results from this process. After this, the Tanimoto's coefficient was applied to measure the similarity among the molecules. Molecules below 0.85 were excluded and 1,500 molecules were considered for the next step. The final step consisted of docking studies, carried out with the GLIDE software and the Induced Fit Docking protocol. Afterward, they selected the three best complexes from the docking and used them as input structures for molecular dynamic studies. Finally, they obtained three compounds with high stability and good binding energies, some of them even better than the reference drugs.

CONCLUDING REMARKS

FBDD has matured to become a key strategy in modern pharmaceutical research. With less requirement for large chemical libraries and the possibility of using a range of biophysical methods for screening, the easier and scalable implementation of this strategy has facilitated its popularization, especially among academic institutions and smaller pharmaceutical companies.

The main reason for the success of the FBDD strategy is because it presents a more efficient and consistent route for optimization of initial screening hits into lead compounds. As reviewed here, many routes are available for expansion of fragment hits and *in silico* methods are key to support or guide the majority of them.

A variety of *in silico* methods have been used in F2L optimization in FBDD, from binding site analysis to *de novo* design of new fragment-derived ligands with synthesizability-aware methods. The case studies highlighted here clearly demonstrate how the different *in silico* methods can be used in integrated form and combined with experimental approaches to successfully develop higher affinity ligands from fragments.

Advances in artificial intelligence methods, such as deep learning, hold a great potential to accelerate the optimization of fragment hits in lead compounds. Recent examples show that these hits can be already optimized automatically taking into consideration several parameters such as bioactivity, solubility, synthetic feasibility, and ADMET properties.

AUTHOR CONTRIBUTIONS

FS, CA, and NF drafted the review topics with the abstract and revised the manuscript. FS drafted the conclusion and contributed to several parts of the manuscript. NF drafted the introduction and one of the case studies. LS drafted the fragment optimization section and one of the case studies. JM-F drafted most of the *in silico* strategies section and one of the case studies. BN designed all figures and revised the manuscript. AG and RM drafted the *de novo* design section and one of the case studies.

ACKNOWLEDGMENTS

The authors would like to thank Brazilian funding agencies CNPq, CAPES, FAPERJ, FAPEG, and FIOCRUZ for financial support and fellowships. This study was also supported by funding from the United Kingdom's Academy of Medical Sciences Newton Fund (NAF\R2\180641).

REFERENCES

Abad-Zapatero, C. (2013). *Ligand Efficiency Indices for Drug Discovery*. Oxford, UK: Elsevier.

Abad-Zapatero, C. (2017). Are SAR tables obsolete? *Drug Discov. Today* 22, 195–198. doi: 10.1016/j.drudis.2016.12.002

Abi Hussein, H., Geneix, C., Petitjean, M., Borrel, A., Flatters, D., and Camproux, A.-C. (2017). Global vision of druggability issues: applications and perspectives. *Drug Discov. Today* 22, 404–415. doi: 10.1016/j.drudis.2016.11.021

Alvarsson, J., Eklund, M., Engkvist, O., Spjuth, O., Carlsson, L., Wikberg, J. E. S., et al. (2014). Ligand-based target prediction with signature fingerprints. *J. Chem. Inf. Model.* 54, 2647–2653. doi: 10.1021/ci500361u

Alves, V., Braga, R., Muratov, E., and Andrade, C. (2018). Development of web and mobile applications for chemical toxicity prediction. *J. Braz. Chem. Soc.* 29, 982–988. doi: 10.21577/0103-5053.20180013

Andrade, C. H., Neves, B. J., Melo-Filho, C. C., Rodrigues, J., Silva, D. C., Braga, R. C., et al. (2018). *In silico* chemogenomics drug repositioning strategies for neglected tropical diseases. *Curr. Med. Chem.* 25, 1–22. doi: 10.2174/0929867325666180309114824

Awale, M., Sirockin, F., Stiefl, N., and Reymond, J.-L. (2019). Drug analogs from fragment-based long short-term memory generative neural networks. *J. Chem. Inf. Model.* 59, 1347–1356. doi: 10.1021/acs.jcim.8b00902

Barril, X. (2013). Druggability predictions: methods, limitations, and applications. *Wiley Interdiscip. Rev. Comput. Mol. Sci.* 3, 327–338. doi: 10.1002/wcms.1134

Benmansour, F., Trist, I., Coutard, B., Decroly, E., Querat, G., Brancale, A., et al. (2017). Discovery of novel dengue virus NS5 methyltransferase non-nucleoside inhibitors by fragment-based drug design. *Eur. J. Med. Chem.* 125, 865–880. doi: 10.1016/j.ejmech.2016.10.007

Berglund, U. W., Sanjiv, K., Gad, H., Kalderén, C., Koolmeister, T., Pham, T., et al. (2016). Validation and development of MTH1 inhibitors for treatment of cancer. *Ann. Oncol.* 27, 2275–2283. doi: 10.1093/annonc/mdw429

Boda, K., Seidel, T., and Gasteiger, J. (2007). Structure and reaction based evaluation of synthetic accessibility. *J. Comput. Aided. Mol. Des.* 21, 311–325. doi: 10.1007/s10822-006-9099-2

Boehr, D. D., Nussinov, R., and Wright, P. E. (2009). The role of dynamic conformational ensembles in biomolecular recognition. *Nat. Chem. Biol.* 5, 789–796. doi: 10.1038/nchembio.232

Boettcher, A., Ruedisser, S., Erbel, P., Vinzenz, D., Schiering, N., Hassiepen, U., et al. (2010). Fragment-based screening by biochemical assays. *J. Biomol. Screen.* 15, 1029–1041. doi: 10.1177/1087057110380455

Bohm, H.-J. (1992). The computer program LUDI: a new method for the *de novo* design of enzyme inhibitors. *J. Comput. Aided. Mol. Des.* 6, 61–78. doi: 10.1007/BF00124387

Bollag, G., Hirth, P., Tsai, J., Zhang, J., Ibrahim, P. N., Cho, H., et al. (2010). Clinical efficacy of a RAF inhibitor needs broad target blockade in BRAF-mutant melanoma. *Nature* 467, 596–599. doi: 10.1038/nature09454

Bollag, G., Tsai, J., Zhang, J., Zhang, C., Ibrahim, P., Nolop, K., et al. (2012). Vemurafenib: the first drug approved for BRAF-mutant cancer. *Nat. Rev. Drug Discov.* 11, 873–886. doi: 10.1038/nrd3847

Braga, R., Alves, V., Silva, A., Nascimento, M., Silva, F., Liao, L., et al. (2014). Virtual screening strategies in medicinal chemistry: the state of the art and current challenges. *Curr. Top. Med. Chem.* 14, 1899–1912. doi: 10.2174/1568026614666140929120749

Braga, R. C., Alves, V. M., Silva, M. F. B., Muratov, E., Fourches, D., Lião, L. M., et al. (2015). Pred-hERG: a novel web-accessible computational tool for predicting cardiac toxicity. *Mol. Inform.* 34, 698–701. doi: 10.1002/minf.201500040

Chen, Y., and Shoichet, B. K. (2009). Molecular docking and ligand specificity in fragment-based inhibitor discovery. *Nat. Chem. Biol.* 5, 358–364. doi: 10.1038/nchembio.155

Cheng, F., Li, W., Zhou, Y., Shen, J., Wu, Z., Liu, G., et al. (2012). admetSAR: a comprehensive source and free tool for assessment of chemical ADMET properties. *J. Chem. Inf. Model.* 52, 3099–3105. doi: 10.1021/ci300367a

Cherkasov, A., Muratov, E. N., Fourches, D., Varnek, A., Baskin, I. I., Cronin, M., et al. (2014). QSAR modeling: where have you been? Where are you going to? *J. Med. Chem.* 57, 4977–5010. doi: 10.1021/jm4004285

Chevillard, F., Rimmer, H., Betti, C., Pardon, E., Ballet, S., van Hilten, N., et al. (2018). Binding-site compatible fragment growing applied to the design of β2 -adrenergic receptor ligands. *J. Med. Chem.* 61, 1118–1129. doi: 10.1021/acs.jmedchem.7b01558

Chung, S., Parker, J. B., Bianchet, M., Amzel, L. M., and Stivers, J. T. (2009). Impact of linker strain and flexibility in the design of a fragment-based inhibitor. *Nat. Chem. Biol.* 5, 407–413. doi: 10.1038/nchembio.163

Ciulli, A. (2013a). Biophysical screening for the discovery of small-molecule ligands. *Methods Mol. Biol.* 1008, 357–388. doi: 10.1007/978-1-62703-398-5_13

Ciulli, A. (2013b). "Biophysical screening for the discovery of small-molecule ligands," in *Methods in Molecular Biology*, eds M. A. Williams and T. Daviter (Totowa, NJ: Humana Press), 357–388.

Coutard, B., Decroly, E., Li, C., Sharff, A., Lescar, J., Bricogne, G., et al. (2014). Assessment of Dengue virus helicase and methyltransferase as targets for fragment-based drug discovery. *Antiviral Res.* 106, 61–70. doi: 10.1016/j.antiviral.2014.03.013

Cox, O. B., Krojer, T., Collins, P., Monteiro, O., Talon, R., Bradley, A., et al. (2016). A poised fragment library enables rapid synthetic expansion yielding the first reported inhibitors of PHIP(2), an atypical bromodomain. *Chem. Sci.* 7, 2322–2330. doi: 10.1039/C5SC03115J

Cukuroglu, E., Engin, H. B., Gursoy, A., and Keskin, O. (2014). Hot spots in protein-protein interfaces: towards drug discovery. *Prog. Biophys. Mol. Biol.* 116, 165–173. doi: 10.1016/j.pbiomolbio.2014.06.003

Daina, A., Michielin, O., and Zoete, V. (2017). SwissADME: a free web tool to evaluate pharmacokinetics, drug-likeness and medicinal chemistry friendliness of small molecules. *Sci. Rep.* 7:42717. doi: 10.1038/srep42717

Davis, B. J., and Roughley, S. D. (2017). "Fragment-based lead discovery," in *Annual Reports in Medicinal Chemistry*, ed R. A. Goodnow (London: Elsevier Inc.), 371–439. doi: 10.1016/bs.armc.2017.07.002

De Fusco, C., Brear, P., Iegre, J., Georgiou, K. H., Sore, H. F., Hyvönen, M., et al. (2017). A fragment-based approach leading to the discovery of a novel binding site and the selective CK2 inhibitor CAM4066. *Bioorg. Med. Chem.* 25, 3471–3482. doi: 10.1016/j.bmc.2017.04.037

Dey, F., and Caflisch, A. (2008). Fragment-based *de novo* ligand design by multiobjective evolutionary optimization. *J. Chem. Inf. Model.* 48, 679–690. doi: 10.1021/ci700424b

Donald, A., McHardy, T., Rowlands, M. G., Hunter, L.-J. K., Davies, T. G., Berdini, V., et al. (2007). Rapid evolution of 6-phenylpurine inhibitors of protein kinase B through structure-based design. *J. Med. Chem.* 50, 2289–2292. doi: 10.1021/jm0700924

Dong, H., Zhang, B., and Shi, P.-Y. (2008). Flavivirus methyltransferase: a novel antiviral target. *Antiviral Res.* 80, 1–10. doi: 10.1016/j.antiviral.2008.05.003

Dong, J., Wang, N.-N., Yao, Z.-J., Zhang, L., Cheng, Y., Ouyang, D., et al. (2018). ADMETlab: a platform for systematic ADMET evaluation based on a comprehensively collected ADMET database. *J. Cheminform.* 10:29. doi: 10.1186/s13321-018-0283-x

Durrant, J. D., Amaro, R. E., and McCammon, J. A. (2009). AutoGrow: a novel algorithm for protein inhibitor design. *Chem. Biol. Drug Des.* 73, 168–178. doi: 10.1111/j.1747-0285.2008.00761.x

Durrant, J. D., Lindert, S., and McCammon, J. A. (2013). AutoGrow 3.0: an improved algorithm for chemically tractable, semi-automated protein inhibitor design. *J. Mol. Graph. Model.* 44, 104–112. doi: 10.1016/j.jmgm.2013.05.006

Erlanson, D. A., Davis, B. J., and Jahnke, W. (2019). Fragment-based drug discovery: advancing fragments in the absence of crystal structures. *Cell Chem. Biol.* 26, 9–15. doi: 10.1016/j.chembiol.2018.10.001

Erlanson, D. A., Fesik, S. W., Hubbard, R. E., Jahnke, W., and Jhoti, H. (2016). Twenty years on: the impact of fragments on drug discovery. *Nat. Rev. Drug Discov.* 15, 605–619. doi: 10.1038/nrd.2016.109

Ertl, P., and Schuffenhauer, A. (2009). Estimation of synthetic accessibility score of drug-like molecules based on molecular complexity and fragment contributions. *J. Cheminform.* 1:8. doi: 10.1186/1758-2946-1-8

Ferreira, L. L. G., and Andricopulo, A. D. (2019). ADMET modeling approaches in drug discovery. *Drug Discov. Today* 24, 1157–1165. doi: 10.1016/j.drudis.2019.03.015

Fukunishi, Y., Kurosawa, T., Mikami, Y., and Nakamura, H. (2014). Prediction of synthetic accessibility based on commercially available compound databases. *J. Chem. Inf. Model.* 54, 3259–3267. doi: 10.1021/ci500568d

Gawehn, E., Hiss, J. A., Brown, J. B., and Schneider, G. (2018). Advancing drug discovery via GPU-based deep learning. *Expert Opin. Drug Discov.* 13, 579–582. doi: 10.1080/17460441.2018.1465407

Giordanetto, F., Jin, C., Willmore, L., Feher, M., and Shaw, D. E. (2019). Fragment hits: what do they look like and how do they bind? *J. Med. Chem.* 62, 3381–3394. doi: 10.1021/acs.jmedchem.8b01855

Godemann, R., Madden, J., Krämer, J., Smith, M., Fritz, U., Hesterkamp, T., et al. (2009). Fragment-based discovery of BACE1 inhibitors using functional assays. *Biochemistry* 48, 10743–10751. doi: 10.1021/bi901061a

Gómez-Bombarelli, R., Wei, J. N., Duvenaud, D., Hernández-Lobato, J. M., Sánchez-Lengeling, B., Sheberla, D., et al. (2018). Automatic chemical design using a data-driven continuous representation of molecules. *ACS Cent. Sci.* 4, 268–276. doi: 10.1021/acscentsci.7b00572

Grove, L. E., Vajda, S., and Kozakov, D. (2016). "Computational methods to support fragment-based drug discovery," in *Fragment-Based Drug Discovery: Lessons and Outlook*, eds D. A. Erlanson and W. Jahnke (Weinheim: Wiley-VCH Verlag GmbH and Co. KGaA), 197–222.

Gupta, A., Müller, A. T., Huisman, B. J. H., Fuchs, J. A., Schneider, P., and Schneider, G. (2018). Generative recurrent networks for *de novo* drug design. *Mol. Inform.* 37:1700111. doi: 10.1002/minf.2017 00111

Hall, D. R., Ngan, C. H., Zerbe, B. S., Kozakov, D., and Vajda, S. (2012). Hot spot analysis for driving the development of hits into leads in fragment-based drug discovery. *J. Chem. Inf. Model.* 52, 199–209. doi: 10.1021/ci200468p

Hall, R. J., Mortenson, P. N., and Murray, C. W. (2014). Efficient exploration of chemical space by fragment-based screening. *Prog. Biophys. Mol. Biol.* 116, 82–91. doi: 10.1016/j.pbiomolbio.2014.09.007

Hall, R. J., Murray, C. W., and Verdonk, M. L. (2017). The fragment network: a chemistry recommendation engine built using a graph database. *J. Med. Chem.* 60, 6440–6450. doi: 10.1021/acs.jmedchem.7b00809

Hann, M. M., Leach, A. R., and Harper, G. (2001). Molecular complexity and its impact on the probability of finding leads for drug discovery. *J. Chem. Inf. Comput. Sci.* 41, 856–864. doi: 10.1021/ci000403i

Harel, S., and Radinsky, K. (2018). Prototype-based compound discovery using deep generative models. *Mol. Pharm.* 15, 4406–4416. doi: 10.1021/acs.molpharmaceut.8b00474

Henzler-Wildman, K., and Kern, D. (2007). Dynamic personalities of proteins. *Nature* 450, 964–972. doi: 10.1038/nature06522

Hoffer, L., Voitovich, Y. V., Raux, B., Carrasco, K., Muller, C., Fedorov, A. Y., et al. (2018). Integrated strategy for lead optimization based on fragment growing: the diversity-oriented-target-focused-synthesis approach. *J. Med. Chem.* 61, 5719–5732. doi: 10.1021/acs.jmedchem.8b00653

Hopkins, A. L., Groom, C. R., and Alex, A. (2004). Ligand efficiency: a useful metric for lead selection. *Drug Discov. Today* 9, 430–431. doi: 10.1016/S1359-6446(04)03069-7

Hubbard, R. (2015). Current perspectives in fragment-based ligand discovery. *Acta Crystallogr. Sect. A Found. Adv.* 71:s37. doi: 10.1107/S2053273315099416

Hubbard, R. E., and Murray, J. B. (2011). *Experiences in Fragment-Based Lead Discovery*, 1st Edn. Oxford, UK: Elsevier Inc.

Hung, A. W., Silvestre, H. L., Wen, S., Ciulli, A., Blundell, T. L., and Abell, C. (2009). Application of fragment growing and fragment linking to the discovery of inhibitors of *Mycobacterium tuberculosis* pantothenate synthetase. *Angew. Chemie Int. Ed.* 48, 8452–8456. doi: 10.1002/anie.200903821

Hussein, H. A., Borrel, A., Geneix, C., Petitjean, M., Regad, L., and Camproux, A.-C. (2015). PockDrug-server: a new web server for predicting pocket druggability on holo and apo proteins. *Nucleic Acids Res.* 43, W436–W442. doi: 10.1093/nar/gkv462

Ichihara, O., Barker, J., Law, R. J., and Whittaker, M. (2011). Compound design by fragment-linking. *Mol. Inform.* 30, 298–306. doi: 10.1002/minf.201000174

Jacquemard, C., Drwal, M. N., Desaphy, J., and Kellenberger, E. (2019). Binding mode information improves fragment docking. *J Cheminform* 11:24. doi: 10.1186/s13321-019-0346-7

Joseph-mccarthy, D., Campbell, A. J., Kern, G., and Moustakas, D. (2013). Fragment-based lead discovery and design. *J. Chem. Inf. Model.* 54, 693–704. doi: 10.1021/ci400731w

Kozakov, D., Grove, L. E., Hall, D. R., Bohnuud, T., Mottarella, S. E., Luo, L., et al. (2015). The FTMap family of web servers for determining and characterizing ligand-binding hot spots of proteins. *Nat Protoc* 10, 733–755. doi: 10.1038/nprot.2015.043

Kumar, A., Voet, A., and Zhang, K. Y. J. (2012). Fragment based drug design: from experimental to computational approaches. *Curr. Med. Chem.* 19, 5128–5147. doi: 10.2174/092986712803530467

Lamoree, B., and Hubbard, R. E. (2017). Current perspectives in fragment-based lead discovery (FBLD). *Essays Biochem.* 61, 453–464. doi: 10.1042/EBC20170028

Li, Y., Zhang, L., and Liu, Z. (2018). Multi-objective *de novo* drug design with conditional graph generative model. *J. Cheminform.* 10, 1–24. doi: 10.1186/s13321-018-0287-6

Lin, F.-Y., Esposito, E. X., and Tseng, Y. J. (2018). LeadOp+R: structure-based lead optimization with synthetic accessibility. *Front. Pharmacol.* 9:96. doi: 10.3389/fphar.2018.00096

Lo, M.-C., Aulabaugh, A., Jin, G., Cowling, R., Bard, J., Malamas, M., et al. (2004). Evaluation of fluorescence-based thermal shift assays for hit identification in drug discovery. *Anal. Biochem.* 332, 153–159. doi: 10.1016/j.ab.2004.04.031

Macarron, R., Banks, M. N., Bojanic, D., Burns, D. J., Cirovic, D. A., Garyantes, T., et al. (2011). Impact of high-throughput screening in biomedical research. *Nat. Rev. Drug Discov.* 10, 188–195. doi: 10.1038/nrd3368

Mak, K. K., and Pichika, M. R. (2019). Artificial intelligence in drug development: present status and future prospects. *Drug Discov. Today* 24, 773–780. doi: 10.1016/j.drudis.2018.11.014

Männel, B., Jaiteh, M., Zeifman, A., Randakova, A., Möller, D., Hübner, H., et al. (2017). Structure-guided screening for functionally selective D 2 dopamine receptor ligands from a virtual chemical library. *ACS Chem. Biol.* 12, 2652–2661. doi: 10.1021/acschembio.7b00493

Matias, P. M., Donner, P., Coelho, R., Thomaz, M., Peixoto, C., Macedo, S., et al. (2000). Structural evidence for ligand specificity in the binding domain of the human androgen receptor: implications for pathogenic gene mutations. *J. Biol. Chem.* 275, 26164–26171. doi: 10.1074/jbc.M004571200

Merk, D., Friedrich, L., Grisoni, F., and Schneider, G. (2018). *De novo* design of bioactive small molecules by artificial intelligence. *Mol. Inform.* 37, 3–6. doi: 10.1002/minf.201700153

Mitcheson, J. S., Chen, J., Lin, M., Culberson, C., and Sanguinetti, M. C. (2000). A structural basis for drug-induced long QT syndrome. *Proc. Natl. Acad. Sci. U.S.A.* 97, 12329–12333. doi: 10.1073/pnas.210244497

Miyake, Y., Itoh, Y., Hatanaka, A., Suzuma, Y., Suzuki, M., Kodama, H., et al. (2019). Identification of novel lysine demethylase 5-selective inhibitors by inhibitor-based fragment merging strategy. *Bioorg. Med. Chem.* 27, 1119–1129. doi: 10.1016/j.bmc.2019.02.006

Mondal, M., Groothuis, D. E., and Hirsch, A. K. H. (2015). Fragment growing exploiting dynamic combinatorial chemistry of inhibitors of the aspartic protease endothiapepsin. *Medchemcomm* 6, 1267–1271. doi: 10.1039/C5MD00157A

Navratilova, I., and Hopkins, A. L. (2010). Fragment screening by surface plasmon resonance. *ACS Med. Chem. Lett.* 1, 44–48. doi: 10.1021/ml900002k

Neves, B. J., Braga, R. C., Melo-Filho, C. C., Moreira-Filho, J. T., Muratov, E. N., and Andrade, C. H. (2018). QSAR-based virtual screening: advances and applications in drug discovery. *Front. Pharmacol.* 9:1275. doi: 10.3389/fphar.2018.01275

Ngan, C. H., Bohnuud, T., Mottarella, S. E., Beglov, D., Villar, E. A., Hall, D. R., et al. (2012). FTMAP: extended protein mapping with user-selected probe molecules. *Nucleic Acids Res.* 40, W271–W275. doi: 10.1093/nar/gks441

Nikiforov, P. O., Surade, S., Blaszczyk, M., Delorme, V., Brodin, P., Baulard, A. R., et al. (2016). A fragment merging approach towards the development of small molecule inhibitors of Mycobacterium tuberculosis EthR for use as ethionamide boosters. *Org. Biomol. Chem.* 14, 2318–2326. doi: 10.1039/C5OB02630J

Nissink, J. W. M. (2009). Simple size-independent measure of ligand efficiency. *J. Chem. Inf. Model.* 49, 1617–1622. doi: 10.1021/ci900094m

Olivecrona, M., Blaschke, T., Engkvist, O., and Chen, H. (2017). Molecular *de-novo* design through deep reinforcement learning. *J. Cheminform.* 9, 1–14. doi: 10.1186/s13321-017-0235-x

Pascoini, A. L., Federico, L. B., Arêas, A. L. F., Verde, B. A., Freitas, P. G., and Camps, I. (2019). *In silico* development of new acetylcholinesterase inhibitors. *J. Biomol. Struct. Dyn.* 37, 1007–1021. doi: 10.1080/07391102.2018.1447513

Patel, D., Bauman, J. D., and Arnold, E. (2014). Advantages of crystallographic fragment screening: functional and mechanistic insights from a powerful platform for efficient drug discovery. *Prog. Biophys. Mol. Biol.* 116, 92–100. doi: 10.1016/j.pbiomolbio.2014.08.004

Pedro, L., and Quinn, R. (2016). Native mass spectrometry in fragment-based drug discovery. *Molecules* 21:E984. doi: 10.3390/molecules21080984

Pegg, S. C. H., Haresco, J. J., and Kuntz, I. D. (2001). A genetic algorithm for structure-based *de novo* design. *J. Comput. Aided. Mol. Des.* 15, 911–933. doi: 10.1023/A:1014389729000

Pérez-Sianes, J., Pérez-Sánchez, H., and Díaz, F. (2018). Virtual screening meets deep learning. *Curr. Comput. Aided. Drug Des.* 15, 6–28. doi: 10.2174/1573409914666181018141602

Pierce, A. C., Rao, G., and Bemis, G. W. (2004). BREED: generating novel inhibitors through hybridization of known ligands. Application to CDK2, P38, and HIV protease. *J. Med. Chem.* 47, 2768–2775. doi: 10.1021/jm030543u

Podolyan, Y., Walters, M. A., and Karypis, G. (2010). Assessing synthetic accessibility of chemical compounds using machine learning methods. *J. Chem. Inf. Model.* 50, 979–991. doi: 10.1021/ci900301v

Polinsky, R. J. (1998). Clinical pharmacology of rivastigmine: a new-generation acetylcholinesterase inhibitor for the treatment of alzheimer's disease. *Clin. Ther.* 20, 634–647. doi: 10.1016/S0149-2918(98)80127-6

Polykovskiy, D., Zhebrak, A., Vetrov, D., Ivanenkov, Y., Aladinskiy, V., Mamoshina, P., et al. (2018). Entangled conditional adversarial autoencoder for *de novo* drug discovery. *Mol. Pharm.* 15, 4398–4405. doi: 10.1021/acs.molpharmaceut.8b00839

Popova, M., Isayev, O., and Tropsha, A. (2018). Deep reinforcement learning for de novo drug design. *Sci. Adv.* 4:eaap7885. doi: 10.1126/sciadv.aap7885

Putin, E., Asadulaev, A., Ivanenkov, Y., Aladinskiy, V., Sanchez-Lengeling, B., Aspuru-Guzik, A., et al. (2018). Reinforced adversarial neural computer for *de novo* molecular design. *J. Chem. Inf. Model.* 58, 1194–1204. doi: 10.1021/acs.jcim.7b00690

Ramsundar, B., Liu, B., Wu, Z., Verras, A., Tudor, M., Sheridan, R. P., et al. (2017). Is multitask deep learning practical for pharma? *J. Chem. Inf. Model.* 57, 2068–2076. doi: 10.1021/acs.jcim.7b00146

Riniker, S., and Landrum, G. A. (2013). Open-source platform to benchmark fingerprints for ligand-based virtual screening. *Riniker Landrum J. Cheminformatics* 5:26. doi: 10.1186/1758-2946-5-26

Rodríguez, D., Chakraborty, S., Warnick, E., Crane, S., Gao, Z.-G., O'Connor, R., et al. (2016). Structure-based screening of uncharted chemical space for atypical adenosine receptor agonists. *ACS Chem. Biol.* 11, 2763–2772. doi: 10.1021/acschembio.6b00357

Rogers, D., and Hahn, M. (2010). Extended-connectivity fingerprints. *J. Chem. Inf. Model.* 50, 742–754. doi: 10.1021/ci100050t

Rudling, A., Gustafsson, R., Almlöf, I., Homan, E., Scobie, M., Warpman Berglund, U., et al. (2017). Fragment-based discovery and optimization of enzyme inhibitors by docking of commercial chemical space. *J. Med. Chem.* 60, 8160–8169. doi: 10.1021/acs.jmedchem.7b01006

Ryan, A., Polycarpou, E., Lack, N. A., Evangelopoulos, D., Sieg, C., Halman, A., et al. (2017). Investigation of the mycobacterial enzyme HsaD as a potential novel target for anti-tubercular agents using a fragment-based drug design approach. *Br. J. Pharmacol.* 174, 2209–2224. doi: 10.1111/bph.13810

Schmidtke, P., and Barril, X. (2010). Understanding and predicting druggability. A high-throughput method for detection of drug binding sites. *J. Med. Chem.* 53, 5858–5867. doi: 10.1021/jm100574m

Schneider, G. (2018). Generative models for artificially-intelligent molecular design. *Mol. Inform.* 37:1880131. doi: 10.1002/minf.201880131

Schneider, G., and Clark, D. E. (2019). Automated *de novo* drug design: are we nearly there yet? *Angew. Chemie Int. Ed.* 58, 10792–10803. doi: 10.1002/anie.201814681

Schneider, G., and Fechner, U. (2005). Computer-based *de novo* design of drug-like molecules. *Nat. Rev. Drug Discov.* 4, 649–663. doi: 10.1038/nrd1799

Schuffenhauer, A., Ruedisser, S., Marzinzik, A., Jahnke, W., Selzer, P., and Jacoby, E. (2005). Library design for fragment based screening. *Curr. Top. Med. Chem.* 5, 751–762. doi: 10.2174/1568026054637700

Schulz, M. N., Landström, J., Bright, K., and Hubbard, R. E. (2011). Design of a fragment library that maximally represents available chemical space. *J. Comput. Aided. Mol. Des.* 25, 611–620. doi: 10.1007/s10822-011-9461-x

Schyman, P., Liu, R., Desai, V., and Wallqvist, A. (2017). vNN web server for ADMET predictions. *Front. Pharmacol.* 8:889. doi: 10.3389/fphar.2017.00889

Segler, M. H. S., Kogej, T., Tyrchan, C., and Waller, M. P. (2018). Generating focused molecule libraries for drug discovery with recurrent neural networks. *ACS Cent. Sci.* 4, 120–131. doi: 10.1021/acscentsci.7b00512

Seo, M.-H., Park, J., Kim, E., Hohng, S., and Kim, H.-S. (2014). Protein conformational dynamics dictate the binding affinity for a ligand. *Nat. Commun.* 5:3724. doi: 10.1038/ncomms4724

Shuker, S. B., Hajduk, P. J., Meadows, R. P., and Fesik, S. W. (1996). Discovering high-affinity ligands for proteins: SAR by NMR. *Science* 274, 1531–1534. doi: 10.1126/science.274.5292.1531

Shultz, M. D. (2013). Setting expectations in molecular optimizations: strengths and limitations of commonly used composite parameters. *Bioorg. Med. Chem. Lett.* 23, 5980–5991. doi: 10.1016/j.bmcl.2013.08.029

Silvestre, H. L., Blundell, T. L., Abell, C., and Ciulli, A. (2013). Integrated biophysical approach to fragment screening and validation for fragment-based lead discovery. *Proc. Natl. Acad. Sci. U.S.A.* 110, 12984–12989. doi: 10.1073/pnas.1304045110

Smits, V. A. J., and Gillespie, D. A. (2014). Cancer therapy: targeting the poison within. *Cell Cycle* 13, 2330–2333. doi: 10.4161/cc.29756

Srinivas Reddy, A., Chen, L., and Zhang, S. (2013). "Structure-based *de novo* drug design," in *De novo Molecular Design*, ed. G. Schneider (Weinheim: Wiley-VCH Verlag GmbH and Co. KGaA), 97–124.

Sterling, T., and Irwin, J. J. (2015). ZINC 15 – ligand discovery for everyone. *J. Chem. Inf. Model.* 55, 2324–2337. doi: 10.1021/acs.jcim.5b00559

Strecker, C., Peters, H., Hackl, T., Peters, T., and Meyer, B. (2019). Fragment growing to design optimized inhibitors for human blood group B Galactosyltransferase (GTB). *ChemMedChem* 1, 1336–1342. doi: 10.1002/cmdc.201900296

Talesa, V. N. (2001). Acetylcholinesterase in Alzheimer's disease. *Mech. Ageing Dev.* 122, 1961–1969. doi: 10.1016/S0047-6374(01)00309-8

Thomas, S. E., Mendes, V., Kim, S. Y., Malhotra, S., Ochoa-Montaño, B., Blaszczyk, M., et al. (2017). Structural biology and the design of new therapeutics: from HIV and cancer to mycobacterial infections. *J. Mol. Biol.* 429, 2677–2693. doi: 10.1016/j.jmb.2017.06.014

Torres, P. H. M., Sodero, A. C. R., Jofily, P., and Silva, F. P. Jr. (2019). Key topics in molecular docking for drug design. *Int. J. Mol. Sci.* 20:4574. doi: 10.3390/ijms20184574

Trevizani, R., Custódio, F. L., dos Santos, K. B., and Dardenne, L. E. (2017). Critical features of fragment libraries for protein structure prediction. *PLoS ONE* 12:e0170131. doi: 10.1371/journal.pone.0170131

Tropsha, A. (2010). Best practices for QSAR model development, validation, and exploitation. *Mol. Inform.* 29, 476–488. doi: 10.1002/minf.201000061

Tversky, A. (1977). Features of similarity. *Psychol. Rev.* 84, 327–352. doi: 10.1037/0033-295X.84.4.327

Vamathevan, J., Clark, D., Czodrowski, P., Dunham, I., Ferran, E., Lee, G., et al. (2019). Applications of machine learning in drug discovery and development. *Nat. Rev. Drug Discov.* 18, 463–477. doi: 10.1038/s41573-019-0024-5

Veber, D. F., Johnson, S. R., Cheng, H.-Y., Smith, B. R., Ward, K. W., and Kopple, K. D. (2002). Molecular properties that influence the oral bioavailability of drug candidates. *J. Med. Chem.* 45, 2615–2623. doi: 10.1021/jm020017n

Verdonk, M. L., Giangreco, I., Hall, R. J., Korb, O., Mortenson, P. N., and Murray, C. W. (2011). Docking performance of fragments and druglike compounds. *J. Med. Chem.* 54, 5422–5431. doi: 10.1021/jm200558u

Verdonk, M. L., and Hartshorn, M. J. (2004). Structure-guided fragment screening for lead discovery. *Curr. Opin. Drug Discov. Devel.* 7, 404–410.

Wang, R., Gao, Y., and Lai, L. (2000). LigBuilder: a multi-purpose program for structure-based drug design. *J. Mol. Model.* 6, 498–516. doi: 10.1007/s0089400060498

Wang, T., Wu, M.-B., Chen, Z.-J., Chen, H., Lin, J.-P., and Yang, L.-R. (2015). Fragment-based drug discovery and molecular docking in drug design. *Curr. Pharm. Biotechnol.* 16, 11–25. doi: 10.2174/1389201015666141122204532

Whitehouse, A. J., Thomas, S. E., Brown, K. P., Fanourakis, A., Chan, D. S.-H., Libardo, M. D. J., et al. (2019). Development of inhibitors against *Mycobacterium abscessus* tRNA (m 1 G37) methyltransferase (TrmD) using fragment-based approaches. *J. Med. Chem.* 62, 7210–7232. doi: 10.1021/acs.jmedchem.9b00809

Willighagen, E. L., Waagmeester, A., Spjuth, O., Ansell, P., Williams, A. J., Tkachenko, V., et al. (2013). The ChEMBL database as linked open data. *J. Cheminform.* 5:23. doi: 10.1186/1758-2946-5-23

Xu, X., Fang, X., Wang, J., and Zhu, H. (2017). Identification of novel ROS inducer by merging the fragments of piperlongumine and dicoumarol. *Bioorg. Med. Chem. Lett.* 27, 1325–1328. doi: 10.1016/j.bmcl.2016.08.016

Yang, H., Lou, C., Sun, L., Li, J., Cai, Y., Wang, Z., et al. (2019a). admetSAR 2.0: web-service for prediction and optimization of chemical ADMET properties. *Bioinformatics* 35, 1067–1069. doi: 10.1093/bioinformatics/bty707

Yang, X., Wang, Y., Byrne, R., Schneider, G., and Yang, S. (2019b). Concepts of artificial intelligence for computer-assisted drug discovery. *Chem. Rev.* 119, 10520–10594. doi: 10.1021/acs.chemrev.8b00728

Yuan, Y., Pei, J., and Lai, L. (2011). LigBuilder 2: a practical *de novo* drug design approach. *J. Chem. Inf. Model.* 51, 1083–1091. doi: 10.1021/ci100350u

13

In silico Druggability Assessment of the NUDIX Hydrolase Protein Family as a Workflow for Target Prioritization

Maurice Michel [1*]***, Evert J. Homan*** [1]***, Elisée Wiita*** [1]***, Kia Pedersen*** [1]***, Ingrid Almlöf*** [1]***, Anna-Lena Gustavsson*** [2]***, Thomas Lundbäck*** [2,3]***, Thomas Helleday*** [1,4] ***and Ulrika Warpman Berglund*** [1*]

[1] Science for Life Laboratory, Department of Oncology-Pathology, Karolinska Institutet, Stockholm, Sweden, [2] Chemical Biology Consortium Sweden (CBCS), Science for Life Laboratory, Department of Medical Biochemistry and Biophysics, Karolinska Institutet, Stockholm, Sweden, [3] Mechanistic Biology and Profiling, Discovery Sciences, R&D, AstraZeneca, Gothenburg, Sweden, [4] Department of Oncology and Metabolism, Sheffield Cancer Centre, University of Sheffield, Sheffield, United Kingdom

***Correspondence:**
Maurice Michel
maurice.grube@scilifelab.se
Ulrika Warpman Berglund
ulrika.warpmanberglund@scilifelab.se

Computational chemistry has now been widely accepted as a useful tool for shortening lead times in early drug discovery. When selecting new potential drug targets, it is important to assess the likelihood of finding suitable starting points for lead generation before pursuing costly high-throughput screening campaigns. By exploiting available high-resolution crystal structures, an *in silico* druggability assessment can facilitate the decision of whether, and in cases where several protein family members exist, which of these to pursue experimentally. Many of the algorithms and software suites commonly applied for *in silico* druggability assessment are complex, technically challenging and not always user-friendly. Here we applied the intuitive open access servers of DoGSite, FTMap and CryptoSite to comprehensively predict ligand binding pockets, druggability scores and conformationally active regions of the NUDIX protein family. In parallel we analyzed potential ligand binding sites, their druggability and pocket parameter using Schrödinger's SiteMap. Then an *in silico* docking cascade of a subset of the ZINC FragNow library using the Glide docking program was performed to assess identified pockets for large-scale small-molecule binding. Subsequently, this initial dual ranking of druggable sites within the NUDIX protein family was benchmarked against experimental hit rates obtained both in-house and by others from traditional biochemical and fragment screening campaigns. The observed correlation suggests that the presented user-friendly workflow of a dual parallel *in silico* druggability assessment is applicable as a standalone method for decision on target prioritization and exclusion in future screening campaigns.

Keywords: druggability, nudix, drug discovery, workflow, malachite green

INTRODUCTION

The nucleoside diphosphates attached to sequence-x (NUDIX) hydrolase protein family was recently comprehensively and exhaustively reviewed by Carreras-Puigvert et al. (2017) NUDIX proteins possess a conserved sequence, called the NUDIX box, i.e., Gx_5Ex_5[UA]$xREx_2EExGU$), which differs little between individual members which are otherwise of low sequence similarity.

Structural and domain analysis revealed three major groups and one outlier, NUDT22, mostly based on their already reported activity against substrate classes such as diphosphoinositol polyphosphates (Caffrey et al., 1999, 2000) and NADH diphosphates (Abdelraheim et al., 2003). Subsequently, a systematical screening against a large set of substrates was performed and painted a rather promiscuous picture of the NUDIX hydrolases, indicating backup functionality or redundancy. Consequently, a global expression analysis was performed and showed a clear dependency on tissue of origin and the corresponding cancer tissue. Interestingly, NUDT1, NUDT5, and NUDT14 amongst others were present in a cluster of highly expressed proteins, confirming a potential role in cancer as reported earlier (Choi et al., 2011; Gad et al., 2014; Huber et al., 2014; Wright et al., 2016). Importantly, when evaluated for epistasis, it became apparent that several NUDIX members sustain relations as measured in cell viability and cell cycle perturbations and that these interactions are more important for cancerous cells. With this overview in structure, expression, substrate specificity and relation, the NUDIX protein family members gained considerable attention as potential drug targets. The original interest in pharmacological modulation of NUDIX members was sparked by the notion that NUDT1 is overexpressed in several cancer cell types, while its role in healthy cells can largely be compensated for as evidenced by the normal life-span of knock-out mice (Tsuzuki et al., 2001). Besides GTP and dGTP, NUDT1 hydrolyzes several oxidatively damaged DNA nucleotides including 8-oxo-dGTP and 2-OH-dATP, thus preventing their incorporation into DNA, which otherwise would lead to DNA damage and ultimately cell death. This led to the hypothesis that increased expression of NUDT1, and hence improved sanitization capacity of oxidatively damaged DNA bases from the nucleotide pool, would enable cancer cells to cope with the increased oxidative stress they are exposed to compared with healthy cells. Gad and coworkers published TH588 (**Figure 1**) as the first small-molecule NUDT1 inhibitor with efficacy in mouse xenograft models (Gad et al., 2014), although subsequent potent and selective NUDT1 inhibitors disclosed by AstraZeneca, MD Anderson, Gilead and Sprint Bioscience/Bayer failed to reproduce these findings with regards to cytotoxicity (**Figure 1**) (Kettle et al., 2016; Petrocchi et al., 2016; Ellermann et al., 2017; Farand et al., 2020). The validity of NUDT1 as an anticancer target has thus been questioned and is still under debate (Warpman Berglund et al., 2016; Samaranayake et al., 2017). Regardless, these studies served to demonstrate significant amenability to small-molecule inhibition of NUDT1, justifying the question as to how this translates to other members of the NUDIX family.

Besides NUDT1, a series of potent, drug-like NUDT5 inhibitors have been described by Page and coworkers (Page et al., 2018). The lead compound TH5427 (**Figure 1**) was shown to block progestin-dependent, PAR-derived nuclear ATP synthesis and subsequent chromatin remodeling, gene regulation and proliferation in breast cancer cells, suggesting that targeting NUDT5 may represent a novel therapeutic approach for breast cancer treatment. Most recently, the covalent NUDT7 inhibitor NUDT7-COV-1 was developed by employing electrophilic fragment screening and a fragment combination approach

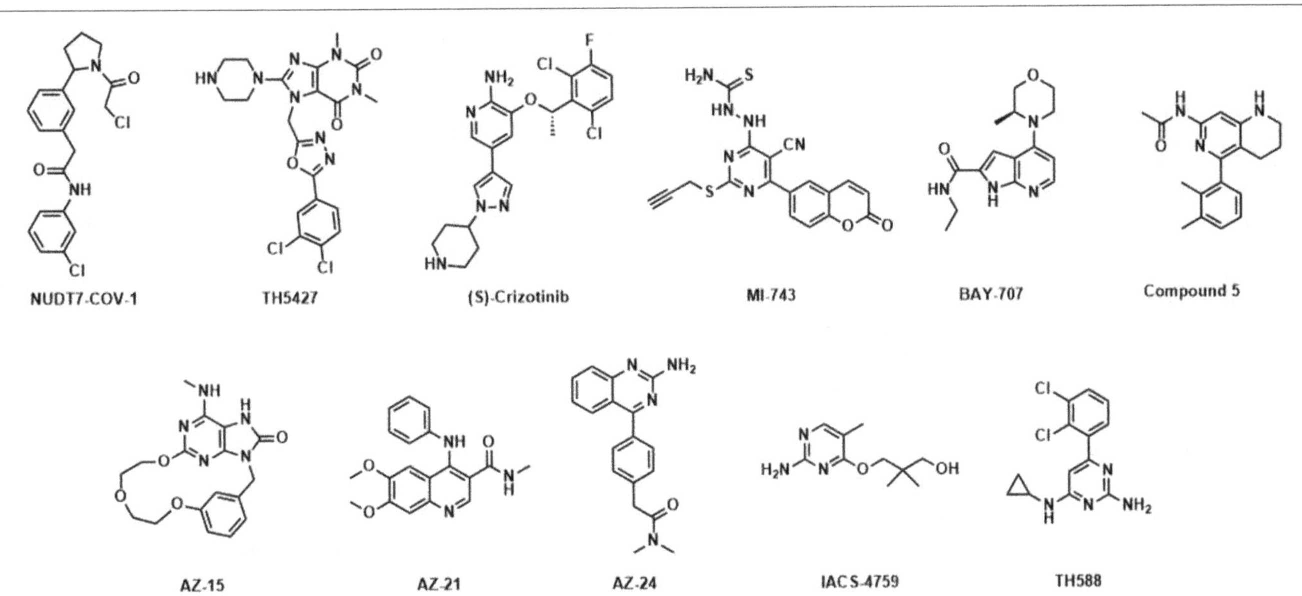

FIGURE 1 | Published NUDIX inhibitors: TH588 was developed as a first in class NUDT1 inhibitor at Science for Life Laboratory and Karolinska Institutet (Gad et al., 2014); (S)-Crizotinib is a potent NUDT1 inhibitor and the enantiomer of (R)-Crizotinib (Huber et al., 2014), a clinically applied tyrosine kinase inhibitor; optimized by Astra-Zeneca; AZ-15, AZ-21 and AZ-24 are distinct chemotype inhibitors targeting NUDT1 (Kettle et al., 2016); BAY-707 (Ellermann et al., 2017) was discovered as a NUTD1 inhibitor by Sprint Bioscience; IACS-4759 (Petrocchi et al., 2016) is a NUDT1 inhibitor developed by MD Anderson; MI-743 is a selective inhibitor of NUDT1 in gastric cancers (Zhou et al., 2019); Compound 5 was reported by Gilead and inhibits NUDT1 (Farand et al., 2020); TH5427 was synthesized as a lead compound against NUDT5 (Page et al., 2018); NUDT7-COV-1 is a covalent inhibitor generated by electrophile screening and fragment combination (Resnick et al., 2019).

(**Figure 1**) (Resnick et al., 2019). To the best of our knowledge no potent inhibitors for any of the other NUDIX hydrolase members have been disclosed to date, although there are public data on hit rates for selected family members on the Structural Genomics Consortium homepage[1, 2].

One aspect not addressed in the recent comprehensive review (Carreras-Puigvert et al., 2017) is an assessment of the potential druggability of the different NUDIX family members, i.e., their amenability to be modulated by drug-like small molecules. With the recent dawn of PROTACs, synthetic neoantigens and biologics, but also established targeting strategies like allosteric modulation or active site inhibition, several scenarios of how to target a protein may be exploited. With that in mind, druggability as such is no longer restricted to active site inhibition of a protein by a small molecule with an optimized small-molecule drug-like profile. Both orthosteric or catalytic sites and secondary, allosteric sites, may be equally interesting to be targeted for the development of small-molecule chemical probes and potential drug candidates. As high-resolution crystal structures of 18 out of the 22 human NUDIX hydrolases are now available, a family-wide *in silico* druggability assessment for available sites is feasible.

Here we use several open-access binding site analysis methods, i.e., DoGSite (Volkamer et al., 2012)[3], CryptoSite (Cimermancic et al., 2016)[4], and FTMap (Kozakov et al., 2015)[5], as well as the commercial SiteMap and *in silico* fragment screening of a fragment library using Glide to probe the NUDIX hydrolase protein structures for potential small-molecule binding sites and assess their druggability and suitability for a prospective drug discovery campaign. This established *in silico* prioritization workflow within the NUDIX family is further supported by results obtained from biochemical screens employing the malachite green assay (Baykov et al., 1988) as well as differential scanning fluorimetry (DSF) (Niesen et al., 2007) fragment screens for some of the family members. This correlation with own experimental results and those published previously highlights the benefit of this comparably low-cost computational assessment workflow prior to applying experimental screening methods for the rapid evaluation of target druggability.

MATERIALS AND METHODS

Protein Preparation and Validation

Available crystal structures of human NUDIX hydrolases with the highest resolution were imported into Maestro (Schrödinger Suite 2019-1, Schrödinger, LLC, New York, NY, 2019.) The structures were then prepared using the Protein Preparation Wizard as implemented in the Schrödinger Suite. Briefly, raw PDB structures were processed by automatically assigning bond orders, adding hydrogens, creating zero-order bonds to metals, converting selenomethionine to methionine, adding missing side-chains, creating possible disulfide bridges, deleting waters beyond 5.0 Å of hetero groups (if present), and generating hetero protonation states at pH 7.0. Residues with alternate positions were locked in the conformations with the highest average occupancy. Small ligands and metal ions originating from crystallization buffer were removed. The hydrogen bonding networks were optimized automatically, by sampling water orientations and optimization of hydroxyls, Asn, Gln, and His residue states using ProtAssign. Any remaining water molecules were subsequently removed. A restrained minimization was then performed using the OPLS3e force field, until an RMSD convergence of 0.30 Å was reached for the heavy atoms. Finally, the minimized NUDIX structures were aligned to the structure of NUDT1 (3Q93) with respect to the backbone atoms of the A chain.

DoGSite

The protein structures as prepared above were exported as PDB files, uploaded to the DoGSite server and assessed for binding sites and their corresponding DrugScores according to the published protocol (Volkamer et al., 2012). Pocket Size and DrugScores were extracted for all identified sites and annotated to pocket numbers.

FTMap

All prepared PDB files were uploaded to the FTMap server and interrogated for number of probes per cluster found according to the published protocols (Kozakov et al., 2015; Vajda et al., 2018).

CryptoSite

All prepared PDB files were uploaded to CryptoSite server and assessed for amino acid flexibility according to the published protocol (Cimermancic et al., 2016). Amino acid residues exceeding a Cryptic Site Score of 0.10 were extracted.

SiteMap

Prepared protein structures were submitted to SiteMap analyses as implemented in Schrödinger Suite 2019-1. The 5 top-ranked potential binding sites were identified. At least 15 site points per reported sites were required. The more restricted definition of hydrophobicity together with a standard grid (0.7 Å) were used. Site maps at 4 Å or more from the nearest site points were cropped. Clustering of the SiteMap parameters was performed using the heatmaply library in R[6]. The SiteMap parameters were transformed using "percentize," and average linking was used for clustering.

Virtual Fragment Screening

1) Fragment subset selection: a subset of the ZINC Frags Now set (Irwin et al., 2012) was created by applying a number of filters implemented in a Knime workflow (Knime 3.5.2, Berthold et al., 2008). Foremost, only fragments available from a list of 19 preferred suppliers, composed by a team of experienced

[1] *Fragment Screening*. Available online at: https://www.thesgc.org/fragment-screening (accessed August 8, 2019).

[2] NUDT15. *Manuscript Submitted*.

[3] *Zentrum für Bioinformatik: Universität Hamburg - Proteins Plus Server*. Available online at: https://proteins.plus/ (accessed June 3, 2019).

[4] *Cryptic binding site*. Available online at: https://modbase.compbio.ucsf.edu/cryptosite/ (accessed June 3, 2019).

[5] *FTMap: A Small Molecule Mapping Server*. Available online at: http://ftmap.bu.edu/login.php (accessed June 3, 2019).

[6] *Introduction to Heatmaply*. Available online at: https://cran.r-project.org/web/packages/heatmaply/vignettes/heatmaply.html (accessed April 16, 2020).

medicinal chemists were considered. These were then filtered using a cascade of structural filters, including REOS (Walters and Murcko, 2002), PAINS (Baell and Holloway, 2010) and a set of in-house filters (ScrapFilter) compiled over the years. Lipinski-type descriptors (SlogP, TPSA, AMW, NumLipinskiHBA, NumLipinskiHBD, NumRotatableBonds, NumHeavyAtoms, NumRings, NumAromaticRings) were then calculated using the RDKit Descriptor Calculation node. An additional descriptor HetRatio was then calculated as the ratio of NumLipinskiHBA and NumHeavyAtoms, and fragments with HetRatio <0.2 or >0.5 were filtered out. Finally, remaining outliers were removed by applying Gaussian Z-score normalization on the descriptor space, and then filtering out fragments with descriptor values deviating more than 3 units from the mean. The entire filtering cascade reduced the original input file of 704,041 structures as downloaded from ZINC to 205,891 fragments (**Supplementary Data Sheet 1**).

2) Ligand preparation: the selected fragment subset was then prepared for docking using LigPrep (Schrödinger): the OPLS3e force field was used for minimizations; possible ionization states at pH 7.0 ± 2.0 were generated using Epik (Shelley et al., 2007; Greenwood et al., 2010), metal binding states were added, and tautomers were generated; specified chiralities were retained and at most 4 stereoisomers were generated per structure. This yielded 345,044 structures for docking.
3) Receptor grid generation: Glide docking grids (Friesner et al., 2004, 2006; Halgren et al., 2004) were generated for each target protein by focusing the grid box on the center of the site with the highest Dscore as determined by SiteMap (Halgren, 2007, 2009). The size of the box enclosing the grid was set to 16 Å. No constraints, rotatable groups or excluded volumes were defined.
4) Virtual screening: The Virtual Screening Workflow as implemented in Schrödinger Suite was used for docking, scoring, and ranking of the top-1,000 fragments against the sites with the highest Dscore as determined by SiteMap. The workflow comprised a cascade of docking steps with increased accuracy (Glide HTVS → SP → XP), where the top-10% ranked ligands are passed on to the next step. After Glide XP docking the top-1,000 ranked fragments were retained for druggability assessment based on their combined docking scores.

Biochemical Screening

Small-molecule screening of NUDT2, NUDT15, and NUDT16 at a compound concentration of 10 μM was conducted using coupled enzymatic assays as already described for NUDT1 (Gad et al., 2014) and NUDT5 (Page et al., 2018). In brief this involved the purification of recombinant proteins following overexpression in *E. coli* and subsequent validation of coupled enzymatic assays based on cognate substrates for each of these [Ap4A for NUDT2, dGTP for NUDT15 and ADP for NUDT16 (Trésaugues et al., 2015)][2]. The assays for NUDT2 and NUDT15 were based on enzymatic release of inorganic pyrophosphate and subsequent degradation to two molecules of inorganic phosphate in the presence of excess inorganic pyrophosphatase. Levels of inorganic phosphate are measured using an established procedure for such measurements in 384-well format in our lab (see e.g., Gad et al., 2014; Page et al., 2018). The screening of NUDT16 was based on enzymatic processing of ADP to release one molecule of inorganic phosphate, such that the coupled enzyme was not needed in this assay. All assays were optimized to allow their application at close to the K_m of each substrate and with an incubation time chosen to ensure consumption of <30% of substrate and near linearity of assay signal increase with time.

Slightly different screening sets have been applied for the family members, with only a smaller subset of 5,500 compounds in common. All screens conducted at Chemical Biology Consortium Sweden have 16 each of negative (DMSO only – 0% inhibition) and positive controls (no enzyme or inhibitor at concentration that gives 100% inhibition). These are located in columns 23 and 24 of the 384-well plates and they are used to normalize the response in each well-containing library compounds to a % inhibition value. Hit limits are defined based on the average plus three standard deviations of the response for all library compounds and hit rates are provided as the percentage of library compounds above this limit. The malachite green assay has been extensively used for screening purposes in our lab as it is associated with low interference rates, as evidenced by the lack of common hits appearing in screens of NUDT1 (Gad et al., 2014), NUDT5 (Page et al., 2018), dCTPase (Llona-Minguez et al., 2016), dUTPase and ITPase besides the herein reported NUDIX proteins (**Supplementary Material** – Screens using malachite green).

DSF Fragment Screening

NUDT1, NUDT2, NUDT5, and NUDT15 druggability was further experimentally assessed through fragment screening by DSF. Different fragments sets were screened over time, reflecting history and development of the available fragment sets. The initial fragment library comprised 450 fragments selected from the Chemical Biology Consortium Sweden reagent store at the Karolinska Institutet, and this set was screened against NUDT1 and NUDT5. Over time this library was complemented with sets of nucleobase analogs acquired from the NCI Developmental Therapeutics Program, which was grown to a subset of 200 compounds. This set, together with the 450-member library, thus totaling 650 fragments, was screened against NUDT2. Subsequently the 450-member library was complemented with 550 additional fragments from the Chemical Biology Consortium Sweden reagent store in order to generate a more diverse generic fragment library of 1,000 compounds. This second version together with the 200 nucleobase analogs acquired from NCI was screened against NUDT15. The proteins were expressed and purified as previously reported (Carreras-Puigvert et al., 2017). Fragment screening by DSF was essentially performed as described in detail by Niesen et al. (2007) All fragments were screened at a final concentration of 500 μM. Positive controls for each target were used at 100 μM. Assay buffer was composed of 100 mM Tris Acetate, 40 mM NaCl, and 10 mM Mg Acetate. Sypro Orange (S6650, Molecular Probes, 5000x) was used as the fluorescent dye. Native melting points of the proteins under the assay conditions were 50.0, 50.0, 76.0, and 57.0°C for NUDT1, NUDT2, NUDT5, and NUDT15, respectively. Screening was performed in 96-well Q-PCR plates using a BioRad 96CFX real-time PCR detection system with temperature increments of 1.0°C. More details of the assay conditions for each target are provided in the **Supplementary Material** – Fragment screen conditions.

RESULTS AND DISCUSSION

Automated Arm - Step 1: DoGSite and FTMap Predict Druggable Catalytic Sites and Potentially Druggable Secondary Sites

We started by compiling a list of available high-resolution crystal structures of human NUDIX proteins (**Table 1**). Due to the systematic work of the Structural Genomics Consortium, the majority of structures were solved with high sequence coverage (**Supplementary Material** – SiteMap secondary sites) and are often available together with screening data[1]. PDBs were imported to Maestro and prepared as described in the Method part. To enable application in the automated workflow, the prepared proteins were exported as new PDB files (**Figure 2**). In a first step, these files were uploaded to the DoGSite server. DoGSite is a web-based open-access algorithm that interrogates rigid protein structures for binding hotspots, including druggability prediction (Volkamer et al., 2012). Initially, a grid covering the protein identifies grid points that overlap with protein atoms. Application of a difference of Gaussian (DoG) filter then screens for preferred binding spots of sphere-like objects. Combination of several hotspots creates subpockets, which, if neighboring, are merged into a pocket. Several geometric and physico-chemical properties are automatically calculated for the predicted pockets and subpockets. A machine learning model trained on a set of known druggable proteins is then used to predict the druggability of the pockets, expressed as DrugScore. Reported as a factor between 0 and 1.0 a DrugScore over 0.5 and closer to 1.0 corresponds to good druggability.

Application of this algorithm to NUDIX crystal structures identified between two and ten pockets with a wide range of DrugScores (**Figure 3** and **Supplementary Material** - DogSite). Between one and four bindings sites were judged druggable by the DoGSite algorithm. For some of the NUDIX hydrolases the natural substrates and their binding sites are yet to be deciphered. In addition, with the broad targeting possibilities provided by PROTACs (An and Fu, 2018) or allosteric inhibitors (Wenthur et al., 2014; Aretz et al., 2018), it is not necessarily required to target a catalytic pocket to convey a desired phenotype. Thus, the single highest-ranking site of each NUDIX structure, often corresponding to the known substrate binding site, was used to calculate a NUDIX druggability score. With an average druggability score of 0.80, the NUDIX family of proteins qualify as good predicted drug targets. As a positive control and validated target when it comes to chemical amenability, NUDT1 (3Q93) reaches a similar score of 0.81. The protein tyrosine phosphatase 1B (PTP1B) was included into the assessment

TABLE 1 | High-resolution crystal structures used in this study.

Protein name	PDB code	References
NUDT1, MTH1	3Q93	Tresaugues et al., 2011a
NUDT2, APAH1	3U53	Ge et al., 2013
NUDT3, DIPP1	2FVV	Thorsell et al., 2009
NUDT4, DIPP2	5LTU	Srikannathasan et al., 2017a
NUDT5, HSPC115	6GRU	Dubianok et al., 2018
NUDT6, FGF2AS	3H95	Tresaugues et al., 2009a
NUDT7	5T3P	Srikannathasan et al., 2017b
NUDT9	1Q33	Shen et al., 2003
NUDT10, DIPP3A	3MCF	Tresaugues et al., 2010
NUDT12	6SCX	Wu et al., 2019
NUDT14, UGPP	3Q91	Tresaugues et al., 2011b
NUDT15, MTH2	5BON	Carter et al., 2015
NUDT16	3COU	Tresaugues et al., 2008
NUDT17	5LF8	Mathea et al., 2017a
NUDT18, MTH3	3GG6	Tresaugues et al., 2009b
NUDT20, DCP2	5MP0	Mathea et al., 2017b
NUDT21	3BAP	Coseno et al., 2008
NUDT22	5LF9	Tallant et al., 2017
PTP1B*	2HNP	Barford et al., 1994

Added as reference protein.

(2HNP) as this is generally known to be a challenging target for classical drug discovery approaches. PTP1B, like other tyrosine phosphatases, contains a relatively polar substrate pocket which can accommodate phosphate isosteres. In the last two decades, small molecules targeting this pocket have been shown to fail eliciting sufficient effects *in vivo* (Zhang and Zhang, 2007; Krishnan et al., 2018). Instead a non-classical approach of allosteric inhibition is currently under evaluation in clinical trials (Mullard, 2018). When interrogated with DoGSite, PTP1B (2HNP) scores 0.72 only by combination of two subpockets through a narrow channel.

An interesting observation is that all NUDIX members, except NUDT4 (0.72, 5LTU) and NUDT18 (0.63, 3GG6), individually score a high DrugScore around 0.80. Furthermore, it can be observed that several members, including NUDT6 (3H95, 0.78), NUDT7 (5T3P, 0.77), NUDT9 (1Q33, 0.82), NUDT17 (5LF8, 0.79), NUDT12 (6SCX, 0.85), and NUDT22 (5LF9, 0.81, **Figure 4**), are predicted to possess a second high-ranking pocket. These sites may increase the potential for pharmacological targeting of the corresponding proteins, for instance by masking a protein-protein interaction or a cofactor binding site. Identification of a second high-ranking pocket remote from the catalytic site, however, may also point toward an artifact in the crystal structure due to the construct used for expression or lack of electron density. For a comparison of resolved and expressed sequences please refer to **Supplementary Material** – SiteMap secondary sites. Thus, when inspected for their location, it became apparent that secondary sites can be distinguished as either neighboring to the top-ranked site or being located more remotely.

The druggability of the identified pockets can be further assessed using FTMap (Kozakov et al., 2015; Yueh et al., 2019). FTMap interrogates the protein surface for contributions

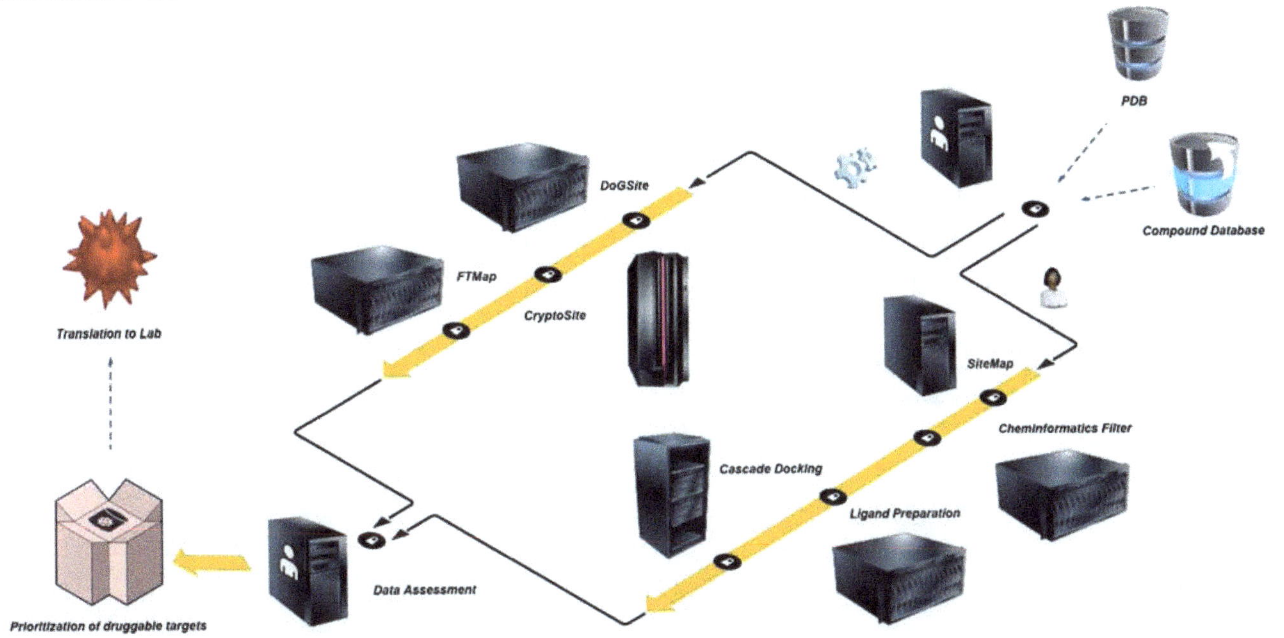

FIGURE 2 | *In silico* druggability prioritization workflow – High-resolution crystal structures and comprehensive commercial space compound databases are freely available. PDBs are prepared by protein preparation wizard (Thorsell et al., 2009), inspected for structural flaws and limitations and exported as new structure files. In a first step, the structures are assessed for binding sites and site druggability by algorithms using rigid proteins or allowing for flexible behavior, i.e. DoGSite (Volkamer et al., 2012) and CryptoSite (Cimermancic et al., 2016). To eliminate artifacts due to protein construct choice, limitations of crystal structure resolution or co-crystallization of additional protein copies, all identified sites are counter-screened by FTMap (Kozakov et al., 2015). In a second and parallel step, the same structures are initially assessed for binding sites, druggability and pocket parameter using SiteMap (Halgren, 2007, 2009). A separate Knime (Berthold et al., 2008) workflow for the elimination of promiscuous functionalities is followed by Ligand Preparation which builds an applicable set of small molecules including a number of tautomers and stereoisomers. In a three-step cascade this set is then docked (Friesner et al., 2004, 2006; Halgren et al., 2004) against the highest-ranking site as identified by SiteMap. The median docking score of the top-1,000 fragments is used to assess druggability based on commercial fragment space. In a final step, prioritization of targets passing both parallel screening schemes may be performed based on published experimental screening data or own future screening efforts during translation to the lab.

to ligand-free energy. Small organic molecules, reflecting the complexity of potential active substances, are scored using a detailed energy function. Some regions bind several clusters of probes and thus identify as a binding hotspot. Earlier, this orthogonal method was applied on pockets identified by CryptoSite (Vajda et al., 2018), where high druggability would correspond to an FTMap cluster populating these sites and containing at least 16 probes. When similarly examined for the number of bound probes, all highest-ranking sites of each NUDIX protein except for NUDT4 (5LTU) and NUDT18 (3GG6), reached more than 16 probes confirming the good druggability of the expected active sites of the enzyme family (**Figure 3** and **Supplementary Material** - FTMap). NUDT4 (5LTU) and NUDT18 (3GG6), which showed a lower DrugScore before, failed to contain more than 16 probes and are the only family members with a lower druggability assessment based on DoGSite and FTMap. Assessment of PTP1B (2HNP) returned all FTMap probe clusters to be located in the smaller of the two sites predicted by DoGSite (DrugScore 0.38). When evaluated with FTMap, secondary sites of NUDT6 (3H95), NUDT7 (5T3P), NUDT9 (1Q33), NUDT17 (5LF8), and NUDT22 (5LF9, **Figure 4**) neighboring the highest-ranking site tend to harbor more probes than those sites found remotely. All remote secondary sites, i.e., NUDT9 (1Q33), NUDT17 (5LF8) and NUDT 12 (6SCX), fail to incorporate the required 16 probes. Of those located much closer to the highest-ranking pocket, only NUDT7 (5T3P) fails to accommodate 16 or more probes underscoring the potential use in pharmacological targeting additionally to the neighboring highest-ranking pocket.

Automated Arm – Step 2: CryptoSite and FTMap Confirm Druggable Active Binding Pockets With High Flexibility

Druggability predictions using DoGSite are based on rigid protein structures, not allowing for flexibility typically induced by larger natural substrates or specifically designed small molecules (Michel et al., 2019). Another aspect is the potential existence of allosteric sites. Typically, a crystal structure of a compound bound to the allosteric site or comprehensive protein dynamics calculations based on several distinct crystal structures are required for their discovery. The CryptoSite algorithm however, can give first insights in whether an already identified active site or a shallow pocket allows for high single amino acid flexibility (Cimermancic et al., 2016). Networks of these flexible cryptic sites could indicate concerted movements of the protein, possibly

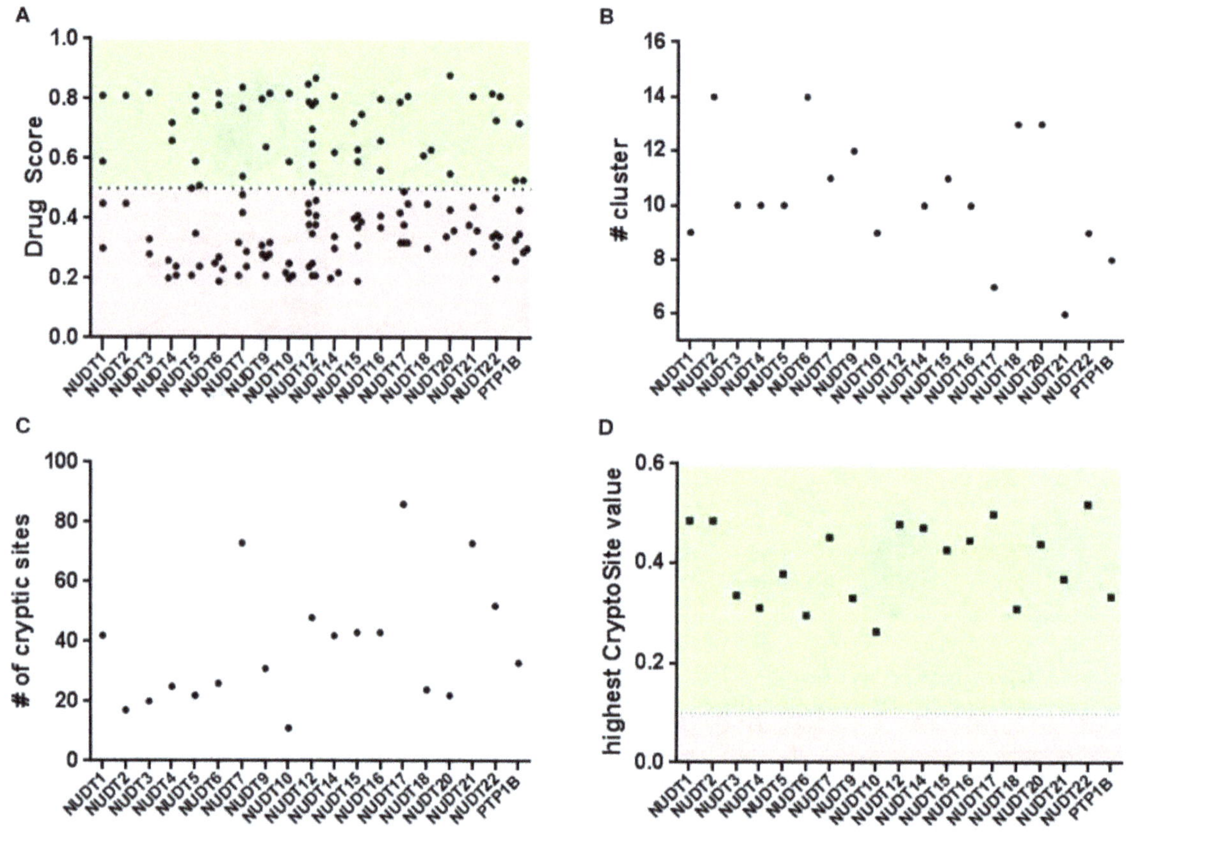

FIGURE 3 | Binding pocket identification and druggability assessment in the automated arm: **(A)** rigid protein assessment with DogSite identifies a number of binding sites within a range of predicted druggability scores; **(B)** FTMap identifies a number of cluster per protein and only NUDT4 and NUDT18 fail to contain enough samples per cluster in the active site; **(C,D)** flexible protein assessment with CryptoSite identifies amino acid residues with different degrees of conformational freedom. Including the top scoring residues these networks largely overlap with pockets identified by DogSite.

forming an allosteric site or conformational changes relevant for substrate binding and protein function. Cryptic scores returned by the algorithm above 0.10 and higher consider a site as cryptic and thus flexible.

When interrogated with CryptoSite, NUDIX hydrolases showed an increased number of cryptic sites around the highest-ranking site as identified before by DoGSite, indicating an extended and flexible three-dimensional network of amino acid residues (**Figure 3** and **Supplementary Material** - CryptoSite). Between 11 and 86 and on average 40 residues scored higher than 0.10 (NUDT1, 42; PTP1B, 33). The highest scoring residues reached values between 0.26 and 0.52 and on average 0.40 (NUDT1, 0.49; PTP1B, 0.33). NUDT10 failed to form a cryptic network while NUDT6, NUDT7 and NUDT22 (**Figure 4**) possessed a second cluster of cryptic sites overlapping with the second highest-ranking sites as identified by DoGSite. Except for NUDT4 (5LTU) and NUDT18 (3GG6), all cryptic networks of the protein family members were populated by more than 16 probes in FTMap (**Figure 3** and **Supplementary Material** – FTMap).

The result of this initial druggability assessment suggest that NUDIX hydrolases are on average good drug targets with regard to their expected or known active sites. Further, only a few members of the family possess a second druggable site as based on DoGSite and FTMap analyses, and even fewer exhibit conformational flexible sites remote from the identified active site.

User Arm – Step 1: SiteMap Binding Site Prediction and Druggability Assessment

In a second parallel approach we assessed druggability using SiteMap and a Glide-based virtual screening workflow applied to a KNIME filtered fragment library (**Figure 2**). SiteMap, an application to identify binding pockets and predict druggability, is implemented in the Schrödinger small-molecule modeling suite. Binding pockets identified on the protein surface are given a score, the Dscore, which is based on pocket parameters such as size, exposure to solvent, enclosure by protein, ratio of hydrogen bond donors and acceptors and importantly hydrophilicity, hydrophobicity and a determined ratio thereof. This druggability score favors proteins with a higher hydrophobic/hydrophilic ratio and thus allows for an early assessment of pocket polarity as required for binding of small-molecule drugs. Typical Dscores for druggable protein pockets are above 1.108 while Dscores below 0.871 suggest a difficult to drug protein (Halgren, 2007, 2009). In addition, comparing individual pocket parameters allows for

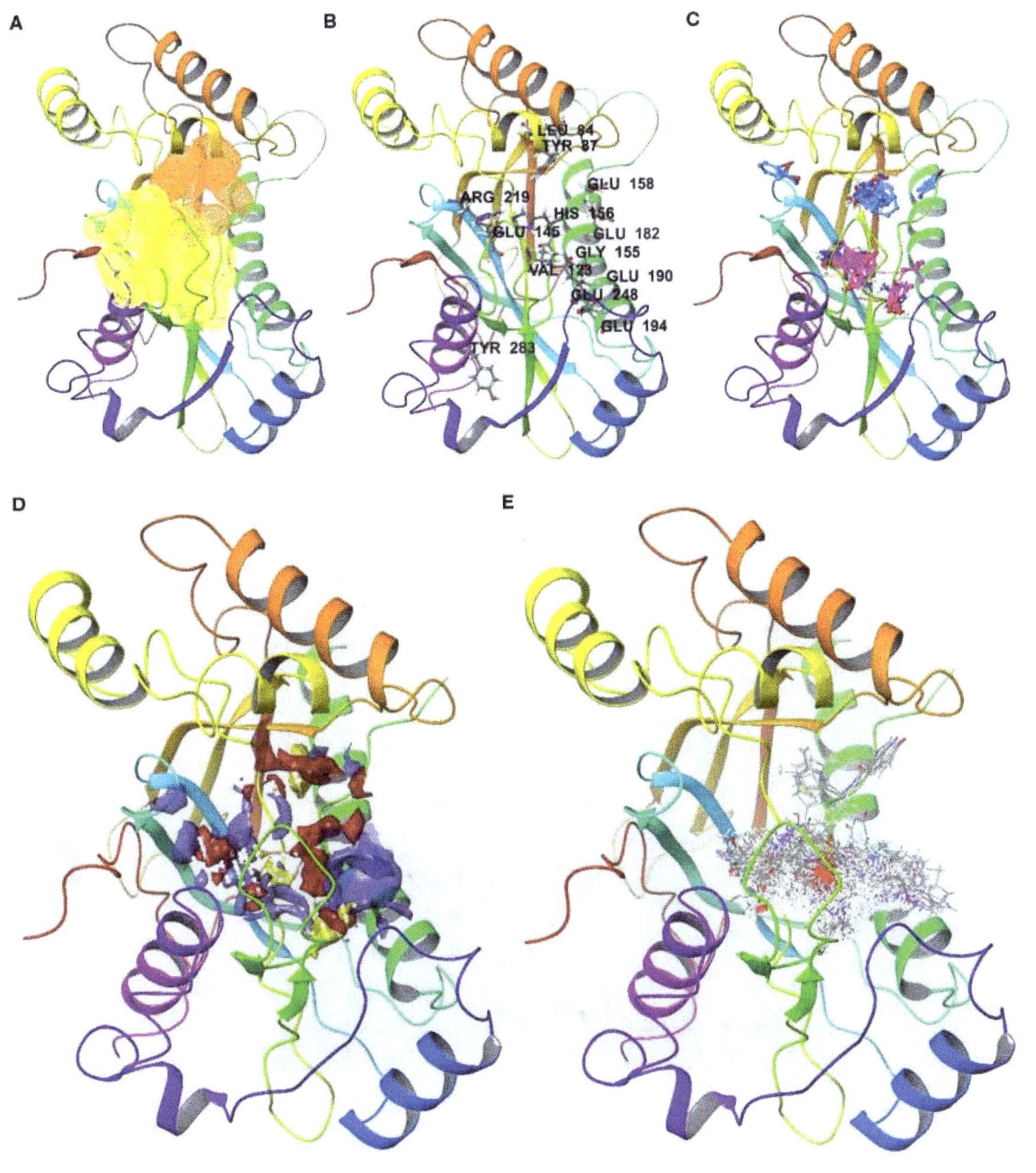

FIGURE 4 | Druggable sites of NUDT22 as identified in the automated and the user arm: **(A)** Rigid assessment with DoGSite identifies a second highly druggable site (orange, DrugScore 0.81) in close proximity to the highest-ranking site (yellow, DrugScore 0.82); **(B)** Flexible assessment with CryptoSite predicts 52 amino acid residues around both pockets as part of an extended 3D network. Highlighted amino acid residues possess cryptic score over 0.2; **(C)** FTMap confirms all cluster hotspots and at least 16 probes within 5 Å radius of either of the binding sites (site 1: pink; site 2: light blue) or high cryptic value sites. **(D)** SiteMap combines the two sites identified by DogSite into a single large binding pocket with an evenly distribution of hydrophobic (yellow) and hydrophilic (red and purple) patches; **(E)** cascade docking of the ZINC fragment library shows a preference for the active site, while the second druggable site is only engaged by members of one chemotype among the top 1000 fragments. The assessment highlights NUDT22 comprising two adjacent druggable sites which in a prospective drug discovery campaign could be targeted separately or in combination.

a detailed picture of druggability and for specific assessment of proteins with similar Dscores and/or sequence.

When SiteMap was applied on the NUDIX hydrolases, the obtained Dscores of the highest-ranking sites were between 0.51 and 1.11 with an average of 0.88 (**Figure 5A** and **Supplementary Material** -SiteMap). Interestingly, except for NUDT4, all identified highest-ranking sites were in overlapping regions or even identical with sites identified with DoGSite

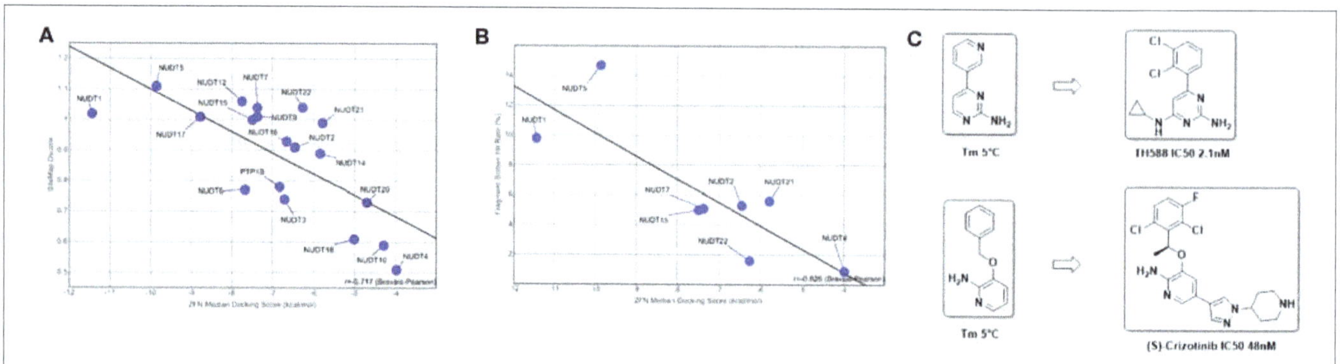

FIGURE 5 | Predictive value of *in silico* assessment and docking for in vitro screening hit rates and suitability of fragment screens for chemical probe generation: **(A)** *in silico* druggability assessment of pockets identified by SiteMap correlates well with the observed ZINC Fragments Now (ZFN) median docking scores of the highest ranking 1000 fragments ($R = -0.717$); **(B)** when translated to *in vitro* to either DSF or X-Ray screens using fragment libraries with overlapping chemical space, a similar correlation can be observed, highlighting the suitability of a purely *in silico* druggability workflow as a standalone method ($R = -0.826$); **(C)** DSF fragment screens reported here yielded strong stabilizing fragment hits that are structural subunits of reported ligands for NUDT1 (Gad et al., 2014; Huber et al., 2014).

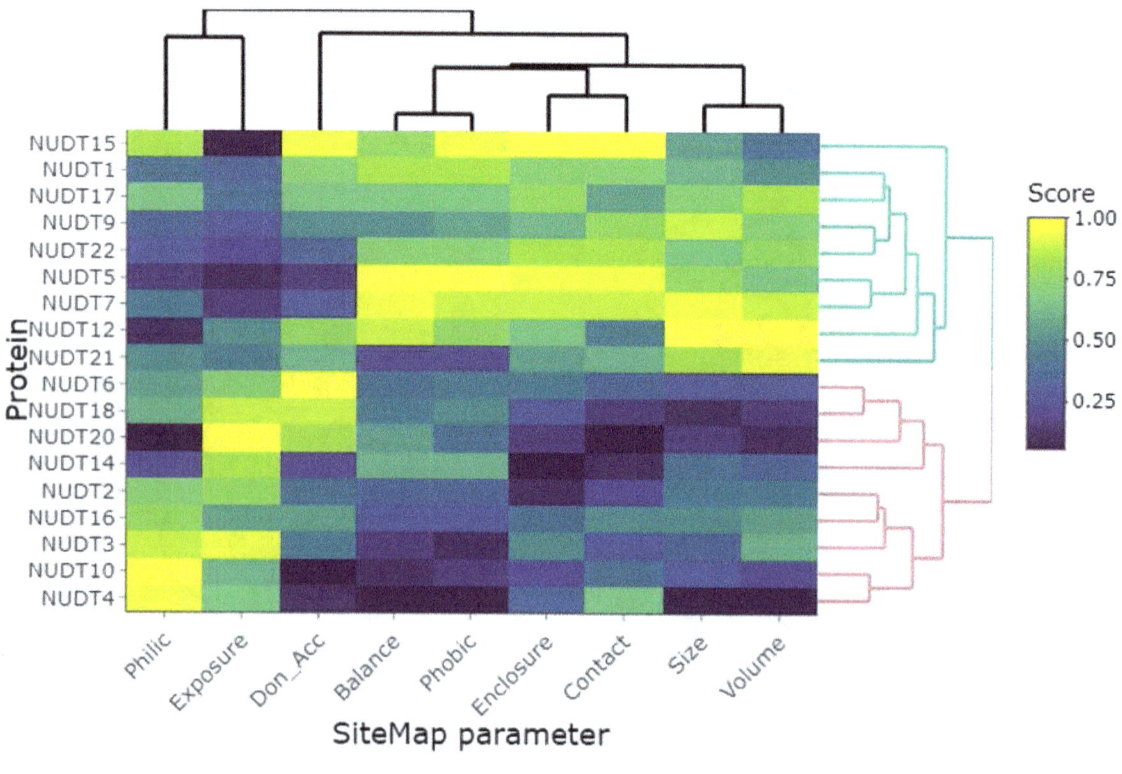

FIGURE 6 | Clustering of investigated NUDIX family members based on the primary SiteMap parameters of the top-ranked sites, resulting in a clear separation of the members deemed druggable (green branches) and those deemed undruggable (red branches).

(**Supplementary Material** - FTMap). Thus, the returned lower Dscore values for NUDT4 (0.51) and NUDT18 (0.61) were consistent between these approaches. In addition, judging by SiteMap, NUDT3 (0.74), NUDT6 (0.77), NUDT10 (0.59), NUDT20 (0.73), and PTP1B (2HNP, 0.78) were classed as difficult drug targets. The highest-ranking members and thus favored drug targets in the family were NUDT1 (1.02), NUDT5 (1.11) NUDT7 (1.04), NUDT9 (1.01), NUDT12 (1.05), NUDT15 (1.00), NUDT17 (1.01), and NUDT22 (1.04, **Figure 3**). Due to the chosen cut-off distance to merge identified pockets (5 Å), SiteMap identified large extended pockets which included several subpockets. Furthermore, as NUDT5, NUDT12, and NUDT15 are functional homodimers, these have two high-ranking pockets. Of these, NUDT12 and NUDT15 contain a third druggable site. NUDT7on the other hand possesses a second high-ranking pocket (Dscore 0.82).

Clustering of the highest-scoring SiteMap pockets using the primary SiteMap parameters shows a clear separation of druggable versus undruggable NUDIX members and allows for comparison of members which are (dis)similar in terms of their active site properties rather than based on sequence (dis)similarities (**Figure 6**). Full-length sequence identity is generally low among the NUDIX family members (see **Supplementary Material**, Percentage Identity), with the exception of NUDT3, NUDT4, NUDT10, and NUDT11. The former 3 being deemed challenging targets and NUDT11 was not evaluated due to lack of structural data. General selectivity issues are thus not anticipated when targeting a specific NUDIX family member. On the other hand, several members have some degree of overlap in their substrate specificity, e.g. NUDT1, 15 and 18 as a subgroup, and NUDT5, NUDT9, NUDT12, and NUDT14 as a second subgroup (Carreras-Puigvert et al., 2017), implying that their active sites share some structural similarity. In this context, the SiteMap parameter profile of NUDT5 is a good reference as it has the highest Dscore of all members. In comparison, NUDT9 has a less favorable balance in hydrophobic and hydrophilic character, while the active site of NUDT12 is somewhat more exposed than NUDT5, but also larger. Although these 3 members have high Dscores, classing them clearly as druggable, they vary in their capacity to accommodate different fragments, as it is reflected by their different median docking scores further down (**Figure 5**). NUDT14 is considered challenging, primarily due to its smaller active site which also is more exposed.

NUDT15 and NUDT18 have been hypothesized to be able to act as back-up enzymes for NUDT1 due to their overlapping substrate specificities. Comparison of their SiteMap parameter profiles shows clear differences despite NUDT1 and NUDT15 being among the NUDIX members with highest Dscores. The active site of NUDT15 is somewhat smaller and more enclosed than for NUDT1 due to an inward movement of a helix (Carter et al., 2015). NUDT18 is considered to be challenging due to its small and more exposed active site. This also results in a poor fragment scoring profile (please see below). Collectively, these differences in site parameters allow for the development of highly selective chemical probes, as witnessed for NUDT1 and NUDT5 (Gad et al., 2014; Page et al., 2018).

User Arm – Step 2: *in silico* Docking of ZINC Library

As a final druggability assessment and potential to identify starting points amenable for a fragment growing-based drug discovery campaign out of commercial fragment space, we performed *in silico* docking campaigns of the ZINC Frag now database (Irwin et al., 2012) against the structures under consideration. The comprehensive fragment library was filtered against unwanted structural motifs and prepared for docking using a KNIME workflow (Berthold et al., 2008). For a detailed description, please refer to the Methods part of this manuscript. Ultimately, 205,891 fragments remained after filtering the original set of 704,041 ZINC fragments. Using the Schrödinger suite, ligand preparation and grid generation for the highest-ranking pocket as identified by SiteMap were performed to enable virtual screening of this subset applying three stages of accuracy. In each stage, the top-ranked 10% of compounds were retained and passed on to the next stage. Finally, the top-ranked 1,000 fragments were used to calculate a median docking score enabling assessment of druggability based on commercially available fragment space. The returned median docking scores, where lower is better, ranged from−4.0 to −11.4 kcal/mol with an average of−6.8 kcal/mol. NUDT1 and NUDT5, both validated drug targets in the literature, scored−11.4 and −9.9 kcal/mol respectively. In addition, and judged by the median docking score, NUDT17 (−8.8 kcal/mol) is a third promising drug target. PTP1B (−6.8 kcal/mol) scores average among the NUDIX family members, while the scores for NUDT4 (−4.0 kcal/mol), NUDT10 (−4.3 kcal/mol), NUDT20 (−4.7 kcal/mol) and NUDT18 (−5.0 kcal/mol) indicate a potentially challenging drug discovery campaign (**Figure 5A**). When using the median docking scores and plotted against their respective SiteMap Dscores, a good inverse correlation ($R = -0.717$, Bravais-Pearson) can be observed (**Figure 5**), suggesting an *in silico*-based prioritization scheme of drug discovery campaigns against NUDIX proteins. Thus, fragment docking against the top-ranked SiteMap pockets recapitulates their druggability potential but additionally provides potential starting points readily accessible for fragment-based drug discovery campaigns.

The hydrophobicity of small-molecule drugs is a property which needs to be delicately balanced since it affects multiple parameters including solubility, permeability, plasma protein binding and metabolism. Druggable binding pockets of target proteins therefore require a certain hydrophobic-hydrophilic balance to accommodate ligands with drug-like properties. When applying a balance of at least 0.5 the SiteMap assessment prefers NUDT1 (3Q93, 0.69), NUDT5 (6GRU, 1.34), NUDT7 (5T3P, 0.72), NUDT15 (5BON, 0.62), NUDT17 (5LF8, 0.50), and NUDT22 (5LF9, 0.58) and disfavors NUDT3 (2FVV, 0.01), NUDT4 (5LTU, 0.00), NUDT10 (3MCF, 0.01), and PTP1B (2HNP, 0.05). With regard to their returned median fragment docking scores, pocket polarity might correlate with either higher or lower scores (**Supplementary Material** - ZINC fragment docking and SiteMap). A possible explanation is, that the library was filtered to fit a drug-like profile and thus preselects for druggable proteins itself, ignoring their respective pocket properties. Importantly, none of the crystal structures used here were bound to high-affinity lead compounds originating from drug discovery campaigns and hence no hydrophobic subpockets induced by such compounds where probed in this study.

When combined, the top-1,000 ranked fragments obtained for the 18 protein targets comprised 13,203 unique fragments, indicating a certain amount of "promiscuity," i.e., fragments binding to 2 or more proteins (36% of fragments). In fact, 73 fragments bound to 6 or more targets (see **Supplementary Material** - Fragment promiscuity), with one fragment hitting 11 out of 18 proteins. It should be noted that the average docking scores were rather poor, ranging from −7.56 to −5.53 kcal/mol. Of interest is the notion that the proteins

TABLE 2 | Summary of NUDIX protein family members in screens against fragment and in biochemical malachite green assays.

Protein	Screening technique	Size screening set	Hit rate
NUDT7	Fragment covalent (Resnick et al., 2019)	993	36 (3.6%)
NUDT4	Fragment diamond Xray[1]	768	7 (0.9%)
NUDT5	Fragment diamond Xray[1]	768	113 (14.7%)
NUDT7	Fragment diamond Xray[1]	768	39 (5.1%)
NUDT21	Fragment diamond Xray[1]	768	43 (5.6%)
NUDT22	Fragment diamond Xray[1]	768	12 (1.6%)
NUDT1	Fragment DSF	450	44 (9.8%)
NUDT2	Fragment DSF	650	35 (5.3%)
NUDT5	Fragment DSF	450	0*
NUDT15	Fragment DSF	1,200	60 (5.0%)
NUDT1	Biochem screen malachite green	5,336	429 (8.0%)
NUDT2	Biochem screen malachite green	5,336 [11,992]	261 (4.9%) [235 (2.0%)**]
NUDT5	Biochem screen malachite green	5,336 [72,004]	3 (0.1%) [527 (0.7%)**]
NUDT15	Biochem screen malachite green	5,336 [17,908]	10 (0.2%) [98 (0.5%)**]
NUDT16	Biochem screen malachite green	5,336	7 (0.1%)

*Please note the biochemical screen library grew over time. For comparison, results beyond the basic set of 5,336 compounds are presented in brackets. *Melting temperature unsuitable for thermal shift screens; **Definition of hit more stringent.*

deemed undruggable by SiteMap appeared to be enriched for promiscuous fragment hits (except NUDT10 and NUDT20), as opposed to druggable proteins (except NUDT15 and NUDT22). A certain degree of promiscuity should be expected when docking 200K fragments to multiple targets, as this is in line with the basic concept of fragment-based drug discovery, i.e., the ability of low-complexity fragments to interact with a multitude of (sub)pockets across a wide range of proteins.

Correlation With Experimental Fragment-Based and Biochemical Screening Data

A number of fragment screens against NUDIX proteins have been performed by others and us[1]. For a list of applied screening techniques, library sets and hit rates, please see **Table 2**. When the hit rates of the fragment screens were compared with the *in silico*-derived median ZFN docking scores a good correlation was observed (Bravais-Pearson 0.826; **Figure 5B**). This underscores the applicability of *in silico* docking for rapid protein druggability assessment. In agreement with most computational assessments, NUDT1 and NUDT5 yield high hit rates of 9.8% and 14.7%, respectively, while the experimental hit rate of 0.9% for NUDT4 confirms its challenging character predicted by computational assessment. Other NUDIX proteins are in the range of common hit rates for fragment screens and between 1.6 and 5.6% (Aretz et al., 2014). This observation holds true for different sets screened by different groups (**Figures 5B**, **7**). Interestingly, the DSF screen against NUDT1 found two structures with a strong thermal stabilization of 5°C. These structures are fragments of the reported NUDT1 inhibitors TH588 (IC50: 2.1 nM) and Crizotinib (IC50: 48 nM) and thus underscore the suitability of DSF to find starting points for lead generation (**Figure 5C**). However, DSF is not feasible for proteins with high native melting points (e.g., NUDT5, 76°C), and here *in silico* fragment screening against druggable sites may be particularly advantageous.

Several biochemical screening campaigns against NUDIX proteins have also been performed in our laboratories. While compound libraries have varied somewhat between targets, reflecting development of the compound libraries over time, there is a small core set of about 5,300 chemically diverse compounds that have been tested for all proteins. It is noteworthy that these screens were performed based on a common screening platform employing a coupled enzymatic assay with a malachite green readout. This cost-effective assay has been frequently employed in our lab, including screens on other nucleotide-processing targets such as dCTPase (Llona-Minguez et al., 2016), ITPase and dUTPase, and with robust performance in compound sets beyond 100,000 compounds (all unpublished). A key reason for this is the low rates of interference with the coupled enzymes and the absorbance readout at 630 nm, as evidenced by a low appearance of common hits. Also, the presence of PAINS and aggregators within hit lists is generally low for this family of proteins (**Supplementary Material** – Screens using malachite green), demonstrating robust screening performance of the recombinantly produced proteins and other assay components. The biochemical screen outcomes are summarized in detail in **Table 2** and in the **Supplementary Material** – Screens using malachite green. In line with assessments of chemical amenability and learnings in the fragment-based screens, the majority of targets generated hits that confirmed activity in follow-up studies, with NUDT1 demonstrating an extreme hit rate in this sub-set. This significant amenability is in line with the publication of hits from multiple groups. A critical outlier in this set was NUDT5, which demonstrated hit rates as low as notoriously challenging targets dUTPase and ITPase, while predictions and fragment-based screening showed the opposite (**Supplementary Material** – Fragment screening hit rates). Already at the time of screening we had a reason to revisit the screening data for NUDT5 and follow-up studies demonstrated competition between active site hits and a structurally important Mg^{2+} (Costa and Dieckmann, 2011; Vardakou et al., 2014). After correction of the assay buffer, by lowering the $MgCl_2$ concentration 10-fold, we observed significantly higher hit rates in the subsequently applied compound sets and identified compounds that could be further optimized to nM potencies (Page et al., 2018). As a general observation and for the five NUDIX protein members screened, no correlation between ZINC fragment docking scores and observed hit rates from biochemical screening can be observed (**Supplementary Material** - Screens using malachite green). In contrast to the covered fragment library chemical space, a rule-of-five compliant library of few thousand compounds may complement the search for a chemical starting point but may be limited in coverage of chemical space itself. However, in the past we have shown, that embarking on drug discovery campaigns from observed hits in both fragment and biochemical screen lead to successful generation of chemical probes for a number of NUDIX protein family members and other pyrophosphatases (Gad et al., 2014; Llona-Minguez et al., 2016; Page et al., 2018)[2].

CONCLUSION AND SUMMARY

Here we presented a dual *in silico* druggability assessment workflow suitable for large-scale evaluation of proteins and protein families, applied to the NUDIX family. Initially, we introduced a hands-on workflow solely based on the protein crystal structure using the open access server of DogSite (Volkamer et al., 2012) and FTMap (Kozakov et al., 2015) for rigid and CryptoSite (Cimermancic et al., 2016) and FTMap for dynamic assessment. Importantly, before using these servers, thorough manual protein structure verification is necessary to exclude artifacts due to crystal packing, construct used and resolution limits. On the one hand, DogSite returns both identity and score of druggable sites, while FTMap docks small organic solvent molecules. Especially in cases of sparsely evaluated proteins or protein complexes this dual assessment may be beneficial for structural assessment and potential chemical probe generation. On the other hand, CryptoSite identifies conformationally active amino acid residues. In the past, the returned cryptic scores have been correlated with FTMap solvent docking and eased decision on whether or where potential allosteric sites may be situated (Vajda et al., 2018). Timewise, this quick computational assessment may be achieved within days for singular proteins and weeks for small protein families. Depending on local load and choice of sever location the return time is usually minutes for DogSite, hours for FTMap, and 1 day for CryptoSite. The detailed assessment and correlation of data from the different algorithms allows for the rationalization of targeting strategies. In case of the NUDIX proteins, NUDT22 for example showed to have high scores in DogSite and FTMap with CryptoSite confirming flexibility around two closely related sites. Further, in the past we have shown that comparing different crystals structures of the same protein can allow for the observation of targetable conformations more suitable small-molecule development (Michel et al., 2019). With the open access deposition of all screening data by the SGC, a similar albeit more time consuming approach is possible for a number of NUDIX proteins[1].

In a second, user-guided arm we assessed protein druggability employing several implemented functions in Schrödinger's commercial small-molecule modeling suite combined with freely available KNIME (Berthold et al., 2008). First, proteins were interrogated for potential binding pockets and the corresponding DScores using SiteMap. The highest ranking pockets were then

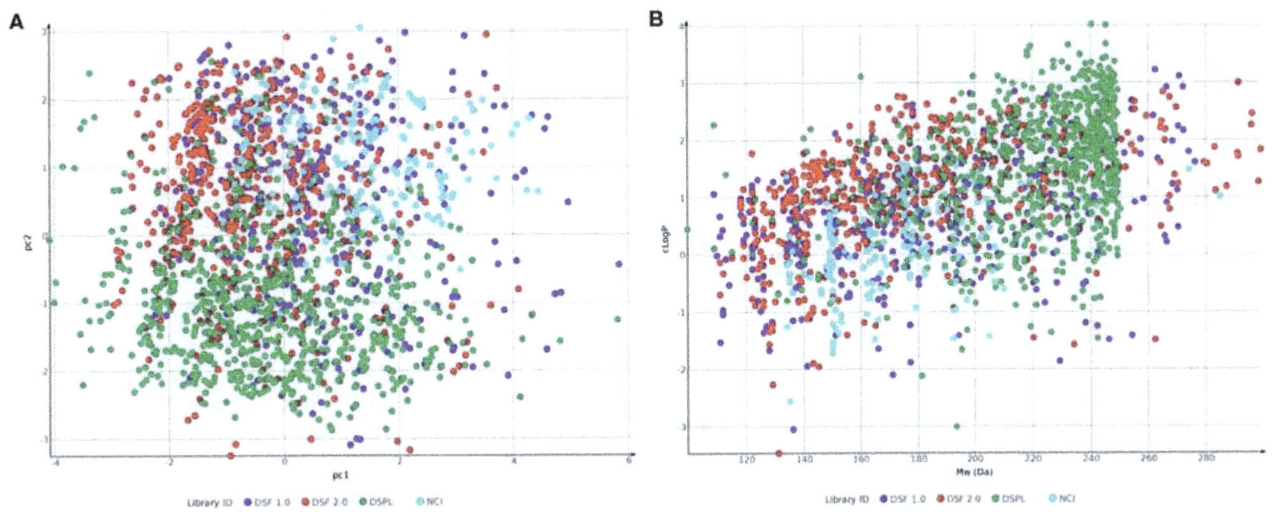

FIGURE 7 | Comparison of fragment libraries used in screens against NUDIX protein family members: Laboratory for Chemical Biology at Karolinska Institutet (LCBKI) DSF fragment library of the first generation (DSF 1.0, blue), additional members of a second generation DSF fragment library (DSF 2.0, red), Nucleobase analogs (NCI, light blue) and Diamond-SGC Poised Library (DSPL, green) with respect to: **(A)** physicochemical property coverage and diversity, expressed as the first two principal components (pc1 and pc2) obtained from a principal component analysis (PCA) on six Lipinski-type properties; **(B)** clogP against Molecular weight.

used to perform cascade docking with a filtered ZINC fragment library (Irwin et al., 2012). Subsequently, the median docking score of the top-1,000 ranked fragments was used as a chemical space-based druggability assessment. Both parameters, DScore and median docking score form the basis of this second *in silico* druggability assessment and require few days per protein, depending on the user set up and the size of the used *in silico* library. The observed docking scores correlate well with predicted DScores (**Figure 5A**) and additionally provide commercially accessible chemical starting points for the development of chemical probes. At last, when compared with experimental fragment screens based on X-ray crystallography, a covalent set and thermal stabilization in DSF, a similar correlation was observed between hit rates and median docking scores (**Figure 5B**), even when using chemically distinct screening sets (**Figure 7**). This supports the applicability of an *in silico* druggability workflow as a standalone method for protein assessment and speaks for the chemical space coverage of fragment libraries generated at CBCS and Diamond/SGC (Michel et al., 2019)[7].

In summary, we report here a fully *in silico* druggability assessment of the NUDIX protein family, that serves as a standalone method and a workflow to identify the most suitable members for a drug discovery campaign. We show that the dual assessment correlates well with experimental results and further allows for the *in silico* identification of secondary druggable sites, alternative targeting strategies and structural basis for fragment growing campaigns. Importantly, the workflow allows for rapid assessment of any protein with reported structures in the protein data bank and as such should be broadly applicable in early drug discovery campaigns.

AUTHOR CONTRIBUTIONS

MM and EH compiled the list of PDB structures and performed protein preparation and validation. MM controlled end stage correlation and assessment and performed tasks in the automated arm. EH performed tasks in the User arm. EW, KP, IA, A-LG, and TL performed assays, fragment, and biochemical high-throughput screens. MM and EH rationalized and designed the project. UW and TH supervised the project. MM, EH, AG, and TL wrote the manuscript. MM coordinated collaborations. All authors commented on the manuscript.

FUNDING

Funding was obtained from the Swedish Cancer Society (TH), the Swedish Children's Cancer Foundation (TH), ERC Tarox-695376 (TH) and Swedish Pain Relief Foundation (TH). Chemical Biology Consortium Sweden received funding from the Swedish Research Council, Karolinska Institutet and SciLifeLab during the course of this work.

ACKNOWLEDGMENTS

The authors gratefully acknowledge the national infrastructure of CBCS and LCBKI for supplying the DSF fragment and HTS library and help during development and performance of the HTS assay for different NUDIX protein family members. The Protein Science Facility of Karolinska Institutet was acknowledged for protein production. Further, the operators of CryptoSite at the University of California, San Francisco, DogSite at the Zentrum für Bioinformatik, University of Hamburg and FTMap at Boston University are acknowledged for their computing set up and the open access to program code. Dana Michel was acknowledged for her critical discussion and proofreading of the manuscript.

REFERENCES

Abdelraheim, S. R., Spiller, D. G., and McLennan, A. G. (2003). Mammalian NADH diphosphatases of the nudix family: cloning and characterization of the human peroxisomal NUDT12 protein. *Biochem. J.* 374(Pt. 2), 329–335. doi: 10.1042/bj20030441

An, S., and Fu, L. (2018). Small-molecule PROTACs: an emerging and promising approach for the development of targeted therapy drugs. *EBioMedicine* 36, 553–562. doi: 10.1016/j.ebiom.2018.09.005

Aretz, J., Anumala, U. R., Fuchsberger, F. F., Molavi, N., Ziebart, N., Zhang, H., et al. (2018). Allosteric inhibition of a mammalian lectin. *J. Am. Chem. Soc.* 140, 14915–14925. doi: 10.1021/jacs.8b08644

Aretz, J., Wamhoff, E.-C., Hanske, J., Heymann, D., and Rademacher, C. (2014). Computational and experimental prediction of human C-type lectin receptor druggability. *Front. Immunol.* 5:323. doi: 10.3389/fimmu.2014.00323

Baell, J. B., and Holloway, G. A. (2010). New substructure filters for removal of pan assay interference compounds (PAINS) from screening libraries and for their exclusion in bioassays. *J. Med. Chem.* 53, 2719–2740. doi: 10.1021/jm901137j

Barford, D., Flint, A. J., and Tonks, N. K. (1994). Crystal structure of human protein tyrosine phosphatase 1B. *Science* 263, 1397–1404. doi: 10.1126/science.8128219

Baykov, A. A., Evtushenko, O. A., and Avaeva, S. M. (1988). A malachite green procedure for orthophosphate determination and its use in alkaline phosphatase-based enzyme immunoassay. *Anal. Biochem.* 171, 266–270. doi: 10.1016/0003-2697(88)90484-8

Berthold, M. R., Cebron, N., Dill, F., Gabriel, T. R., Kötter, T., Meinl, T., et al. (2008). "KNIME: The Konstanz Information Miner," in *Data Analysis, Machine Learning and Applications; Studies in Classification, Data Analysis, and Knowledge Organization*, eds C. Preisach, H. Burkhardt, L.

Schmidt-Thieme, and R. Decker (Berlin; Heidelberg: Springer). p. 319–326. doi: 10.1007/978-3-540-78246-9_38

Caffrey, J. J., Hidaka, K., Matsuda, M., Hirata, M., and Shears, S. B. (1999). The human and rat forms of multiple inositol polyphosphate phosphatase: functional homology with a histidine acid phosphatase up-regulated during endochondral ossification. *FEBS Lett.* 442, 99–104. doi: 10.1016/S0014-5793(98)01636-6

Caffrey, J. J., Safrany, S. T., Yang, X., and Shears, S. B. (2000). Discovery of molecular and catalytic diversity among human diphosphoinositol-polyphosphate phosphohydrolases. an expanding nudt family. *J. Biol. Chem.* 275, 12730–12736. doi: 10.1074/jbc.275.17.12730

Carreras-Puigvert, J., Zitnik, M., Jemth, A.-S., Carter, M., Unterlass, J. E., Hallström, B., et al. (2017). A comprehensive structural, biochemical and biological profiling of the human NUDIX hydrolase family. *Nat. Commun.* 8:1541. doi: 10.1038/s41467-017-01642-w

Carter, M., Jemth, A.-S., Hagenkort, A., Page, B. D. G., Gustafsson, R., Griese, J. J., et al. (2015). Crystal structure, biochemical and cellular activities demonstrate separate functions of MTH1 and MTH2. *Nat. Commun.* 6:7871. doi: 10.1038/ncomms8871

Choi, S.-Y., Jang, J. H., and Kim, K. R. (2011). Analysis of Differentially Expressed Genes in Human rectal carcinoma using suppression subtractive hybridization. *Clin. Exp. Med.* 11, 219–226. doi: 10.1007/s10238-010-0130-5

Cimermancic, P., Weinkam, P., Rettenmaier, T. J., Bichmann, L., Keedy, D. A., Woldeyes, R. A., et al. (2016). CryptoSite: expanding the druggable proteome by characterization and prediction of cryptic binding sites. *J. Mol. Biol.* 428, 709–719. doi: 10.1016/j.jmb.2016.01.029

Coseno, M., Martin, G., Berger, C., Gilmartin, G., Keller, W., and Doublié, S. (2008). Crystal structure of the 25 KDa subunit of human cleavage factor I_m. *Nucleic Acids Res.* 36, 3474–3483. doi: 10.1093/nar/gkn079

Costa, J. B. D., and Dieckmann, T. (2011). Entropy and Mg2+ control ligand affinity and specificity in the malachite green binding RNA aptamer. *Mol. BioSyst.* 7, 2156–2163. doi: 10.1039/c1mb05075c

Dubianok, Y., Collins, P., Krojer, T., Fairhead, M., MacLean, E., Diaz, S., et al. (2018). *LPDB 6gru Structure Summary ‹ Protein Data Bank in Europe (PDBe) ‹ EMBL-EBI.* Available online at: https://www.ebi.ac.uk/pdbe/entry/pdb/6gru (accessed June 3, 2019).

Ellermann, M., Eheim, A., Rahm, F., Viklund, J., Guenther, J., Andersson, M., et al. (2017). Novel class of potent and cellularly active inhibitors devalidates MTH1 as broad-spectrum cancer target. *ACS Chem. Biol.* 12, 1986–1992. doi: 10.1021/acschembio.7b00370

Farand, J., Kropf, J. E., Blomgren, P., Xu, J., Schmitt, A. C., Newby, Z. E., et al. (2020). Discovery of potent and selective MTH1 inhibitors for oncology: enabling rapid target (In)validation. *ACS Med. Chem. Lett.* 11, 358–364. doi: 10.1021/acsmedchemlett.9b00420

Friesner, R. A., Banks, J. L., Murphy, R. B., Halgren, T. A., Klicic, J. J., Mainz, D. T., et al. (2004). Glide: a new approach for rapid, accurate docking and scoring. 1. method and assessment of docking accuracy. *J. Med. Chem.* 47, 1739–1749. doi: 10.1021/jm0306430

Friesner, R. A., Murphy, R. B., Repasky, M. P., Frye, L. L., Greenwood, J. R., Halgren, T. A., et al. (2006). Extra precision glide: docking and scoring incorporating a model of hydrophobic enclosure for protein–ligand complexes. *J. Med. Chem.* 49, 6177–6196. doi: 10.1021/jm051256o

Gad, H., Koolmeister, T., Jemth, A.-S., Eshtad, S., Jacques, S. A., Ström, C. E., et al. (2014). MTH1 inhibition eradicates cancer by preventing sanitation of the DNTP pool. *Nature* 508, 215–221. doi: 10.1038/nature13181

Ge, H., Chen, X., Yang, W., Niu, L., and Teng, M. (2013). Crystal structure of wild-type and mutant human Ap4A hydrolase. *Biochem. Biophys. Res. Commun.* 432, 16–21. doi: 10.1016/j.bbrc.2013.01.095

Greenwood, J. R., Calkins, D., Sullivan, A. P., and Shelley, J. C. (2010). Towards the comprehensive, rapid, and accurate prediction of the favorable tautomeric states of drug-like molecules in aqueous solution. *J. Comput. Aided Mol. Des.* 24, 591–604. doi: 10.1007/s10822-010-9349-1

Halgren, T. (2007). New method for fast and accurate binding-site identification and analysis. *Chem Biol Drug Des.* 69, 146–148. doi: 10.1111/j.1747-0285.2007.00483.x

Halgren, T. A. (2009). Identifying and characterizing binding sites and assessing druggability. *J. Chem. Inf. Model* 49, 377–389. doi: 10.1021/ci800324m

Halgren, T. A., Murphy, R. B., Friesner, R. A., Beard, H. S., Frye, L. L., Pollard, W. T., et al. (2004). Glide: a new approach for rapid, accurate docking and scoring. 2. enrichment factors in database screening. *J. Med. Chem.* 47, 1750–1759. doi: 10.1021/jm030644s

Huber, K. V. M., Salah, E., Radic, B., Gridling, M., Elkins, J. M., Stukalov, A., et al. (2014). Stereospecific targeting of MTH1 by (S)-crizotinib as an anticancer strategy. *Nature* 508, 222–227. doi: 10.1038/nature13194

Irwin, J. J., Sterling, T., Mysinger, M. M., Bolstad, E. S., and Coleman, R. G. (2012). ZINC: a free tool to discover chemistry for biology. *J. Chem. Inf. Model* 52, 1757–1768. doi: 10.1021/ci3001277

Kettle, J. G., Alwan, H., Bista, M., Breed, J., Davies, N. L., Eckersley, K., et al. (2016). Potent and selective inhibitors of MTH1 probe its role in cancer cell survival. *J. Med. Chem.* 59, 2346–2361. doi: 10.1021/acs.jmedchem.5b01760

Kozakov, D., Grove, L. E., Hall, D. R., Bohnuud, T., Mottarella, S. E., Luo, L., et al. (2015). The FTMap family of web servers for determining and characterizing ligand-binding hot spots of proteins. *Nat. Protoc.* 10, 733–755. doi: 10.1038/nprot.2015.043

Krishnan, N., Konidaris, K. F., Gasser, G., and Tonks, N. K. (2018). A potent, selective, and orally bioavailable inhibitor of the protein-tyrosine phosphatase PTP1B improves insulin and leptin signaling in animal models. *J. Biol. Chem.* 293, 1517–1525. doi: 10.1074/jbc.C117.819110

Llona-Minguez, S., Höglund, A., Jacques, S. A., Johansson, L., Calderón-Montaño, J. M., Claesson, M., et al. (2016). Discovery of the first potent and selective inhibitors of human DCTP pyrophosphatase 1. *J. Med. Chem.* 59, 1140–1148. doi: 10.1021/acs.jmedchem.5b01741

Mathea, S., Salah, E., Velupillai, S., Tallant, C., Pike, A. C. W., Bushell, S. R., et al. (2017b). *PDB 5mp0 Structure Summary ‹ Protein Data Bank in Europe (PDBe) ‹ EMBL-EBI.* Available online at: https://www.ebi.ac.uk/pdbe/entry/pdb/5mp0 (accessed June 3, 2019).

Mathea, S., Tallant, C., Salah, E., Wang, D., Velupillai, S., Nowak, R., et al. (2017a). *PDB 5lf8 Structure Summary ‹ Protein Data Bank in Europe (PDBe) ‹ EMBL-EBI.* Available online at: https://www.ebi.ac.uk/pdbe/entry/pdb/5lf8 (accessed June 3, 2019).

Michel, M., Visnes, T., Homan, E. J., Seashore-Ludlow, B., Hedenström, M., Wiita, E., et al. (2019). Computational and experimental druggability assessment of human DNA glycosylases. *ACS Omega* 4, 11642–11656. doi: 10.1021/acsomega.9b00162

Mullard, A. (2018). Phosphatases start shedding their stigma of undruggability. *Nat. Rev. Drug Discov.* 17, 847–849. doi: 10.1038/nrd.2018.201

Niesen, F. H., Berglund, H., and Vedadi, M. (2007). The use of differential scanning fluorimetry to detect ligand interactions that promote protein stability. *Nat. Protoc.* 2, 2212–2221. doi: 10.1038/nprot.2007.321

Page, B. D. G., Valerie, N. C. K., Wright, R. H. G., Wallner, O., Isaksson, R., Carter, M., et al. (2018). Targeted NUDT5 inhibitors block hormone signaling in breast cancer cells. *Nat. Commun.* 9:250. doi: 10.1038/s41467-017-02293-7

Petrocchi, A., Leo, E., Reyna, N. J., Hamilton, M. M., Shi, X., Parker, C. A., et al. (2016). Identification of potent and selective MTH1 inhibitors. *Bioorg. Med. Chem. Lett.* 26, 1503–1507. doi: 10.1016/j.bmcl.2016.02.026

Resnick, E., Bradley, A., Gan, J., Douangamath, A., Krojer, T., Sethi, R., et al. (2019). Rapid covalent-probe discovery by electrophile-fragment screening. *J. Am. Chem. Soc.* 141:8951–8968. doi: 10.1021/jacs.9b02822

Samaranayake, G. J., Huynh, M., and Rai, P. (2017). MTH1 as a chemotherapeutic target: the elephant in the room. *Cancers* 9:47. doi: 10.3390/cancers9050047

Shelley, J. C., Cholleti, A., Frye, L. L., Greenwood, J. R., Timlin, M. R., and Uchimaya, M. (2007). Epik: a software program for PK prediction and protonation state generation for drug-like molecules. *J. Comput. Aided. Mol. Des.* 21, 681–691. doi: 10.1007/s10822-007-9133-z

Shen, B. W., Perraud, A.-L., Scharenberg, A., and Stoddard, B. L. (2003). The crystal structure and mutational analysis of human NUDT9. *J. Mol. Biol.* 332, 385–398. doi: 10.1016/S0022-2836(03)00954-9

Srikannathasan, V., Nunez, C. A., Tallant, C., Siejka, P., Mathea, S., Kopec, J., et al. (2017b). *PDB 5t3p Structure Summary ‹ Protein Data Bank in Europe (PDBe) ‹ EMBL-EBI.* Available online at: https://www.ebi.ac.uk/pdbe/entry/pdb/5t3p (accessed June 3, 2019).

Srikannathasan, V., Nunez, C. A., Tallant, C., Siejka, P., Mathea, S., Newman, J., et al. (2017a). *PDB 5ltu Structure Summary ‹ Protein Data Bank in Europe (PDBe) ‹ EMBL-EBI.* Available online at: https://www.ebi.ac.uk/pdbe/entry/pdb/5ltu (accessed June 3, 2019).

Tallant, C., Siejka, P., Mathea, S., Shrestha, L., Krojer, T., Srikannathasan, V., et al. (2017). *PDB 5lf9 structure summary ‹ Protein Data Bank in Europe (PDBe) ‹ EMBL-EBI*. Available online at: https://www.ebi.ac.uk/pdbe/entry/pdb/5lf9 (accessed June 3, 2019).

Thorsell, A.-G., Persson, C., Gräslund, S., Hammarström, M., Busam, R. D., and Hallberg, B. M. (2009). Crystal structure of human diphosphoinositol phosphatase 1. *Proteins* 77, 242–246. doi: 10.1002/prot.22489

Trésaugues, L., Lundbäck, T., Welin, M., Flodin, S., Nyman, T., Silvander, C., et al. (2015). Structural basis for the specificity of human nudt16 and its regulation by inosine monophosphate. *PLoS ONE* 10:e0131507. doi: 10.1371/journal.pone.0131507

Tresaugues, L., Moche, M., Arrowsmith, C. H., Berglund, H., Bountra, C., Collinsm, R., et al. (2009a). *PDB 3h95 Structure Summary ‹ Protein Data Bank in Europe (PDBe) ‹ EMBL-EBI*. Available online at: https://www.ebi.ac.uk/pdbe/entry/pdb/3h95 (accessed June 3, 2019).

Tresaugues, L., Moche, M., Arrowsmith, C. H., Berglund, H., Busam, R. D., and Collins, R. (2008). *PDB 3cou Structure Summary ‹ Protein Data Bank in Europe (PDBe) ‹ EMBL-EBI*. Available online at: https://www.ebi.ac.uk/pdbe/entry/pdb/3cou (accessed June 3, 2019).

Tresaugues, L., Siponen, M. I., Arrowsmith, C. H., Berglund, H., Bountra, C., Collins, R., et al. (2011a). *PDB 3q93 structure summary ‹ Protein Data Bank in Europe (PDBe) ‹ EMBL-EBI*. Available online at: https://www.ebi.ac.uk/pdbe/entry/pdb/3q93 (accessed June 3, 2019).

Tresaugues, L., Siponen, M. I., Arrowsmith, C. H., Berglund, H., Bountra, C., Collins, R., et al. (2011b). *PDB 3q91 Structure Summary ‹ Protein Data Bank in Europe (PDBe) ‹ EMBL-EBI*. Available online at: https://www.ebi.ac.uk/pdbe/entry/pdb/3q91 (accessed June 3, 2019).

Tresaugues, L., Siponen, M. I., Lehtio, L., Arrowsmith, C. H., Berglund, H., Bountra, C., et al. (2009b). *PDB 3gg6 Structure Summary ‹ Protein Data Bank in Europe (PDBe) ‹ EMBL-EBI*. Available online at: https://www.ebi.ac.uk/pdbe/entry/pdb/3gg6 (accessed June 3, 2019).

Tresaugues, L., Welin, M., Arrowsmith, C. H., Berglund, H., Bountra, C., Collins, R., et al. (2010). *PDB 3mcf structure summary ‹ Protein Data Bank in Europe (PDBe) ‹ EMBL-EBI*. Available online at: https://www.ebi.ac.uk/pdbe/entry/pdb/3mcf (accessed June 3, 2019).

Tsuzuki, T., Egashira, A., and Kura, S. (2001). Analysis of MTH1 gene function in mice with targeted mutagenesis. *Mutat. Res.* 477, 71–78. doi: 10.1016/S0027-5107(01)00108-7

Vajda, S., Beglov, D., Wakefield, A. E., Egbert, M., and Whitty, A. (2018). Cryptic binding sites on proteins: definition, detection, and druggability. *Curr. Opin. Chem. Biol.* 44, 1–8. doi: 10.1016/j.cbpa.2018.05.003

Vardakou, M., Salmon, M., Faraldos, J. A., and O'Maille, P. E. (2014). Comparative analysis and validation of the malachite green assay for the high throughput biochemical characterization of terpene synthases. *MethodsX* 1, 187–196. doi: 10.1016/j.mex.2014.08.007

Volkamer, A., Kuhn, D., Rippmann, F., and Rarey, M. (2012). DoGSiteScorer: a web server for automatic binding site prediction, analysis and druggability assessment. *Bioinformatics* 28, 2074–2075. doi: 10.1093/bioinformatics/bts310

Walters, W. P., and Murcko, M. A. (2002). Prediction of "drug-likeness". *Adv. Drug Deliv. Rev.* 54, 255–271. doi: 10.1016/S0169-409X(02)00003-0

Warpman Berglund, U., Sanjiv, K., Gad, H., Kalderén, C., Koolmeister, T., Pham, T., et al. (2016). Validation and development of MTH1 inhibitors for treatment of cancer. *Ann. Oncol.* 27, 2275–2283. doi: 10.1093/annonc/mdw429

Wenthur, C. J., Gentry, P. R., Mathews, T. P., and Lindsley, C. W. (2014). Drugs for allosteric sites on receptors. *Annu Rev Pharmacol Toxicol* 54, 165–184. doi: 10.1146/annurev-pharmtox-010611-134525

Wright, R. H. G., Lioutas, A., Le Dily, F., Soronellas, D., Pohl, A., Bonet, J., et al. (2016). ADP-ribose-derived nuclear ATP synthesis by NUDIX5 is required for chromatin remodeling. *Science* 352, 1221–1225. doi: 10.1126/science.aad9335

Wu, H., Li, L., Chen, K.-M., Homolka, D., Gos, P., Fleury-Olela, F., et al. (2019). Decapping enzyme NUDT12 partners with BLMH for cytoplasmic surveillance of NAD-capped RNAs. *Cell Rep.* 29, 4422–4434.e13. doi: 10.1016/j.celrep.2019.11.108

Yueh, C., Rettenmaier, T. J., Xia, B., Hall, D. R., Alekseenko, A., Porter, K. A., et al. (2019). Kinase atlas: druggability analysis of potential allosteric sites in kinases. *J. Med. Chem.* 62, 6512–6524. doi: 10.1021/acs.jmedchem.9b00089

Zhang, S., and Zhang, Z.-Y. (2007). PTP1B as a drug target: recent developments in PTP1B inhibitor discovery. *Drug Discov. Today* 12, 373–381. doi: 10.1016/j.drudis.2007.03.011

Zhou, W., Ma, L., Yang, J., Qiao, H., Li, L., and Guo, Q., et al. (2019). Potent and specific MTH1 inhibitors targeting gastric cancer. *Cell Death Dis.* 10:434. doi: 10.1038/s41419-019-1665-3

14

Competition Between Phenothiazines and BH3 Peptide for the Binding Site of the Antiapoptotic BCL-2 Protein

Aline Lagoeiro do Carmo [1], *Fernanda Bettanin* [2], *Michell Oliveira Almeida* [3], *Simone Queiroz Pantaleão* [1], *Tiago Rodrigues* [1], *Paula Homem-de-Mello* [1*] and *Kathia Maria Honorio* [1,2*]

[1] Centro de Ciências Naturais e Humanas, Universidade Federal do ABC, Santo André, Brazil, [2] Escola de Artes, Ciências e Humanidades, Universidade de São Paulo (USP), São Paulo, Brazil, [3] Instituto de Química de São Carlos, Universidade de São Paulo (USP), São Paulo, Brazil

***Correspondence:**
Paula Homem-de-Mello
paula.mello@ufabc.edu.br
Kathia Maria Honorio
kmhonorio@usp.br

The study of proteins and mechanisms involved in the apoptosis and new knowledge about cancer's biology are essential for planning new drugs. Tumor cells develop several strategies to gain proliferative advantages, including molecular alterations to evade from apoptosis. Failures in apoptosis could contribute to cancer pathogenesis, since these defects can cause the accumulation of dividing cells and do not remove genetic variants that have malignant potential. The apoptosis mechanism is composed by proteins that are members of BCL-2 and cysteine-protease families. BH3-only peptides are the "natural" intracellular ligands of BCL-2 family proteins. On the other hand, studies have proved that phenothiazine compounds influence the induction of cellular death. To understand the characteristics of phenothiazines and their effects on tumoral cells and organelles involved in the apoptosis, as well as evaluating their pharmacologic potential, we have carried out computational simulation with the purpose of relating the structures of the phenothiazines with their biological activity. Since the tridimensional (3D) structure of the target protein is known, we have employed the molecular docking approach to study the interactions between compounds and the protein's active site. Hereafter, the molecular dynamics technique was used to verify the temporal evolution of the BCL-2 complexes with phenothiazinic compounds and the BH3 peptide, the stability and the mobility of these molecules in the BCL-2 binding site. From these results, the calculation of binding free energy between the compounds and the biological target was carried out. Thus, it was possible to verify that thioridazine and trifluoperazine tend to increase the stability of the BCL-2 protein and can compete for the binding site with the BH3 peptide.

Keywords: apoptosis, cancer, BCL-2, BH3, phenothiazines, docking, molecular dynamics, binding free energy calculations

INTRODUCTION

Apoptosis is a highly regulated form of programmed cell death occurring physiologically in living organisms. However, alterations and defects in this process are also involved in the pathogenesis of several diseases, such as cancer, AIDS, Parkinson and Alzheimer diseases, amyotrophic lateral sclerosis and others (Thompson, 1995). Apoptotic cells exhibit morphological alterations, including plasma membrane blebbing, chromatin condensation, internucleosomal DNA, and formation of apoptotic bodies. Such features result from the action of complex machinery, involving the regulation and execution by BCL-2 family proteins and also by cysteine proteases (initiator or executioner caspases) (Kalkavan and Green, 2018). Particularly regarding cancer, the unlimited proliferative capacity of tumor cells is due to several genetic and molecular alterations, including mechanisms for evading apoptosis (Brown and Attardi, 2005; Hanahan and Weinberg, 2011). One of these mechanisms is the altered expression and function of pro- and antiapoptotic members of B-cell lymphoma-2 (BCL-2) family proteins, directly involved with tumorigenesis and tumor progression/malignance (Coustan-Smith et al., 1996; Gobé et al., 2002). Thus, there are a plenty of molecular studies and clinical trials in course to target BCL-2 proteins to cancer therapy (Adams et al., 2019).

The BCL-2 family is currently divided in proapoptotic members, including BAX and BAK, antiapoptotic members, such as BCL-2, BCL-xL, and MCL-1, and BH3-only proteins (BIM, BID, PUMA, NOXA, and others), which are potent activators of apoptosis (Letai et al., 2002; Youle and Strasser, 2008). Structural characteristics are defined by sequence homology analysis, which allowed identifying four domains (BH1-BH4) involved in protein-protein interactions among members of the BCL-2 family. A hydrophobic slit is formed by BH1, BH2, and BH3 domains, which participates in the uptake of the BH3 domain of pro-apoptotic proteins via heterodimerization; the BH4 domain is present in antiapoptotic activity. The BH3-only proteins just possess the BH3 motif. There are complex interactions among the BCL-2 family members, which comprise a regulatory mechanism of control of cell fate in response to different stimuli. The recruitment of proapoptotic by antiapoptotic proteins occurs through the interaction between the highly conserved helical BH3 domain of the proapoptic protein and a binding groove in the antiapoptotic protein. Considering the homology and structural similarities with the BH3 domain of proapoptotic proteins, BH3-only proteins interact with the binding groove, releasing the proapoptotic proteins and neutralizing the antiapoptotic proteins. In this scenario, BH3-only members have a crucial role in the initiation of apoptotic cell death, since they can bind to the specific domains in anti- or proapoptotic BCL-2 proteins (Lomonosova and Chinnadurai, 2008). It was proposed that BH3-only members can activate directly proapoptotic BAX and BAK. Also, the interaction of BH3-only proteins with antiapoptotic BCL-2 members can disrupts their inhibitory interaction with the proapoptotic members triggering apoptosis (Du et al., 2011; Shamas-Din et al., 2011). As a result, the comprehension of the interaction of BH3-only proteins with other BCL-2 members acting as apoptosis activators resulted in the development of BH3-only mimetic molecules as a strategy to cancer therapy (Merino et al., 2018; Ewald et al., 2019).

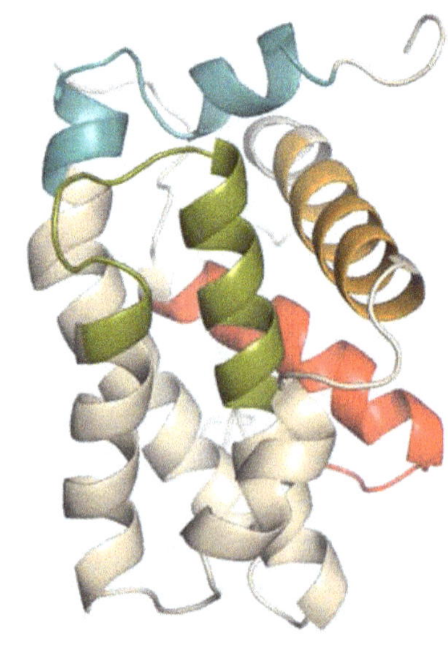

FIGURE 1 | Antiapoptotic BCL-2 protein domains (PDB_ID: 2O22): BH1 (green), BH2 (blue), BH3 (orange), BH4 (red).

Currently, chemicals are under development to inhibit the interactions of pro-apoptotic proteins with the hydrophobic slit of the antiapoptotic protein BCL-2, enabling the imitation of the action of pro-apoptotic proteins with the BH3 domain (Degterev et al., 2001; Delbridge and Strasser, 2015; Zacarías-Lara et al., 2016). Thus, proposals for small molecule interactions with BCL-2 proteins have enabled the development of cancer therapies, including BH3 domain mimetic molecules that bind to the BH3 binding domain in antiapoptotic BCL-2 members such as BCL-2 and BCL-xL (**Figure 1** PDB ID: 2O22). As example of these compounds, one may cite ABT-737, navitoclax (ABT-263), obatoclax mesylate (GX15-070), venetoclax (ABT-199), and gossypol and its derivatives (the structures of these compounds are presented in **Figures S1A–E**) (Oltersdorf et al., 2005; Bajwa et al., 2012; Souers et al., 2013; Pan et al., 2014; Kalkavan and Green, 2018). Thus, several studies are being conducted to identify novel small molecules or peptides able to act as BH3-only mimetics.

In this regards, a class of substances that has potential against BCL-2 refers to phenothiazines (**Figure 2**), as interactions between these compounds and BCL-2 protein may be favored due to the presence of a polycyclic ring system and different substituents modulating the BCL-2 biological activity. The ability of phenothiazines to interact with hydrophobic slits

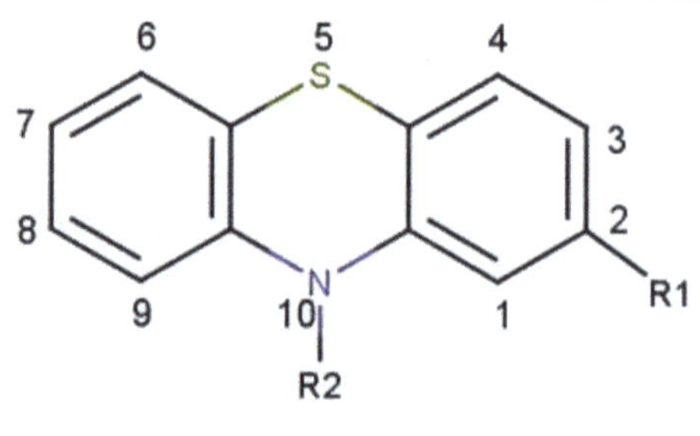

FIGURE 2 | Chemical structure of thiazine nucleus.

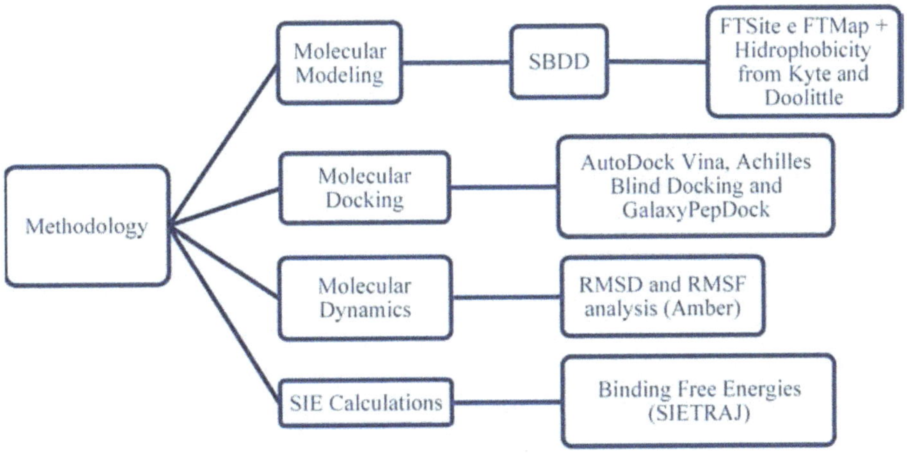

FIGURE 3 | Sequence of methods applied to study the interactions of phenothiazines and the BH3 peptide with BCL-2 protein.

was previously shown by the interactions of thioridazine with putative binding sites of human thioredoxin 1 (Philot et al., 2016). The interaction between phenothiazines and biological membranes occurs because there is amphipathic character of the molecules. The thiazine nucleus is relatively hydrophobic and its side chain can be hydrophilic and even positively charged depending on the pH of the environment (Homem-de-Mello et al., 2005, 2007; Rodrigues et al., 2006; Perussi, 2007; Rodrigues, 2007; Bettanin et al., 2015; de Faria et al., 2015; Nuñez et al., 2015). Additionally, it has been shown that antipsychotic phenothiazine derivatives possess potent cytotoxicity against several types of tumor cells by triggering of apoptosis, with involvement of mitochondrial permeabilization (de Faria et al., 2015; de Mello et al., 2016; Wu et al., 2016; Chu et al., 2019).

Thus, considering that drug design methods have been employed to understand the interactions between small molecules and biological targets, a study via computational techniques and experimental data of BCL-2 and antipsychotic phenothiazine derivatives was developed applying drug design methods to describe a relationship between chemical structure and biological activity of the selected compounds to propose new drug candidates. Bioinformatics tools were used to characterize possible binding sites and regions for anchoring compounds to the target protein (BCL-2). Molecular docking was also employed to identify the interactions of phenothiazines with the BCL-2 antiapoptotic protein, as well as comparing these results with the interactions of BCL-2 with the BH3 peptide.

MATERIALS AND METHODS

The workflow used to study the interactions between phenothiazines (and the BH3 peptide) and BCL-2 protein is presented in **Figure 3**.

To study the relationship between chemical structure and biological activity, as well as evaluating the interactions between bioactive ligands and biological targets, molecular modeling tools can be employed to plan new drug candidates (Andricopulo et al., 2009; Sant'Anna, 2009). The strategy employed in this work is known as Structure-Based Drug Design (SBDD), in which three-dimensional biological receptor structures (obtained from experimental techniques such as X-ray diffraction or nuclear magnetic resonance) are used to propose ligand modifications to improve target affinity and specificity (Andricopulo et al., 2009). In this study, the BCL-2 structures obtained from X-ray and nuclear magnetic resonance (NMR), available in the PDB database (PDB_ID: 1YSW, 2O2F, 2O21, 2O22, 2W3L, 4AQ3, 4IEH, 4LVT, 4LXD, 4MAN, 5AGW, 5AGX, 5JSN) were compared to verify significant differences by aligning these structures (**Figure S2**). The overlap of the structures (**Figure S3**) was performed in the MUSTANG v3.2.2—Multiple Structural Alignment Algorithm program (Konagurthu et al., 2006).

Given this set of alo-protein structures, multiple alignment was obtained using the Cα atom spatial information with the following steps: (I) calculation of root-mean-square deviation (RMSD) taking into account the distances between the Cα atoms for all structures to detect similar substructures between two structures and obtain a quality value for each possible residue-residue match between the two structures; (II) compute the scores of the corresponding residue-residue pairs; (III) structural alignments in pairs; (IV) recalculation of the scores of the corresponding residue-residue pairs in the context of multiple structures; (V) progressive alignment by using the Mustang algorithm (Konagurthu et al., 2006).

Some sequence failures were observed in all BCL-2 structures, so we have selected the structure obtained via NMR (PDB ID: 2O22) (Bruncko et al., 2007; Rose et al., 2018) because it preserves the loop region. Moreover, besides it is an uncut structure, the backbone alignment is similar to the X-ray structures (**Figures S2, S4**).

After choosing the more suitable 3D structure, a study was performed to detect the possible binding sites of human BCL-2, followed by the characterization of these regions, using FTSite (Brenke et al., 2009; Ngan et al., 2012; Kozakov et al., 2015) and FTMap (Brenke et al., 2009; Kozakov et al., 2011, 2015;

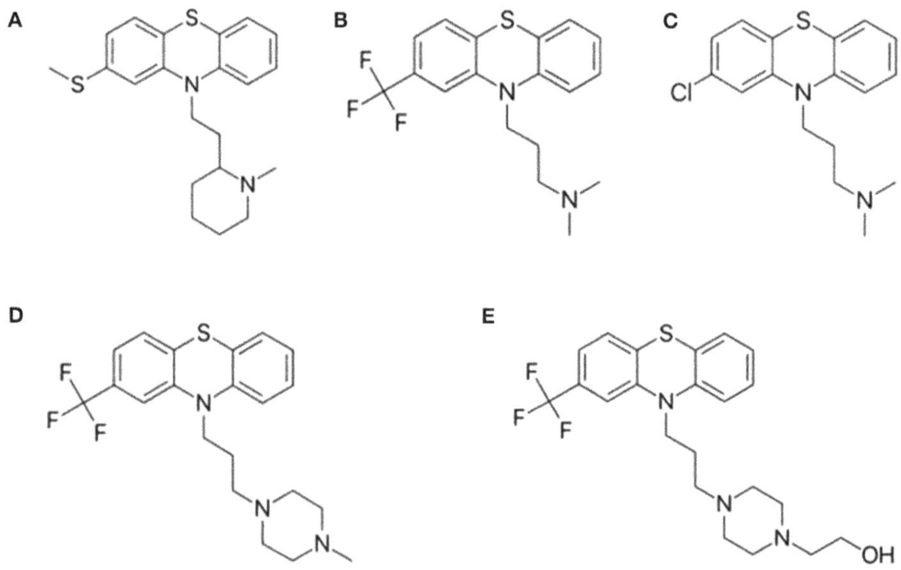

FIGURE 4 | Structure of phenothiazine derivatives analyzed in this study. **(A)** thioridazine; **(B)** triflupromazine; **(C)** chlorpromazine; **(D)** trifluoperazine, and **(E)** fluphenazine.

Bohnuud et al., 2012). FTMap is a server that identifies regions in the macromolecule that have important contributions to the ligand-binding free energy (hot spots). For this, the FTMap algorithm uses 16 probe molecules (**Table S1**) with different shapes, sizes and polarities, which run across the entire surface of the protein looking for the best "positions" for these probes. FTMap is capable of sampling billions of positions for the probe molecules, as well as clustering and ranking them according to an average energy. Consensus sites (CS) are generated, which can be defined as regions at the macromolecule that bind clusters containing different probe molecules, suggesting possible binding hot spots. It is important to highlight that FTMap serves as basis for other algorithms, for example, FTSite that is used to identify ligand binding sites. The main idea of FTSite is ranking the consensus clusters based on the number of non-bonded interactions between the protein and all probe molecules contained in the consensus cluster. So, the amino acid residues interacting with the probe molecules in the top ranked consensus cluster are considered as a possible binding site.

In addition, to better understand the main protein-phenothiazine interactions, the protein hydrophobicity surface was obtained using the UCSF Chimera 1.12 (Pettersen et al., 2004).

The phenothiazine derivatives studied here include thioridazine, triflupromazine, chlorpromazine, trifluoperazine, and fluphenazine (**Figure 4**), which yield relevant *in vitro* cytotoxicity in hepatoma HTC cells (de Faria et al., 2015).

From molecular docking simulations, information on the interaction mode and physicochemical characteristics that affect the affinity of the ligand for the macromolecule is obtained (Wang et al., 2004; Sanchez-Linares et al., 2012). Molecular docking study was performed targeting BCL-2 protein and phenothiazine compounds using the AutoDock Vina 1.5.7. For this, we employed the BCL-2 crystallographic structure (PDB 2O22) with the maximum generation of 10 conformations of each compound. The following parameters were employed in the docking simulations: grid center_x = 4.255, center_y = 1.45, center_z = −5.0, size_x = 25, size_y = 3 and size_z = 34, and exhaustiveness = 20. To validate the docking procedure, redocking analyses were performed in order to recover the original position of the ligand found in the 3D structure of the biological target (Moraes and de Azevedo, 2010).

Visual inspection of the best ligand poses at the target binding site was performed using the PyMOL 2.0, also analyzing the RMSD values calculated by the UCSF Chimera 1.12 and the representation of interactions provided by the Poseview server. It is noteworthy that the RMSD value refers to the average deviation of atoms of an initial structure from the proposed structures and generally the fit is considered successful if the value is below 2.0 Å (Verdonk et al., 2003).

In addition to the AutoDock Vina program, the Achilles Blind Docking server was used to verify molecular interactions in various regions of BCL-2, corroborating the molecular interactions established by phenothiazines in hot spots, where ligands can potentially interact (Brenke et al., 2009; Sanchez-Linares et al., 2012; Kozakov et al., 2015).

For molecular docking and analysis of the interactions between BCL-2 and the BH3 domain, the GalaxyPepDock server was used to analyze protein-protein interactions and better understand cell functions and organization (Lee et al., 2015). In this approach, one of the proteins (or receptor) refers to the origin of the fixed grid coordinate system, and the second protein (or ligand) is defined in a movable grid; interaction energy is defined as a scoring function (Kozakov et al., 2017). To verify the accuracy of the GalaxyPepDock server, redocking analyses with calculation of RMSD values was performed.

The best poses generated by each docking program were selected based on the interactions and binding energies that were generated by the scoring functions, in order to complement the analysis of interactions obtained from the BINANA 1.2.0. This one is able to characterize hydrogen bonding, hydrophobic contact, close contacts, electrostatic interactions, π interactions and salt bridge between receptor—ligand.

After the molecular docking analyses for the five ligands and the BH3 peptide interacting with BCL-2, the next step to be carried out was the preparation of the systems for molecular dynamics (MD) simulations from the calculation of restrained electrostatic potential charges (Wang et al., 2000) of each ligand (from the conformations obtained from molecular docking). For this, we used the Hartree-Fock methodology (Echenique and Alonso, 2007), as implemented in Gaussian09 (Frisch et al., 2009), with 6-31G* basis set (Ditchfield et al., 1971).

Afterwards, the next step related to the preparation of the systems was the solvent box analysis for the target. In this step, we aim to establish the most suitable solvent box for the BCL-2 protein, where the visual analysis was performed in Chimera 1.62 (Pettersen et al., 2004) and the chosen parameters were: periodic octahedral box with a distance of 12 Å between the target and the walls of the box.

From the obtained solvent parameters, the next steps involved in the preparation of the six systems for the MD simulations were: (I) preparation of the topology of the five phenothiazines in the Antechamber module implemented in Ambertools 12 (Salomon-Ferrer et al., 2013) using the RESP charges (charges for BH3 peptide were obtained from the force field); (II) insertion of the FF99SB force field for the coordinates of the six complexes with the Tleap program; (III) total charge calculation of the six systems (the total charge obtained for the six complexes was −9, so 9 sodium ions were inserted to neutralize the system); (IV) inclusion of TIP3P-type water molecules to fill the simulation box; (V) preparation of MD scripts: isothermal-isobaric or NPT ensemble, Langevin thermostat (ntt = 3) and Monte Carlo barostat (Case et al., 2012).

Simulations were then performed following the following steps: (i) four minimizations to eliminate very close contacts between atoms; in the first minimization, the system was kept fixed (without degrees of freedom); in the second and third simulations, only ligands and peptide were kept fixed and in

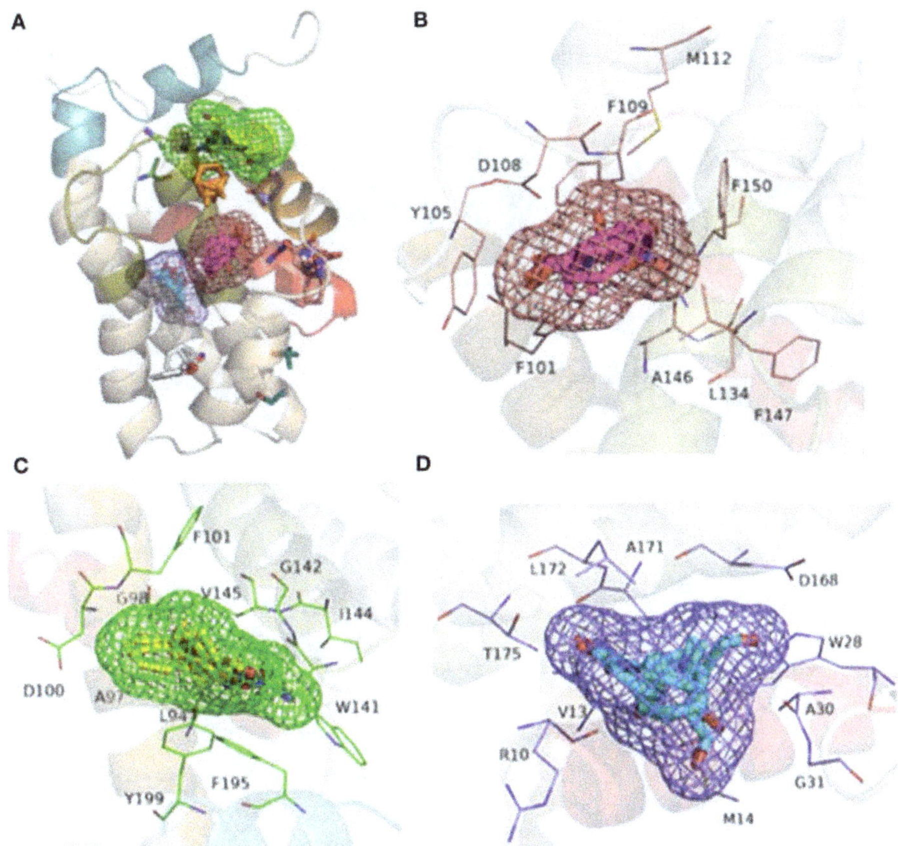

FIGURE 5 | Representation of the BH1-BH4 domains with the presence of the binding sites detected from FTSite and the coupling of probe molecules (in clusters) by the FTMap server produced in the PyMOL 2.0 program: **(A)** the three binding sites with their respective probes; **(B)** Site 1: residues (light pink) with FTSite probes (light pink mesh) and 001 cluster probes (pink); **(C)** Site 2: residues (green) with FTSite probes (green mesh) and 002 cluster probes (yellow) and **(D)** Site 3: residues (blue) with FTSite probes (blue mesh) and 000 cluster probes (light blue).

the last minimization, the whole system was free; (ii) heating (thermal bath) from 0 to 300 K, and a time period of 0.5 ns; the purpose of this step was to control the temperature and adjust the kinetic energy of the system; (iii) 10 ns for equilibration of the system, and it is finalized with the thermal equilibrium of the system; (iv) production step to obtain time subtrajectories. In this final step, the system moves freely and, in addition to simulating thermodynamic properties, a lower energy conformation is obtained for each system under study. This last step was performed over a time period of 100 ns; (v) subtrajectory RMSD value analysis (trajectory stability analysis); (vi) analysis of root-mean-square fluctuation (RMSF) values in order to verify the fluctuations that occur between BCL-2 residues in the presence of the ligands.

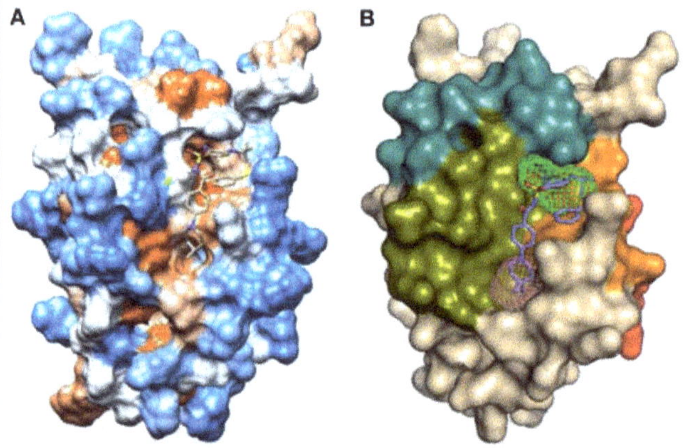

FIGURE 6 | (A) Hydrophobicity surface from Kyte and Doolittle (1982) (**Table S2**): hydrophobic orange-red; neutral white; hydrophilic blue, obtained from UCSF Chimera 1.12 with the crystallographic ligand of protein BCL-2 (PDB_ID: 2O22); **(B)** Representation of the domains: BH1 (green), BH2 (blue), BH3 (orange), BH4 (red), and binding site 1 (pink) and site 2 (green) in the human BCL-2 enzyme - crystallographic structure (PDB_ID: 2O22).

Finally, SIE (Solvated Interaction Energy) methodology was employed to estimate the binding free energy related to the ligand-receptor complex by applying the boundary element method (BEM) to solve the Poisson-Boltzmann equation. This method also uses implicit solvation in the study of protein-ligand complexes (Naïm et al., 2007; Silva et al., 2016). For this, SIE was used in this study to estimate the binding free energy between BCL-2 and the five phenothiazine derivatives, or the BH3 peptide, from the most stable subtrajectories generated by the MD simulations. Thus, for the SIE method to be implemented, the following steps were performed: (I) solvent removal using the cpptraj program, generating a file without periodic solvation coordinates (SIE uses implicit solvation); (II) elaboration of the file containing the initial and final coordinates of the dynamics trajectory; (III) choice of frame range over start and end frames (each sub-trajectory of molecular dynamics has 500 frames),

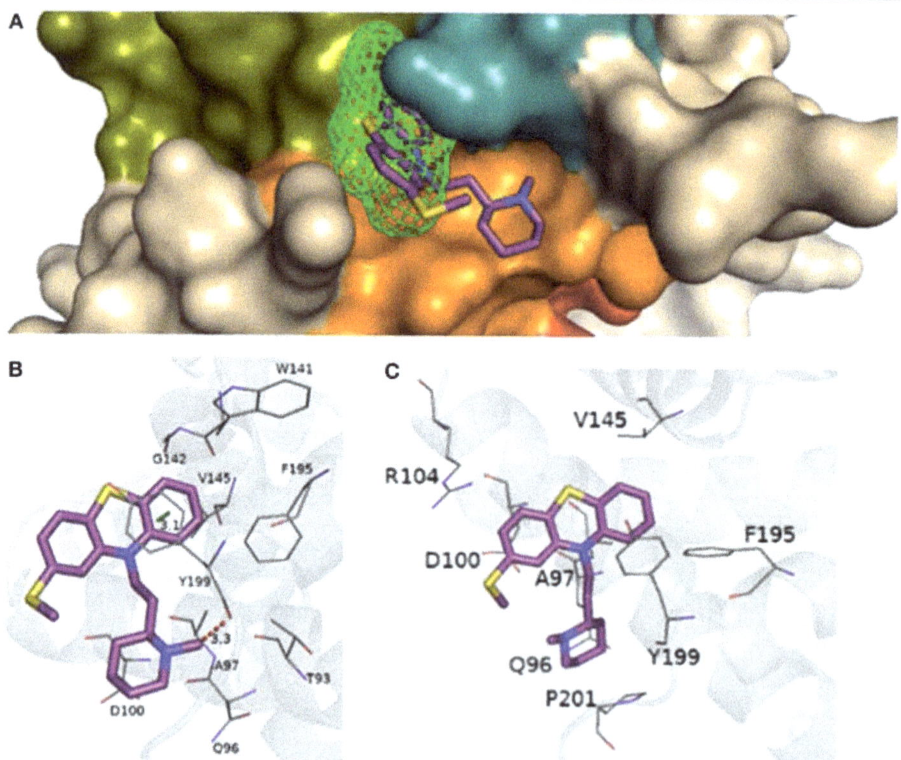

FIGURE 7 | (A) Representation of the BH1-BH4 domains with the presence of the site 2 detected from FTSite and the molecular docking of thioridazine, piperidine subclass, EC_{50} = (45.5 ± 1.0) μmol.L^{-1}, performed at AutoDock Vina 1.5.7. Representation of hydrogen bonding (red) from the molecular docking performed in AutoDock Vina 1.5.7, **(B)** in the Achilles Blind Docking Server, **(C)** and the additional interactions and/or confirmed by BINANA 1.2.0.

from frame 1 to 250; (IV) specify the number of atoms of the target, the five ligands and the peptide; (V) output file definition (sie.log), which contains the results obtained; (VI) calculations by the SIETRAJ program and analysis of the estimated free energy values for the six complexes (BCL-2 + phenothiazines and BCL-2 + BH3 peptide).

RESULTS AND DISCUSSION

Structural Analysis of BCL-2 Structure

Three binding site candidates were located on the BCL-2 protein (PDB_ID: 2W3L) using the FTSite and FTMap servers. The detected sites have the following residues: **site 1**—Phe101, Tyr105, Asp108, Phe109, Met112, Leu134, Ala146, Phe147, Glu149, Phe150; **site 2**—Leu94, Ala97, Gly98, Asp100, Phe101, Trp141, Gly142, Ile144, Val145, Phe195, Tyr199; e **site 3**—Arg10, Val13, Met14, Trp28, Ala30, Gly31, Asp168, Ala171, Leu172 e Thr175. Different probe molecules were used to determine which had the highest affinity for each binding site. The results indicate that the three sites have affinity for polar molecules, hydrogen bond donors and acceptors, hydrophobic and aromatic groups. The representation of the detected binding sites containing the clusters of probe molecules according to the affinity of the molecular interaction on the protein is illustrated in **Figure 5A**. Some probes may also have small contacts with the protein or be in small buried sites, but large CSs occur at the binding site hot spots, also depicted in **Figure 5A**, where the FTMap probes are not in place connection sites determined by FTSite. Residues of the sites 1, 2, and 3 are also shown in **Figures 5B–D**, respectively.

The hydrophobicity scale of the BCL-2 protein was used to complement the results obtained from FTMap and FTSite. **Figure 6** indicates that the crystallographic ligand interacts with the sites 1 and 2 due to its structural size and hydrophobic characteristics. In order to understand the position and the

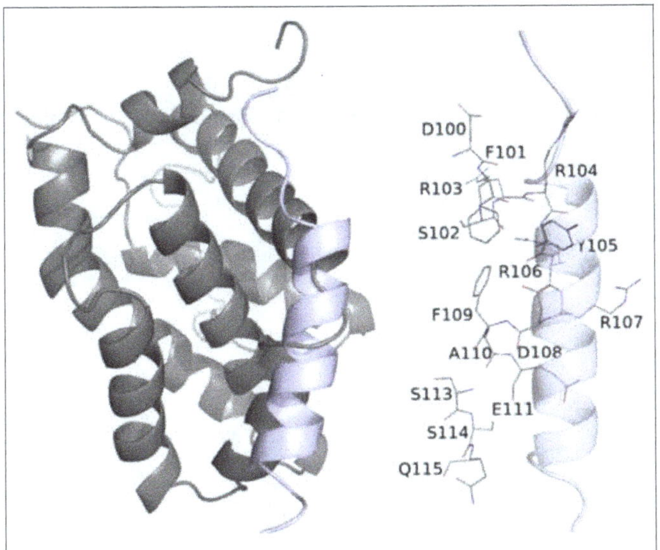

FIGURE 8 | Representation of BCL-2 protein residues with BH3 peptide obtained from molecular docking performed in the GalaxyPepDock server with additional interactions, confirmed by BINANA 1.2.0.

TABLE 1 | Description on the interactions between the main residues of BCL-2 and phenothiazines.

AutoDock Vina 1.5.7		Achilles blind docking server	
Residue	**Interaction**	**Residue**	**Interaction**
Chlorpromazine			
Ala97	Hydrogen Bond	Ala97	Hydrophobic contact
Asp100	Salt Bridge	Asp100	Salt bridge
Phe101	Hydrophobic contact	Phe101	Hydrophobic contact
Arg104	Hydrophobic contact	Arg104	Hydrophobic contact
Trp141	Hydrophobic contact	Trp141	Hydrophobic contact
Val145	Hydrophobic contact	Val145	Hydrophobic contact
Phe195	π-stacking	Phe195	Hydrophobic contact
		Tyr199	Hydrophobic contact
Triflupromazine			
Gln96	Hydrophobic contact	Leu94	Hydrophobic contact
Ala97	Hydrophobic contact	Ala97	Hydrophobic contact
Asp100	Hydrophobic contact	Phe101	Hydrophobic contact
Phe101	Hydrophobic contact	Trp141	Hydrophobic contact
Arg104	Cation-π	Val145	Hydrophobic contact
Val145	Hydrophobic contact	Phe195	Cátion-π
Phe195	Hydrophobic contact	Tyr199	π-stacking
Tyr199	Hydrogen Bond		
Pro201	Hydrophobic contact		
Fluphenazine			
Ala97	Hydrophobic contact	Gln96	Hydrophobic contact
Asp100	Hydrophobic contact	Ala97	Hydrophobic contact
Phe101	Hydrophobic contact	Asp100	Hydrophobic contact
Arg104	Cátion-π	Phe101	Hydrophobic contact
Tyr105	Hydrophobic contact	Arg104	Hydrophobic contact
Gly142	Hydrogen Bond	Val145	Hydrophobic contact
Phe195	Hydrophobic contact	Pro201	Hydrophobic contact
Tyr199	π-stacking	Ser202	Hydrogen Bond
Trifluoperazine			
Leu94	Hydrogen bond	Thr93	Hydrophobic contact
Ala97	Hydrogen bond	Leu94	Hydrophobic contact
Asp100	Salt bridge	Gln96	Hydrophobic contact
Phe101	Hydrophobic contact	Ala97	Hydrophobic contact
Arg104	Hydrophobic contact	Phe101	Hydrophobic contact
Trp141	Hydrophobic contact	Arg104	Hydrophobic contact
Val145	Hydrophobic contact	Trp141	Hydrophobic contact
Phe195	π-stacking	Val145	Hydrophobic contact
Tyr199	Hydrogen Bond	Phe195	Hydrophobic contact
		Tyr199	Hydrophobic contact
Thioridazine			
Thr93	Hydrophobic contact	Gln96	Hydrophobic contact
Gln96	Hydrophobic contact	Ala97	Hydrophobic contact
Ala97	Hydrophobic contact	Asp100	Hydrophobic contact
Asp100	Hydrophobic contact	Arg104	Hydrophobic contact
Trp141	Hydrophobic contact	Val145	Hydrophobic contact
Gly142	Hydrophobic contact	Phe195	Hydrophobic contact
Val145	Hydrophobic contact	Tyr199	Hydrophobic contact
Phe195	Hydrophobic contact	Pro201	Hydrophobic contact
Tyr199	π-stacking and hydrogen Bond		

interactions of phenothiazines with BCL-2, molecular redocking was required.

Next, the molecular docking procedure was performed with the maximum number of poses to be generated at the defined binding site. Thus, the ligand structure found in the tridimensional structure of BCL-2 was superimposed with the ligand pose obtained via molecular docking (**Figure S5**). This overlap generated a RMSD value of 1.327 Å, indicating that the parameters used for the redocking analysis reliably reproduce the experimental conformation of the ligand and can be used to dock the phenothiazine derivatives. An analysis of the images generated by the Poseview program shows that the interactions of the ligand (via redocking) with BCL-2 protein are very similar to those observed in the experimental structure (**Figure S6**).

Molecular Docking

Once the parameters were validated from the redocking analyses, molecular docking studies between BCL-2 and phenothiazine derivatives were performed. It is noteworthy that, according to the experimental data (de Faria et al., 2015), it is possible to establish the following ascending order for cytotoxicity: chlorpromazine < triflupromazine < fluphenazine < trifluoperazine < thioridazine.

The interaction of the most cytotoxic phenothiazine derivative thioridazine with BCL-2 is depicted in **Figure 7** (docking data for the other phenothiazine derivatives are presented in **Figures S7–S10**). In addition, considering the possible competition between a BH3-only peptide and the thioridazine for BCL-2 binding site, the interaction of BCL-2 and a BH3 domain was evaluated. The docking results considering the interaction between BCL-2 and the BH3 domain obtained from the GalaxyPepDock server are presented in **Figure 8**. Validation of the docking procedure between BCL-2 and BH3 peptide resulted in a satisfactory RMSD (root-mean-square deviation) value of 1.962 Å and preservation of the alpha helix structure (**Figure S11**).

From the docking results, it was possible to verify that phenothiazine derivatives showed similar interactions at BCL-2 protein, since we can see that the thiazine nucleus is located at the site 2 recognized by the FTSite server, which has favorable affinities by aromatic and hydrophobic groups.

Both strategies employed to predict the interactions between phenothiazines and BCL-2 are in reasonable agreement with regard to energies and interactions, as can be seen in **Tables 1, 2**. The ligand-target complexes obtained from the AutoDock Vina program proved to be adequate and confirmed by the Achilles

TABLE 3 | Description of the interactions between BCL-2 residues and the BH3 peptide.

GalaxyPepDock Server	
Residue	**Interaction**
Asp100	Hydrophobic contact
Phe101	Hydrophobic contact
Ser102	Hydrophobic contact
Arg103	Hydrophobic contact
Arg104	Hydrophobic contact
Tyr105	Hydrophobic contact
Arg106	Hydrophobic contact
Arg107	Hydrogen Bond and Salt Bridge
Asp108	Hydrophobic contact
Phe109	Hydrophobic contact
Ala110	Hydrophobic contact
Glu111	Hydrophobic contact
Met112	Hydrophobic contact
Ser114	Hydrophobic contact
Gln115	Hydrophobic contact

TABLE 2 | EC_{50} values (± 1.0 μmol.L^{-1}), interaction energies (kcal.mol^{-1}) and number (#) of interactions obtained from AutoDock Vina and Achilles Blind Docking for phenothiazines and BCL-2.

		Chlorpromazine	Triflupromazine	Fluphenazine	Trifluoperazine	Thioridazine
	EC^{*}_{50}	125.3	105.9	63.2	56.2	45.5
AutoDock Vina 1.5.7	Interaction energy (kcal.mol^{-1})	−6.4	−6.6	−6.6	−7.1	−6.0
	#hydrophobic contacts	4	7	5	4	8
	#hydrogen bonds	1	1	1	3	1
	# π-stacking	1	0	1	1	1
	#other interactions**	1	1	1	1	0
	Total #interactions	7	9	8	9	10
Achilles Blind Docking	Energy (kcal.mol^{-1})	−6.3	−7.1	−7.4	−7.5	−6.8
	#hydrophobic contacts	7	5	7	10	8
	#hydrogen bonds	0	0	1	0	0
	# π-stacking	0	1	0	0	0
	# other interactions**	1	1	0	0	0
	Total #interactions	8	7	8	10	8

*(de Faria et al., 2015).

**salt bridge or cation- π.

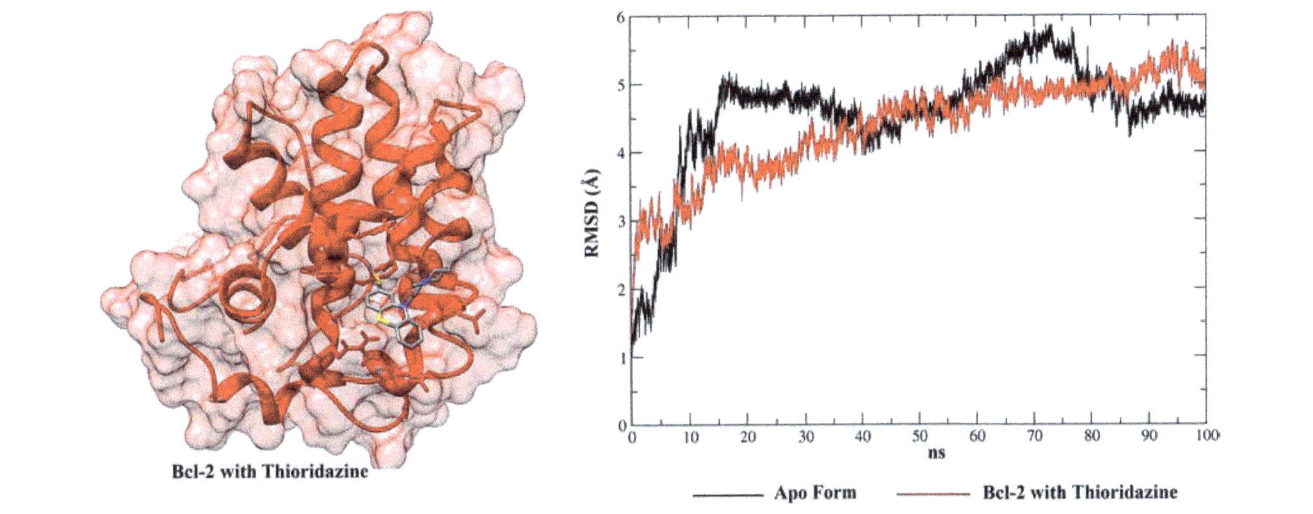

FIGURE 9 | RMSD values of BCL-2 in the apo form (black), BCL-2 with thioridazine (red) and 3D conformation obtained from the clustering of all structures obtained from the MD simulation.

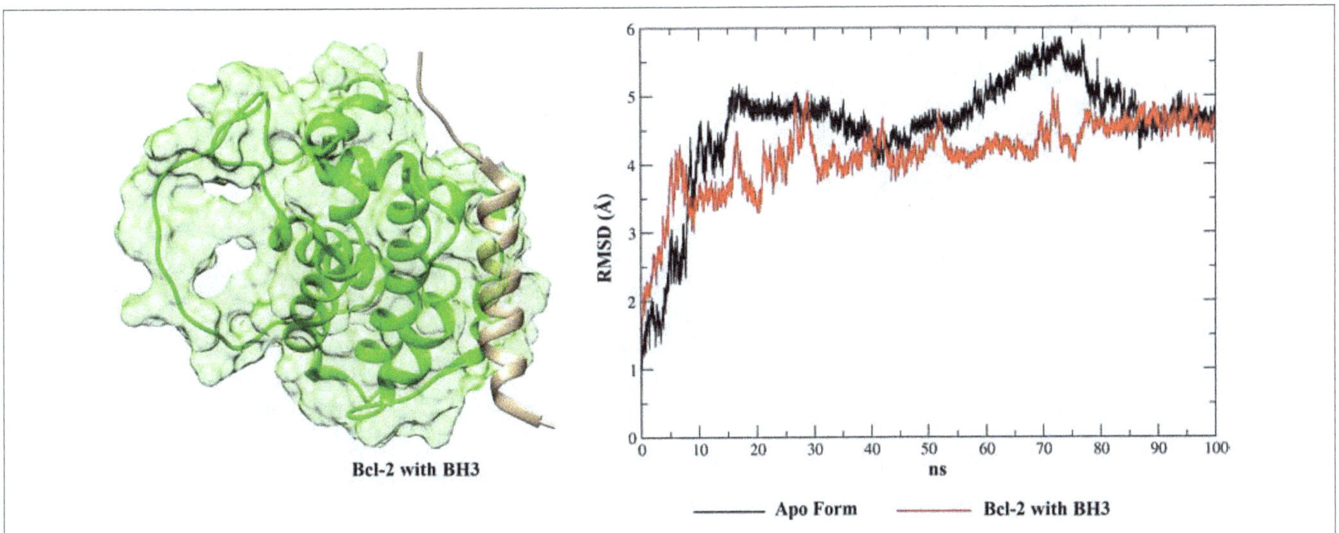

FIGURE 10 | RMSD values of BCL-2 in the apo form (black), BCL-2 with the BH3 peptide (red) and 3D conformation obtained from the clustering of all structures obtained from the MD simulation.

Blind Docking Server, and then, they were used for the molecular dynamics simulations. The main interactions between BCL-2 and the BH3-only peptide are displayed in **Table 3**, and we can see that the main interactions observed were hydrophobic contacts. This simulation was possible only with the GalaxyPepDock Server, which is specific to identify protein-peptide interactions.

Through the analysis of the bioactive conformations obtained from both programs, it was observed that the thiazine nucleus present in the studied ligands showed affinity by BCL-2, possibly due to the presence of aromatic and hydrophobic groups, which was also suggested by the FTSite server. In order to understand dynamic and energetic factors involved in the interaction between the phenothiazines and BCL-2, molecular dynamics simulations and calculations of binding free energy (ΔG) were performed.

Molecular Dynamics

From the molecular docking between phenothiazines and BCL-2 (and between the peptide BH3 and BCL-2), the possible conformations of the phenothiazine derivatives and, additionally the BH3 peptide to evaluate competition, were chosen to perform MD simulations. Then, after the end of the simulations, the RMSD plots were generated from the Cpptraj platform (Amber 12). This analysis was performed to verify the temporal evolution of the complexes BCL-2 + phenothiazines and BCL-2 + BH3, as well as the stability and the mobility of the formed systems. MD simulations were also performed with the apo BCL-2 target (no ligand at its binding site) and, in addition to the RMSD plots, the structures observed along 100 ns of MD simulations were clustered for all complexes and the protein in the form apo using Chimera 1.13.1. **Figures 9, 10** show the RMSD plots for

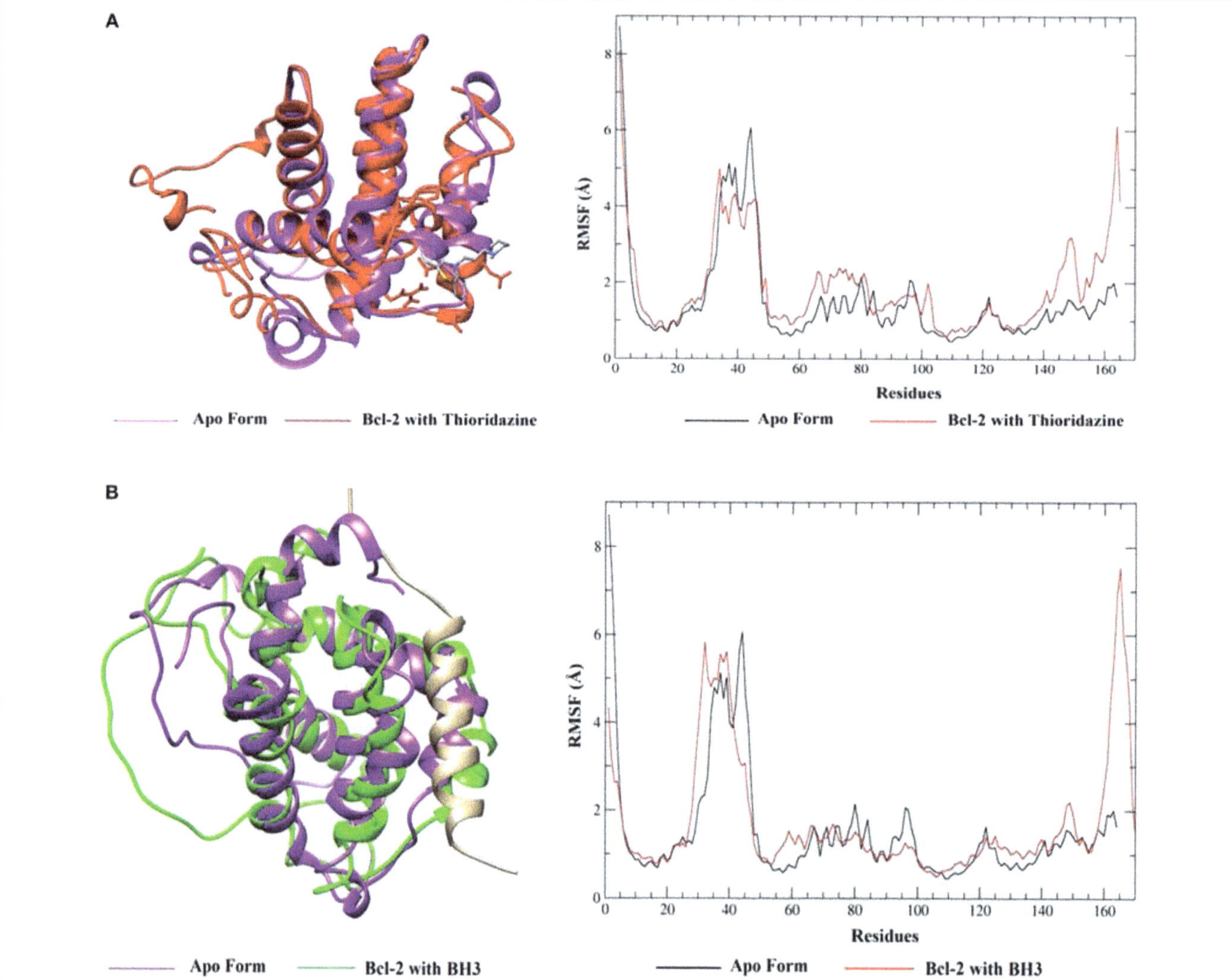

FIGURE 11 | RMSF values of BCL-2 in the presence of **(A)** thioridazine and **(B)** BH3-only peptide.

the complexes formed by BCL-2 + thioridazine and BCL-2 + BH3. The results obtained from the MD simulations for the other phenothiazines are presented in **Figures S12–S15**.

From the RMSD plots for the BCL-2 trajectories, the five phenothiazine compounds and the BH3 peptide, an analysis of trajectory stability and mobility can be performed. Thus, **Figure 9** shows that thioridazine increases the level of stability of the complex, because BCL-2 with this molecule coupled at its binding site exhibits lower RMSD variations. The second complex with the smallest variations is shown in **Figure S12** (**Supplementary Material**—BCL-2 + trifluoperazine). These two phenothiazine compounds have the lowest EC_{50} values for cytotoxicity against HTC cells (45.5 ± 1.0 and 56.2 ± 1.0 $\mu mol.L^{-1}$, respectively) and these results showed that BCL-2 has greater stability in the presence of these two ligands. Compared to other phenothiazine compounds (**Figures S13–S15**), RMSD results show greater variations, i.e., suggesting that fluphenazine, trifluopromazine and chlorpromazine decreased the target stability.

With respect to the peptide BH3, **Figure 10** shows that the receptor exhibits smaller RMSD variations than for the phenothiazines, suggesting that the peptide BH3 assists in increasing the target stability. However, **Figure 10** also shows that BH3 is the ligand that exhibits greater variations in RMSD and this can be explained by the size of this peptide relative to the phenothiazine compounds.

When these RMSD values are compared with the apo form, thioridazine and the BH3 peptide cause structural changes in the BCL-2 target; however, when this receptor has the thioridazine molecule in its binding site, the complex is more stable. It is also noted that in all cases the RMSD variations for the receptors are >4 Å and this can be explained by loops on the BCL-2 chains, which increase their mobility. These results are corroborated by the RMSF plots, which are displayed in **Figure 11** for thioridazine

TABLE 4 | Half maximal effective concentration (EC50) number of interactions obtained with the different softwares (Total #interactions), binding free energy (ΔG) and binding free energy divided by the number of interactions (ΔG/#interactions) calculated for the six complexes (BCL-2 + phenothiazines and BCL-2 + BH3).

Ligand	EC_{50} ($\pm$ 1.0 $\mu mol.L^{-1}$)*	Total #interactions (Vina/Achilles)	ΔG ($kcal.mol^{-1}$)	ΔG/ #interactions ($kcal.mol^{-1}$)	
				Vina	Achilles
Thioridazine	45.5	10/8	−7.00	−0.70	−0.88
Trifluoperazine	56.2	9/10	−6.47	−0.72	−0.65
Fluphenazine	63.2	8/8	−5.51	−0.69	−0.69
Triflupromazine	105.69	9/7	−4.93	−0.55	−0.70
Chlorpromazine	125.3	7/8	−4.05	−0.58	−0.51
BH3	-	16**	−12.81	−0.80	

*de Faria et al. (2015).
** Obtained from Galaxy PepDock Server.

and the BH3 peptide, respectively. RMSF plots for the other phenothiazines can be viewed in **Figures S16–S19**.

RMSF plots were generated in order to verify the flexibility and the mobility of the backbone atoms at the complexes. The plots show the different amplitudes of fluctuations in the apo and holo forms (**Figure 11A** and **Figure S16**) and indicate that the complexes with thioridazine and trifluoperazine have the smallest fluctuations in the main residues, relative to the other phenothiazine derivatives. It is also noted that there is a large fluctuation of residues in the loop regions. For the BH3 peptide (**Figure 11B**), the fluctuations of the amino acid residues are smaller, confirming the RMSD values. Some loop regions of both BCL-2 and the peptide structure show higher fluctuations, suggesting that the peptide is more mobile compared to other compounds because it has a larger number of atoms in its structure and has side chains and a loop.

Therefore, from the results obtained from MD simulations (RMSD and RSMF values) it was possible to verify that thioridazine and trifluoperazine tend to increase the stability of the BCL-2 protein. From **Figure 11**, we can also verify the alignment of the conformations generated after the clustering, the differences in the fluctuations of the apo-BCL-2 residues and the complexes (BCL-2 + ligands). Thus, from these results, the next step of this work involved the calculation of the binding free energy between BCL-2 and the phenothiazine derivatives or the BH3-only peptide using the SIE method.

Free Energy Calculation via SIE Method

After choosing the sub-trajectories that presented the smallest variations (from RMSD values derived from MD simulations), it was possible to estimate the binding free energy (ΔG) of BCL-2 and the molecules under study, using the SIE method. These simulations were performed in order to analyze the stability of BCL-2 in relation to the six ligands. Thus, the ΔG values calculated by the SIE method are presented in **Table 4**.

The EC_{50} values of phenothiazines were directly proportional to the binding ΔG values. The interaction of BCL-2 with thioridazine has a ΔG^{SIE} value of -7.00 $kcal.mol^{-1}$, while chlorpromazine (the highest EC_{50} value) has the lowest binding free energy value when interacts with BCL-2 (-4.05 $kcal.mol^{-1}$). As expected from its physiological role, the ΔG value for the BH3 peptide was the highest (-12.81 $kcal.mol^{-1}$) that corroborates the RMSD/RSMF analysis and reinforces that BCL-2 presents a strong interaction with the peptide, increasing its stability.

The results obtained from the SIE method also showed that thioridazine and trifluoperazine could inhibit the target BCL-2, just like BH3 peptide, because complexes are favorable and stable since its ΔG values are the most negative. Since most of the interactions between ligands and protein are hydrophobic, one can estimate the free energy of interaction per site (ΔG/#interactions in **Table 4**) by combining SIE free energies and the number of interactions obtained from docking. This analysis is proposed here since the molecules are smaller than the peptide, and so are the number of possible interactions. Then, if one ligand can interact in the same intensity per site of interaction as BH3 peptide, this ligand can compete for the binding site. Of course, this is a simplistic analysis because each interaction may be stronger or weaker, but it is insightful to verify that thioridazine and trifluoperazine have interaction energy per binding site comparable to BH3 peptide.

CONCLUSIONS

From this study on the BCL-2 protein (involved in the apoptosis process) and some phenothiazine derivatives that have pharmacological properties, we can concluded that phenothiazines may compete with pro-apoptotic proteins. These results were obtained from molecular docking, RMSD and RMSF values and binding free energy.

Docking simulations were important to understand the main interactions between the target (BCL-2) and the phenothiazine compounds. RMSD results for the complex formed between BCL-2 and the two most active phenothiazine compounds (thioridazine and trifluoperazine) suggest that BCL-2 has a higher stability in the presence of these two ligands. Compared to other phenothiazine compounds, RMSD results show greater variations, i.e., the results suggest that fluphenazine, triflupromazine and chlorpromazine decrease the target stability. RMSF plots for the trajectories of BCL-2 and the five phenothiazine compounds showed that thioridazine and trifluoperazine have the smallest fluctuations considering the major residues compared to other phenothiazine compounds.

The binding free energy between BCL-2, the phenothiazine compounds and the BH3 peptide was calculated using the SIE method and the results obtained indicated that the phenothiazine compounds with lower EC_{50} values presented greater affinity (measured by means of ΔG). The net binding energy for BH3 peptide is larger than the net binding energy obtained for the phenothiazines, since BH3 is a larger compound, with many different points for interaction with BCL-2. Moreover, BH3 is the natural ligand of BCL-2, selected evolutionarily to bind. However, our data indicate that the interactions are quite specific for the compounds with greater EC_{50}; this interaction can generate competition in specific situations, including chemotherapy in tumor cells, which would induce cell death, and can act as co-adjuvants by this mechanism. Thus, the results obtained in this study can help to better understand the mechanisms involved in the interaction of BCL-2 and phenothiazine compounds and, consequently, may help the design of new substances with improved activity against BCL-2. It should be noted that the inhibition of the antiapoptotic protein BCL-2 by phenothiazines may help explain its apoptosis-inducing effect on tumor cells.

AUTHOR CONTRIBUTIONS

AC and SP carried out calculations (characterization of the protein and docking). MO performed molecular dynamics and SIE calculations, TR was the experimental collaborator (proposed the problem and obtained EC50 data). FB participated on discussions and writing the manuscript. PH-d-M and KH proposed and supervised all the computational simulations, organized discussions with experimental collaborator and wrote/revised the manuscript.

ACKNOWLEDGMENTS

The authors thank FAPESP (2006/00995-9, 2016/07367-5, 2017/23416-9, 2016/24524-7, and 2017/10118-0), CNPq (#306177/2016-1, 306585/2019-7, and 312020/2019-8) and CAPES (Finance Code 001 and fellowship EACH/CPG 027/2019). The authors are grateful to the Multiuser Central Facilities (UFABC) for the computational facility.

REFERENCES

Adams, C. M., Clark-Garvey, S., Porcu, P., and Eischen, C. M. (2019). Targeting the BCL-2 family in B cell lymphoma. *Front Oncol.* 8:636. doi: 10.3389/fonc.2018.00636

Andricopulo, A. D., Salum, L. B., and Abraham, D. J. (2009). Structure-based drug design strategies in medicinal chemistry. *Curr. Top. Med. Chem.* 9, 771–790. doi: 10.2174/156802609789207127

Bajwa, N., Liao, C., and Nikolovska-Coleska, Z. (2012). Inhibitors of the anti-apoptotic BCL-2 proteins: a patent review. *Expert Opin. Ther. Pat.* 22, 37–55. doi: 10.1517/13543776.2012.644274

Bettanin, F., de Carvalho Fontinelles, T. A., Maciel, C. D., Dias, L. G., Coutinho-Neto, M. D., and Homem-de-Mello, P. (2015). Aggregation of photosensitizers: the role of dispersion and solvation on dimer formation energetics. *Theor. Chem. Acc.* 134,152. doi: 10.1007/s00214-015-1732-5

Bohnuud, T., Beglov, D., Ngan, C. H., Zerbe, B., Hall, D. R., Brenke, R., et al. (2012). Computational mapping reveals dramatic effect of Hoogsteen breathing on duplex DNA reactivity with formaldehyde. *Nucleic Acids Res.* 40, 7644–7652. doi: 10.1093/nar/gks519

Brenke, R., Kozakov, D., Chuang, G-Y., Beglov, D., Hall, D., Landon, M. R., et al. (2009). Fragment-based identification of druggable 'hot spots' of proteins using Fourier domain correlation techniques. *Bioinformatics* 25, 621–627. doi: 10.1093/bioinformatics/btp036

Brown, M. J., and Attardi, L. D. (2005). The role of apoptosis in cancer development and treatment response. *Nat. Rev. Cancer* 5, 231–237. doi: 10.1038/nrc1560

Bruncko, M., Oost, T. K., Belli, B. A., Ding, H., Joseph, M. K., Kunzer, A., et al. (2007). Solution structure of the anti-apoptotic protein BCL-2 in complex with an acyl-sulfonamide-based *ligand. J. Med. Chem.* 50, 641–662. doi: 10.2210/pdb2o2f/pdb

Case, D. A., Darden, T., Cheatham, T. E., Simmerling, C., Wang, J., Duke, R. E., et al. (2012). *AMBER 12.* São Francisco, CA: University of California.

Chu, C-W, Ko, H-J., Chou, C-H., Cheng, T-S., Cheng, H-W., Liang, Y-H., et al. (2019). Thioridazine enhances P62-mediated autophagy and apoptosis through Wnt/β-catenin signaling pathway in glioma cells. *Int. J. Mol. Sci.* 20:473. doi: 10.3390/ijms20030473

Coustan-Smith, E., Kitanaka, A., Pui, C. H., McNinch, L., Evans, W. E., Raimondi, S. C., et al. (1996). Clinical relevance of BCL-2 overexpression in childhood acute lymphoblastic leukemia. *Blood* 87, 1140–1146. doi: 10.1182/blood.V87.3.1140.bloodjournal8731140

de Faria, P. A., Bettanin, F., Cunha, R. L. O. R., Paredes-Gamero, E. J., Homem-de-Mello, P., Nantes, I. L., et al. (2015). Cytotoxicity of phenothiazine derivatives associated with mitochondrial dysfunction: a structure-activity investigation. *Toxicology* 330, 44–54. doi: 10.1016/j.tox.2015.02.004

de Mello, J. C., Moraes, V. W. R., Watashi, C. M., da Silva, D. C., Cavalcanti, L. P., Franco, M. K. K. D., et al. (2016). Enhancement of chlorpromazine antitumor activity by pluronics F127/L81 nanostructured system against human multidrug resistant leukemia. *Pharmacol. Res.* 111, 102–112. doi: 10.1016/j.phrs.2016.05.032

Degterev, A., Lugovskoy, A., Cardone, M., Mulley, B., Wagner, G., Mitchison, T., et al. (2001). Identification of small-molecule inhibitors of interaction between the BH3 domain and BCL-XL. *Nat. Cell Biol.* 3, 173–182. doi: 10.1038/35055085

Delbridge, A. R. D., and Strasser, A. (2015). The BCL-2 protein family, BH3-mimetics and cancer therapy. *Cell Death Differ.* 22, 1071–1080. doi: 10.1038/cdd.2015.50

Ditchfield, R., Hehre, W. J., and Pople, J. A. (1971). Self-consistent molecular-orbital methods. IX. an extended gaussian-type basis for molecular-orbital studies of organic molecules. *J. Chem. Phys.* 54:724. doi: 10.1063/1.1674902

Du, H., Wolf, J., Schafer, B., Moldoveanu, T., Chipuk, J. E., and Kuwana, T. (2011). BH3 domains other than bim and bid can directly activate Bax/Bak. *J. Biol. Chem.* 286:491–501. doi: 10.1074/jbc.M110.167148

Echenique, P., and Alonso, J. L. (2007). A mathematical and computational review of hartree-fock SCF methods in quantum chemistry. *Mol. Phys.* 105, 3057–3098. doi: 10.1080/00268970701757875

Ewald, L., Dittmann, J., Vogler, M., and Fulda, S. (2019). Side-by-side comparison of BH3-mimetics identifies MCL-1 as a key therapeutic target in AML. *Cell Death Dis.* 10:917. doi: 10.1038/s41419-019-2156-2

Frisch, M. J., Trucks, G. W., Schlegel, H. B., Scuseria, G. E., Robb, M. A., Cheeseman, J. R., et al. (2009). *Gaussian 09.* Wallingford, CT: Gaussian, Inc.

Gobé, G., Rubin, M., Williams, G., Sawczuk, I., and Buttyan, R. (2002). Apoptosis and expression of BCL-2, BCL-XL, and bax in renal cell carcinomas. *Cancer Invest.* 20, 324–332. doi: 10.1081/CNV-120001177

Hanahan, D., and Weinberg, R. A. (2011). Hallmarks of cancer: the next generation. *Cell* 144, 646–674. doi: 10.1016/j.cell.2011.02.013

Homem-de-Mello, P., Mennucci, B., Tomasi, J., and da Silva, A. B. F. (2005). The effects of solvation in the theoretical spectra of cationic dyes. *Theor. Chem. Acc.* 113, 274–280. doi: 10.1007/s00214-005-0668-6

Homem-de-Mello, P., Mennucci, B., Tomasi, J., and da Silva, A. B. F. (2007). Cationic dye dimers: a theoretical study. *Theor. Chem. Acc.* 118, 305–314. doi: 10.1007/s00214-007-0261-2

Kalkavan, H., and Green, D. R. (2018). MOMP, cell suicide as a BCL-2 family business. *Cell Death Diff.* 25, 46–55. doi: 10.1038/cdd.2017.179

Konagurthu, A. S., Whisstock, J. C., Stuckey, P. J., and Lesk, A. M. (2006). MUSTANG: a multiple structural alignment algorithm. *Proteins* 64, 559–574. doi: 10.1002/prot.20921

Kozakov, D., David, R. H., Xia, B., Porter, K. A., Padhorny, D., Yueh, C., et al. (2017). The ClusPro web server for protein-protein docking. *Nat. Protoc.* 12, 255–278. doi: 10.1038/nprot.2016.169

Kozakov, D., Grove, L. E., Hall, D. R., Bohnuud, T., Mottarella, S. E., Luo, L., et al. (2015). The FTMap family of web servers for determining and characterizing ligand-binding hot spots of proteins. *Nat. Protoc.* 10, 733–755. doi: 10.1038/nprot.2015.043

Kozakov, D., Hall, D. R., Chuang, G. Y., Cencic, R, Brenke, R., Grove, L. E., et al. (2011). Structural conservation of druggable hot spots in protein- protein interfaces. *Proc. Natl. Acad. Sci. U.S.A.* 108, 13528–13533. doi: 10.1073/pnas.1101835108

Kyte, J., and Doolittle, R. F. (1982). A simple method for displaying the hydropathic character of a protein. *J. Mol. Biol.* 157, 105–132. doi: 10.1016/0022-2836(82)90515-0

Lee, H., Heo, L., Lee, M. S., and Seok, C. (2015). GalaxyPepDock: a protein-peptide docking tool based on interaction similarity and energy optimization. *Nucleic Acids Res.* 43, W431–W435. doi: 10.1093/nar/gkv495

Letai, A., Bassik, M. C., Walensky, L. D., Sorcinelli, M. D., Weiler, S., and Korsmeyer, S. J. (2002). Distinct BH3 domains either sensitize or activate mitochondrial apoptosis, serving as prototype cancer therapeutics. *Cancer Cell.* 2, 183–192. doi: 10.1016/S1535-6108(02)00127-7

Lomonosova, E., and Chinnadurai, G. (2008). BH3-only proteins in apoptosis and beyond: an overview. *Oncogene.* 27(Suppl. 1):S2–19. doi: 10.1038/onc.2009.39

Merino, D., Kelly, G. L., Lessene, G., Wei, A. H., Roberts, A. W., and Strasser, A. (2018). BH3-mimetic drugs: blazing the trail for new cancer medicines. *Cancer Cell.* 34, 879–891. doi: 10.1016/j.ccell.2018.11.004

Moraes, F. P., and de Azevedo, W. F., Jr. (2010). *Computação Biologicamente Inspirada Aplicada Ao Estudo Da Interação Proteína-Ligante.* Porto Alegre: PUCRS.

Naïm, M., Bhat, S., Rankin, K. N., Dennis, S., Chowdhury, S., F., and Siddiqi, I., et al. (2007). Solvated Interaction Energy (SIE) for scoring protein-ligand binding affinities. 1. exploring the parameter space. *J. Chem. Inform. Model.* 47, 122–133. doi: 10.1021/ci600406v

Ngan, C-H., Hall, D. R., Zerbe, B., Grove, L. E., Kozakov, D., Vajda, S. (2012). FTSite: high accuracy detection of ligand binding sites on unbound protein structures. *Bioinformatics* 28, 286–287. doi: 10.1093/bioinformatics/btr651

Nuñez, S. C., Yoshimura, T. M., Ribeiro, M. S., Junqueira, H. C., Maciel, C., Coutinho-Neto, M. D., and Baptista, M. S. (2015). Urea enhances the photodynamic efficiency of methylene blue. *J. Photochem. Photobiol. B* 50, 31–37. doi: 10.1016/j.jphotobiol.2015.03.018

Oltersdorf, T., Elmore, S. W., Shoemaker, A. R., Armstrong, R. C., Augeri, D. J., Belli, B. A., et al. (2005). An inhibitor of BCL-2 family proteins induces regression of solid tumours. *Nature* 435, 677–681. doi: 10.1038/nature03579

Pan, R., Hogdal, L. J., Benito, J. M., Bucci, D., Han, L., Borthakur, G., et al. (2014). Selective BCL-2 inhibition by ABT-199 causes on-target cell death in acute myeloid leukemia. *Cancer Discov.* 4, 362–375. doi: 10.1158/2159-8290.CD-13-0609

Perussi, J. R. (2007). Inativação fotodinâmica de microrganismos. *Química Nova* 30, 988–994. doi: 10.1590/S0100-40422007000400039

Pettersen, E. F., Goddard, T. D., Huang, C. C., Couch, G. S., Greenblatt, D. M., Meng, E. C., et al. (2004). UCSF chimera–a visualization system for exploratory research and analysis. *J. Comput. Chem.* 25, 1605–1612. doi: 10.1002/jcc.20084

Philot, E. A., da Mata Lopes, D., de Souza, A. T., Braz, A. S. K., Nantes, I. L., Rodrigues, T., et al. (2016). Binding of phenothiazines into allosteric hydrophobic pocket of human thioredoxin 1. *Eur. Biophys. J.* 45, 279–286. doi: 10.1007/s00249-016-1113-6

Rodrigues, T. (2007). *Chemical and Photochemical Behavior of Phenothiazines in Heterogeneous Media Related to a Diversity of Biological Effects.* Kerala: Catalysis and Photochemistry in Heterogeneous Media. Research Signpost.

Rodrigues, T., dos Santos, C. G., Riposati, A., Barbosa, L. R. S., Di Mascio, P., Itri, R., et al. (2006). Photochemically generated stable cation radical of phenothiazine aggregates in mildly acid buffered solutions. *J. Phys. Chem. B* 110, 12257–12265. doi: 10.1021/jp0605404

Rose, A. S., Bradley, A. R., Valasatava, Y., Duarte, J. M., Prlic, A., and Rose, P. W. (2018). NGL viewer: web-based molecular graphics for large complexes. *Bioinformatics* 34, 3755–3758. doi: 10.1093/bioinformatics/bty419

Salomon-Ferrer, R., Case, D. A., and Walker, R. C. (2013). An overview of the amber biomolecular simulation package. *Comp. Mol. Sci.* 3, 198–210. doi: 10.1002/wcms.1121

Sanchez-Linares, I., Perez-Sanchez, H., Cecilia, J. M., and Garcia, J. M. (2012). High-throughput parallel blind virtual screening using BINDSURF. *BMC Bioinformatics* 13(Suppl. 14):S13. doi: 10.1186/1471-2105-13-S14-S13

Sant'Anna, C. M. R. (2009). Molecular modeling methods in the study and design of bioactive compounds: an introduction. *Rev Virtual de Química* 1, 49–57. doi: 10.5935/1984-6835.20090007

Shamas-Din, A., Brahmbhatt, H., Leber, B., and Andrews, D. W. (2011). BH3-only proteins: orchestrators of apoptosis. *Biochim Biophys Acta.* 1813:508–20. doi: 10.1016/j.bbamcr.2010.11.024

Silva, J. R. A., Bishai, W. R., Govender, T., Lamichhane, G., Maguire, G. E. M., Kruger, H. G., et al. (2016). Targeting the cell wall of *mycobacterium tuberculosis*: a molecular modeling investigation of the interaction of imipenem and meropenem with L,D-transpeptidase 2. *J. Biomol. Struct. Dyn.* 34, 304–317. doi: 10.1080/07391102.2015.1029000

Souers, A. J., Leverson, J. D., Boghaert, E. R., Ackler, S. L., Catron, N. D., Chen, J., et al. (2013). ABT-199, a Potent and selective BCL-2 inhibitor, achieves antitumor activity while sparing platelets. *Nat. Med.* 19, 202–208. doi: 10.1038/nm.3048

Thompson, C. B. (1995). Apoptosis in the pathogenesis and treatment of disease. *Science* 267, 1456–1462. doi: 10.1126/science.7878464

Verdonk, M. L., Cole, J. C., Hartshorn, M. J., Murray, C. W., and Taylor, R. D. (2003). Improved protein-ligand docking using GOLD. *Proteins.* 52, 609–623. doi: 10.1002/prot.10465

Wang, J., Cieplak, P., and Kollman, P. A. (2000). How Well does a Restrained Electrostatic Potential (RESP) model perform in calculating conformational energies of organic and biological molecules? *J. Comput. Chem.* 21, 1049–74. doi: 10.1002/1096-987X(200009)21:12<1049::AID-JCC3>3.0.CO;2-F

Wang, R., Lu, Y., Fang, X., and Wang, S. (2004). An extensive test of 14 scoring functions using the PDBbind refined set of 800 protein-ligand complexes. *J. Chem. Inf. Comput. Sci.* 44, 2114–2125. doi: 10.1021/ci049733j

Wu, C. H., Bai, L. Y., Tsai, M. H., Chu, P-C., Chiu, C. F., Chen, M. Y., et al. (2016). Pharmacological exploitation of the phenothiazine antipsychotics to develop novel antitumor agents-a drug repurposing strategy. *Sci. Rep.* 6:27540. doi: 10.1038/srep27540

Youle, R. J., and Strasser, A. (2008). The BCL-2 protein family: opposing activities that mediate cell death. *Nat. Rev. Mol. Cell Biol.* 9, 47–59. doi: 10.1038/nrm2308

Zacarías-Lara, O. J., Correa-Basurto, J., and Bello, M. (2016). Exploring the conformational and binding properties of unphosphorylated/phosphorylated monomeric and trimeric BCL-2 through docking and molecular dynamics simulations. *Biopolymers* 105, 393–413. doi: 10.1002/bip.22839

15

High-Throughput Docking Using Quantum Mechanical Scoring

Claudio N. Cavasotto [1,2,3]* *and M. Gabriela Aucar* [1]

[1] Computational Drug Design and Biomedical Informatics Laboratory, Translational Medicine Research Institute (IIMT), CONICET-Universidad Austral, Pilar, Argentina, [2] Facultad de Ciencias Biomédicas and Facultad de Ingeniería, Universidad Austral, Pilar, Argentina, [3] Austral Institute for Applied Artificial Intelligence, Universidad Austral, Pilar, Argentina

***Correspondence:**
Claudio N. Cavasotto
ccavasotto@austral.edu.ar;
cnc@cavasotto-lab.net

Today high-throughput docking is one of the most commonly used computational tools in drug lead discovery. While there has been an impressive methodological improvement in docking accuracy, docking scoring still remains an open challenge. Most docking programs are rooted in classical molecular mechanics. However, to better characterize protein-ligand interactions, the use of a more accurate quantum mechanical (QM) description would be necessary. In this work, we introduce a QM-based docking scoring function for high-throughput docking and evaluate it on 10 protein systems belonging to diverse protein families, and with different binding site characteristics. Outstanding results were obtained, with our QM scoring function displaying much higher enrichment (screening power) than a traditional docking method. It is acknowledged that developments in quantum mechanics theory, algorithms and computer hardware throughout the upcoming years will allow semi-empirical (or low-cost) quantum mechanical methods to slowly replace force-field calculations. It is thus urgently needed to develop and validate novel quantum mechanical-based scoring functions for high-throughput docking toward more accurate methods for the identification and optimization of modulators of pharmaceutically relevant targets.

Keywords: high-throughput docking, structure-based drug design, molecular docking, quantum mechanics, semi-empirical methods

INTRODUCTION

The cost to bring a new drug to the market could be as high as 2.6 billion US dollars, and can take up to 15 years (DiMasi et al., 2016). For many years, both the identification and optimization of novel drug lead compounds were accomplished within the drug discovery process by the experimental high-throughput screening of large chemical libraries. In spite of multiple efforts to improve its performance, drug discovery remains a costly and time consuming technique (Phatak et al., 2009). However, for the last 25 years, theoretical developments, better computational algorithms, faster computing resources, and improved visualization tools enabled the routine use of computational methods to model and visualize protein-ligand (PL) interactions, calculate binding free energy to different degrees of accuracy, and *in silico* screen chemical libraries using ligand-based and structure-based approaches. Today, computational chemistry is firmly established as a valuable tool in any drug lead discovery endeavor, aimed at saving time, effort, resources, and reducing costs (Cavasotto and Orry, 2007; Jorgensen, 2009, 2012; Spyrakis and Cavasotto, 2015; Pagadala et al., 2017).

During the last three decades, molecular docking has been one of the most commonly used computational methods in drug lead discovery (for review, cf., Kitchen et al., 2004; Rognan, 2011; Ciancetta and Moro, 2015; Sotriffer, 2015; Spyrakis and Cavasotto, 2015; Sulimov et al., 2019b). The aim of protein-small-molecule docking is the characterization of the optimal binding modes (poses) of a molecule within the binding site, and an estimation of its binding free energy. In high-throughput docking (HTD), where the protein is usually considered rigid or with very few degrees of freedom, and thousands to millions of molecules from a chemical library are screened, the goal is to generate a sub-library enriched with potential ligands, which will be prioritized for further experimental evaluation. In HTD, two different stages can be distinguished: the assessment of the best binding mode(s) of each molecule of the library ("docking stage"), and, on each *in silico* generated protein-small-molecule complex, the calculation of a score reflective of the likelihood that the molecule will actually bind to the target ("scoring stage") (Cavasotto and Orry, 2007; Guedes et al., 2018). In the docking stage, the docking energy (DE) is used to select, for each molecule, the lowest-energy pose(s) from a large amount of conformations generated, while the docking score (DS) is generally calculated as a fast approximation to the binding free energy ($\Delta G_{binding}$), and depends on several factors, such as the energy representation of the system, the model used to represent the aqueous environment and the consideration of explicit water molecules within the active site (Cozzini et al., 2006; Amadasi et al., 2008), and the degree of consideration of receptor flexibility (Cavasotto and Singh, 2008; Spyrakis et al., 2011; Spyrakis and Cavasotto, 2015). Thus, DE discriminates among poses of the same molecule, while the DS characterizes each molecule of the docked chemical library and is used to rank them according to the likelihood of binding. Many docking programs, however, use a single function as DE and DS.

It should be stressed that one of the main advantages of docking is that *in silico* generated poses usually serve as the starting point for *in silico* ligand optimization, using for example molecular dynamics-based calculation of binding free energies, such as Molecular Mechanics-Poisson Boltzmann Surface Area (MM-PBSA) and MM-Generalized Born Surface Area (MM-GBSA) methods (Kerrigan, 2013; Reddy et al., 2014; Genheden and Ryde, 2015; Sun et al., 2018; Wang et al., 2019).

While docking accuracy depends on the program, it is acknowledged that most of them are usually successful in identifying the correct pose (RMSD < 2 Å) with respect to the native structure (Warren et al., 2006; Wang et al., 2016). Moreover, an extensive recent benchmark of the Comparative Assessment of Scoring Functions (CASF) (Su et al., 2019) highlighted that docking programs display a better performance in terms of docking accuracy than in any of these three scoring-related metrics: correlation with experimental binding data (scoring power), ranking of ligands by their binding affinity data provided their correct poses are known (ranking power), and identification of actual ligands from a sub-library of top-ranking small-molecules (screening power). This was in agreement with other works (Cavasotto and Abagyan, 2004; Slater and Kontoyianni, 2019).

Most docking developments have been mainly rooted in molecular mechanics (MM) force-fields (FF). However, to better characterize protein-ligand interactions, at least in some cases, the use of a quantum mechanical (QM) description would be necessary (Cavasotto et al., 2019). The QM formulation is theoretically exact, as in principle, it accounts for all contributions to the energy (including terms or effects usually missing in FFs, such as electronic polarization, charge transfer, halogen bonding, and covalent-bond formation). Moreover, the QM framework is general across the chemical space so that all elements and interactions can be considered on equal footing, thus avoiding MM parameterizations.

Following the pioneering work of Raha and Merz (2004, 2005) where a QM-based score was used to discriminate ligand from decoy poses, there have been recently some applications of QM methods in docking, mainly aiming for accurate ligand binding mode assessment (for a survey of recent related works cf., Mucs and Bryce, 2013; Cavasotto et al., 2018; Aucar and Cavasotto, 2020). In a significant step forward, Pecina et al. obtained impressive results on the discrimination of native from decoy docking poses on four challenging systems (Pecina et al., 2016) using a docking energy function (Lepšík et al., 2013) based on the semi-empirical QM PM6 Hamiltonian (Stewart, 2007) supplemented with the D3H4X correction for dispersion, hydrogen- and halogen-bonding interactions (Řezáč and Hobza, 2012). In a follow-up contribution (Pecina et al., 2017), an even superior performance was achieved for accurate pose assessment using a self-consistent-charge density-functional tight-binding method (SCC-DFTB) formulation coupled with D3H4 corrections for dispersion and hydrogen-bond interactions, though at a higher computational cost. This docking energy score function was further used to obtain a reliable ranking on 10 inhibitors binding to carbonic anhydrase II (CAII) (Pecina et al., 2018).

However, the development of QM-based docking scoring functions aiming at the ranking of molecules within HTD (screening power) has progressed at a significantly slower pace. Only very recently, a QM-based approach was presented displaying a very good performance on discriminating ligands and decoys on a single system (heat shock protein 90, HSP90) (Eyrilmez et al., 2019). In fact, the development of fast yet accurate docking scoring functions still constitutes an area of active research (Cavasotto, 2012; Guedes et al., 2018). Moreover, the blind challenges ran by the Drug Design Data Resource (D3R) for ligand-pose and affinity prediction in 2015 (Gathiaka et al., 2016), 2016 (Gaieb et al., 2018), and 2018 (Gaieb et al., 2019), have shown the importance of method development and benchmarking in pose prediction and binding affinity ranking of ligands.

In this work, we introduce a QM-based docking scoring function and evaluate it in terms of ligand enrichment on 10 protein systems belonging to diverse protein families in terms of different binding site characteristics, the presence of co-factors and water molecules, and the enrichment factors computed with a standard HTD method. Excellent results were obtained by displaying our QM-based scoring function a much higher enrichment (screening power) than a traditional docking method. We stress that our goal is to present and to validate an initial straightforward approach, which could serve as a starting point for further developments and improvement. A wider and extensive benchmarking on more systems and a systematic comparison with most of the standard docking programs, and the assessment of the optimal combination of the different components of our approach (QM formalism and continuum solvent model, energy minimization strategies, use of single or multiple docking poses for scoring, and entropy contribution) are considerations of their importance. However, they exceed the purpose of our work and will be published in due course.

Assuming a continuous development in QM theory, algorithms and computer hardware, it is likely that semi-empirical methods [or low-cost Density Functional Theory (DFT) methods] will replace FF over the next 25 years (Grimme and Schreiner, 2018). Therefore, it is absolutely justified and there is an urgent need to start developing the next generation of QM-based scoring functions for HTD toward better methods for the identification of small-molecule modulators of pharmaceutically relevant targets.

TABLE 1 | Target proteins used in the evaluation of QM-based scoring functions.

Receptor name	Receptor code	PDB code	Co-factor[a]	Number of water molecules[b]	*EF*(1)[c]
Cyclin-dependent Kinase 2	CDK2	1FVV	–	–	8.0
Estrogen receptor α	ESR1	3ERT	–	–	16.5
Cyclooxygenase-1	COX1	2OYU	–	–	1.3
Neuraminidase	NRAM	1B9V	Ca^{2+}	–	0.
Heat shock protein 90 α	HSP90a	1UYG	–	4	0.
Hexokinase type IV	HXK4	3F9M	–	–	1.1
Coagulation factor VII	FA7	1W7X	–	1	20.2
Thymidine kinase	KITH	2B8T	–	–	35.1
Fatty acid binding protein adipocyte	FABP4	2NNQ	–	4	31.9
Phospholipase A2	PA2GA	1KVO	Ca^{2+}	–	2.0

[a] *Within 8 Å of the cyrstallographic ligand.*
[b] *Within 4 Å of the cyrstallographic ligand.*
[c] *Enrichment factor at 1% corresponding to docking with AutoDock Vina.*

MATERIALS AND METHODS

Protein Systems Preparation

The following targets were downloaded from the PDB (cf. **Table 1**): Cyclin-dependent Kinase 2 (CDK2, PDB 1FVV), Estrogen Receptor α (ESR1, PDB 3ERT), Cyclooxygenase-1 (COX1, PDB 2OYU), Neuraminidase (NRAM, PDB 1B9V), Heat Shock Protein 90 α (HSP90a, PDB 1UYG), Hexokinase Type IV (HXK4, PDB 3F9M), Coagulation Factor VII (FA7, PDB 1W7X), Thymidine kinase (KITH, PDB 2B8T), Fatty Acid Binding Protein Adipocyte (FABP4, PDB 2NNQ), and Phospholipase A2 (PA2GA, PDB 1KVO). All water molecules and co-factors were deleted, except in the following cases: NRAM and PA2GA, the Ca^{2+} atom within 8 Å of the bound ligand; HSP90a, water molecules 2059, 2121, 2123, and 2236; FA7, water molecule 2440; FABP4 water molecules 303, 623, 634, 665.

Each target was prepared using ICM software (MolSoft, San Diego, CA, 2019; Abagyan et al., 1994) in a similar fashion as in earlier works (Phatak et al., 2010). Succinctly, hydrogen atoms were added, followed by a local energy minimization of the complete system, and polar and water hydrogen positions were determined by optimizing the hydrogen bonding network within the torsional coordinates space. All Asp and Glu residues were assigned a -1 charge, and all Arg and Lys residues were assigned a $+1$ charge. Histidine tautomers were chosen according to their corresponding hydrogen bonding pattern. For docking with AutoDock Vina (Trott and Olson, 2010), the systems were pre-processed with AutoDock Tools (Morris et al., 2009).

Docking Library Preparation

For each target, the docking libraries were built by merging a set of ligands and a set of decoys, where the latter had similar physico-chemical properties to the ligands, but dissimilar 2-D topology. This has been shown to be necessary to ensure unbiased results when benchmarking docking programs (Huang et al., 2006; Gatica and Cavasotto, 2012). Ligands and decoys were extracted from the Directory of Useful Decoys (DUD, Huang et al., 2006), the NRLiSt binding data base for nuclear receptors (Lagarde et al., 2014), or the Directory of Useful Decoys- Enhanced (DUD-E, Mysinger et al., 2012), according to: CDK2, DUD (72, 2074) (number of ligands, number of decoys); ESR1, NRLiSt (133, 6555); COX1, DUD-E (210, 6955); NRAM, DUD-E (222, 6227); HSP90a (125, 4942); HXK4, DUD-E (127, 4802); FA7, DUD-E (185, 6300); KITH, DUD-E (132, 2866); FABP4, DUD-E (57, 2855); PA2GA (127, 5215). The protonation state and chirality of all molecules were conserved as in their original database.

High-Throughput Docking With AutoDock Vina

Molecular docking of the chemical libraries onto the associated targets using AutoDock Vina (Trott and Olson, 2010) was performed in a similar fashion as in our recent work (Palacio-Rodriguez et al., 2019).

Protein-Molecule Complex Generation, Structural Relaxation, and Unbound Protein and Ligand States Characterization

Protein-molecule complexes for QM-scoring were generated using the ICM docking module, keeping for each molecule its lowest DE conformation (docking RMSD values of native ligands are shown in **Table 2**). These protein-molecule complexes were also relaxed through cycles of local energy minimization in ICM according to the following procedure: (i) For each protein, the collected dihedral angles of amino-acids within 4 Å of any docked ligand of the corresponding chemical library were considered free; (ii) For each protein-molecule complex, five cycles of local energy minimization were performed restraining the heavy atoms with a harmonic potential with respect to their initial conformation; in each cycle the weight of this added potential

TABLE 2 | RMSD values of docked native ligands.

Receptor name	Receptor code	PDB ligand ID	RMSD (Å)	
			ICM	AD Vina
Cyclin-dependent Kinase 2	CDK2	107	0.74	2.68
Estrogen receptor α	ESR1	oht	1.48	4.69
Cyclooxygenase-1	COX1	ims	1.40	0.36
Neuraminidase	NRAM	ra2	0.54	0.91
Heat shock protein 90 α	HSP90a	pu2	0.52	0.26
Hexokinase type IV	HXK4	mrk	0.47	7.56
Coagulation factor VII	FA7	413	0.31	0.60
Thymidine kinase	KITH	thm	0.22	0.70
Fatty acid binding protein adipocyte	FABP4	t4b	0.37	0.79
Phospholipase A2	PA2GA	oap	0.54	1.37

was reduced in the following way: 50, 10, 5, 1, and 0 kcal/mol (no restraint). During this local energy minimization, the protein system was optimized in the torsional space (Abagyan et al., 1994), and the small-molecule in the Cartesian space.

To generate the unbound states, local energy minimization was performed on both protein and small-molecule in isolation from the crystallographic structure and the docked conformation, respectively.

System Cutout

For each target, a reduced-system was defined by first listing all the amino-acids within 8 Å of any docked molecule with ICM (only heavy atoms were considered in this threshold). Then, upon visual inspection, other amino-acids were eventually added to the list in order to avoid intra-helix or intra-β-sheet fragmentation, or loop fragments with just one amino-acid. A reduced-system was then built by deleting from the structure all amino-acids not included in the list, capping the N- and C-terminal of each fragment with hydrogens.

Entropy Calculation

Binding small-molecule conformational entropy was estimated as

$$\Delta S = -R \ln \Omega \tag{1}$$

where it is assumed that, upon binding, the molecule adopts a single conformation state (thus $S_{bound} = 0$), and Ω is the number of conformations in the free state, which was estimated in two different ways: i) by assigning each of the N free torsional bonds three rotational degrees of freedom (and thus $\Omega = 3^N$); ii) by performing a Monte-Carlo (MC) sampling with local energy minimization in the torsional space using ICM (Abagyan and Totrov, 1994; Abagyan et al., 1994), collecting all distinct conformations within the lowest 3 kcal/mol energy, and assuming all conformers are equally probable (a similar low-level sampling approach was used to explore the conformational flexibility of small-molecules, Forti et al., 2012). The MC approach was considered since rotamer count is known to overestimate the number of low-energy conformations, and thus the entropy (Anisimov and Cavasotto, 2011).

Quantum Mechanical Calculations

All QM calculations were performed using the QM package MOPAC2016 (Stewart, 2016) and its linear-scaling module MOZYME (Stewart, 1996), using the semi-empirical PM7 Hamiltonian (Stewart, 2013). In agreement with other authors (Sulimov et al., 2017a), we selected PM7 since it accounts for dispersion interactions, and hydrogen and halogen bonding have been taken into consideration at the paramterization stage, while it also includes several corrections to the PM6 Hamiltonian. Moreover, PM7 exhibited a very good performance on energy calculations aimed at discriminating native ligand positions in crystallographic complexes (Sulimov et al., 2017b). The solvation energy contribution in aqueous environment was calculated using the Conductor Like Screening Model (COSMO, Klamt and Schüürmann, 1993) continuum solvent model, with default atomic radii and surface tension parameters. The solvent-accessible surface area was taken from the program output [cf. (Stewart, 2016) for details on how the surface is built]. Those molecules which did not complete the QM calculation were excluded when computing the enrichment.

Evaluation Metrics

The enrichment factor (*EF*) measures the enrichment of actual ligands in a docked hit-list given a specific percentage of the dataset (threshold). The *EF* is defined as the ratio between actual number ligands (hits) found at the top $x\%$ of the screened database ($Hits_{x\%}$) and the number of molecules at that threshold $N_{x\%}$, normalized by the ratio between the total number of actual ligands within the entire dataset ($Hits_{\text{total}}$) and the total number of molecules of the latter (N_{total}).

$$EF(x) = \frac{Hits_{x\%}}{N_{x\%}} / \frac{Hits_{total}}{N_{total}} \tag{2}$$

Thus, the EF represents the probability of finding an actual ligand within the $x\%$ of the screened database with respect to the probability of finding an actual ligand at random. Whenever a molecule is represented within a chemical library with different states according to its protonation or chirality, each state is assigned an individual score, and the lowest score is used in the hit-list, and thus to calculate the *EF*. Throughout this work we report *EF*(1) and *EF*(2), since they are more representative of early enrichment.

We also report receiver operating characteristics (ROC) curves for each of the studied systems, measuring the area under the curve (AUC).

THEORETICAL FRAMEWORK

The binding free energy ($\Delta G_{binding}$) corresponding to Protein-Ligand (PL) association is expressed within the end-point molecular mechanics-quantum mechanics surface area method

(MM-QMSA) (Anisimov and Cavasotto, 2011; Anisimov et al., 2011) as

$$\Delta G_{binding} = \Delta \langle G^{QM} \rangle - T\Delta S \quad (3)$$

where the difference in the first term is calculated between the bound (PL) and unbound (P, L) states, <...> represents the average over QM-minimized classical molecular dynamics (MD) trajectories, G^{QM} is the QM energy including a continuum solvation term in an aqueous environment, and the second term represents the entropy change of P and L upon binding. We prefer to note the first term as a free energy, since it also includes the change in solvation free energy.

Since $\Delta G_{binding}$ in Equation (3) is obviously too costly to be used to score and rank large chemical libraries of small-molecules in HTD, a reasonable QM docking scoring function (*QMDS*) can be defined as an approximation to Equation (3), namely

$$QMDS = \Delta G^{QM} - T\Delta S \quad (4)$$

where averages over MD trajectories have been replaced by single-point QM calculations on the docked PL structure, and the free unbound L and P structures. The L and P deformation penalty contributions due to changes in L and P conformations upon binding are expressed as

$$\Delta G^{QM}_{conf}(X) = G^{QM}_{o}(X) - G^{QM}(X)\,,\ \text{with}\ X = \text{L}, \text{P} \quad (5)$$

where $G_o(X)$ is the energy of the isolated X in the conformation of the docked PL complex, and $G(X)$ is the energy of X in the free unbound state. Considering Equation (5), Equation (4) can be now be written out making the deformation contributions explicit as

$$QMDS = \Delta G^{QM}_{o} + \Delta G^{QM}_{conf}(P) + \Delta G^{QM}_{conf}(L) - T\Delta S \quad (6)$$

where the "o" subscript in the first term refers to calculations using the PL, P, and L conformations from the docked complex. It should be pointed out that Equation 6 is formally identical to another formulation (Eyrilmez et al., 2019).

Two types of QM docking scoring functions were defined according to the relaxation of the reference docked PL complexes: (i) $QMDS_1$, with no relaxation, that is, the QM calculations are performed directly on the docked PL complex, and (ii) $QMDS_2$, where docked PL complexes are relaxed through local energy minimization (see Methods). When the deformation contributions (second and third terms in Equation 6) were included, the suffix "d" is added ($QMDS_{1d}$ and $QMDS_{2d}$).

RESULTS AND DISCUSSION

Improved HTD Enrichment Using QM-Based Scoring

Ten target proteins were selected based on different characteristics such as protein family, binding site properties, presence of co-factors and water molecules (within or close to the binding site), and enrichment factor at 1% calculated after docking with AutoDock Vina (**Table 1**). Only crystallographic and/or conserved water molecules within 4 Å of the native ligand were included.

TABLE 3 | Comparison of the enrichment factors [*EF*(1)] for docking and scoring ($QMDS_1$) using a complete and reduced protein systems.

Receptor	Complete system	Reduced system
CDK2	20.1	24.2
ESR1	33.7	36.4

Throughout all this work, the *QMDS* was calculated in all its variants on PL complexes generated with ICM docking, since it is acknowledged to generate high quality protein-molecule poses (Bursulaya et al., 2003; Neves et al., 2012), as confirmed by the RMSD values of the docked native ligands in **Table 2**). Clearly, better enrichment is strongly coupled to scoring over correct docking poses. In this regard, the use of multiple docked conformations for each molecule, stemming from the same docking program or not, might clearly enhance the results of our QM-scoring scheme. However, we preferred to use a single pose from a single program, to keep our methodology straightforward, and to establish a clear baseline from which to start looking for improvement.

Since a target receptor protein is usually very large for QM calculations, to calculate the *QMDS* we used a reduced system by cutting out amino acids farther than ~8 Å from any docked molecule (cf. the Methods section for full details on the cutout process), since a threshold of <6 Å has been reported to seriously deteriorate the results (Ehrlich et al., 2017); moreover, it should be highlighted that the smaller the threshold, the greater the impact of the continuous solvent surface replacing the cutout amino-acids. To further validate our approach, quantum mechanical docking scores *QMDS* considering the complete protein and its associated reduced system were calculated on CDK2 and ESR1 (**Table 3**). We observe that using a cutout system has no impact on the calculation. Thus, throughout this work, a reduced representation of the target protein will be used for all QM calculations.

In **Table 4**, we display the enrichment factors *EF*(1) for the 10 target systems comparing AutoDock Vina with four schemes of QM docking scoring (for HSP90a, enrichment values including and excluding the 19 macrocycle containing ligands are shown). The conformational entropy change upon ligand binding was estimated in two ways: (i) ΔS^{rot}, based on a term proportional to the number of N free rotatable bonds of the molecule ($\Omega_{conf} = 3^N$), and (ii) ΔS^{conf}, by estimating Ω_{conf} as the number of low-energy diverse conformations generated using Monte-Carlo sampling with local energy minimization (cf. Methods). We found that the use of S^{rot} deteriorates the *EF* (data not shown), so S^{conf} is used in all calculations. In $QMDS_2$ and $QMDS_{2d}$ the reference docked PL complexes were local energy minimized using MM (see Methods). Obviously, a QM minimization would have been desirable, but this would render any QM docking scoring function useless due to the computational times involved,

TABLE 4 | Enrichment factors calculated at 1% [$EF(1)$] and 2% [$EF(2)$] (in parenthesis) for AutoDock Vina and QM docking scoring.

Receptor	AD Vina	$QMDS_1$	$QMDS_{1d}$	$QMDS_2$	$QMDS_{2d}$
CDK2	8.0 (5.0)	24.2 (15.1)	26.2 (18.1)	26.3 (16.2)	26.3 (18.2)
ESR1	16.5 (11.0)	36.4 (26.1)	30.6 (22.4)	44.0 (29.2)	43.2 (26.4)
COX1	1.3 (0.7)	2.8 (2.8)	3.5 (3.9)	2.8 (1.4)	3.5 (3.5)
NRAM	0. (0.)	9.3 (8.7)	9.3 (10.2)	21.4 (15.8)	21.4 (16.3)
HSP90a	0. (0.)	15.3 (11.9)	16.7 (11.9)	28.3 (16.1)	31.1 (16.1)
HSP90a[a]	0. (0.)	14.1 (10.5)	15.2 (10.5)	23.3 (14.5)	26.8 (14.0)
HXK4	1.1 (1.1)	11.4 (7.9)	9.1 (6.2)	15.6 (8.8)	15.6 (9.9)
FA7	20.2 (20.2)	49.0 (42.5)	47.0 (42.5)	54.0 (41.0)	52.0 (41.0)
KITH	35.1 (21.1)	35.4 (23.8)	31.7 (22.9)	34.1 (24.2)	30.5 (26.9)
FABP4	31.9 (16.0)	33.9 (18.9)	36.2 (20.9)	32.8 (18.6)	32.8 (23.0)
PA2GA	2.0 (2.0)	6.5 (7.5)	10.9 (8.6)	18.2 (12.9)	16.1 (12.9)

[a] *Excluding the macrocycle containing molecules for calculating the EF.*

even for reduced systems. Moreover, in this case further caution should be exerted not to artificially deform the molecular system.

As stated before, a wide range of enrichment factors calculated from docking with AD Vina was taken into account for selecting the target proteins for this benchmark. It can be readily seen from **Table 4** that using any variant of QM docking scoring has an impressive improvement over AD Vina, especially in those cases with low AD Vina *EF*. This happens even in the simplest case of $QMDS_1$, where no relaxation is performed on the PL complexes.

It is clear that PL relaxation, even using a MM-based approach, has on average a positive effect for calculating the QM docking score. Moreover, in those cases where the $EF(1)$ slightly decreases (KITH, FABP4), the $EF(2)$ is conserved. Focusing in the analysis of $QMDS_2$ and $QMDS_{2d}$, inclusion of the deformation contribution (second and third term in Equation 6) slightly deteriorates the results in ESR1, FA7, KITH, and PA2GA. However, in all but ESR1, $EF(2)$ improves after inclusion of the deformation term (as it also happens in the other cases where $EF(1)$ increases or is constant, CDK2, COX1, NRAM, HSP90a, HXK4, and FABP4). Considering that the effect on $EF(1)$ is in no way dramatic, and that $EF(2)$ (which also refers to early enrichment), improves except in one case, we state that the deformation terms are necessary to obtain better enrichment factors, though this should obviously be validated in a larger-scale benchmark. We hypothesize that this slight deterioration might be related to a small noise introduced upon energy minimization, which is canceled out in the $QMDS_2$ case. In the special case of HSP90a, the consideration of 19 macrocycle containing molecules has a negative effect in the *EF* calculation. We hypothesize that the strong performance of QM-scoring is due to a better representation of intra- and inter-molecular interactions, though of course further validation and benchmarking is still needed to confirm this.

In **Figure 1**, the ROC plots of $QMDS_2$ and AD Vina for the 10 systems are shown, including the corresponding AUC values. Analysis of the curves confirm what has been noted above based on *EF*, exhibiting the QM-score excellent results.

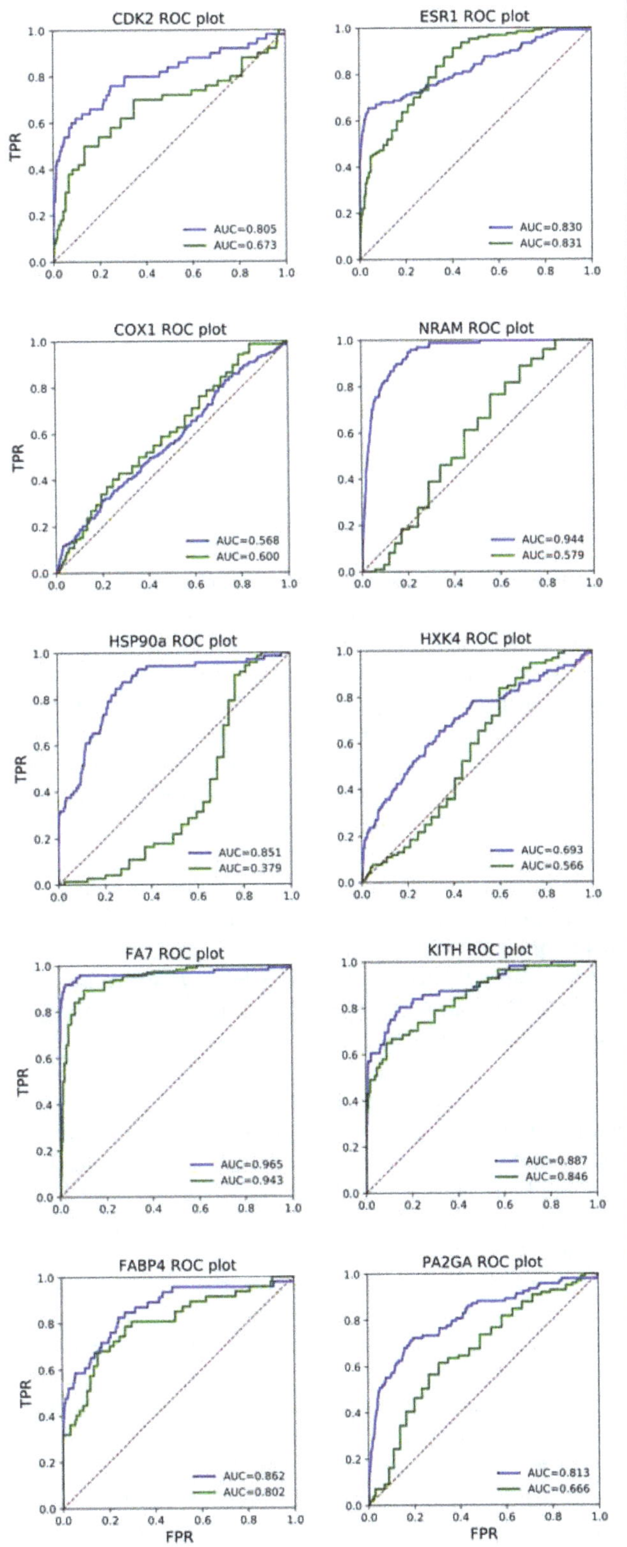

FIGURE 1 | Receiver operating characteristic (ROC) plots of AutoDock Vina (red line) and QM-scoring $QMDS_{2d}$ (blue line) for the 10 systems studied. The dotted line corresponds to random selection (AUC = 0.5). FPR, False Positive Rate; TPR, True Positive Rate; AUC, Area under the curve.

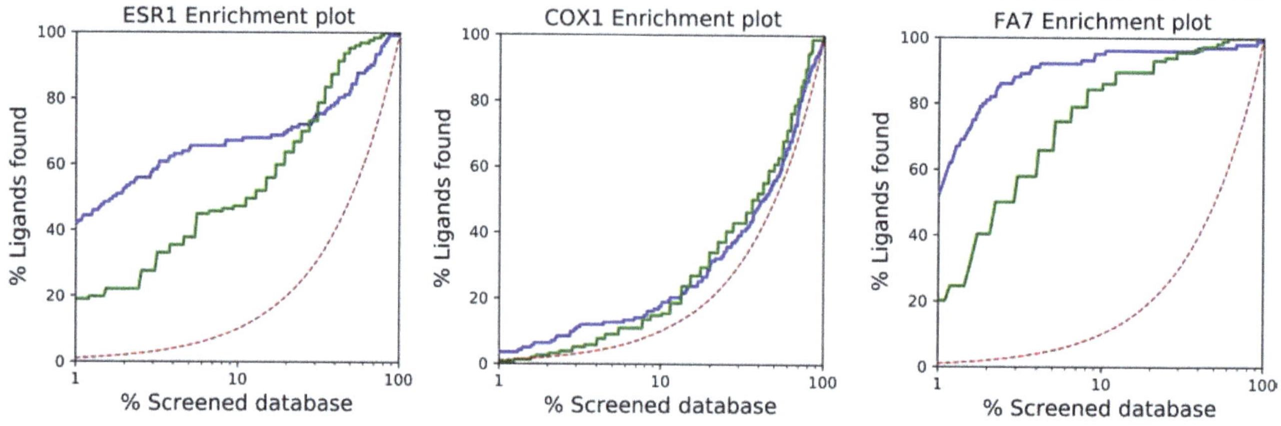

FIGURE 2 | Enrichment plots for ESR1, COX1, and FA7 using AutoDock Vina (red line) and QM-scoring $QMDS_{2d}$ (blue line). The dotted line corresponds to random selection.

Interestingly, in ESR1 both scoring methods show basically the same AUC, which is in conflict with the large difference in EF values reported in **Table 4**. To clarify this issue, in **Figure 2** we show the enrichment plot associated to ESR1. It can be seen that AD out-performs $QMDS_2$ after 30% of the screened database, a region of no importance for drug discovery; for early enrichment, the enrichment plot in **Figure 2** confirms the trend observed in **Table 4** that $QMDS_2$ is remarkable superior in the initial part of the ranking. A similar behavior is observed for FA7 (cf. **Table 4** and **Figures 1, 2**). In the case of COX1, while the AUC of the QM-score is slightly less than AD Vina, the enrichment plot in **Figure 2** shows that for early enrichment, QM-scoring out-performs AD Vina.

While our QM-score appears to be a very promising for HTD, and QM calculations are in principle more accurate than classical ones to describe molecular interactions, there are still a number of approximations which prevent the direct use of *QMDS* as a measure of actual absolute binding free energy. We mention three, among many: (i) QM local energy minimization was not performed (for computational efficiency, as said above); (ii) Vibrational entropies were not included; (iii) PM7 has not been parameterized to reproduce binding free energies. Our QM calculations were in the order of −70 kcal/mol, in agreement with recent binding enthalpy calculations on protein-ligand complexes using a PM7+COSMO approach (Sulimov et al., 2019a), where in spite of the difference between experimental and calculated absolute binding enthalpies, very good correlation with experimental values was obtained. It should be added that it is also well-known that traditional scoring functions correlate poorly with binding energy (cf. Enyedy and Egan, 2008, among others). Moreover, among traditional scoring functions there is no uniform scale: While AutoDock and Glide (Friesner et al., 2004; Halgren et al., 2004) are roughly in the range of −10 kcal/mol and higher, others are around −60 kcal/mol. Moreover, even end-point methods such as MM/PBSA or MM/GBSA exhibited calculated binding free energies in the order of −60 kcal/mol, or even lower when changes in vibrational entropy are not included (Zhong and Carlson, 2005), and even when including those terms (Woo and Roux, 2005; Anisimov and Cavasotto, 2011; Anisimov et al., 2011). Thus, we stress that *QMDS* should be considered a score, not a measure of absolute binding energy. It is aimed for relative binding energy estimation, and thus for compound ranking.

On average, the computing time of this QM docking score on a single core is ~6–8 minutes (depending on the size of the system, and on whether the deformation energy term is considered), around an order of magnitude slower than a MM-based DS.

CONCLUSIONS AND PERSPECTIVES

Docking programs have been so far based on molecular mechanics force-fields. However, a better description of protein-ligand interactions could be achieved, in principle, with quantum mechanical methods, which are theoretically exact, capture the underlying physics of the molecular system, and account for all contributions to the energy, including those effects usually missing in force-fields, such as electronic polarization, covalent-bond formation, and charge transfer. Moreover, a quantum mechanical formulation is generally valid across the chemical space, thus avoiding the force-field parameterizations.

We present a new QM-based high-throughput docking scoring function, which has been evaluated on 10 protein systems belonging to different protein families, displaying diverse binding site properties, and covering a wide range of enrichment factors computed with a traditional docking program. As shown in **Table 4**, even the simplest QM docking scoring function (where no relaxation is performed on the reference docked protein-small-molecule complex) shows excellent results in terms of enrichment (screening power). In fact, the improvement over AutoDock Vina on all systems is remarkable, especially in those cases with very low AD Vina enrichment. Upon complex relaxation, the improvement is even larger, regardless of whether the protein and ligand deformation terms are included or not.

We highlight that our main aim is to develop and validate a simple, straightforward approach for QM docking scoring, from which further developments can be built. Clearly, to further improve this methodology, several aspects should be analyzed: (i) a wider and extensive benchmark on many more target systems; (ii) comparison with other MM-based standard docking scoring functions; (iii) evaluation of other QM formalisms, continuum solvent models and their associated parameters (atomic radii and surface tension parameters); (iv) structural relaxation strategies; (v) use of single or multiple poses for scoring; (vi) the vibrational entropy changes upon binding. All of these considerations are important. They are currently being investigated and will be published in due course. Considering the outstanding improvements to our methods, we highlight that the *QMDS* should be used as a score and not an estimation to the absolute binding energy.

In terms of CPU time, our QM docking scoring function is approximately 10 times slower than MM-based standard scores on a single core. In spite of this, our impressive results on a set of 10 different protein targets highlight the huge potential of QM-based scoring. Moreover, considering future developments in QM theory, algorithms and computer hardware, it can be hypothesized that semi-empirical methods (or low-cost DFT methods) will replace FF over the following years (Grimme and Schreiner, 2018). We thus believe it is fully justified and of the utmost importance to develop the next generation of QM-based scoring functions for HTD toward highly accurate methods for the identification and optimization of small-molecule modulators of pharmaceutically relevant targets.

AUTHOR CONTRIBUTIONS

CC conceived and designed the research, performed simulations, analysis, interpretation, and wrote the paper. MA performed quantum mechanical simulations and enrichment calculations and contributed with interpretation and analysis. All authors approved the manuscript for publication.

FUNDING

This work was supported by the National Agency for the Promotion of Science and Technology (ANPCyT) (PICT-2014-3599 and PICT-2017-3767).

ACKNOWLEDGMENTS

The Authors thank Prof. F. Javier Luque for helpful discussions. CNC thanks Molsoft LLC (San Diego, CA) for providing an academic license for the ICM program. The authors thank the National System of High Performance Computing (Sistemas Nacionales de Computación de Alto Rendimiento, SNCAD), the Centro de Computación de Alto Rendimiento (Computational Centre of High Performance Computing, CeCAR), and the Centro de Cálculo de Alto Desempeño (Universidad Nacional de Córdoba) for granting the use of their computational resources.

REFERENCES

Abagyan, R., and Totrov, M. (1994). Biased probability monte carlo conformational searches and electrostatic calculations for peptides and proteins. *J. Mol. Biol.* 235, 983–1002. doi: 10.1006/jmbi.1994.1052

Abagyan, R., Totrov, M., and Kuznetsov, D. (1994). ICM - a new method for protein modeling and design - applications to docking and structure prediction from the distorted native conformation. *J. Comput. Chem.* 15, 488–506. doi: 10.1002/jcc.540150503

Amadasi, A., Surface, J. A., Spyrakis, F., Cozzini, P., Mozzarelli, A., and Kellogg, G. E. (2008). Robust classification of "relevant" water molecules in putative protein binding sites. *J. Med. Chem.* 51, 1063–1067. doi: 10.1021/jm701023h

Anisimov, V. M., and Cavasotto, C. N. (2011). Quantum mechanical binding free energy calculation for phosphopeptide inhibitors of the Lck SH2 domain. *J. Comput. Chem.* 32, 2254–2263. doi: 10.1002/jcc.21808

Anisimov, V. M., Ziemys, A., Kizhake, S., Yuan, Z., Natarajan, A., and Cavasotto, C. N. (2011). Computational and experimental studies of the interaction between phospho-peptides and the C-terminal domain of BRCA1. *J. Comput. Aided Mol. Des.* 25, 1071–1084. doi: 10.1007/s10822-011-9484-3

Aucar, M. G., and Cavasotto, C. N. (2020). Molecular docking using quantum mechanical-based methods. *Methods Mol. Biol.* 2114, 269–284. doi: 10.1007/978-1-0716-0282-9_17

Bursulaya, B. D., Totrov, M., Abagyan, R., and Brooks, C. L. 3rd. (2003). Comparative study of several algorithms for flexible ligand docking. *J. Comput. Aided Mol. Des.* 17, 755–763. doi: 10.1023/B:JCAM.0000017496.76572.6f

Cavasotto, C. N. (2012). "Binding free energy calculations and scoring in small-molecule docking," in *Physico-Chemical and Computational Approaches to Drug Discovery*, eds F. J. Luque and X. Barril (London: Royal Society of Chemistry), 195–222.

Cavasotto, C. N., and Abagyan, R. A. (2004). Protein flexibility in ligand docking and virtual screening to protein kinases. *J. Mol. Biol.* 337, 209–225. doi: 10.1016/j.jmb.2004.01.003

Cavasotto, C. N., Adler, N. S., and Aucar, M. G. (2018). Quantum chemical approaches in structure-based virtual screening and lead optimization. *Front. Chem.* 6:188. doi: 10.3389/fchem.2018.00188

Cavasotto, C. N., Aucar, M. G., and Adler, N. S. (2019). Computational chemistry in drug lead discovery and design. *Int. J. Quantum Chem.* 119:e25678. doi: 10.1002/qua.25678

Cavasotto, C. N., and Orry, A. J. (2007). Ligand docking and structure-based virtual screening in drug discovery. *Curr. Top. Med. Chem.* 7, 1006–1014. doi: 10.2174/156802607780906753

Cavasotto, C. N., and Singh, N. (2008). Docking and high throughput docking: successes and the challenge of protein flexibility. *Curr. Comput. Aided Drug Design* 4, 221–234. doi: 10.2174/157340908785747474

Ciancetta, A., and Moro, S. (2015). "Protein-ligand docking: virtual screening and applications to drug discovery," in *In silico Drug Discovery and Design: Theory, Methods, Challenges, and Applications*, ed C.N. Cavasotto (Boca Raton, FL: CRC Press, Taylor & Francis Group), 189–213.

Cozzini, P., Fornabaio, M., Mozzarelli, A., Spyrakis, F., Kellogg, G. E., and Abraham, D. J. (2006). Water: how to evaluate its contribution in protein-ligand interactions. *Int. J. Quantum Chem.* 106, 647–651. doi: 10.1002/qua.20812

DiMasi, J. A., Grabowski, H. G., and Hansen, R. W. (2016). Innovation in the pharmaceutical industry: new estimates of R&D costs. *J. Health Econ.* 47, 20–33. doi: 10.1016/j.jhealeco.2016.01.012

Ehrlich, S., Goller, A. H., and Grimme, S. (2017). Towards full quantum-mechanics-based protein-ligand binding affinities. *ChemPhysChem* 18, 898–905. doi: 10.1002/cphc.201700082

Enyedy, I. J., and Egan, W. J. (2008). Can we use docking and scoring for hit-to-lead optimization? *J. Comput. Aided Mol. Des.* 22, 161–168. doi: 10.1007/s10822-007-9165-4

Eyrilmez, S. M., Kopruluoglu, C., Rezac, J., and Hobza, P. (2019). Impressive enrichment of semiempirical quantum mechanics-based scoring function: HSP90 protein with 4541 inhibitors and decoys. *ChemPhysChem* 20, 2759–2766. doi: 10.1002/cphc.201900628

Forti, F., Cavasotto, C. N., Orozco, M., Barril, X., and Luque, F. J. (2012). A multilevel strategy for the exploration of the conformational flexibility of small molecules. *J. Chem. Theor. Comput.* 8, 1808–1819. doi: 10.1021/ct300097s

Friesner, R. A., Banks, J. L., Murphy, R. B., Halgren, T. A., Klicic, J. J., Mainz, D. T., et al. (2004). Glide: a new approach for rapid, accurate docking and scoring. 1. method and assessment of docking accuracy. *J. Med. Chem.* 47, 1739–1749. doi: 10.1021/jm0306430

Gaieb, Z., Liu, S., Gathiaka, S., Chiu, M., Yang, H., Shao, C., et al. (2018). D3R grand challenge 2: blind prediction of protein-ligand poses, affinity rankings, and relative binding free energies. *J. Comput. Aided Mol. Design* 32, 1–20. doi: 10.1007/s10822-017-0088-4

Gaieb, Z., Parks, C. D., Chiu, M., Yang, H., Shao, C., Walters, W. P., et al. (2019). D3R grand challenge 3: blind prediction of protein-ligand poses and affinity rankings. *J. Comput. Aided Mol. Design* 33, 1–18. doi: 10.1007/s10822-018-0180-4

Gathiaka, S., Liu, S., Chiu, M., Yang, H., Stuckey, J. A., Kang, Y. N., et al. (2016). D3R grand challenge 2015: evaluation of protein-ligand pose and affinity predictions. *J. Comput. Aided Mol. Design* 30, 651–668. doi: 10.1007/s10822-016-9946-8

Gatica, E. A., and Cavasotto, C. N. (2012). Ligand and decoy sets for docking to g protein-coupled receptors. *J. Chem. Inf. Model* 52, 1–6. doi: 10.1021/ci200412p

Genheden, S., and Ryde, U. (2015). The MM/PBSA and MM/GBSA methods to estimate ligand-binding affinities. *Expert Opin. Drug Discov.* 10, 449–461. doi: 10.1517/17460441.2015.1032936

Grimme, S., and Schreiner, P. R. (2018). Computational chemistry: the fate of current methods and future challenges. *Angew. Chem. Int. Ed. Engl.* 57, 4170–4176. doi: 10.1002/anie.201709943

Guedes, I. A., Pereira, F. S. S., and Dardenne, L. E. (2018). Empirical scoring functions for structure-based virtual screening: applications, critical aspects, and challenges. *Front. Pharmacol.* 9:1089. doi: 10.3389/fphar.2018.01089

Halgren, T. A., Murphy, R. B., Friesner, R. A., Beard, H. S., Frye, L. L., Pollard, W. T., et al. (2004). Glide: a new approach for rapid, accurate docking and scoring. 2. enrichment factors in database screening. *J. Med. Chem.* 47, 1750–1759. doi: 10.1021/jm030644s

Huang, N., Shoichet, B. K., and Irwin, J. J. (2006). Benchmarking sets for molecular docking. *J. Med. Chem.* 49, 6789–6801. doi: 10.1021/jm0608356

Jorgensen, W. L. (2009). Efficient drug lead discovery and optimization. *Acc. Chem. Res.* 42, 724–733. doi: 10.1021/ar800236t

Jorgensen, W. L. (2012). Challenges for academic drug discovery. *Angew. Chem. Int. Ed. Engl.* 51, 11680–11684. doi: 10.1002/anie.201204625

Kerrigan, J. E. (2013). Molecular dynamics simulations in drug design. *Methods Mol. Biol.* 993, 95–113. doi: 10.1007/978-1-62703-342-8_7

Kitchen, D. B., Decornez, H., Furr, J. R., and Bajorath, J. (2004). Docking and scoring in virtual screening for drug discovery: methods and applications. *Nat. Rev. Drug Discov.* 3, 935–949. doi: 10.1038/nrd1549

Klamt, A., and Schüürmann, G. (1993). COSMO: a new approach to dielectric screening in solvents with explicit expressions for the screening energy and its gradient. *J. Chem. Soc. Perkin Trans.* 2, 799–805. doi: 10.1039/P29930000799

Lagarde, N., Ben Nasr, N., Jeremie, A., Guillemain, H., Laville, V., Labib, T., et al. (2014). NRLiSt BDB, the manually curated nuclear receptors ligands and structures benchmarking database. *J. Med. Chem.* 57, 3117–3125. doi: 10.1021/jm500132p

Lepšík, M., Řezáč, J., Kolár, M., Pecina, A., Hobza, P., and Fanfrlík, J. (2013). The semiempirical quantum mechanical scoring function for *in silico* drug design. *ChemPlusChem* 78, 921–931. doi: 10.1002/cplu.201300199

Morris, G. M., Huey, R., Lindstrom, W., Sanner, M. F., Belew, R. K., Goodsell, D. S., et al. (2009). AutoDock4 and AutoDockTools4: automated docking with selective receptor flexibility. *J. Comput. Chem.* 30, 2785–2791. doi: 10.1002/jcc.21256

Mucs, D., and Bryce, R. A. (2013). The application of quantum mechanics in structure-based drug design. *Expert Opin. Drug Discov.* 8, 263–276. doi: 10.1517/17460441.2013.752812

Mysinger, M., Carchia, M., Irwin, J. J., and Shoichet, B. K. (2012). Directory of useful decoys, enhanced (DUD-E) - better ligands and decoys for better benchmarking. *J. Med. Chem.* 55, 6582–6594. doi: 10.1021/jm300687e

Neves, M. A., Totrov, M., and Abagyan, R. (2012). Docking and scoring with ICM: the benchmarking results and strategies for improvement. *J. Comput. Aided Mol. Design* 26, 675–686. doi: 10.1007/s10822-012-9547-0

Pagadala, N. S., Syed, K., and Tuszynski, J. (2017). Software for molecular docking: a review. *Biophys. Rev.* 9, 91–102. doi: 10.1007/s12551-016-0247-1

Palacio-Rodriguez, K., Lans, I., Cavasotto, C. N., and Cossio, P. (2019). Exponential consensus ranking improves the outcome in docking and receptor ensemble docking. *Sci. Rep.* 9:5142. doi: 10.1038/s41598-019-41594-3

Pecina, A., Brynda, J., Vrzal, L., Gnanasekaran, R., Horejsi, M., Eyrilmez, S., et al. (2018). Ranking power of the SQM/COSMO scoring function on carbonic anhydrase II-inhibitor complexes. *ChemPhysChem* 19, 873–879. doi: 10.1002/cphc.201701104

Pecina, A., Haldar, S., Fanfrlik, J., Meier, R., Rezac, J., Lepsik, M., et al. (2017). SQM/COSMO scoring function at the DFTB3-D3H4 level: unique identification of native protein-ligand poses. *J. Chem. Infor. Model.* 57, 127–132. doi: 10.1021/acs.jcim.6b00513

Pecina, A., Meier, R., Fanfrlik, J., Lepsik, M., Rezac, J., Hobza, P., et al. (2016). The SQM/COSMO filter: reliable native pose identification based on the quantum-mechanical description of protein-ligand interactions and implicit COSMO solvation. *Chem. Commun.* 52, 3312–3315. doi: 10.1039/C5CC09499B

Phatak, S. S., Gatica, E. A., and Cavasotto, C. N. (2010). Ligand-steered modeling and docking: a benchmarking study in class A G-protein-coupled receptors. *J. Chem. Inf. Model.* 50, 2119–2128. doi: 10.1021/ci100285f

Phatak, S. S., Stephan, C. C., and Cavasotto, C. N. (2009). High-throughput and *in silico* screenings in drug discovery. *Exp. Opin. Drug Discov.* 4, 947–959. doi: 10.1517/17460440903190961

Raha, K., and Merz, K. M. Jr. (2004). A quantum mechanics-based scoring function: study of zinc ion-mediated ligand binding. *J. Am. Chem. Soc.* 126, 1020–1021. doi: 10.1021/ja038496i

Raha, K., and Merz, K. M. Jr. (2005). Large-scale validation of a quantum mechanics based scoring function: predicting the binding affinity and the binding mode of a diverse set of protein-ligand complexes. *J. Med. Chem.* 48, 4558–4575. doi: 10.1021/jm048973n

Reddy, M. R., Reddy, C. R., Rathore, R. S., Erion, M. D., Aparoy, P., Reddy, R. N., et al. (2014). Free energy calculations to estimate ligand-binding affinities in structure-based drug design. *Curr. Pharm. Des.* 20, 3323–3337. doi: 10.2174/13816128113199990604

Řezáč, J., and Hobza, P. (2012). Advanced corrections of hydrogen bonding and dispersion for semiempirical quantum mechanical methods. *J. Chem. Theor. Comput.* 8, 141–151. doi: 10.1021/ct200751e

Rognan, D. (2011). "Docking methods for virtual screening: principles and recent advances," in *Virtual Screening. Principles, Challenges and Practical Guidelines, ed C. Sotriffer* (Weinheim: Wiley-VCH Verlag), 153–176.

Slater, O., and Kontoyianni, M. (2019). The compromise of virtual screening and its impact on drug discovery. *Expert Opin. Drug Discov.* 14, 619–637. doi: 10.1080/17460441.2019.1604677

Sotriffer, C. A. (2015). "Protein-ligand docking: from basic principles to advanced applications," in *In silico Drug Discovery and Design: Theory, Methods, Challenges, and Applications*, ed C.N. Cavasotto (Boca Raton, FL: CRC Press, Taylor & Francis Group), 155–188.

Spyrakis, F., Bidon-Chanal, A., Barril, X., and Luque, F. J. (2011). Protein flexibility and ligand recognition: challenges for molecular modeling. *Curr. Top. Med. Chem.* 11, 192–210. doi: 10.2174/156802611794863571

Spyrakis, F., and Cavasotto, C. N. (2015). Open challenges in structure-based virtual screening: Receptor modeling, target flexibility consideration and active site water molecules description. *Arch. Biochem. Biophys.* 583, 105–119. doi: 10.1016/j.abb.2015.08.002

Stewart, J. J. (2013). Optimization of parameters for semiempirical methods VI: more modifications to the NDDO approximations and re-optimization of parameters. *J. Mol. Model.* 19, 1–32. doi: 10.1007/s00894-012-1667-x

Stewart, J. J. P. (1996). Application of localized molecular orbitals to the solution of semiempirical self-consistent field equations. *Int. J. Quant. Chem.* 58, 133–146.

Stewart, J. J. P. (2007). Optimization of parameters for semiempirical methods V: modification of NDDO approximations and application to 70 elements. *J. Mol. Model.* 13, 1173–1213. doi: 10.1007/s00894-007-0233-4

Stewart, J. J. P. (2016). *"MOPAC2016"*. Colorado Spring, CO: Stewart Computational Chemistry. Available online at: www.OpenMOPAC.net

Su, M., Yang, Q., Du, Y., Feng, G., Liu, Z., Li, Y., et al. (2019). Comparative assessment of scoring functions: the CASF-2016 update. *J. Chem. Inform. Model.* 59, 895–913. doi: 10.1021/acs.jcim.8b00545

Sulimov, A., Kutov, D., Gribkova, A., Ilin, I., Tashchilova, A., and Sulimov, V. (2019a). "Search for approaches to supercomputer quantum-chemical docking," in *Supercomputing,* eds V. Voevodin and S. Sobolev (Cham: Springer International Publishing), 363–378.

Sulimov, A. V., Kutov, D. C., Katkova, E. V., Ilin, I. S., and Sulimov, V. B. (2017a). New generation of docking programs: supercomputer validation of force fields and quantum-chemical methods for docking. *J. Mol. Graph. Model.* 78, 139–147. doi: 10.1016/j.jmgm.2017.10.007

Sulimov, A. V., Kutov, D. C., Katkova, E. V., and Sulimov, V. B. (2017b). Combined docking with classical force field and quantum chemical semiempirical method PM7. *Adv. Bioinformatics* 2017:7167691. doi: 10.1155/2017/7167691

Sulimov, V. B., Kutov, D. C., and Sulimov, A. V. (2019b). Advances in docking. *Curr. Med. Chem.* 26, 7555–7580. doi: 10.2174/0929867325666180904115000

Sun, H., Duan, L., Chen, F., Liu, H., Wang, Z., Pan, P., et al. (2018). Assessing the performance of MM/PBSA and MM/GBSA methods. 7. entropy effects on the performance of end-point binding free energy calculation approaches. *Phys. Chem. Chem. Phys.* 20, 14450–14460. doi: 10.1039/C7CP07623A

Trott, O., and Olson, A. J. (2010). AutoDock vina: improving the speed and accuracy of docking with a new scoring function, efficient optimization, and multithreading. *J. Comput. Chem.* 31, 455–461. doi: 10.1002/jcc.21334

Wang, E., Sun, H., Wang, J., Wang, Z., Liu, H., Zhang, J. Z. H., et al. (2019). End-point binding free energy calculation with MM/PBSA and MM/GBSA: strategies and applications in drug design. *Chem. Rev.* 119, 9478–9508. doi: 10.1021/acs.chemrev.9b00055

Wang, Z., Sun, H., Yao, X., Li, D., Xu, L., Li, Y., et al. (2016). Comprehensive evaluation of ten docking programs on a diverse set of protein-ligand complexes: the prediction accuracy of sampling power and scoring power. *Phys. Chem. Chem. Phys.* 18, 12964–12975. doi: 10.1039/C6CP01555G

Warren, G. L., Andrews, C. W., Capelli, A. M., Clarke, B., LaLonde, J., Lambert, M. H., et al. (2006). A critical assessment of docking programs and scoring functions. *J. Med. Chem.* 49, 5912–5931. doi: 10.1021/jm050362n

Woo, H. J., and Roux, B. (2005). Calculation of absolute protein-ligand binding free energy from computer simulations. *Proc. Natl. Acad. Sci. U.S.A.* 102, 6825–6830. doi: 10.1073/pnas.0409005102

Zhong, H., and Carlson, H. A. (2005). Computational studies and peptidomimetic design for the human p53-MDM2 complex. *Proteins* 58, 222–234. doi: 10.1002/prot.20275

Exploring the RNA-Recognition Mechanism Using Supervised Molecular Dynamics (SuMD) Simulations: Toward a Rational Design for Ribonucleic-Targeting Molecules?

*Maicol Bissaro, Mattia Sturlese and Stefano Moro**

Molecular Modeling Section, Department of Pharmaceutical and Pharmacological Sciences, University of Padova, Padua, Italy

***Correspondence:**
Stefano Moro
stefano.moro@unipd.it*

Although proteins have represented the molecular target of choice in the development of new drug candidates, the pharmaceutical importance of ribonucleic acids has gradually been growing. The increasing availability of structural information has brought to light the existence of peculiar three-dimensional RNA arrangements, which can, contrary to initial expectations, be recognized and selectively modulated through small chemical entities or peptides. The application of classical computational methodologies, such as molecular docking, for the rational development of RNA-binding candidates is, however, complicated by the peculiarities characterizing these macromolecules, such as the marked conformational flexibility, the singular charges distribution, and the relevant role of solvent molecules. In this work, we have thus validated and extended the applicability domain of SuMD, an all-atoms molecular dynamics protocol that allows to accelerate the sampling of molecular recognition events on a nanosecond timescale, to ribonucleotide targets of pharmaceutical interest. In particular, we have proven the methodological ability by reproducing the binding mode of viral or prokaryotic ribonucleic complexes, as well as that of artificially engineered aptamers, with an impressive degree of accuracy.

Keywords: nucleic acids, RNA, SMIRNA, molecular recognition, molecular dynamics (MD), supervised molecular dynamics (SuMD), structure-based drug design (SBDD)

INTRODUCTION

Ribonucleic acid (RNA) is a polymer whose biological importance has increased progressively over the last 50 years. Despite the central dogma of molecular biology considering this nucleic acid simply as a functional messenger between DNA genetic information storage and protein biosynthesis, RNA has recently been reappraised as an ancestral molecule of primary importance in the abiogenesis process. At the origin of life, RNA probably encompassed both an informational role, which progressively evolved toward involving the more stable and easily replicable DNA polymer, and a catalytic function, which was gradually flanked by more versatile proteins

(Morris and Mattick, 2014). The complexity hiding behind RNA's biological functions is intuitable by taking into consideration the human organism, which genetic heritage could quite entirely be transcribed into RNA, despite coding only in a minimal portion (about 3%) for proteins (Warner et al., 2018). A great majority of these transcripts therefore remain untranslated, originating non-coding genomic portions. RNA revolution has thus shed light on the regulatory activity of this widely different class of macromolecules that, along with some proteins, cooperate to control and finely orchestrate the genome expression (Connelly et al., 2016).

RNA polymer lengths range from small hairpins composed of a few tens of nucleobases to long non-coding RNAs sequences (lncRNAs) that can reach up to a few thousands nucleotides (Connelly et al., 2016). Differently from DNA, RNA usually exists as a single-stranded molecule that is not strictly limited by a Watson-Crick base pairing. In solution, ribonucleic acids explore a wide landscape of three-dimensional structures, characterizable by the presence of peculiar functional domains able to specifically recognize other nucleic acids, polypeptides, glyco-derivates, or cognates of small organic molecules (Draper, 1995; Cruz and Westhof, 2009; Salmon et al., 2014; Flynn et al., 2019).

From a topological point of view, the tertiary and quaternary structures that distinguish ribonucleic acids from their deoxyribonucleic counterpart make them more similar to proteins, a consideration that has paved the way for an attempt to pharmacologically modulate their biological functions through the discovery of small molecules interacting with RNA (SMIRNA) (Sucheck and Wong, 2000; Connelly et al., 2016). Interestingly, in recent research work, it has been estimated that pharmacologically modulating RNA would allow us to expanding—by more than an order of magnitude—the universe of targetable macromolecules, and this would thus considerably extend the portion of the druggable genome (Ecker and Griffey, 1999; Warner et al., 2018). Although RNA has been historically considered as an "undruggable" pharmaceutical target, the discovery that many drugs of undeniable therapeutic importance, especially antibiotics, act at this level has attracted the interest of the scientific community, resulting in greater effort being made toward the development of new tools for this purpose (Donlic and Hargrove, 2018; Disney, 2019). Furthermore, the orthogonality characterizing RNA homologous transcripts belonging to virus, prokaryote, and eukaryote genomes make RNA an interesting target for the purpose of achieving selectivity, especially in the field of anti-infectives compound development (Ecker and Griffey, 1999; Connelly et al., 2016). All these aspects, therefore, make the discovery of SMIRNAs extremely intriguing. A first pioneering approach to rationally design new RNA-targeting compounds, simply starting from the knowledge of the oligonucleotide sequence of pathological interest, was developed by the Disney research group and was successfully applied to a plethora of expanded repeating RNAs that are known to cause microsatellite disorders (Velagapudi et al., 2014; Disney et al., 2016). In addition, the quantitative structure-activity relationship (QSAR) model and chemical similarity search were initially exploited to *in-silico* identify or optimize new chemical probes targeting RNA (Disney et al., 2014). Since X-ray crystallography, NMR spectroscopy and, recently, Cryo-EM techniques have unveiled with an atomistic level of detail a multitude of three-dimensional RNA structures, the scientific community has begun to evaluate the applicability of structure-based drug design strategies (SBDD). These approaches, until now mainly validated on proteins targets, could enhance the rational design of SMIRNAs. Molecular docking represents one of the electives of *in silico* techniques, exploited both in the academic and industrial world, to accelerate the discovery and optimization of new drug candidates by evaluating the putative small molecules' binding mode and providing a way to perform a ranking of vast compound libraries. There are however many peculiarities of ribonucleic acids that affect both performance and accuracy of docking protocols, and this makes its application challenging. The polyanionic backbone of RNA determines a peculiar charge distribution on the polymer surface—quite different from the one characterizing proteins—to which the scoring functions were traditionally calibrated (Disney, 2019). Furthermore, docking protocols do not explicitly consider the role of solvent during the molecular recognition process, whereas structural data have highlighted how water molecules can stabilize RNA-ligand complexes, often mediating hydrogen bonds networks (Fulle and Gohlke, 2009). However, the aspect that mostly affects RNA-docking accuracy is the flexibility and the dynamic behavior characterizing ribonucleic acids, which are usually neglected by docking algorithms, thus limiting the discovery of compounds targeting a narrow region of the conformational space (Hermann, 2002; Fulle and Gohlke, 2009; Disney et al., 2014). An attempt to overcome these limitations was conducted by Stelzer et al., who performed a docking-based virtual screening on an RNA dynamic ensemble constructed by combining molecular dynamics simulations (MD) with NMR spectroscopy and reported the discovery of six molecules able to bind HIV-1 TAR with quite good affinity. MD simulations would represent a valuable computational tool with which to investigate different ligand–RNA recognition processes, fully considering both target flexibility and the solvent presence. Interestingly, molecular mechanics force fields (FF), such as AMBER or CHARMM, were revisited and refined during the last year to improve ribonucleotide simulation accuracy (Pérez et al., 2007; Denning et al., 2011). Nevertheless, the use of MD is mostly limited to the fluctuation exploration in the post-docking procedure since ligand–target associations are rare events that can be sampled only through long-timescale computationally expensive simulations. An implementation of classical MD, called supervised molecular dynamics (SuMD), was recently developed in our research group. SuMD is able to speed up the exploration of the ligand–receptor recognition pathways on a nanosecond timescale through the implementation of a tabu-like supervision algorithm (Sabbadin and Moro, 2014). The protocol was so far validated in different scenarios, including ion–protein, ligand–protein, and peptide–protein bound complexes, proving that it could reproduce the experimental determined final state with great geometric accuracy (Cuzzolin et al., 2016; Salmaso et al., 2017; Bissaro et al., 2019).

In this work, SuMD simulations were applied for the first time to investigate the recognition mechanism involving ribonucleic acid macromolecules with the aim to extend the methodology applicability domain. This pilot study, which provided encouraging results, took into account a plethora of different ribonucleic complexes of pharmaceutical interest, the three-dimensional structures of which are known and available on the Protein Data Bank archive (Berman et al., 2000). SuMD methodology proved its ability in describing, with a reduced computational effort, the whole process of ligand–RNA recognition (from the unbound to the bound state), independently by the target topological complexity. As far as we know, this represents the first attempt to overcome methodological limitations within molecular docking when applied to ribonucleic acids, describing binding events through an all-atoms MD-based approach. This study confirms the possible use of SuMD as an innovative computational tool that can accelerate the discovery of new drug candidates and with peculiar attention to SMIRNAs.

MATERIALS AND METHODS

Software Overview

MOE suite (Molecular Operating Environment, version 2018.0101) was used to perform most of the general molecular modeling operations, such as RNA and ligand preparation. All these operations have been performed on an 8 CPU (Intel® Xeon® CPU E5-1620 3.50 GHz) Linux workstation. Molecular dynamics (MD) simulations were performed with an ACEMD engine (Harvey et al., 2009) on a GPU cluster composed of 18 NVIDIA drivers whose models go from GTX 980 to Titan V. For all the simulations, the ff14SB force field with χ modification tuned for RNA (χOL3) was adopted to describe ribonucleic acids, while a general Amber force field (GAFF) was adopted to parameterize small organic molecules (Wang et al., 2006; Sprenger et al., 2015; Tan et al., 2018).

Structures Preparation

The three-dimensional coordinates of each RNA–SMIRNA complex investigated were retrieved from the RCSB PDB database and prepared for SuMD simulations as herein described (Cuzzolin et al., 2016). For structures solved by NMR, which contain multiple conformations of the same complex, the one with the lowest potential energy (usually the first) was selected and then used. All complexes were then processed by means of an MOE protein structure preparation tool: missing atoms in nucleotide bases were built according to AMBER14 force field topology. Missing hydrogen atoms were added to X-Ray-derived complexes, and appropriate ionization states were assigned by Protonate-3D tool (Labute, 2009). Ligand coordinates (both small molecules and peptides) were moved at least 30 Å away from RNA binding cleft, a distance bigger than the electrostatic cut-off term used in the simulation (9 Å with Amber force field) to avoid premature interaction during the initial phases of the SuMD simulations.

Solvated System Setup and Equilibration

Each system investigated by means of SuMD contained an RNA target macromolecule, and the respective ligand, which was a SMIRNA or a peptide, moved far away from the binding site as previously described. The systems were explicitly solvated by a cubic water box with cell borders placed at least 15 Å away from any RNA/ligand atom, using TIP3P as a water model. To neutralize the total charge of each system, Na^+/Cl^- counterions were added to a final salt concentration of 0.154 M. The systems were energy minimized by 500 steps with the conjugate-gradient method, then 500,000 steps (1 ns) of NVT followed by 500,000 steps (1 ns) of NPT simulations were carried out, both using 2 fs as time step and applying harmonic positional constraints on RNA and ligand heavy atoms by a force constant of 1 kcal mol^{-1} $Å^{-2}$, gradually reducing with a scaling factor of 0.1. During this step, the temperature was maintained at 310 K by a Langevin thermostat with low dumping of 1 ps^{-1} and the pressure at 1 atm by a Berendsen barostat (Berendsen et al., 1984; Loncharich et al., 1992). The M-SHAKE algorithm was applied to constrain the bond lengths involving hydrogen atoms. The particle-mesh Ewald (PME) method was exploited to calculate electrostatic interactions with a cubic spline interpolation and 1 Å grid spacing, and a 9.0 Å cutoff was applied for Lennard–Jones interactions (Essmann et al., 1995).

Supervised Molecular Dynamics (SuMD) Simulations

Molecular dynamics simulations represent a well-validated computational tool that, through the numerical solution of the Newton equation of motion, makes it possible to describe the time-dependent evolution of a molecular system. Despite the impressive temporal resolution characterizing the technique, to capture pharmaceutically relevant events, such as the molecular recognition between a drug and its biological target, huge computational efforts are required. The SuMD protocol instead improves the efficiency with which a binding event is sampled, from a microsecond to a nanosecond timescale, by applying a tabu-like algorithm. In detail, short (600 ps long) unbiased MD trajectories are collected, and these monitor, during the entire simulation, the distance between the ligand center of mass with respect to the ribonucleic acid binding site; then, those distance points are fitted into a linear function. Only productive MD steps in which the computed slope is negative are maintained, thus indicating a ligand approach toward the RNA binding site. Otherwise, the simulation is restarted by randomly assigning the atomic velocities from the previous set of coordinates. The supervision algorithm controlled the sampling until the distance between the ligand and the ribonucleic binding site dropped below 5 Å, at which point it was disabled, and a short classical MD simulation was performed, allowing the system to relax. For each case study, up to a maximum of 10 SuMD binding simulations were collected, of which only the best was thoroughly analyzed and discussed in the manuscript. A detailed report on SuMD protocol performance can be found in the **Supplementary Material**. The three-dimensional RNA structures investigated in this study, along with the nucleotides selected for the computation of the respective binding cleft center of mass, are reported in **Figure 1**. In this implementation, the SuMD code is written in

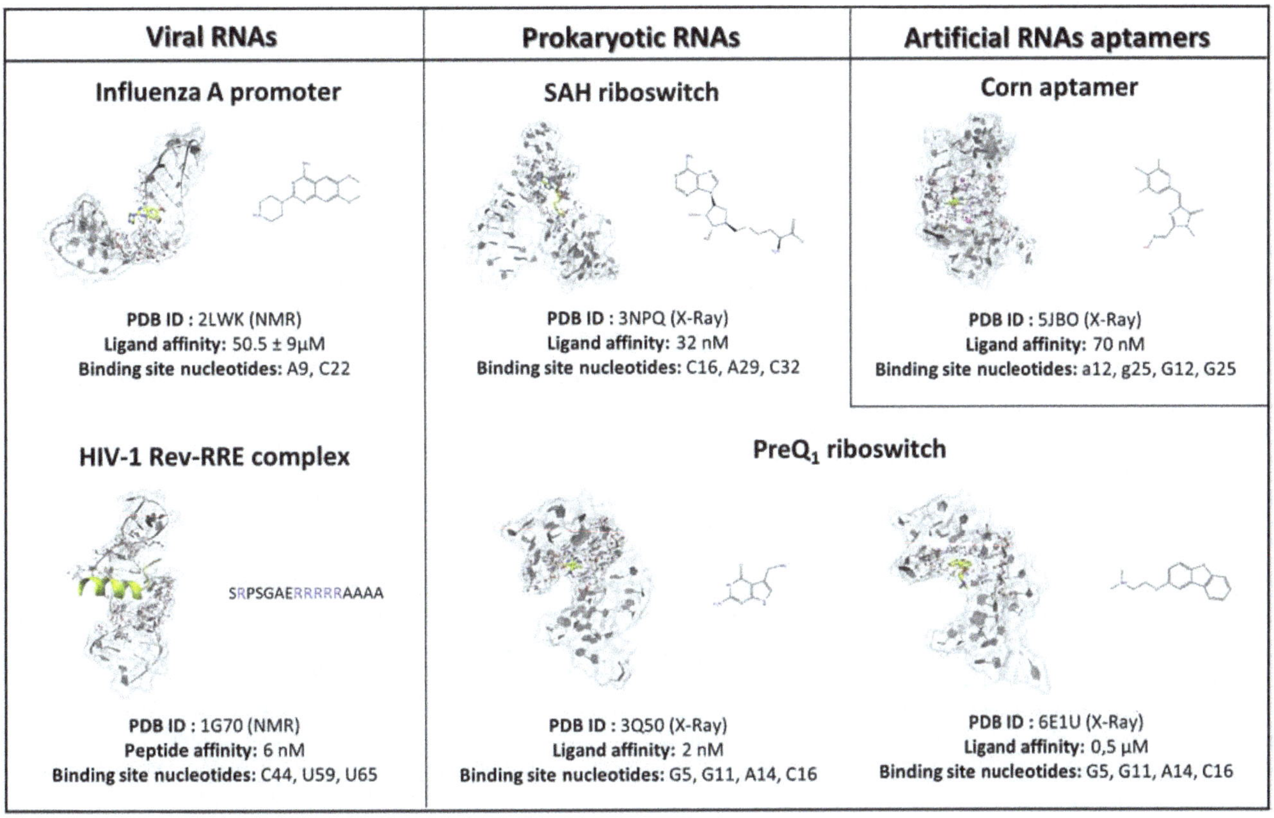

FIGURE 1 | The case studies selected for the SuMD methodological validation are herein summarized and subdivided into RNA of viral origin, prokaryotic origin, or artificially engineered aptamers. For each complex investigated, the three-dimensional structure is depicted, representing with a green color the reference ligand, together with the nucleobases selected to define the binding site position in the SuMD simulations. Finally, the chemical structures of each ligand are reported, along with the experimental datum of binding affinity. In the case of the peptide, the primary sequence is reported, highlighting the basic residues constituting the arginine reach motif (ARM) in a blue color.

Python programming languages and exploits the ProDy python package to perform the geometrical ligand–target supervision process (Bakan et al., 2011).

SuMD Trajectory Analysis

All the SuMD trajectories collected were analyzed by an in-house tool written in tcl and python languages, as described in the original publication (Salmaso et al., 2017). Briefly, the dimension of each trajectory was reduced, saving MD frames at a 20 ps interval; each trajectory was then superposed and aligned on the RNA phosphate atoms of the first frames and wrapped into an image of the system simulated under periodic boundary conditions. The geometric performance of SuMD methodology was evaluated, and it computed the ligand RMSD (Root mean square deviation) along with the entire simulation with respect to the experimental resolved three-dimensional complex. Furthermore, the RMSD of RNA structures were computed on the P atoms of the backbone and plotted over time, and these can be viewed in the **Supplementary Figures S1–S6A**. A ligand–RNA interaction energy estimation during the recognition process was calculated using an MMGBSA protocol, as implemented in AMBER 2014, and it plotted MMGBSA values over time (Miller et al., 2012). The MMGBSA values were also arranged according to the distances between ligand and ribonucleic target mass centers in the Interaction Energy Landscape plots (**Supplementary Figures S1–S6B**). Here, the distances between mass centers are reported on the x-axis, while the MMGBSA values are plotted on the y-axis, and these are rendered by a colorimetric scale going from blue to red for negative to positive energetic values. These graphs allow for the evaluation of the variation of the interaction energy profile at different ligand–RNA distances; this helps to individuate meta-stable binding states during the binding process. Furthermore, for each target investigated in this work, the nucleotides within a distance of 4 Å from the respective ligand atoms were dynamically selected to qualitatively and quantitatively evaluate the number of contacts during the entire binding process. The most contacted nucleotides were thus selected, to compute a per-nucleotide electrostatic and vdW interaction, and energy contribution, with the ribonucleic target. NAMD was used for post-processing computation of electrostatic interactions using an AMBER ff14SB force field. The cumulative electrostatic interactions were computed for the same target nucleotides by summing the energy values frame by frame along the trajectory, and the resulting graphs were reported to the lower-right of movies provided as **Supplementary Videos 1–6**. Representations of the molecular structures were prepared with VMD software (Humphrey et al., 1996).

RESULTS AND DISCUSSION

To investigate the SuMD applicability domain and accuracy in the context of ribonucleic acid molecular recognition, a retrospective validation approach was selected, and it stressed the computational methodology ability in geometrically reproducing experimental binding modes of SMIRNA or small folded peptides. The three-dimensional structures of six ligand–RNA complexes solved both through X-Ray and NMR spectroscopy were retrieved from the RCSB PDB database and prepared for subsequent SuMD simulations moving ligands far away from the ribonucleic binding clefts, as accurately described in materials and methods section. The RNA structures, reported in **Figure 1**, were selected to span a vast plethora of pharmaceutically interesting ribonucleic targets, which vary between being of viral and bacterial origin, up to artificially engineered aptamers. Furthermore, the selected structures provide an overview of different peculiar three-dimensional RNA motifs, from a small stem-loop to a riboswitch characterized by a complex architecture. The results collected through SuMD simulations are then reported herein along with the geometric and interactives analysis performed. A summary of all the statistics regarding the simulation performances are reported in the **Supplementary Information.**

Targeting Viral RNAs (vRNAs)

The discovery and design of new antiviral compounds targeting viral proteins are complicated by the enormous variability affecting these macromolecules, an aspect representing the core of the drug resistance phenomenon. On the other hand, lncRNA regions belonging to viral genomes, being less affected by genetic mutations and having no counterpart in human organisms, are becoming attractive pharmaceutical targets. Aminoglycosides, antibacterial drugs known to inhibit protein synthesis acting at the level of the prokaryotic ribosome, have proven to be promiscuous molecules that are also able to bind lncRNA structural elements of viral genomes (Bernacchi et al., 2007). This experimental evidence has paved the way for the discovery of drug-like small molecules able to inhibit the replication for a plethora of pathological viral diseases, such as human immunodeficiency virus (HIV), hepatitis C virus (HCV), severe respiratory syndrome coronavirus (SARS CoV), and influenza A virus (Hermann, 2016).

Influenza a Virus Promoter

Influenza A represents a group of viruses differing from virulence and pathogenicity profiles that all belong to the Orthomyxoviridae family. The Influenza A genome comprises eight negative-sense single-stranded RNA segments (vRNA) encoding for 13 proteins (Coloma et al., 2009). The 5′-end and 3′-end terminal portions of each vRNA segment in the physiological condition fold together in a partial duplex, forming an arrangement called a promoter, which controls RNA-dependent RNA polymerase (RdRp) recognition and, thus, genome transcription and replication (Desselberger et al., 1980). Since the promoter sequences are highly conserved among Influenza A viruses and marginally affected by genetic variation that can enhance the onset of drug resistance, they represent a promising pharmaceutical target. The Varani research group, exploiting an NMR-based fragments screening approach, has identified 6,7-dimethoxy-2-(1-piperazinyl)-4-quinazolinamine (DPQ) as a promising scaffold for antiviral drug development as it is able to bind the Influenza A promoter region with a low micromolar affinity (K_d 50.5 ± 9 μM) and is also able to inhibit the virus replication in a comparable range of concentration (Lee et al., 2014). The SMIRNA binding mode was experimentally elucidated by means of NMR, as depicted in **Figure 1**, confirming DPQ recognition within the RNA major groove at the (A-A)-U internal loop level.

The SuMD algorithm was then applied to this first case study, in an attempt to investigate the entire DPQ binding mechanism, stressing at the same time the methodology accuracy in reproducing the experimental solved complex. A first interesting aspect is represented by the reduced time window of 30 ns required to sample a putative molecular recognition event between DPQ and its ribonucleic target (**Supplementary Video 1**). This result is quite impressive, especially if compared with classical MD simulations, which otherwise would require extensive computational efforts. At the end of the simulation, as depicted in the **Figure 2** graph, the SMIRNA has converged both from a geometrical and interactive point of view toward the NMR structure binding mode. The low $RMSD_{min}$ value of 2.6 Å, computed on DPQ heavy atoms, confirm, also in the case of nucleic acids, SuMD ability in predicting a reasonable binding hypothesis. This value must not be evaluated with excessive severity, having been calculated only with respect to one of the 16 conformations of the complex deposited on the PDB database. The solution NMR structure has indeed highlighted an important variability in the DPQ positioning within the RNA binding site, with an $RMSD_{max}$, computed on ligand-heavy atoms of 1.4 Å. Moreover, this approach makes it possible to peek at the entire molecular recognition process and to not focus merely on the final state. **Figure 2C** reports a time-dependent analysis performed on the nucleotides most frequently contacted during the simulation, reporting their cumulative contribution to binding, which is defined as the sum of each nucleotide electrostatic and van der Waals (vdW) interaction energy. It is encouraging to note how the nucleotides that computationally have shown a primary role in stabilizing the DPQ complex (A9–A11 and C21–G24) also correspond to those that have experimentally experienced the greatest chemical shift perturbations during NMR experiments. In addition, as reported in **Figures 2B,C** and on **Supplementary Figure S1**, SuMD simulation allows us to decipher the different role played by aforementioned nucleotides, some of them (A9–A11) participating only during the early phases of SMIRNA recognition (until 10 ns) and the other (C21–G24) stabilizing the complex within the ribonucleic cleft (after 10 ns). These results appear even more interesting if we consider the high flexibility characterizing the small RNA duplex. Despite the reduced time window explored by SuMD methodology, the

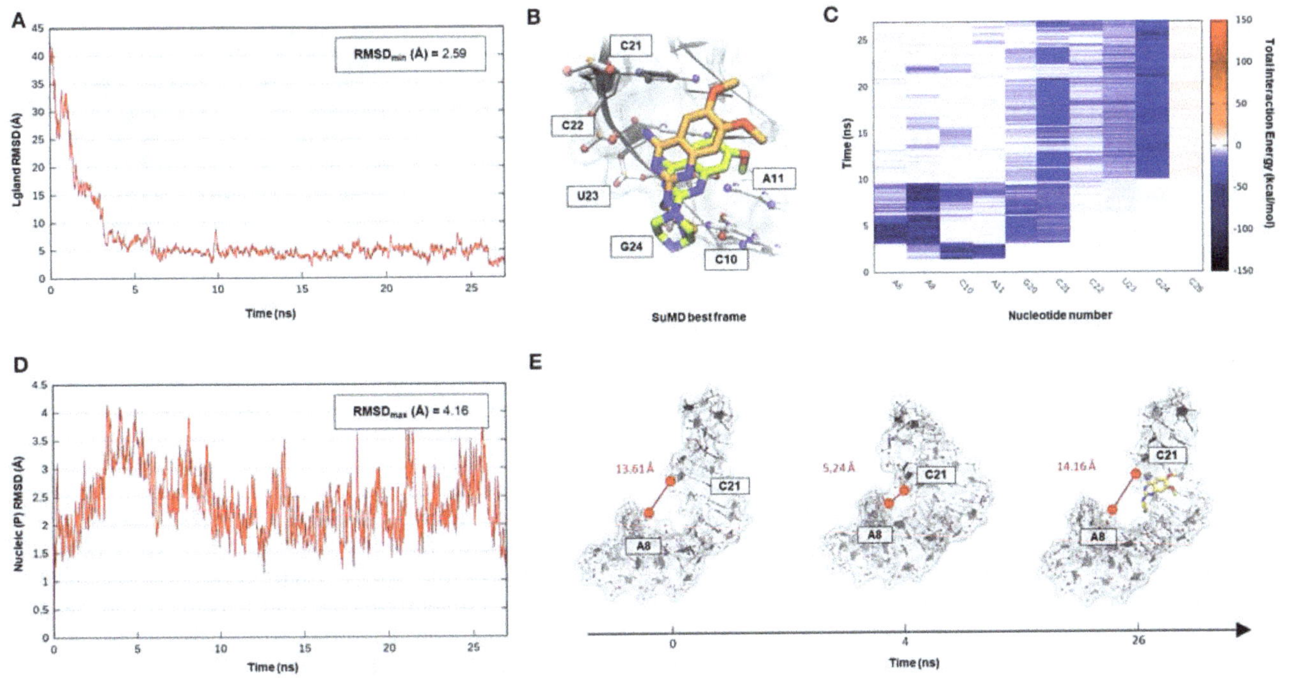

FIGURE 2 | This panel summarizes the recognition pathway of the DPQ fragment with the Influenza A promoter region. **(A)** RMSD of DPQ heavy atoms against the PDB reference. **(B)** Superimposition between the experimental NMR complex (PDB ID 2LWK, green-colored DPQ molecule) and the SuMD conformation with lowest RMSD along the trajectory (orange-colored molecule). The nucleotides surrounding the binding site are reported. **(C)** Dynamic total interaction energy (electrostatic + vdW) computed for most contacted RNA nucleobase. **(D)** RMSD of RNA phosphate atoms belonging to the backbone, computed against the PDB reference. **(E)** Flexibility characterizing the RNA structure during DPQ binding event, binding clef dimension was monitored as the distance dynamically occurring between two key nucleotides (A8 and C21).

structure has indeed shown a relevant $RMSD_{max}$ of 4.2 Å from the initial experimental coordinates (**Figure 2D**). In detail, after a few ns of simulation, the promoter duplex in the ligand-free form folds back on itself, and only DPQ binding allows the structure to return to the experimental linear conformation (**Figure 2E**). The same behavior was coherently captured also by NMR experiments, which previously highlighted how the RNA helical axis curvature changes upon ligand binding, enlarging the dimension of the binding cleft (Lee et al., 2014).

HIV-1 Rev-RRE Complex

The human immunodeficiency virus of type 1 (HIV-1) is a retrovirus belonging to the Lentivirus family, and it is responsible for acquired immunodeficiency syndrome (AIDS). RNA–protein interactions play a fundamental role in controlling the HIV replication cycle and, consequently, virulence profile (Battiste et al., 1996). HIV-1 Rev, in particular, is a small regulatory protein that drives the nuclear export of unspliced and partially spliced viral mRNAs transcripts. Rev protein mediated its function, recognizing a purine-rich bulge within stem-loop IIb of the Rev response element (RRE), a highly structured mRNA region within an *env* intron (DiMattia et al., 2010). The minimal binding domain in the Rev protein is constituted by a short α-helix folded peptide, which contains an arginine-rich binding motif (ARM), a domain known to be important also for tat-TAR (trans-acting region) interactions in HIV. Harada et al., exploiting an *in-vivo* strategy, have identified a class of specific RNA-binding peptides able to target HIV-1 Rev-RRE complex. Specifically, RSG-1.2, an α-helical peptide of 22 amino acids, was selected among a combinatorial library and subsequently engineered, providing a 7-fold increase in binding affinity and a 15-fold increase in selectivity toward the ribonucleic target, further resulting in an *in vivo* ability to completely disrupt the RNA–Rev protein interaction (Harada et al., 1996, 1997). The solution structure of an oligonucleotide portion derived from HIV-1 RRE-IIb stem domain in a complex with an RSG-1.2 peptide was solved through NMR, providing structural details about vRNA targeting by means of the small peptide (Gosser et al., 2001). We have therefore chosen this case study to validate SuMD performance in one of the most complex methodological scenarios, namely the molecular recognition between two highly flexible partners: a small α-helix folded peptide and a portion of ribonucleic acid. In addition, the predominant electrostatic component that both characterizes the RNA polyanionic backbone and the small polycationic peptide, which contain six Arg residues, makes the prediction of the binding mode even more complex. Despite the unfavorable premises, a few tens of ns proved to be sufficient for the SuMD protocol to sample a binding hypothesis for the RSG-1.2 peptide. During the simulation, as observable on **Supplementary Video 1**, the peptide was accommodated with the correct orientation within the HIV-1 RRE-IIb major groove reaching, as reported in **Figure 3A**, an $RMSD_{min}$ value

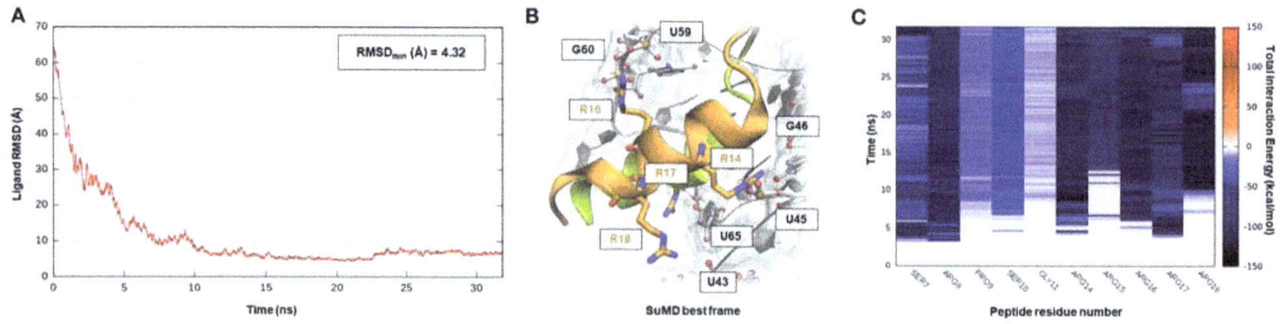

FIGURE 3 | This panel summarizes the recognition pathway of RSG-1.2 peptide with HIV-1 REE. **(A)** RMSD of RSG-1.2 Cα atoms against the PDB reference. **(B)** Superimposition between the experimental NMR complex (PDB ID 1G70, green-colored peptide) and the SuMD conformation with lowest RMSD along the trajectory (orange-colored peptide). The nucleotides surrounding the binding site, along with R residues belonging to ARM, are reported. **(C)** Dynamic total interaction energy (electrostatic + vdW) computed for most contacted RNA nucleobase.

of 4.3 Å, computed on Cα peptide atoms. Although the geometric accuracy is lower than the previous example, the SuMD simulation has allowed us to identify the main interactive hotspots stabilizing the complex. As hypothesized and confirmed by **Figure 3C**, the ARM motif plays a fundamental role in anchoring the RSG-1.2 peptide, with charged residue R 16, R17, and R18 mediating fork electrostatic interactions with the phosphate atoms of the ribonucleic backbone, in a coherent way with the experimentally solved structure. Furthermore, the analysis performed on the trajectory (**Supplementary Figure S2**) has highlighted the peculiar behavior of R14; its guanidinium side chain is deeply buried within the RNA groove, where, differently from the other charged residues, it stabilizes the peptide through a solvent-shielded hydrogen bond and vdW interactions, an aspect in great agreement with the experimental NMR data (Gosser et al., 2001).

Targeting Prokaryotic RNAs

In the last decades, the discovery that many aminoglycoside compounds clinically exploited to treat severe bacterial infections mediated their action by affecting the ribosome machinery confirmed the initial hypothesis of considering RNA, especially prokaryotic ones, as an appetible pharmaceutical target (Disney, 2019). However, the drugs that target ribosomes represent an exception, rather than a model: the abundance of ribosome macromolecules in the cytoplasmic compartment means, therefore, that even modest drug-binding affinity could result in acceptable therapeutic efficacy (Warner et al., 2018). Apart from ribosomes, a putative regulatory role of lncRNAs in bacterial systems has recently become increasingly clear. From a mechanistic point of view, it is possible to distinguish regulatory RNAs acting in *trans*, either by base-pairing with a complementary region in the target mRNA or by sequestration of an RNA-binding protein and regulatory sequences that, in contrast, are encoded as part of the mRNA for the gene they regulate, thus acting in *cis* (Sherwood and Henkin). Riboswitches, which are structured elements typically found in the 5′ untranslated regions (UTR) of mRNAs, represent an interesting example of the latter case (Tucker and Breaker, 2005). These RNA elements, through an aptameric portion, directly sense a physiological signal (ions, cofactors, or metabolites) and transmit the information to the gene expression machinery via a signal-dependent RNA conformational change (Sherwood and Henkin, 2016). The discovery that clinically approved antibacterial Roseflavin exerts part of its therapeutic action by binding the flavin mononucleotide (FMN) riboswitch, together with the increasing availability of structural data on riboswitches, has made these targets very interesting pharmaceutically (Pedrolli et al., 2012).

S-Adenosylhomocysteine Riboswitch

S-adenosyl-(L)-methionine (SAM) is a fundamental cofactor that serves as the primary methyl group donor in a large set of biochemical reactions. In bacteria, SAM homeostasis is so important to the point that at least six classes of RNA riboswitch regulatory elements have since now been characterized (Weinberg et al., 2010). Following SAM-mediated methylation, the by-product S-adenosyl-(L)-homocysteine (SAH) that is released, due to its high toxicity, must be readily degraded by SAH hydrolase (ahcY) enzymes. Recently, a new type of riboswitch was discovered, and it is able to sense and be responsible for the intracellular SAH concentration, upregulating the expression of ahcY enzymes in prokaryotes (Wang et al., 2008). The aptameric portion of the SAH riboswitch recognizes its cognate ligand with a quite high binding affinity of 32 nM and, surprisingly, also provides a discrete selectivity profile toward the original cofactor SAM (1,000-fold lower affinity), ensuring a fine regulation of the SAM/SAH metabolic cycle. The high-resolution crystal structure of the SAH riboswitch aptameric domain in complex with its cognate ligand was recently solved, elucidating the molecular basis for SAH substrate specificity (Edwards et al., 2010). This case study not only represents a pharmaceutical appealing prokaryotic RNA target but also provides the opportunity to stress the SuMD performance in a more complex binding site recognition, if compared to the simple duplex structures until now investigated. The SAH molecule indeed binds a small cleft located in the minor groove of the SAH riboswitch, which adopts an unusual "LL-type" pseudoknot conformation. Also, in this case, around 20 ns were sufficient for the SuMD

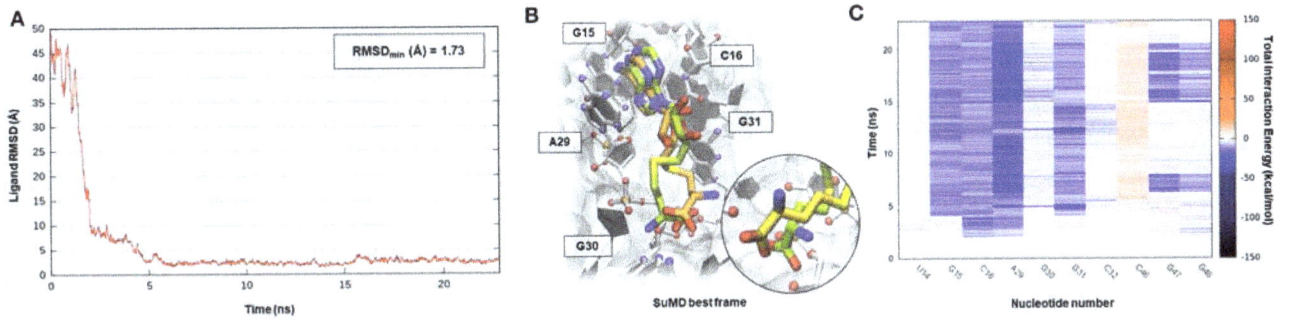

FIGURE 4 | This panel summarizes the recognition pathway of the SAH molecule with SAH riboswitch. **(A)** RMSD of SAH heavy atoms against the PDB reference. **(B)** Superimposition between the experimental X-Ray complex (PDB ID 3NPQ, green-colored SAH molecule) and the SuMD conformation with lowest RMSD along the trajectory (orange-colored molecule). The nucleotides surrounding the binding site are reported. Within the circular window, the SuMD conformation sampled for SAH tail is compared to a different crystallographic reference (PDB ID 3NPN). **(C)** Dynamic total interaction energy (electrostatic + vdW) computed for most contacted RNA nucleobase.

protocol to sample a putative molecular recognition trajectory (**Supplementary Video 3**). In detail, as reported in **Figure 4**, after only a few nanoseconds, SAH reached the riboswitch binding cleft reproducing the crystallographic complex with a notable geometric accuracy ($RMSD_{min}$ 1.7 Å). Then, the ligand conformation remained stable until the end of the simulation. From an interactive point of view, as reported in **Figure 4C** and also in **Supplementary Figure S3**, the SuMD trajectory analysis correctly highlighted the stabilizing role played by nucleotide C16 and A29, among which the adenine core of SAH is intercalated, providing the greatest vdW interactions. In contrast, the electrostatic contribution to binding analysis has revealed a divergent situation. Indeed, nucleobase G15, mediating a hydrogen bond network with an SAH adenine scaffold, is responsible for a great stabilizing contribution, whereas nucleotide C46 has shown during the entire simulation an unexpected repulsive contribution. The reason for this can be found in the conformation sampled by SuMD for the SAH homocysteine terminal tail. As depicted by **Figure 4B**, the carboxylic moiety of the ligand spatially approaches the C46 pyrimidine carbonyl, whereas in the crystallographic structure (green representation), through a simple bond rotation, the interaction is instead mediated by the vicinal amino group. Curiously, the same research group also deposited on the PDB database a worst resolution structure of the complex under investigation (PDB ID 3NPN), reporting the same apparently energetic unfavored SAH conformation described by the SuMD protocol (**Figure 4B**, circular window), thus validating the goodness of the sampling and the flexibility characterizing the ligand tail.

Pre-queuosine$_1$ Riboswitch

Pre-queosine$_1$ ($PreQ_1$), or 7-aminomethyl-7-deazaguanine, is a metabolic intermediate in the synthetic pathway that, starting from guanosine-5′-triphosphate (GTP) nucleotide, originates the hypermodified guanine derivate queuosine (Q). Q has been detected both in eubacteria and eukaryotic organisms where it occupies the anticodon wobble position of tRNAs specific for the amino acid asparagine, aspartate, histidine, and tyrosine (Roth et al., 2007). Q modification has been related to an improvement in translation fidelity as well as bacterial pathogenicity. Interestingly, only prokaryotes can synthesize Q via a multistep reaction, whereas eukaryotes are obliged to assimilate the nucleoside through the diet (Eichhorn et al., 2014). In bacteria like *Bacillus subtilis (Bs)* or *Thermoanaerobacter tengcongenesis (Tt)*, the expression of genes responsible for Q biosynthesis is negatively modulated by the intermediate $PreQ_1$ intracellular concentration. $PreQ_1$, binding to a small aptameric RNA motif composed of 34 nucleotides determines the folding of the $PreQ_1$ riboswitch in an "H-type" pseudoknot structure in which more than half of the nucleobases engage in triplet or quartet interactions (Rieder et al., 2010; Jenkins et al., 2011). The three-dimensional structure of the class I $PreQ_1$ riboswitch in complex with its cognate ligand was solved by X-ray crystallography (PDB ID 3Q50), and this allowed us to speculate about the quite impressive binding affinity characterizing this endogenous precursor ($K_d = 2$ nM) (Edwards et al., 2010). Even in this case, <40 ns of SuMD simulation proved to be sufficient in describing a binding event between the metabolic intermediate $PreQ_1$ and its related riboswitch (**Supplementary Video 4**). As observable in **Figure 5A**, $PreQ_1$ recognition mainly articulates in three well-distinguishable phases. In the beginning, the ligand approaches the riboswitch binding site vestibule where it negotiates for about 15 ns the accommodation in the deep cleft before converging, with great geometric accuracy ($RMSD_{min}$ 1.3 Å), toward the solved crystallographic conformation. This behavior has also been captured by the interaction energy graph (**Supplementary Figure S4B**), highlighting the presence of two major sites visited during the recognition trajectory, i.e., the canonical binding cleft and the aforementioned external vestibular region, located about 10 Å apart. It is interesting to note the comparable interaction energy characterizing these two distal sites, which are distinguishable for their different degrees of solvent exposition. In addition, the dynamic interaction fingerprint reported in **Figure 5C**, elucidates the role played by the binding site nucleotides during recognition in a coherent way with respect to the results reported on the original publication.

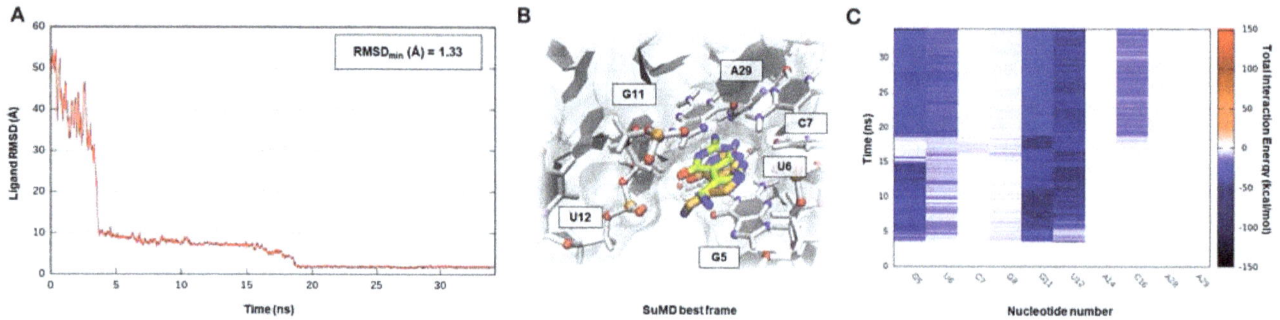

FIGURE 5 | This panel summarizes the recognition pathway of the PreQ$_1$ molecule with PreQ$_1$-1 riboswitch. **(A)** RMSD of PreQ$_1$ heavy atoms against the PDB reference. **(B)** Superimposition between the experimental X-Ray complex (PDB ID 3Q50, green-colored PreQ$_1$ molecule) and the SuMD conformation with lowest RMSD along the trajectory (orange-colored molecule). The nucleotides surrounding the binding site are reported. **(C)** Dynamic total interaction energy (electrostatic + vdW) computed for most contacted RNA nucleobase.

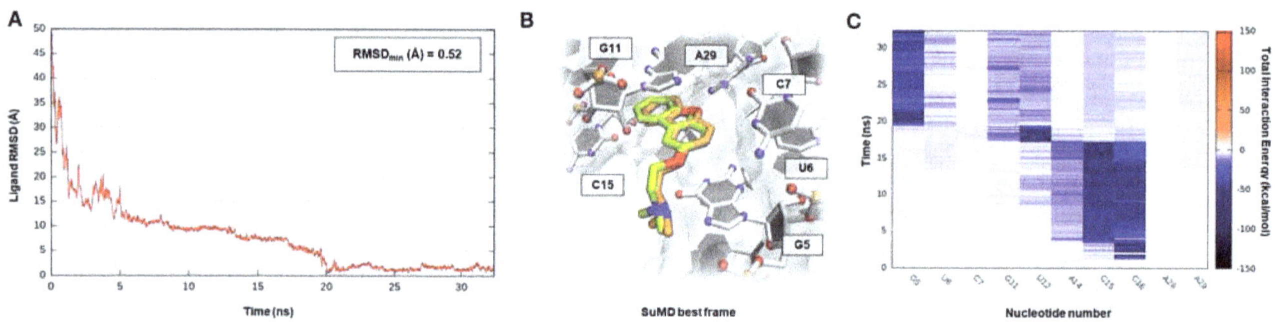

FIGURE 6 | This panel summarizes the recognition pathway of HMJ molecule with PreQ$_1$-1 riboswitch. **(A)** RMSD of HMJ heavy atoms against the PDB reference. **(B)** Superimposition between the experimental X-Ray complex (PDB ID 6E1U, green-colored HMJ molecule) and the SuMD conformation with lowest RMSD along the trajectory (orange-colored molecule). The nucleotides surrounding the binding site are reported. **(C)** Dynamic total interaction energy (electrostatic + vdW) computed for most contacted RNA nucleobase.

All the cases considered so far have confirmed the ability of SuMD to predict reasonable binding hypotheses for different ligands when exploiting as starting point the experimental structures of the ribonucleic targets in which each of these ligands were originally co-crystallized. From a pharmaceutical and applicative perspective, however, it is often required to rationalize the binding mode of compounds that are in most of the cases different from the ones now co-crystallized. It has thus become crucial to understand how the choice of the initial RNA target conformation could affect SuMD performance. The studies performed by the Schneekloth Jr. group in the attempt to experimentally asses the druggability profile of PreQ$_1$-I riboswitch through synthetic organic molecules have then given us an opportunity to further explore this question. In a recent scientific work, it the discovery of HMJ was indeed reported; this is a dibenzofuran derivative that, despite the not obvious chemical similarity with PreQ$_1$, exhibits a sub-micromolar affinity to the RNA target (K_d = 0.5 μM) and the ability to induce premature transcriptional termination (Connelly et al., 2019). The three-dimensional structure determination of the complex was, however, quite difficult and was achieved only by designing a hybrid riboswitch aptamer sequence in which the nucleobase A14, as well as the two vicinal ones, were removed (PDB ID 6E1U). Since this structure lacked a key binding site nucleotides, it represent a non-optimal starting point for a computational study; we therefore decided to investigate the HMJ binding mechanism, exploiting the high-quality riboswitch structure originally solved in the presence of PreQ$_1$ and then comparing the accuracy of the prediction with the experimental solved data. Encouragingly, even for such a system, the SuMD protocol has succeeded in sampling, in about 30 ns, an extremely accurate binding hypothesis for HMJ, whose $RMSD_{min}$ was computed with respect to reference structure (PDB ID 3Q50) and has reached the impressive value of 0.5 Å (**Figure 6A, Supplementary Video 5**). From the analysis of the trajectory, it was furthermore possible to confirm how the benzofuran ligand competes with PreQ$_1$ for the riboswitch binding site. As depicted by **Figure 6C**, and as is coherent with experimental evidence, HMJ makes a strong stabilizing interaction with the nucleobases G5, G11, and C16, which define the "floor" and the "ceiling" of the binding cleft where the aromatic core stacks, and nucleobase U6, C15, and A29, which shape instead the binding cavity borders. Moreover, the Interaction Energy Landscape (**Supplementary Figure S5B**) highlights a binding profile similar to the one previously described for the cognate ligand PreQ$_1$, confirming the vestibular region's role in recruiting the riboswitch binding partners.

Targeting Artificial RNA Aptamers Containing G-Quadruplex Motifs

The discovery, made in 1994, that the green fluorescent protein (GFP) from the jellyfish *Aequorea victoria* could be used as a marker for protein localization and expression has revolutionized molecular biology to the point that, in 2008, the discovery earned a Nobel prize (Swaminathan, 2009). However, since a minimal portion of the human genome is translated into proteins while most of it is transcribed into RNA, being able to investigate the dynamic and spatial properties of the human transcriptome has become essential. As there are no known naturally fluorescent RNAs, a series of *in vitro* engineered ribonucleic tags able to fold into peculiar three-dimensional structures were selected (Trachman and Ferré-D'Amaré, 2019). These RNAs, through an aptameric domain, can bind fluorophore molecules, increasing their spectroscopic signal and hence allowing for the dynamic monitoring of nucleic acid expression and localization in cells. Most of the fluorophore RNA binding sites, despite the different overall architecture, have evolutionarily converged on G-quadruplex motifs, supporting their important role in enhancing the fluorescence phenomenon, in a similar way to how the β-barrel domains characterize GFPs (Warner et al., 2014).

Corn Aptamer

Corn is one recently developed RNA aptamer engineered *in vitro* to bind 3,5-difluoro-4-hydroxybenzylidene imidazolinone-2-oxime (DFHO), a fluorophore analogous of red fluorescent protein (RFP) (Warner et al., 2017). Corn-DFHO differs from other similar RNA tags for its limited light-induced cytotoxicity, its minimal background fluorescence, and its increased photostability, thus representing a valuable imaging tool. Corn aptamer is characterized by an atypical three-dimensional structure elucidated by X-ray crystallography and biophysical experiments. How it is observable in **Figure 1** that two RNA segments join together in a quasi-symmetric homodimer structure (1:2 chromophore:RNA stoichiometry) at the interfaces where a single DFHO molecule is tightly bound (K_d = 70 nM), stacking between two G-quadruplex planes stabilized by the presence of K^+ ions (Warner et al., 2017). Despite the lack of therapeutic application for this aptamer, which is instead more suitable for molecular biology studies, the investigation of such a complex binding site recognition can be considered as a proof of concept to validate G-quadruplex motif targeting through an SuMD approach. Nucleotide quartet structures, which presence have been extensively characterized in the telomeric terminal portion of eukaryotes chromosomes and within gene promoter regions, are indeed acquiring increasing attention, as they could represent promising pharmaceutical targets (Balasubramanian and Neidle, 2009). As shown in **Supplementary Video 6**, SuMD methodology has produced a putative binding trajectory for DFHO in <30 ns, converging with an impressive geometrical accuracy toward the experimental solved complex ($RMSD_{min}$ 0.34 Å) (**Figure 7A**). Moreover, the Dynamic Total Interaction Energy plot reported on **Figure 7C**, strongly retraces the interactive pattern already described on the original scientific work, highlighting the role played by nucleotide G12, G25 (first protomer), and g25 (second protomer) in circumscribing the sandwich cavity within which the aromatic chromophore stacks. Nucleobase A14 (first protomer) and a11 (second protomer) instead mediated a hydrogen bond network with oxime and imine moieties of the DFHO ligand, respectively. SuMD simulation has also illuminated how the entire binding process is not driven by the electrostatic contribution, as often it happens for SMIRNA, but is instead controlled by the vdW interactions (**Supplementary Figure S6**). From this perspective, Corn aptamer represents an unusual, but potentially revolutionary case study, as it distorts an old paradigm that has now since affected the identification of putative RNA binders. DFHO has indeed demonstrated how even apolar or anionic molecules can target ribonucleic acids reaching a nanomolar binding affinity. This provides the opportunity to expand the chemical space explorable by SMIRNA beside that of the well-known, but often problematic, polycationic compounds.

CONCLUSION

Over the last decades, among all the biological macromolecules, proteins have represented the target of choice for the

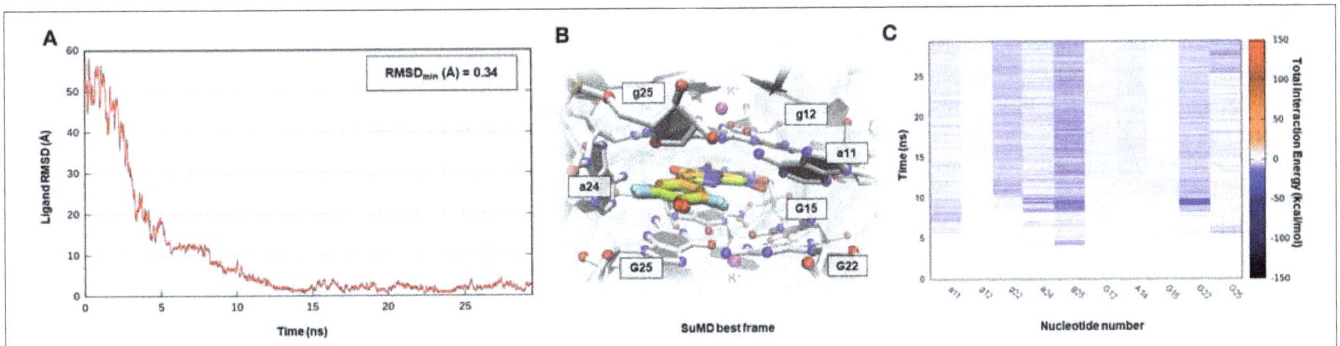

FIGURE 7 | This panel summarizes the recognition pathway of DFHO molecules with the Corn aptamer. **(A)** RMSD of DFHO heavy atoms against the PDB reference. **(B)** Superimposition between the experimental X-Ray complex (PDB ID 5BJO, green-colored DFHO molecule) and the SuMD conformation with lowest RMSD along the trajectory (orange-colored molecule). The nucleotides surrounding the binding site are reported. **(C)** Dynamic total interaction energy (electrostatic + vdW) computed for most contacted RNA nucleobase.

development of new drug candidates. Nucleic acids, on the other hand, have so far represented a less attractive target due to the difficulty in guaranteeing a selective recognition mechanism. The recent discovery of peculiar and physiologically stable three-dimensional conformation characterizing RNAs oligomers has, however, paved the way for the investigation of SMIRNA. The increasing availability of structural data for a wide range of relevant therapeutic ribonucleic targets has promoted the application of well-validated SBDD computational approaches, such as molecular docking, also in this field. However, the remarkable flexibility and the peculiar electrostatic potential, which distinguish nucleic acids from proteins, have readily highlighted the limitation of many of these methodologies. MD simulations would allow us to overcome some of the aforementioned problems; however, the computational cost required to capture rare events such as ligand binding has so far limited their routine utilization.

In this work, we have investigated the applicability domain of SuMD in the field of pharmaceutically relevant RNA polymers. The performances of the protocol were measured as the geometrical accuracy, expressed in terms of RMSD, with which an experimentally solved complex is predicted by the SuMD simulation. Case studies in this research were chosen in such a way as to span very different ribonucleic secondary, tertiary, and even quaternary structures, starting from small duplex stem-loops up to pseudoknot or aptameric homodimers, which contain G-quadruplex motifs. Furthermore, the recognition of different ligands was investigated, both small organic molecules and folded α-helical peptides.

Although this work must be considered as a preliminary investigation and the number of examples taken into consideration cannot guarantee statistical robustness, it is encouraging to note how, in all the six ribonucleic complexes simulated, SuMD correctly reproduced the experimentally solved final state starting from the unbound state in few hours of simulation. The accuracy of the protocol varies significantly in a system-dependent manner, but, in all the cases, it was possible to collect valuable interactive and energetic information about the nucleotides dynamically involved in the recognition process. Curiously, the RNA target in which the architecture of the binding site is not very complex, such as the stem-loop domain of Influenza A promoter and HIV-1 RRE, are those in which the computational protocol experienced the poorest geometric accuracy in reproducing the ligand-binding mode. A separate consideration must be made for the latter complex (PDB ID 1G70) since the recognition between two extremely flexible entities, i.e., the small peptide and the RNA duplex, represents a very challenging case. However, the results obtained, with an $RMSD_{min}$ lower than 5 Å, are in line with those previously described when applying SuMD methodology to peptide–protein recognition. Moving toward more complex binding sites, such as the one that characterizes pseudoknot riboswitch structures or G-quadruple-shaped clefts, the geometric accuracy of the method progressively improves, with the best results obtained in the artificial aptameric structure ($RMSD_{min}$ 0.34 Å). These findings are in agreement with a recent perspective work that assessed how the complexity of an RNA binding site, measured in terms of information content, could represent a valuable discriminant to individuate druggable oligonucleotides (Warner et al., 2018). Indeed, the three-dimensional complexity of a binding site makes ribonucleic pocket more similar to a protein-like environment rather than an ordered and repetitive structure like that characterizing DNA.

Furthermore, the high conformational flexibility that has characterized all the investigated ribonucleic structures (RMSD computed on RNA backbone are reported on **Supplementary Material**) during SuMD simulations has evidenced the importance of adopting techniques able to consider the flexibility of both macromolecules and ligands to better describe such complex molecular recognition. In conclusion, we have shown how SuMD can be a valid computational method to generate binding hypothesis for ribonucleic targets in a nanosecond timescale, explicitly considering both the role of the solvent and the flexibility of the macromolecule. SuMD simulation results could not only help with the interpretation and investigation of the complex mechanism of recognition characterizing SMIRNA, especially when structural information is not available, but they could also guide the rational discovery and optimization of these compounds.

AUTHOR CONTRIBUTIONS

MB carried out the experiment. MB wrote the manuscript with support from MS. MS and SM supervised the project. MB and SM conceived the original idea.

ACKNOWLEDGMENTS

We are very grateful to Chemical Computing Group, OpenEye, and Acellera for the scientific and technical partnership, and we thank NVIDIA for the donation of the Titan Xp and Titan V GPUs used to perform the computational studies.

REFERENCES

Bakan, A., Meireles, L. M., and Bahar, I. (2011). ProDy: protein dynamics inferred from theory and experiments. *Bioinformatics* 27, 1575–1577. doi: 10.1093/bioinformatics/btr168

Balasubramanian, S., and Neidle, S. (2009). G-quadruplex nucleic acids as therapeutic targets. *Curr. Opin. Chem. Biol.* 13, 345–353. doi: 10.1016/j.cbpa.2009.04.637

Battiste, J. L., Mao, H., Rao, N. S., Tan, R., Muhandiram, D. R., Kay, L. E., et al. (1996). α helix-RNA major groove recognition in an HIV-1 rev peptide-RRE RNA Complex. *Science* 273, 1547–1551. doi: 10.1126/science.273.5281.1547

Berendsen, H. J. C., Postma, J. P. M., van Gunsteren, W. F., DiNola, A., and Haak, J. R. (1984). Molecular dynamics with coupling to an external bath. *J. Chem. Phys.* 81, 3684–3690. doi: 10.1063/1.448118

Berman, H. M., Westbrook, J., Feng, Z., Gilliland, G., Bhat, T. N., Weissig, H., et al. (2000). The protein data bank. *Nucleic Acids Res.* 28, 235–242. doi: 10.1093/nar/28.1.235

Bernacchi, S., Freisz, S., Maechling, C., Spiess, B., Marquet, R., Dumas, P., et al. (2007). Aminoglycoside binding to the HIV-1 RNA dimerization initiation site: thermodynamics and effect on the kissing-loop to duplex conversion. *Nucleic Acids Res.* 35, 7128–7139. doi: 10.1093/nar/gkm856

Bissaro, M., Bolcato, G., Deganutti, G., Sturlese, M., and Moro, S. (2019). Revisiting the allosteric regulation of sodium cation on the binding of adenosine at the human A2A adenosine receptor: insights from supervised molecular dynamics (SuMD) simulations. *Molecules* 24:2752. doi: 10.3390/molecules24152752

Coloma, R., Valpuesta, J. M., Arranz, R., Carrascosa, J. L., Ortín, J., and Martín-Benito, J. (2009). The structure of a biologically active influenza virus ribonucleoprotein complex. *PLoS Pathog.* 5:e1000491. doi: 10.1371/journal.ppat.1000491

Connelly, C. M., Moon, M. H., and Schneekloth, J. S. (2016). The emerging role of RNA as a therapeutic target for small molecules. *Cell Chem. Biol.* 23, 1077–1090. doi: 10.1016/j.chembiol.2016.05.021

Connelly, C. M., Numata, T., Boer, R. E., Moon, M. H., Sinniah, R. S., Barchi, J. J., et al. (2019). Synthetic ligands for $PreQ_1$ riboswitches provide structural and mechanistic insights into targeting RNA tertiary structure. *Nat. Commun.* 10:1501. doi: 10.1038/s41467-019-09493-3

Cruz, J. A., and Westhof, E. (2009). The dynamic landscapes of RNA architecture. *Cell* 136, 604–609. doi: 10.1016/j.cell.2009.02.003

Cuzzolin, A., Sturlese, M., Deganutti, G., Salmaso, V., Sabbadin, D., Ciancetta, A., et al. (2016). Deciphering the complexity of ligand–protein recognition pathways using supervised molecular dynamics (SuMD) simulations. *J. Chem. Inf. Model.* 56, 687–705. doi: 10.1021/acs.jcim.5b00702

Denning, E. J., Priyakumar, U. D., Nilsson, L., and Mackerell, A. D. (2011). Impact of 2′-hydroxyl sampling on the conformational properties of RNA: update of the CHARMM all-atom additive force field for RNA. *J. Comput. Chem.* 32, 1929–1943. doi: 10.1002/jcc.21777

Desselberger, U., Racaniello, V. R., Zazra, J. J., and Palese, P. (1980). The 3′ and 5′-terminal sequences of influenza A, B and C virus RNA segments are highly conserved and show partial inverted complementarity. *Gene* 8, 315–328. doi: 10.1016/0378-1119(80)90007-4

DiMattia, M. A., Watts, N. R., Stahl, S. J., Rader, C., Wingfield, P. T., Stuart, D. I., et al. (2010). Implications of the HIV-1 Rev dimer structure at 3.2 Å resolution for multimeric binding to the Rev response element. *Proc. Natl. Acad. Sci. U.S.A.* 107, 5810–5814. doi: 10.1073/pnas.0914946107

Disney, M. D. (2019). Targeting RNA with small molecules to capture opportunities at the intersection of chemistry, biology, and medicine. *J. Am. Chem. Soc.* 141, 6776–6790. doi: 10.1021/jacs.8b13419

Disney, M. D., Winkelsas, A. M., Velagapudi, S. P., Southern, M., Fallahi, M., and Childs-Disney, J. L. (2016). Inforna 2.0: a platform for the sequence-based design of small molecules targeting structured RNAs. *ACS Chem. Biol.* 11, 1720–1728. doi: 10.1021/acschembio.6b00001

Disney, M. D., Yildirim, I., and Childs-Disney, J. L. (2014). Methods to enable the design of bioactive small molecules targeting RNA. *Org. Biomol. Chem.* 12, 1029–1039. doi: 10.1039/C3OB42023J

Donlic, A., and Hargrove, A. E. (2018). Targeting RNA in mammalian systems with small molecules. *Wiley Interdiscip. Rev. RNA* 9:e1477. doi: 10.1002/wrna.1477

Draper, D. E. (1995). Protein-RNA recognition. *Annu. Rev. Biochem.* 64, 593–620. doi: 10.1146/annurev.bi.64.070195.003113

Ecker, D. J., and Griffey, R. H. (1999). RNA as a small-molecule drug target: doubling the value of genomics. *Drug Discov. Today* 4, 420–429. doi: 10.1016/S1359-6446(99)01389-6

Edwards, A. L., Reyes, F. E., Héroux, A., and Batey, R. T. (2010). Structural basis for recognition of S-adenosylhomocysteine by riboswitches. *RNA* 16, 2144–2155. doi: 10.1261/rna.2341610

Eichhorn, C. D., Kang, M., and Feigon, J. (2014). Structure and function of $preQ_1$ riboswitches. *Biochim. Biophys. Acta - Gene Regul. Mech.* 1839, 939–950. doi: 10.1016/j.bbagrm.2014.04.019

Essmann, U., Perera, L., Berkowitz, M. L., Darden, T., Lee, H., and Pedersen, L. G. (1995). A smooth particle mesh Ewald method. *J. Chem. Phys.* 103, 8577–8593. doi: 10.1063/1.470117

Flynn, R. A., Smith, B. A. H., Johnson, A. G., Pedram, K., George, B. M., Malaker, S. A., et al. (2019). Mammalian Y RNAs are modified at discrete guanosine residues with N-glycans. *bioRxiv[Preprint]* 787614. doi: 10.1101/787614

Fulle, S., and Gohlke, H. (2009). Molecular recognition of RNA: challenges for modelling interactions and plasticity. *J. Mol. Recognit.* 23, 220–231. doi: 10.1002/jmr.1000

Gosser, Y., Hermann, T., Majumdar, A., Hu, W., Frederick, R., Jiang, F., et al. (2001). Peptide-triggered conformational switch in HIV-1 RRE RNA complexes. *Nat. Struct. Biol.* 8, 146–150. doi: 10.1038/84138

Harada, K., Martin, S. S., and Frankel, A. D. (1996). Selection of RNA-binding peptides *in vivo*. *Nature* 380, 175–179. doi: 10.1038/380175a0

Harada, K., Martin, S. S., Tan, R., and Frankel, A. D. (1997). Molding a peptide into an RNA site by *in vivo* peptide evolution. *Proc. Natl. Acad. Sci. U.S.A.* 94, 11887–11892. doi: 10.1073/pnas.94.22.11887

Harvey, M. J., Giupponi, G., and Fabritiis, G., De (2009). ACEMD: accelerating biomolecular dynamics in the microsecond time scale. *J. Chem. Theory Comput.* 5, 1632–1639. doi: 10.1021/ct9000685

Hermann, T. (2002). Rational ligand design for RNA: the role of static structure and conformational flexibility in target recognition. *Biochimie* 84, 869–875. doi: 10.1016/S0300-9084(02)01460-8

Hermann, T. (2016). Small molecules targeting viral RNA. *Wiley Interdiscip. Rev. RNA* 7, 726–743. doi: 10.1002/wrna.1373

Humphrey, W., Dalke, A., and Schulten, K. (1996). VMD: Visual molecular dynamics. *J. Mol. Graph.* 14, 33–38. doi: 10.1016/0263-7855(96)00018-5

Jenkins, J. L., Krucinska, J., McCarty, R. M., Bandarian, V., and Wedekind, J. E. (2011). Comparison of a $PreQ_1$ riboswitch aptamer in metabolite-bound and free states with implications for gene regulation. *J. Biol. Chem.* 286, 24626–24637. doi: 10.1074/jbc.M111.230375

Labute, P. (2009). Protonate3D: assignment of ionization states and hydrogen coordinates to macromolecular structures. *Proteins* 75, 187–205. doi: 10.1002/prot.22234

Lee, M.-K., Bottini, A., Kim, M., Bardaro, M. F., Zhang, Z., Pellecchia, M., et al. (2014). A novel small-molecule binds to the influenza A virus RNA promoter and inhibits viral replication. *Chem. Commun.* 50, 368–370. doi: 10.1039/C3CC46973E

Loncharich, R. J., Brooks, B. R., and Pastor, R. W. (1992). Langevin dynamics of peptides: the frictional dependence of isomerization rates of N-acetylalanyl-N′-methylamide. *Biopolymers* 32, 523–535. doi: 10.1002/bip.360320508

Miller, B. R., McGee, T. D., Swails, J. M., Homeyer, N., Gohlke, H., and Roitberg, A. E. (2012). MMPBSA.py: an efficient program for end-state free energy calculations. *J. Chem. Theory Comput.* 8, 3314–3321. doi: 10.1021/ct300418h

Morris, K. V., and Mattick, J. S. (2014). The rise of regulatory RNA. *Nat. Rev. Genet.* 15, 423–437. doi: 10.1038/nrg3722

Pedrolli, D. B., Matern, A., Wang, J., Ester, M., Siedler, K., Breaker, R., et al. (2012). A highly specialized flavin mononucleotide riboswitch responds differently to similar ligands and confers roseoflavin resistance to *Streptomyces davawensis*. *Nucleic Acids Res.* 40, 8662–8673. doi: 10.1093/nar/gks616

Pérez, A., Marchán, I., Svozil, D., Sponer, J., Cheatham, T. E., Laughton, C. A., et al. (2007). Refinement of the AMBER force field for nucleic acids: improving the description of alpha/gamma conformers. *Biophys. J.* 92, 3817–3829. doi: 10.1529/biophysj.106.097782

Rieder, U., Kreutz, C., and Micura, R. (2010). Folding of a transcriptionally acting $PreQ_1$ riboswitch. *Proc. Natl. Acad. Sci. U.S.A.* 107, 10804–10809. doi: 10.1073/pnas.0914925107

Roth, A., Winkler, W. C., Regulski, E. E., Lee, B. W. K., Lim, J., Jona, I., et al. (2007). A riboswitch selective for the queuosine precursor $preQ_1$ contains an unusually small aptamer domain. *Nat. Struct. Mol. Biol.* 14, 308–317. doi: 10.1038/nsmb1224

Sabbadin, D., and Moro, S. (2014). Supervised molecular dynamics (SuMD) as a helpful tool to depict GPCR–ligand recognition pathway in a nanosecond time scale. *J. Chem. Inf. Model.* 54, 372–376. doi: 10.1021/ci400766b

Salmaso, V., Sturlese, M., Cuzzolin, A., and Moro, S. (2017). Exploring protein-peptide recognition pathways using a supervised molecular dynamics approach. *Structure 25,* 655–662.e2. doi: 10.1016/j.str.2017.02.009

Salmon, L., Yang, S., and Al-Hashimi, H. M. (2014). Advances in the determination of nucleic acid conformational ensembles. *Annu. Rev. Phys. Chem.* 65, 293–316. doi: 10.1146/annurev-physchem-040412-110059

Sherwood, A. V., and Henkin, T. M. (2016). Riboswitch mediated gene regulation: novel RNA architectures dictate gene expression responses. *Annu. Rev. Microbiol.* 70, 361–374. doi: 10.1146/annurev-micro-091014-104306

Sprenger, K. G., Jaeger, V. W., and Pfaendtner, J. (2015). The general AMBER force field (GAFF) can accurately predict thermodynamic and transport properties of many ionic liquids. *J. Phys. Chem. B* 119, 5882–5895. doi: 10.1021/acs.jpcb.5b00689

Sucheck, S. J., and Wong, C.-H. (2000). RNA as a target for small molecules. *Curr. Opin. Chem. Biol.* 4, 678–686. doi: 10.1016/S1367-5931(00)00142-3

Swaminathan, S. (2009). GFP: the green revolution. *Nat. Cell Biol.* 11:S20. doi: 10.1038/ncb1953

Tan, D., Piana, S., Dirks, R. M., and Shaw, D. E. (2018). RNA force field with accuracy comparable to state-of-the-art protein force fields. *Proc. Natl. Acad. Sci. U.S.A.* 115, E1346–E1355. doi: 10.1073/pnas.1713027115

Trachman, R. J., and Ferré-D'Amaré, A. R. (2019). Tracking RNA with light: selection, structure, and design of fluorescence turn-on RNA aptamers. *Q. Rev. Biophys.* 52:e8. doi: 10.1017/S0033583519000064

Tucker, B. J., and Breaker, R. R. (2005). Riboswitches as versatile gene control elements. *Curr. Opin. Struct. Biol.* 15, 342–348. doi: 10.1016/j.sbi.2005.05.003

Velagapudi, S. P., Gallo, S. M., and Disney, M. D. (2014). Sequence-based design of bioactive small molecules that target precursor microRNAs. *Nat. Chem. Biol.* 10, 291–297. doi: 10.1038/nchembio.1452

Wang, J., Wang, W., Kollman, P. A., and Case, D. A. (2006). Automatic atom type and bond type perception in molecular mechanical calculations. *J. Mol. Graph. Model.* 25, 247–260. doi: 10.1016/j.jmgm.2005.12.005

Wang, J. X., Lee, E. R., Morales, D. R., Lim, J., and Breaker, R. R. (2008). Riboswitches that sense S-adenosylhomocysteine and activate genes involved in coenzyme recycling. *Mol. Cell* 29, 691–702. doi: 10.1016/j.molcel.2008.01.012

Warner, K. D., Chen, M. C., Song, W., Strack, R. L., Thorn, A., Jaffrey, S. R., et al. (2014). Structural basis for activity of highly efficient RNA mimics of green fluorescent protein. *Nat. Struct. Mol. Biol.* 21, 658–663. doi: 10.1038/nsmb.2865

Warner, K. D., Hajdin, C. E., and Weeks, K. M. (2018). Principles for targeting RNA with drug-like small molecules. *Nat. Rev. Drug Discov.* 17, 547–558. doi: 10.1038/nrd.2018.93

Warner, K. D., Sjekloa, L., Song, W., Filonov, G. S., Jaffrey, S. R., and Ferré-D'Amaré, A. R. (2017). A homodimer interface without base pairs in an RNA mimic of red fluorescent protein. *Nat. Chem. Biol.* 13, 1195–1201. doi: 10.1038/nchembio.2475

Weinberg, Z., Wang, J. X., Bogue, J., Yang, J., Corbino, K., Moy, R. H., et al. (2010). Comparative genomics reveals 104 candidate structured RNAs from bacteria, archaea, and their metagenomes. *Genome Biol.* 11:R31. doi: 10.1186/gb-2010-11-3-r31

Permissions

All chapters in this book were first published by Frontiers; hereby published with permission under the Creative Commons Attribution License or equivalent. Every chapter published in this book has been scrutinized by our experts. Their significance has been extensively debated. The topics covered herein carry significant findings which will fuel the growth of the discipline. They may even be implemented as practical applications or may be referred to as a beginning point for another development.

The contributors of this book come from diverse backgrounds, making this book a truly international effort. This book will bring forth new frontiers with its revolutionizing research information and detailed analysis of the nascent developments around the world.

We would like to thank all the contributing authors for lending their expertise to make the book truly unique. They have played a crucial role in the development of this book. Without their invaluable contributions this book wouldn't have been possible. They have made vital efforts to compile up to date information on the varied aspects of this subject to make this book a valuable addition to the collection of many professionals and students.

This book was conceptualized with the vision of imparting up-to-date information and advanced data in this field. To ensure the same, a matchless editorial board was set up. Every individual on the board went through rigorous rounds of assessment to prove their worth. After which they invested a large part of their time researching and compiling the most relevant data for our readers.

The editorial board has been involved in producing this book since its inception. They have spent rigorous hours researching and exploring the diverse topics which have resulted in the successful publishing of this book. They have passed on their knowledge of decades through this book. To expedite this challenging task, the publisher supported the team at every step. A small team of assistant editors was also appointed to further simplify the editing procedure and attain best results for the readers.

Apart from the editorial board, the designing team has also invested a significant amount of their time in understanding the subject and creating the most relevant covers. They scrutinized every image to scout for the most suitable representation of the subject and create an appropriate cover for the book.

The publishing team has been an ardent support to the editorial, designing and production team. Their endless efforts to recruit the best for this project, has resulted in the accomplishment of this book. They are a veteran in the field of academics and their pool of knowledge is as vast as their experience in printing. Their expertise and guidance has proved useful at every step. Their uncompromising quality standards have made this book an exceptional effort. Their encouragement from time to time has been an inspiration for everyone.

The publisher and the editorial board hope that this book will prove to be a valuable piece of knowledge for researchers, students, practitioners and scholars across the globe.

List of Contributors

Pavel Sidorov, Jérémy Ariey-Bonnet, Eddy Pasquier and Pedro J. Ballester
CRCM, INSERM, Cancer Research Center of Marseille, Institut Paoli-Calmettes, Aix-Marseille Univ, CNRS, Marseille, France

Stefan Naulaerts
CRCM, INSERM, Cancer Research Center of Marseille, Institut Paoli-Calmettes, Aix-Marseille Univ, CNRS, Marseille, France
Department of Tumor Immunology, Institut de Duve, Bruxelles, Belgium

Sven Bühlmann and Jean-Louis Reymond
Department of Chemistry and Biochemistry, University of Bern, Bern, Switzerland

Lucas N. Alberca, Sara R. Chuguransky and Alan Talevi
Laboratory of Bioactive Compounds Research and Development (LIDeB), Department of Biological Sciences, Exact Sciences College, Universidad Nacional de La Plata, La Plata, Argentina

Cora L. Álvarez
Departamento de Biodiversidad y Biología Experimental, Facultad de Farmacia y Bioquímica, Facultad de Ciencias Exactas y Naturales, Consejo Nacional de Investigaciones Científicas y Técnicas, Instituto de Química y Fisico-Química Biológicas (IQUIFIB) "Prof. Alejandro C. Paladini", Universidad de Buenos Aires, Buenos Aires, Argentina

Emir Salas-Sarduy
Instituto de Investigaciones Biotecnológicas "Dr. Rodolfo Ugalde", Universidad Nacional de San Martín, CONICET, Buenos Aires, Argentina

Juan Francisco Sánchez-Tejeda, Juan Rodrigo Salazar and Marco A. Loza-Mejía
Facultad de Ciencias Químicas, Universidad La Salle, Mexico City, Mexico

Juan F. Sánchez-Ruiz
Ciencia y Estrategia S.A. de C.V., Mexico City, Mexico

Anders Wallqvist
Department of Defense Biotechnology High Performance Computing Software Applications Institute, Telemedicine and Advanced Technology Research Center, U.S. Army Medical Research and Development Command, Fort Detrick, MD, United States

Andrés González Barrios
Grupo de Diseño de Productos y Procesos (GDPP), School of Chemical Engineering, Universidad de los Andes, Bogotá, Colombia

Andrés Felipe Vásquez
Grupo de Diseño de Productos y Procesos (GDPP), School of Chemical Engineering, Universidad de los Andes, Bogotá, Colombia
Laboratorio de Fisiología Molecular, Instituto Nacional de Salud, Bogotá, Colombia

Ruifeng Liu and Mohamed Diwan M. AbdulHameed
Department of Defense Biotechnology High Performance Computing Software Applications Institute, Telemedicine and Advanced Technology Research Center, U.S. Army Medical Research and Development Command, Fort Detrick, MD, United States
The Henry M. Jackson Foundation for the Advancement of Military Medicine, Inc., Bethesda, MD, United States

Danfeng Shi and Xiaoli An
State Key Laboratory of Applied Organic Chemistry, Department of Chemistry, Lanzhou University, Lanzhou, China

Qifeng Bai
School of Basic Medical Science, Lanzhou University, Lanzhou, China

Zhitong Bing
School of Basic Medical Science, Lanzhou University, Lanzhou, China
Institute of Modern Physics of Chinese Academy of Sciences, Lanzhou, China

Shuangyan Zhou
State Key Laboratory of Applied Organic Chemistry, Department of Chemistry, Lanzhou University, Lanzhou, China
School of Pharmacy, Lanzhou University, Lanzhou, China

Xiaojun Yao
State Key Laboratory of Applied Organic Chemistry, Department of Chemistry, Lanzhou University, Lanzhou, China
State Key Laboratory of Quality Research in Chinese Medicine, Macau Institute for Applied Research in Medicine and Health, Macau University of Science and Technology, Macau, China

Letícia Cristina Assis and Alex Gutterres Taranto
Laboratory of Pharmaceutical Medicinal Chemistry, Federal University of São João Del Rei, Divinópolis, Brazil

Eduardo Habib Bechelane Maia
Laboratory of Pharmaceutical Medicinal Chemistry, Federal University of São João Del Rei, Divinópolis, Brazil
Federal Center for Technological Education of Minas Gerais—CEFET-MG, Belo Horizonte, Brazil

Tiago Alves de Oliveira and Alisson Marques da Silva
Federal Center for Technological Education of Minas Gerais—CEFET-MG, Belo Horizonte, Brazil

Lucas de Azevedo Santos and Ingrid G. Prandi
Department of Chemistry, Federal University of Lavras, Lavras, Brazil

Teodorico C. Ramalho
Department of Chemistry, Federal University of Lavras, Lavras, Brazil
Department of Chemistry, Faculty of Science, University of Hradec Kralove, Hradec Kralove, Czechia

José Luis Velázquez-Libera, Carlos Navarro-Retamal and Julio Caballero
Centro de Bioinformática y Simulación Molecular, Facultad de Ingeniería, Universidad de Talca, Talca, Chile

Giacomo Rossino and Simona Collina
Pharmaceutical and Medicinal Chemistry Section, Drug Sciences Department, Università di Pavia, Pavia, Italy

Zarko Gagic
Department of Pharmaceutical Chemistry, Faculty of Medicine, University of Banja Luka, Banja Luka, Bosnia and Herzegovina

Dusan Ruzic, Nemanja Djokovic, Teodora Djikic and Katarina Nikolic
Department of Pharmaceutical Chemistry, Faculty of Pharmacy, University of Belgrade, Belgrade, Serbia

Lauro Ribeiro de Souza Neto and Floriano Paes Silva Jr.
LaBECFar - Laboratório de Bioquímica Experimental e Computacional de Fármacos, Instituto Oswaldo Cruz, Fundação Oswaldo Cruz, Rio de Janeiro, Brazil

Ana Carolina Ramos Guimarães
Laboratório de Genômica Funcional e Bioinformática, Instituto Oswaldo Cruz, Fundação Oswaldo Cruz, Rio de Janeiro, Brazil

Rocío Lucía Beatriz Riveros Maidana
LaBECFar - Laboratório de Bioquímica Experimental e Computacional de Fármacos, Instituto Oswaldo Cruz, Fundação Oswaldo Cruz, Rio de Janeiro, Brazil
Laboratório de Genômica Funcional e Bioinformática, Instituto Oswaldo Cruz, Fundação Oswaldo Cruz, Rio de Janeiro, Brazil

José Teófilo Moreira-Filho and Carolina Horta Andrade
LabMol - Laboratory for Molecular Modeling and Drug Design, Faculdade de Farmácia, Universidade Federal de Goiás, Goiânia, Brazil

Bruno Junior Neves
LabMol - Laboratory for Molecular Modeling and Drug Design, Faculdade de Farmácia, Universidade Federal de Goiás, Goiânia, Brazil
Laboratory of Cheminformatics, Centro Universitário de Anápolis - UniEVANGÉLICA, Anápolis, Brazil

Nicholas Furnham
Department of Infection Biology, London School of Hygiene and Tropical Medicine, London, United Kingdom

Maurice Michel, Evert J. Homan, Elisée Wiita, Kia Pedersen, Ingrid Almlöf and Ulrika Warpman Berglund
Science for Life Laboratory, Department of Oncology-Pathology, Karolinska Institutet, Stockholm, Sweden

Anna-Lena Gustavsson
Chemical Biology Consortium Sweden (CBCS), Science for Life Laboratory, Department of Medical Biochemistry and Biophysics, Karolinska Institutet, Stockholm, Sweden

Thomas Lundbäck
Chemical Biology Consortium Sweden (CBCS), Science for Life Laboratory, Department of Medical Biochemistry and Biophysics, Karolinska Institutet, Stockholm, Sweden
Mechanistic Biology and Profiling, Discovery Sciences, R&D, AstraZeneca, Gothenburg, Sweden

Thomas Helleday
Science for Life Laboratory, Department of Oncology-Pathology, Karolinska Institutet, Stockholm, Sweden
Department of Oncology and Metabolism, Sheffield Cancer Centre, University of Sheffield, Sheffield, United Kingdom

Aline Lagoeiro do Carmo, Simone Queiroz Pantaleão, Tiago Rodrigues and Paula Homem-de-Mello
Centro de Ciências Naturais e Humanas, Universidade Federal do ABC, Santo André, Brazil

Kathia Maria Honorio
Centro de Ciências Naturais e Humanas, Universidade Federal do ABC, Santo André, Brazil
Escola de Artes, Ciências e Humanidades, Universidade de São Paulo (USP), São Paulo, Brazil

M. Gabriela Aucar
Computational Drug Design and Biomedical Informatics Laboratory, Translational Medicine Research Institute (IIMT), CONICET-Universidad Austral, Pilar, Argentina

Claudio N. Cavasotto
Computational Drug Design and Biomedical Informatics Laboratory, Translational Medicine Research Institute (IIMT), CONICET-Universidad Austral, Pilar, Argentina
Facultad de Ciencias Biomédicas and Facultad de Ingeniería, Universidad Austral, Pilar, Argentina
Austral Institute for Applied Artificial Intelligence, Universidad Austral, Pilar, Argentina

Leticia T. Ferreira, Tatyana A. Tavella, Gustavo C. Cassiano, Fabio T. M. Costa and Kaira C. P. Tomaz
Laboratory of Tropical Diseases—Prof. Dr. Luiz Jacintho da Silva, Department of Genetics, Evolution, Microbiology and Immunology, Institute of Biology, University of Campinas (UNICAMP), Campinas, Brazil

Fernanda Bettanin
Escola de Artes, Ciências e Humanidades, Universidade de São Paulo (USP), São Paulo, Brazil

Michell Oliveira Almeida
Instituto de Química de São Carlos, Universidade de São Paulo (USP), São Paulo, Brazil

Index

www.ingramcontent.com/pod-product-compliance
Lightning Source LLC
LaVergne TN
LVHW082158200926
848484LV00008B/2179
* 9 7 9 8 8 8 7 4 0 2 5 5 0 *